Atlas of
Vitreoretinal Surgery

H. MacKenzie Freeman
and
Felipe I. Tolentino

Atlas of Vitreoretinal Surgery

538 Illustrations
Illustrated by Rudolf Brammer

1990

Georg Thieme Verlag
Stuttgart · New York

Thieme Medical Publishers, Inc.
New York

H. MacKenzie Freeman, M.D., P.C.
Felipe I. Tolentino, M.D., P.C.
Retina Associates, Inc.
100 Charles River Plaza
Cambridge Street
Boston, MA 02114
USA

Atlas of Ophthalmic Surgery, Vol. III
Edited by Klaus Heilmann and David Paton

Library of Congress Cataloging-in-Publication Data
(Revised for volume 3)

Atlas of ophthalmic surgery.

Includes bibliographies and index.
Contents: v. 1. Lids, orbits, extraocular muscles / editors, Charles K. Beyer-Machule, Gunter K. von Noorden – –v. 3. Atlas of Vitreoretinal Surgery / H. MacKenzie Freeman and Felipe I. Tolentino.
1. Eye–Surgery–Atlases. 2. Eyelids–Surgery–Atlases. 3. Eye–sockets–Surgery–Atlases.
I. Heilmann, Klaus. II. Paton, David.
RE80.A87 1989 617.7'1 84-52205

Thieme Medical Publishers, Inc., 381 Park Avenue South, New York, N.Y. 10016
Printed in Germany by Grammlich, Pliezhausen
Typesetting: Hurler, Notzingen (Linotronic 300)

ISBN 3-13-656601-7 (Georg Thieme Verlag, Stuttgart)
ISBN 0-86577-331-9 (Thieme Medical Publishers, Inc., New York)

2 3 4 5 6

Important Note: Medicine is an ever-changing science. Research and clinical experience are continually broadening our knowledge, in particular our knowledge of proper treatment and drug therapy. Insofar as this book mentions any dosage or application, readers may rest assured that the authors, editors and publishers have made every effort to ensure that such references are strictly in accordance with the **state of knowledge at the time of production of the book. Nevertheless, every user is requested** to examine carefully the manufacturer's leaflets accompanying each drug to check on his own responsibility whether the dosage schedules recommended therein or the contraindications stated by the manufacturers differ from the statements made in the present book. Such examination is particularly important with drugs that are either rarely used or have been newly released on the market.

Dedication

To our patients, past and present. We hope that the knowledge we have gained in our association with you and are passing on in this book will benefit many other vitreoretinal surgeons and their patients.

Preface

We hope that this Atlas of Vitreoretinal Surgery will provide the resident, fellow and vitreoretinal surgeon with a concise description of clinically proven surgical techniques used to manage vitreoretinal disorders, including penetrating ocular trauma.

The main thrust of the book is to describe surgical techniques in a step-by-step series of detailed illustrations accompanied by brief text. We trust that this Atlas may serve as a reference, a refresher and a practical guide to treatment of cases of varying degrees of severity. In addition, an effort was made to deal with the prevention and management of complications.

The initial chapters describe the basic techniques of vitrectomy and such ancillary techniques as preretinal and subretinal membrane surgery; internal drainage of subretinal fluid; exchanges of air, gas, silicone or fluorosilicone oil; retinotomy and retinectomy; and bimanual vitreoretinal surgery.

Chapters 10–16 deal with the management of intraoperative and late complications of cataract surgery. Simple and complex tractional and rhegmatogenous retinal detachments, including anterior and posterior proliferative vitreoretinopathy, are described in Chapters 25–27. Vitrectomy in children is in Chapter 28.

The management of anterior and posterior segment trauma, including persistent hyphema, vitreous hemorrhage, corneoscleral laceration, double perforating injury, and posterior segment intraocular foreign bodies, is described in Chapters 25–32.

It is our wish that this Atlas will contribute to the improvement of the care of vitreoretinal disorders. If one complication is prevented, it will have been well worth our efforts. We will welcome your observations, criticisms or suggestions, both for our edification and for inclusion in a possible future edition.

August 1989 *Hal Freeman and Felipe Tolentino*

Acknowledgments

We are very grateful to Dr. Charles Schepens who has, as in all the years of our association, generously contributed time and effort to reviewing this and other manuscripts. We are especially appreciative and greatly indebted to Mr. Frank Shelton for his editing and his untiring efforts to bring together the myriad of details necessary in publishing a book. It has been a pleasure and a privilege to work with such a gifted and patient medical illustrator as Mr. Rudolf Brammer. We appreciate the encouragement of Dr. Klaus Heilmann, who stimulated us to undertake this endeavor. We are grateful to Dr. Tatsuo Hirose for advice in the chapter on retinopathy of prematurity; to Dr. Ann Baker for her assistance in the chapter on endophthalmitis; and to Dr. Miguel Refojo for checking the section on silicone oil.

We gratefully acknowledge the work of Leona Greenhill and the staff of the editorial services unit of the Eye Research Institute of Retina Foundation, offer our special thanks to Judy Cerone and Marilyn Glick for assisting in typing the manuscript, and thank Mr. Tom Monego and Mr. Bill Fischer for the instrument photographs.

The authors have made the Eye Research Institute of Retina Foundation the beneficiary of all royalties paid on the sale of this book.

Hal Freeman and Felipe Tolentino

Contents

Abbreviations

EER Electrically evoked response
ERG Electroretinography
MVR Microvitreoretinal
PHPV Persistent hyperplastic primary vitreous
PVR Proliferative vitreoretinopathy
ROP Retinopathy of prematurity
VEP Visually evoked potential
VER Visually evoked response

1

Surgical Anatomy

This chapter deals with the ocular and periocular structures that may be involved in vitreoretinal surgery. The emphasis has been placed on the relevant vascular and nervous systems, the surface anatomy of the sclera, and the topography of the vitreous base.

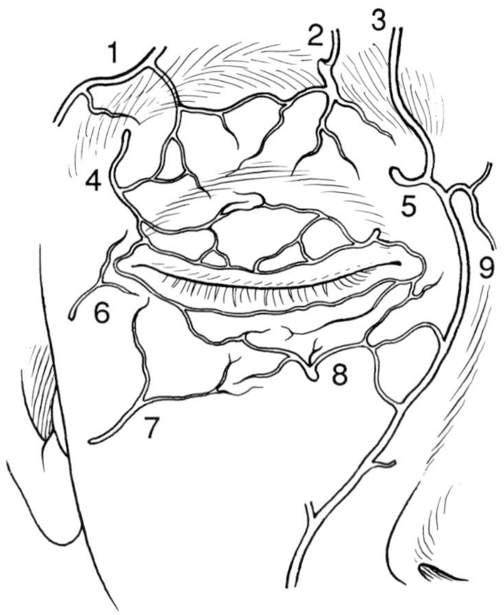

1.**1a Arteries of the eyelids.** 1 Frontal branch of the superficial temporal; 2 supraorbital; 3 frontal branch of the ophthalmic; 4 lacrimal; 5 ophthalmic; 6 zygomatico-orbital; 7 transverse facial; 8 infraorbital; 9 angular.

1. *Frontal branch of the superficial temporal:* a terminal branch of the external carotid artery which supplies the outer and upper parts of the orbicularis muscle.

2. *Supraorbital:* arises from the ophthalmic artery to pass through the supraorbital foramen and anastomose with the superficial temporal and frontal arteries to supply the upper eyelid and levator muscle.

3. *Frontal branch of the ophthalmic:* pierces the septum orbitale, passing upward around the inner end of the supraorbital margin to supply the skin, muscle, and periosteum of the mesial part of the forehead.

4. *Lacrimal:* arises from the ophthalmic artery and courses anteriorly at the upper border of the lateral rectus muscle to supply the lacrimal gland with branches to form arcades in the lids and conjunctiva.

5. *Ophthalmic:* arises as a branch of the internal carotid and traverses the optic canal to enter the orbit through the optic foramen. Near the orbital end of the canal, the artery leaves the dural sheath, and, lying within the muscle cone and the lateral rectus muscle, it crosses the nerve on its superior aspect and runs toward the medial wall of the orbit. It runs forward between the superior oblique and the medial rectus muscles to end behind the septum orbitale, where it divides into two branches, the central artery of the retina and the lacrimal artery.

6. *Zygomatico-orbital:* a branch of the superficial temporal artery which runs above the zygoma to supply branches to the lateral parts of the upper and lower lids and the orbit.

7. *Transverse facial:* a branch of the superficial temporal artery running below the zygoma to the lateral border of the eyelid.

8. *Infraorbital:* a terminal branch of the internal maxillary artery which enters the orbit through the inferior orbital fissure and appears on the face through the infraorbital foramen. In the orbit, it supplies branches to the inferior rectus and inferior oblique muscles, the lower lid, and lacrimal gland; on the face, it breaks up into terminal palpebral, nasal, and labial branches.

9. *Angular:* the facial artery, which is derived from the external carotid artery, passes over the mandible, travelling up the face and the side of the nose to reach the inner canthus, where it becomes the angular artery.

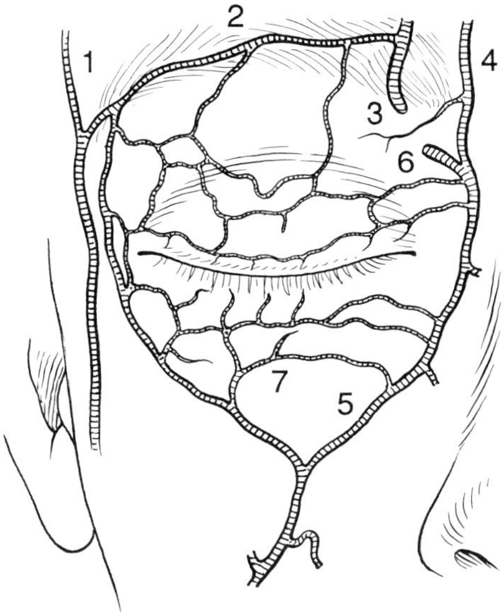

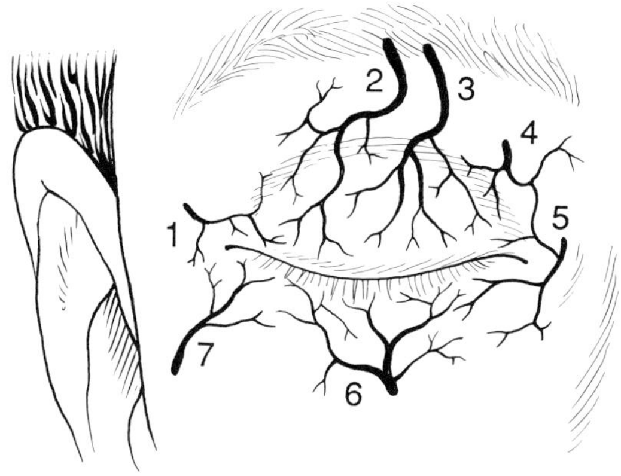

b Veins of the eyelids. 1 Superficial temporal; 2 supraorbital; 3 supraorbital branch to the superior ophthalmic; 4 frontal; 5 anterior facial; 6 angular branch to the superior ophthalmic; 7 inferior palpebral.

1. *Superficial temporal:* arises from a plexus of veins below the ear which includes the external and internal jugular veins. It courses over the skull to unite with the superficial temporal veins of the other side and communicates with the supraorbital vein.

2. *Supraorbital:* runs horizontally along the orbital margin deep to the orbicularis, which it pierces under the inner end of the eyebrow to join the frontal and form the angular vein.

3. *Supraorbital branch to the superior ophthalmic:* the supraorbital vein communicates with the superior ophthalmic vein through the supraorbital notch, at which point it receives a vein from the frontal sinus and the diploë.

4. *Frontal:* runs down the forehead accompanying the supraorbital artery.

5. *Anterior facial:* the angular vein continues down the face as the anterior facial vein, uniting with the anterior branch of the posterior facial vein to form the common facial vein, which empties into the internal jugular vein in the neck.

6. *Angular branch to the superior ophthalmic:* a branch of the anterior facial vein which unites with a branch of the supraorbital vein to form the commencement of the superior ophthalmic vein.

7. *Inferior palpebral:* a branch of the angular vein running medially from the lid.

c Nerves to the eyelids. 1 Lacrimal; 2, 3 supraorbital from frontal; 4 supratrochlear from frontal; 5 infratrochlear from nasociliary; 6 infraorbital from maxillary; 7 temporal branch of orbital.

1. *Lacrimal:* smallest branch of the terminal branch of the ophthalmic nerve. It supplies the conjunctiva and the skin of the outer part of the upper and lower lids.

2. *Supraorbital:* terminal branch of the frontal nerve, supplying the upper eyelid and conjunctiva.

3. *Frontal:* largest branch of the ophthalmic nerve, it branches into the supraorbital and supratrochlear.

4. *Supratrochlear:* supplies branches to the skin, lower part of the forehead, upper lid, and conjunctiva.

5. *Infratrochlear:* branch of the nasociliary nerve supplying the skin and conjunctiva around the inner angle of the eye, root of the nose, lacrimal sac, and caruncle.

6. *Infraorbital:* branch of the superior maxillary nerve which runs in the infraorbital canal to emerge on the face through the infraorbital foramen.

7. *Zygomaticofacial:* branch of the superior maxillary nerve supplying the skin over the malar bone.

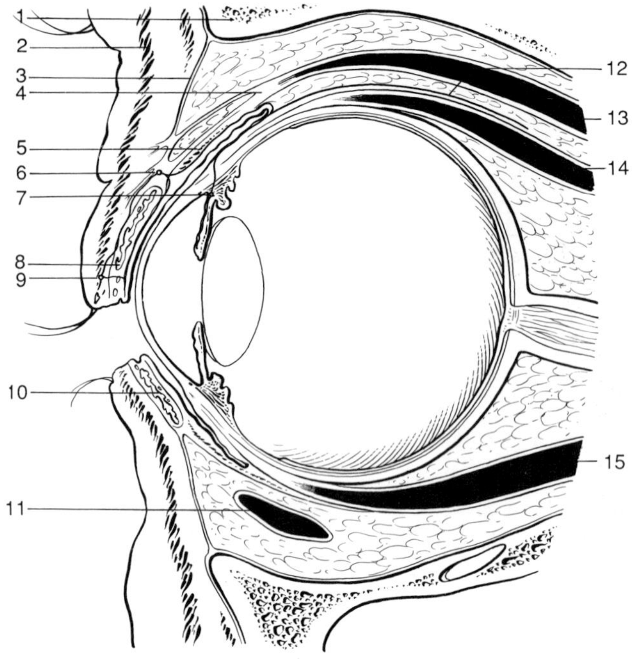

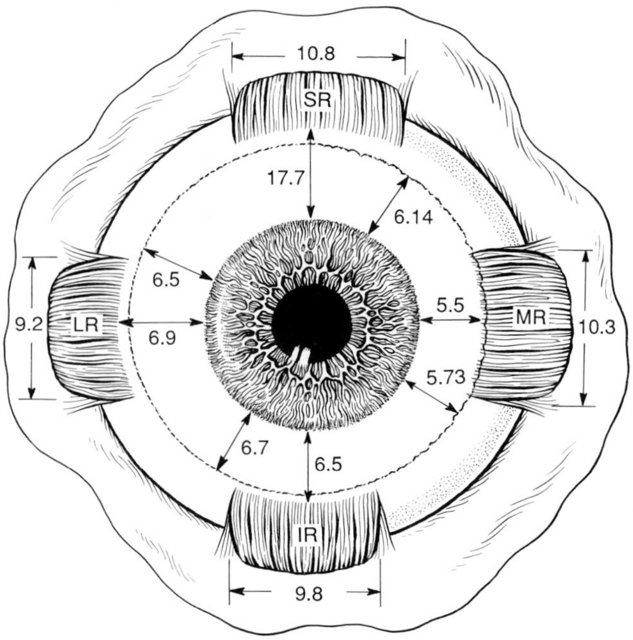

1.2 Cross section of the orbit and eyeball through the optic nerve.
1 Supraorbital bone;
2 orbicularis muscle;
3 orbital septum;
4 levator aponeurosis muscle;
5 superior tarsal muscle;
6 superior tarsal arcade;
7 greater circle of iris;
8 superior tarsal plate;
9 inferior tarsal arcade;
10 inferior tarsal plate;
11 inferior oblique muscle;
12 anterior ciliary artery;
13 levator muscle;
14 superior rectus muscle;
15 inferior rectus muscle.

1.3 Distance from the limbus and width of insertion of the recti muscles. The broken line corresponds to the ora serrata which is located nearer to the nasal than to the temporal limbus, and closer to the limbus superiorly than inferiorly. The arrows indicate the distance (in mm) from the limbus to the ora serrata in the four quadrants, and from the limbus to the insertion of the recti muscles.
SR: superior rectus muscle;
IR: inferior rectus muscle;
LR: lateral rectus muscle;
MR: medial rectus muscle.

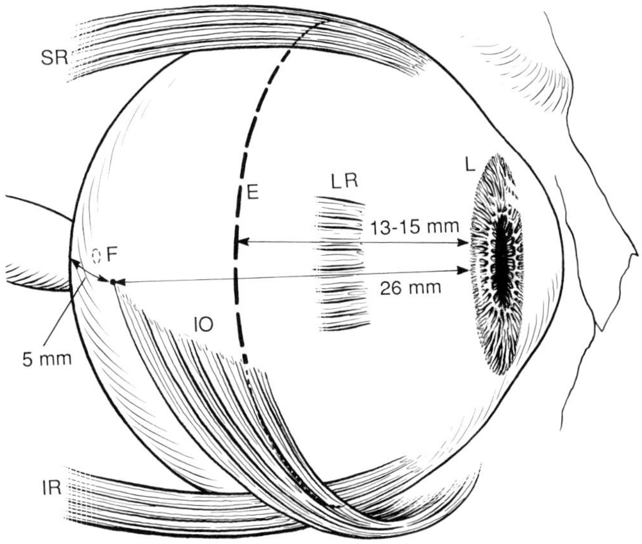

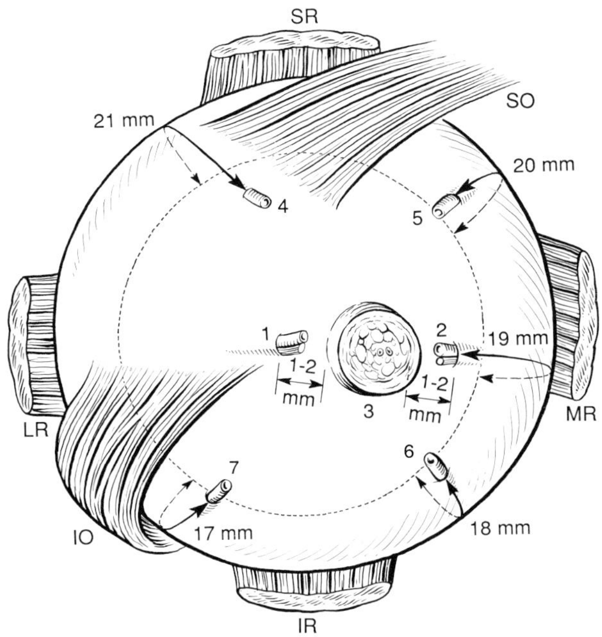

1.4 **Insertion and relationship of the inferior oblique muscle** (IO). The distance from the limbus (L) to the equator (E) varies from 13 to 15 mm. The insertion of the inferior oblique muscle is concave anteriorly; its posterior end is approximately 26 mm from the temporal limbus, 5 mm from the edge of the optic nerve, 1 mm inferior to it, and 1–2 mm from the point on the sclera corresponding to the retinal fovea (F).
SR: superior rectus muscle;
IR: inferior rectus muscle;
LR: lateral rectus muscle.

1.5 **Posterior aspect of the globe,** showing the distance from the limbus (broken line) to the vortex veins. The long posterior ciliary arteries and nerves enter the globe approximately 1–2 mm from the edge of the optic nerve, which averages 3 mm in diameter.
SR: superior rectus muscle;
SO: superior oblique muscle;
IO: inferior oblique muscle;
LR: lateral rectus muscle;
MR: medial rectus muscle;
1 and 2: long ciliary arteries and nerves;
3: optic nerve;
4, 5, 6, and 7: vortex veins.

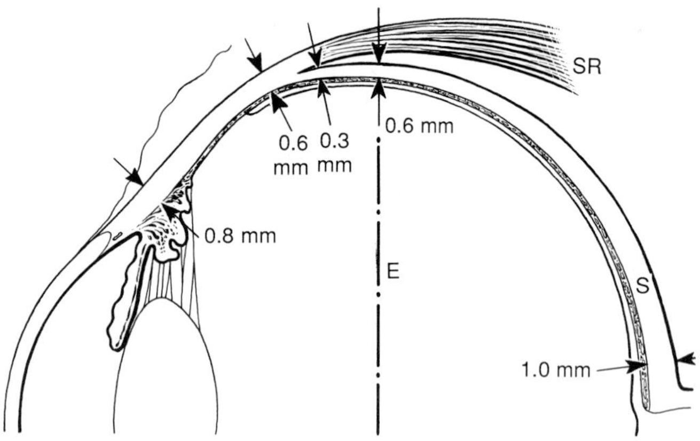

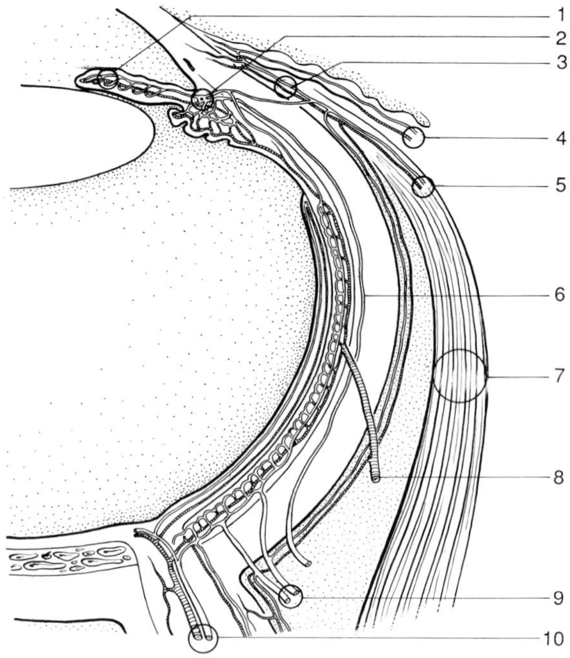

1.6 Cross-section showing the approximate thickness of the sclera from the anterior to the posterior aspect of the eyeball and at the equator (E). The sclera varies in thickness. It is 0.8 mm thick near the limbus, 0.6 mm near the ora serrata, at its thinnest (0.3 mm) at the insertion of the recti muscles, and at its thickest (1.0 mm) near the optic nerve.

1.7 Uveal circulation.
1 Minor arterial circle of the iris;
2 major arterial circle of the iris;
3 anterior conjunctival artery and vein;
4 posterior conjunctival artery and vein;
5 anterior ciliary artery and vein,
6 long posterior ciliary artery;
7 medial rectus muscle;
8 vortex vein;
9 short posterior ciliary vessels;
10 central retinal artery and vein.

Long posterior ciliary arteries. Vitreoretinal surgery frequently involves the region of the long posterior ciliary arteries; familiarization with their anatomy is therefore important. The lateral and medial arteries arise from the ophthalmic artery in the posterior region of the orbit. They pass forward in the orbit in the horizontal meridian, one on either side of the optic nerve, maintaining this position so that they perforate the sclera in the horizontal meridian on the lateral and medial sides of the nerve head slightly beyond the perforating short posterior ciliary arteries. They pass through the sclera obliquely forward along a canal about 3–7 mm in length, and on entering the suprachoroidal space, they run forward in the horizontal plane, one in the lateral, the other in the medial aspect of the globe beside one of the ciliary nerves. During this part of their course, they do not give off any branches, but on entering the outer aspect of the posterior portion of the ciliary body, each artery divides into two main divisions from which other, smaller branches may arise and spread out to anastomose with branches of the anterior ciliary artery to form the major arterial circle of the iris, which runs around the anterior part of the ciliary body just behind the root of the iris. Two or three branches from each main artery pass backward as recurrent arteries through the ciliary body into the anterior part of the choroid as far as the region of the equator.

Anterior ciliary arteries. As a general rule, one should try to avoid detaching the recti muscles for exposure during vitreoretinal surgery, because of possible impairment of the vascular supply of the anterior segment by the anterior ciliary arteries. The anterior ciliary arteries are continuations of the muscular arteries of the four recti muscles, and are derived from the opthalmic artery. They leave the tendons of the muscles at their insertions; two are usually associated with each muscle except the lateral rectus, which contributes only one. On the sclera, they terminate in branches to form an episcleral limbal plexus, or branches that pass into the canal of Schlemm. Large perforating branches run perpendicularly through the sclera near the limbus to enter the ciliary body and ciliary muscle to terminate in the anterior part of the ciliary body by anastomosing with the lateral and medial long posterior ciliary arteries to form the major arterial circle of the iris.

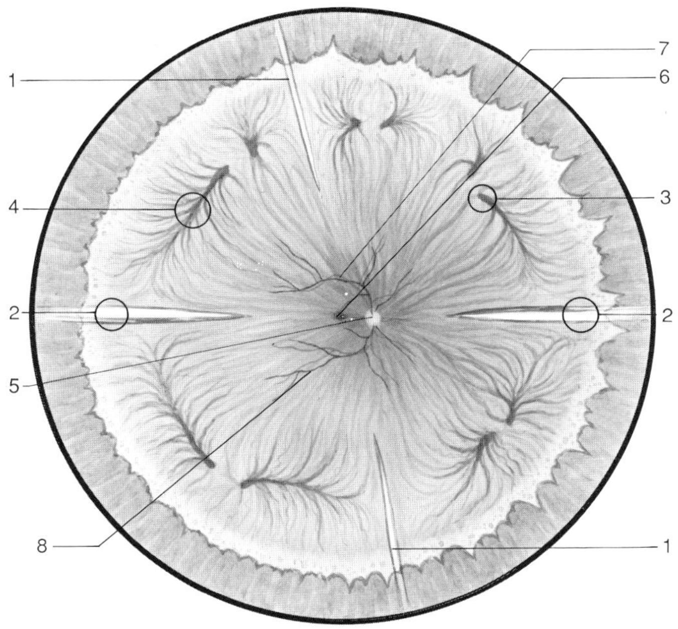

1.8 Ophthalmoscopic landmarks of the fundus.
1 Short ciliary nerve;
2 long posterior ciliary artery and nerve;
3 vortex vein ampulla;
4 vortex vein with anterior and posterior tributaries;
5 optic nerve;
6 macula;
7 superior temporal vascular arcade;
8 inferior temporal vascular arcade.

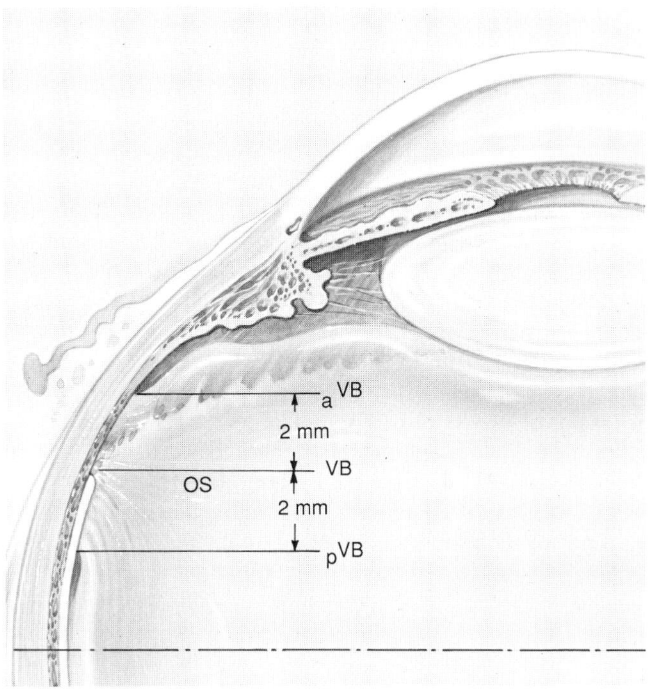

1.9 **Anatomy of the vitreous base.** Cross-section of the anterior segment to illustrate the vitreous base. The width of the vitreous base is irregular, varying from 3 to 4 mm.
VB: vitreous base;
OS: ora serrata;
aVB: anterior border of vitreous base;
pVB: posterior border of vitreous base.

The long posterior ciliary artery is usually superior to the long ciliary nerve nasally and inferior to it temporally. The vortex systems consist of whirling anterior and posterior tributaries that flow into a larger vein (vortex) which may widen into a vortex ampulla. The vortex vein leaves the eye through a scleral canal that varies in length from 1.5 to 8 mm.

The attachment of the vitreous to the fundus periphery and pars plana ciliaris is termed the vitreous base. The vitreous base straddles the ora serrata and has an overall anteroposterior dimension of approximately 3–4 mm in the temporal horizontal meridian. The anterior border of the vitreous base is approximately 2 mm anterior to the ora serrata with protrusions in an irregular pattern into the valleys between ciliary processes. The location cannot be measured with great precision; however, gross observations indicate that it extends approximately 1.5 mm posterior to the mean contour of the ora serrata in the temporal and nasal horizontal meridians. The posterior margin has a relatively smooth circular contour, parallel to the ora serrata, with occasional irregular protrusions posterior. It is these protrusions that are responsible for tearing the retina at the time of posterior vitreous detachment (1–6).

References

1. Michels RG. Vitreous surgery. St. Louis: C V Mosby, 1980: 6–14.
2. Peyman GA, Schulman JA. Intravitreal surgery: principles and practice. New York: Appleton-Century-Crofts, 1986: 1–13.
3. Straatsma BS, Foos RY, Spencer LM. The retina: topography and clinical correlations. In: Symposium on retina and retinal surgery: transactions of the New Orleans Academy of Ophthalmology. St. Louis, C V Mosby, 1969: 1–26.
4. Sigelman J. Retinal diseases: pathogenesis, laser therapy and surgery. Boston: Little, Brown, 1984: 3–65.
5. Tasman W, Shields JA. Disorders of the peripheral fundus. Hagerstown: Harper and Row, 1980: 7–11.
6. Tolentino FI, Schepens CL, Freeman HM. Vitreoretinal disorders: diagnosis and management. Philadelphia: W B Saunders, 1976: 12–13.

2

Preoperative Considerations

Ocular History

To provide the most thorough care, it is mandatory to obtain a detailed and accurate ocular history from the patient. The history should include the onset of symptoms, such as light flashes and their location, sudden changes in vision, location and progression of field loss, previous ocular surgery and complications, ocular medications, response and tolerance to eye medications, and information about associated eye diseases.

Medical History and Systemic Review

Many patients requiring vitreoretinal surgery are in the older age group, and are therefore likely to have medical problems. For this reason, a thorough medical history and systemic review should be obtained. The history should cover the patient's cardiovascular, pulmonary, renal and urinary, hepatic, and nervous systems. Specific information about a family history of diabetes and allergies should be obtained from the patient or from medical records. We have a preoperative medical consultation on all patients over the age of 60 who are to undergo general anesthesia (3).

Ocular Examination

Visual acuity. An accurate visual acuity measurement is a basic preoperative requirement in all patients.

Color perception. Blood in the vitreous cavity may alter color perception. A positive response to color is meaningful; a negative response is not conclusive. Perception of color suggests that the macula is attached.

Entoptic phenomenon. A light probe is applied to the patient's closed lids with the eyes looking down. Shadows cast by retinal blood vessels are perceived as branches or cracks, and suggest that the posterior retina is attached (10).

Biomicroscopy. Clarity of the cornea and crystalline lens is essential during closed vitrectomy. The presence of cells and flare in aqueous fluid indicates intraocular inflammation that will require administration of systemic or topical steroids prior to vitreous or retinal surgery. Cells in the anterior chamber that appear as tiny brownish or khaki-colored particles that have gravitated in layers may be the result of longstanding vitreous hemorrhage. Such cells are capable of producing erythroclastic glaucoma. In diabetic patients, a careful biomicroscopic and gonioscopic examination is important to detect early rubeosis iridis, alerting one to consider panretinal photocoagulation of the peripheral retina intraoperatively. In brown irides, early rubeosis iridis is difficult to detect, and may be suspected only in the presence of an irregular pupil, posterior synechiae, and ectropion uveae. When cataractous changes are present in an eye requiring vitreoretinal surgery, an effort should be made to determine the degree of hardness of the nucleus. A white cataract is usually soft and may be amenable to aspiration. A brown cataract indicates a hard nucleus requiring phacoemulsification or extracapsular or intracapsular lens extraction.

Gonioscopy. It is important to know the status of the iridocorneal angle before performing scleral buckling or vitreous surgery. In some eyes, extensive scleral buckling or postoperative choroidal detachment may compromise a narrow angle and provoke angle-closure glaucoma. In eyes with a narrow angle, a laser iridectomy may be indicated prior to the buckling procedure. An early diagnosis of rubeosis iridis may be revealed by small vessels that begin in the iridocorneal angle. Photocoagulation of these vessels may be attempted before subjecting the eye to surgery that may accelerate rubeosis.

Indirect ophthalmoscopy and scleral depression. A patient with a retinal break or retinal detachment must be examined thoroughly with scleral depression and indirect ophthalmoscopy (9). This examination is best done with the patient in the supine position. A +20D condensing lens is used, and if the pupil is small or the media are hazy, a +27D lens is helpful. The +14D lens is used to study fine details. The fundus chart is held on a clipboard resting on the patient's chest, with the chart oriented upside down so that 12 o'clock on the chart is toward the patient's feet and 6 o'clock toward the chin. The observer sees the inverted image of the fundus through the indirect ophthalmoscope, and simply records on the chart what he sees, as he sees it. The following color code is used to represent fundus details:

Blue for detached retina and retinal veins.

Red for attached retina, retinal arteries, and hemorrhage in retina.

Red lined with blue for retinal breaks.

Black for retinal pigmentation and choroidal pigmentation seen through attached retina.

Brown for choroidal pigmentation seen through detached retina.

Green for opacities in the media, including vitreous hemorrhage.

Yellow for choroidal exudation and macular edema.

Biomicroscopy of the posterior segment is important in evaluating vitreoretinal relationships and vitreous and preretinal membranes and for examining suspicious areas of the fundus with high magnification. The Goldmann three-mirror contact lens is particularly suited for studying retinal breaks or detachments. The slit beam of the slit lamp microscope can be particularly helpful in detecting or confirming a retinal break that appears as a discontinuity of the beam.

Ancillary Tests

Ultrasonography. This technique has greatly improved the surgeon's ability to assess the posterior segment structures preoperatively (1, 2, 5, 7). In cases of ocular trauma associated with cataract or vitreous hemorrhage, a finding of a partial retinal detachment indicates early vitreoretinal surgery. Extensive cyclitic membranes in a hypotonous eye suggest an unfavorable prognosis. Ultrasonographic configuration of a retinal detachment may differentiate a tractional from a rhegmatogenous retinal detachment. Ultrasonography can be helpful in predicting the outcome of vitreoretinal surgery in eyes with retinopathy of prematurity. An open-funnel configuration of retinal detachment carries a better prognosis than a closed funnel. Ultrasonography can help in establishing a diagnosis of choroidal tumor in an eye with vitreous hemorrhage and a secondary retinal detachment.

Electrophysiology tests. These tests include bright-flash electroretinography (ERG), visually evoked response or potential (VER or VEP), and electrically evoked response (EER) (4, 6, 8). The findings can be useful when correlated with those of ultrasonography, and help the surgeon to assess the functional potential of the retina and optic nerve in eyes with opaque media and poor light perception. VER tests the function of the macula and optic nerve. EER uses an electrical stimulus and records conduction responses of the retina and optic nerve.

References

1. Charles S. Vitreous microsurgery. 2nd ed. Baltimore: Williams and Wilkins, 1987: 11–22.
2. Coleman DJ, Lizzi FL, Jack RL. Ultrasonography of the eye and orbit. Philadelphia: Lea and Febiger, 1977: 196–201.
3. Dyole GJ, Schepens CL. Medical management of the patient. In: Schepens CL, ed. Retinal detachment and allied diseases. Philadelphia: W B Saunders, 1983: 233–276.
4. Fuller D, Knighton R, Machemer R. Bright-flash ERG. In: Irvine AR, O'Malley C, eds. Advances in vitreous surgery. Springfield, IL: Charles C Thomas, 1976: 97–99.
5. Goldberg RE, Sarin LK. Experiences with ultrasonography, part I: the posterior segment of the globe. Am I Opththalmol 1966; 61: 1497–1502.
6. Matsuhashi M, Nagai M, Hirose T, Miyake Y. Prognostic value of electrophysiologic tests in vitrectomy in diabetics with vitreous hemorrhage. In: Henkind P, ed. Acta: XXIV International Congress of Ophthalmology, San Francisco, 1982. Philadelphia: J B. Lippincott, 1983, vol 2: 795–799.
7. Michels RG. Vitreous surgery. St. Louis: C V Mosby, 1980.
8. Miyake Y, Hirose T, Hara A. Electrophysiologic testing of visual functions for vitrectomy candidates, I: results in eyes with known fundus diseases. Retina 1983; 3: 86–94.
9. Schepens CL. Retinal detachment and allied diseases. Philadelphia: W B Saunders, 1983: 103–119.
10. Tolentino FI, Freeman HM, Schepens CL, Hirose T. Preoperative evaluation. (Symposium: Pars plana vitrectomy) Trans Am Acad Ophthalmol Otolaryngol 1976; 81: OP 358–370.

3

Equipment and Instrumentation

Instrumentation for Intravitreous Surgery

3.**1 a, b** Vitreoretinal surgery requires a microscope with special features such as gross and fine focus; zoom adjustment, X-Y movement; and a binocular observer's scope for the surgeon's assistant. In addition, the microscope should be able to have a filter assembly for an endolaser attached to it. These features are offered in many commercially available microscopes, including the Zeiss OPM 1-6 (**a**), Wild (**b**), Moeller-Wedel, Olympus, and others.

a

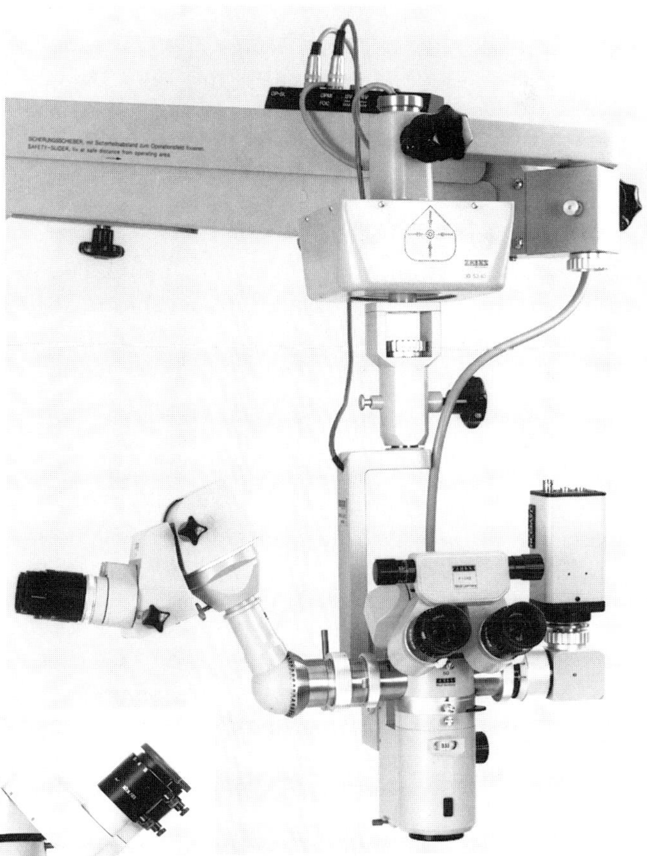

Zeiss, Oberkochen, West Germany

b

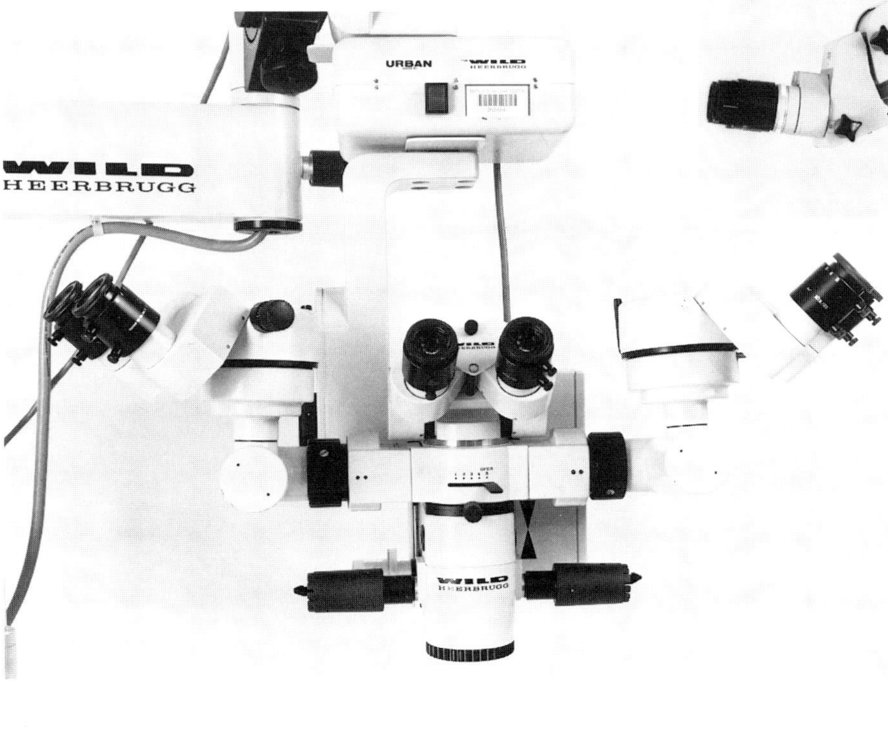

Wild Leitz, Heerbrogg, Switzerland

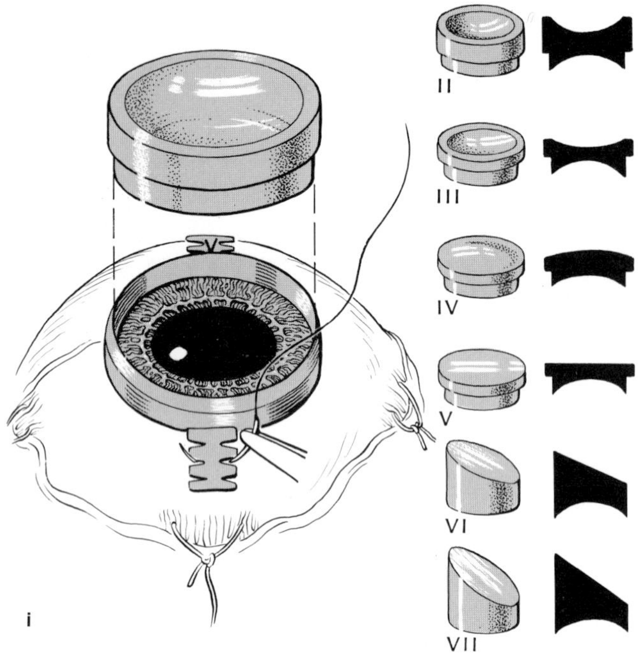

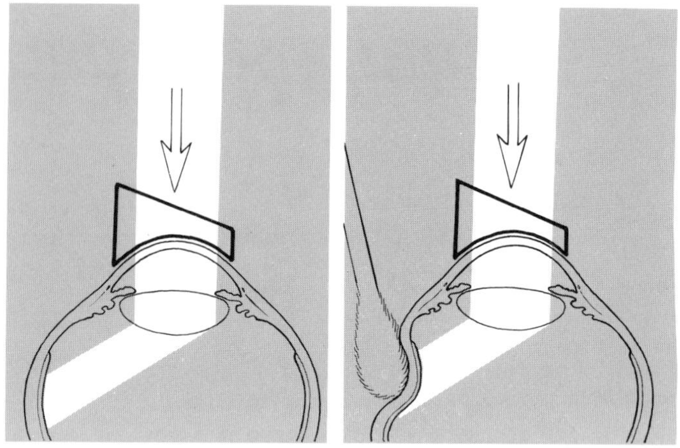

Contact lenses for vitreoretinal surgery. A contact lens is necessary to visualize the mid- and posterior portions of the vitreous cavity (12, 17). A variety of lenses are available; some are fixed to the globe, others are held in contact with the cornea by the assistant (8).

3.**2a** i. One method utilizes a set of contact lenses held in contact with the cornea by a retaining ring. This ring is sutured to the episclera adjacent to the limbus in the 12 and 6 o'clock meridians using 6-0 polyglactin (Vicryl) suture which is tied over each scleral strut. The well created by the ring is filled with hyaluronic acid or methylcellulose. The appropriate lens is selected and placed into the ring. The Landers vitrectomy ring system contains the following lenses:

ii. Landers biconcave lens, which allows the fundus to be visualized when the vitreous cavity is filled with air (10).

iii. Machemer magnifying lens for examining details on the surface of the retina.

iv. Peyman wide-field lens for visualizing the equatorial portion of the vitreous cavity (15).

v. Planoconcave lens, suitable for "core" vitrectomy.

vi. Tolentino 20° prism lens for visualizing the periphery of the vitreous cavity.

vii. Tolentino 30° prism lens for visualizing the extreme periphery of the vitreous cavity.

3.**2b** **Use of the Prism lenses.** Left: The 20° and 30° prism lenses allow the surgeon to extend the peripheral view through the microscope (20). The base of the prism is rotated to the meridian of the globe to be viewed.

Right: A more peripheral view can be obtained with scleral depression.

3.2c **Irrigating vitrectomy contact lenses.** Different lenses may be mounted in a lens holder with an irrigating capability (14). The handle is connected to intravenous tubing attached to the BSS Plus bottle. The lens is held in place by an assistant who visualizes the eye through a beam splitter on the operating microscope.

The lens at the upper left is biconcave, with a small degree of concavity in front, and provides slight minification of the image in the vitreous. The lens at the lower left is planconcave, and gives a standard image. The lens at the (upper right) is biconcave, with equal concavity on each side resulting in a great minification of the image. It is used to visualize the vitreous cavity filled with air or gas. The lens at the (lower right) is convex in front an concave on the back. It provides a magnified image, suitable for posterior segment membrane dissection in cases of macular pucker.

Charles has designed a glass irrigating-type lens with a handle for the assistant (2). The irrigation system washes away blood that may accumulate between the lens and the cornea.

Instruments for exploring, isolating, and peeling preretinal membranes. The goal in preretinal membrane surgery is to separate the membrane as thoroughly as possible without producing a retinal break. To accomplish this, it is helpful to have an array of instruments of varying thickness, sharpness, and angulation for peeling membranes of varying thickness, adherence, and orientation.

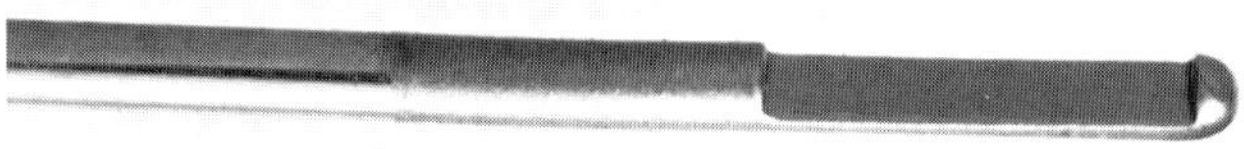

Dorc, Geervliet, Holland

3.3 **Membrane Peeler.** The blunt, rounded tip of the membrane peeler is well suited for separating weakly adherent preretinal membranes (25). The notch near the tip is useful for engaging the edge of a membrane as the peeler passes over the surface of a steep, funnel-shaped retinal detachment. The rounded tip is helpful for atraumatic exploration of a membrane between deep retinal folds.

A variety of spatulas with blades of varying thickness, curvature, sharpness, and abrasiveness is helpful in separating surface membranes of varying thickness and varying degrees of adherence to the retina (9).

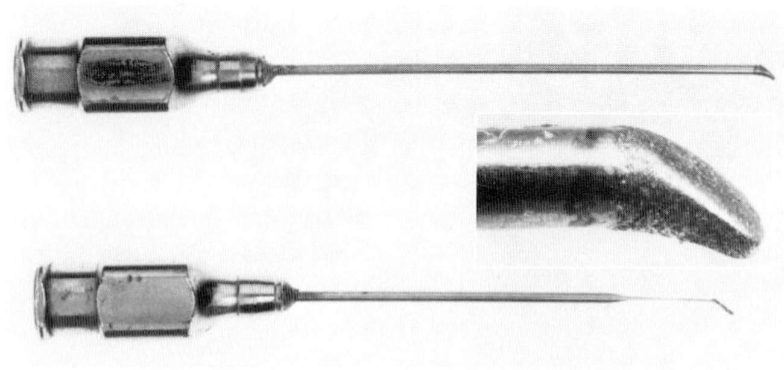

Stortz, St. Louis, USA

3.4a **Diamond-dusted microspatulas.** The spatula set consists of four tips and a universal handle (21). The range of tip angulation is 30°, 45°, 60°, and 80°. The bottom surface of the spatula tip is covered with fine diamond dust (inset), which provides an abrasive surface to rub against a preretinal membrane to separate its edge. The edge can then be grasped with end-gripping forceps.

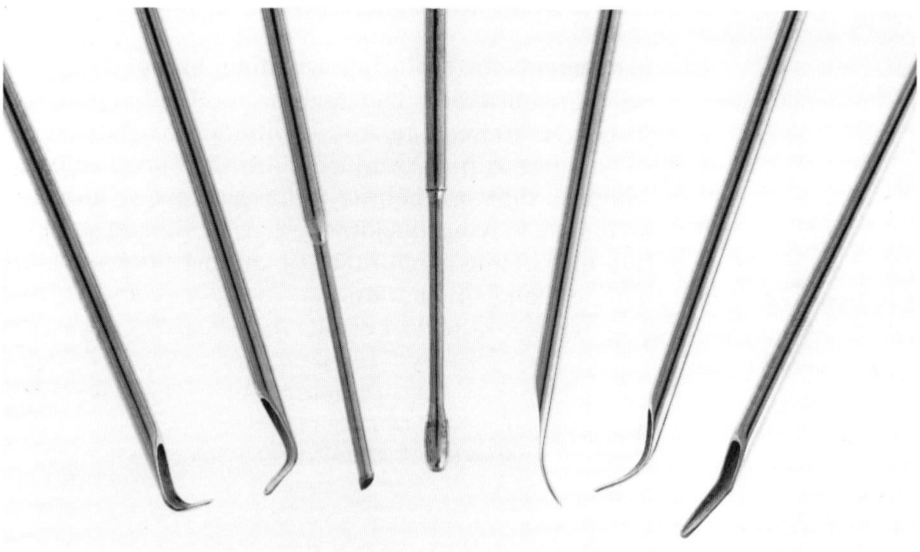

Storz, MIRA, Waltham, MA, USA or Visatec, Bradentor, FL, USA

3.4b **Membrane microdissection set.** The set includes 6 spatulas and a matchhead-shaped irrigating-dissecting tip (middle). The angle between spatula and shaft varies from 60° to 160°. The spatulas have a spearhead shape and a blunt edge (9). Normally, they have an opening in front, but a special spatula (third from the left) opens at the back. These openings allow aspirations or irrigation of fluid. The irrigation capability makes it possible to use the spatula for dissection in the presence of bleeding and for gentle hydraulic membrane dissection of preretinal membranes. The matchhead-shaped tip is used for blunt dissection and irrigation.

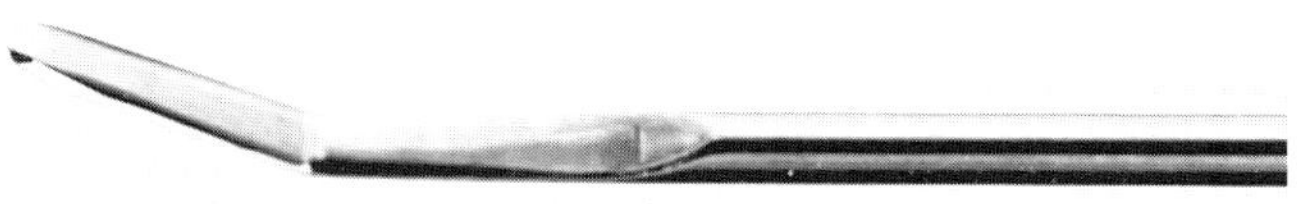

Dorc

3.4c **Hooked membrane spatula.** The blade of this spatula is dull and bent at an angle of 45° 5 mm from the rounded tip. The thin spatula blade is useful for separating fibrovascular membranes and adhesions between deep retinal folds.

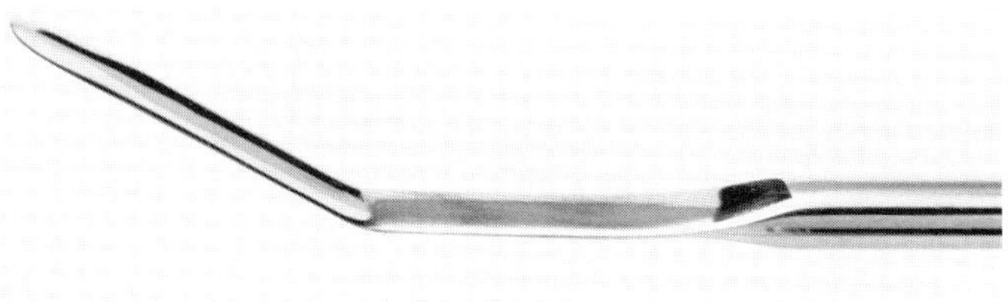

Dorc

3.4d **Membrane spatula knife.** This spatula has sharp edges for undermining and cutting adherent surface membranes.

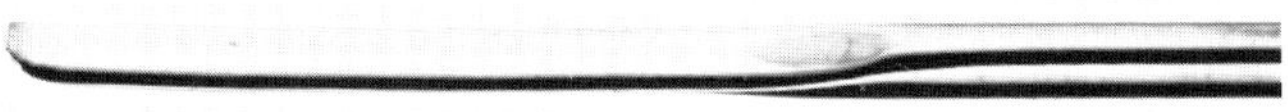

Dorc

3.4e **Curved membrane spatula.** The tip of this blunt, thick spatula is curved at an angle of 45°, which makes it useful for picking up and isolating preretinal membranes lining a steep, funnel-shaped retinal detachment.

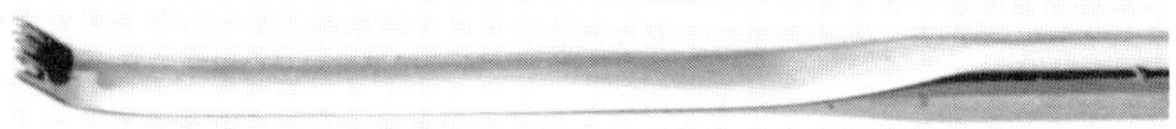

Dorc

3.4f **Membrane scratcher.** This spatula has the configuration of a rake, with four small teeth 0.15 mm wide and 0.4 mm long bent at an angle of 45° (25: 31–32). The scratcher is useful for scraping and clearing friable membranes and clusters of pigmented cells from the surface of the retina. The small, smooth, rounded teeth at each end of the rake can be especially effective in engaging and lifting the edge of a thin preretinal membrane.

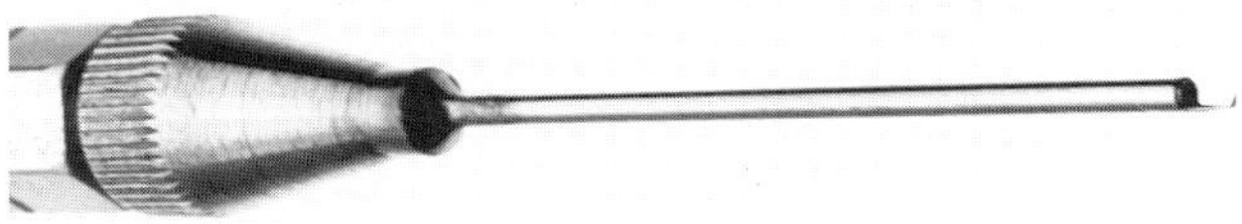

3.5a **Lighted membrane pick.** The pick is located at the end of a 25 mm, 19-gauge hollow sleeve containing a solid 20-gauge fiber-optic light cable. This lighted pick is useful in bimanual delamination of preretinal membranes.

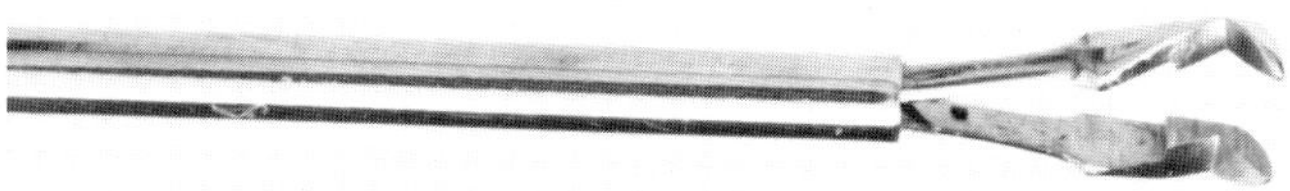

Grieshaber, Schaffhausen, Switzerland

3.5b **Pick forceps.** The wedge-shaped tip of the pick forceps makes it possible to peel and grip a membrane with the same instrument. This lighted pick is helpful in membrane delamination with vitreous scissors. The pick is a hollow sleeve, 25 mm long, that is inserted onto a solid 20-gauge light pipe.

Membrane forceps. It is helpful to have a variety of forceps to aid in removing preretinal and subretinal membranes. Forceps with jaws of various lengths and angulation with the shaft allow an optimal approach to the membrane (25).

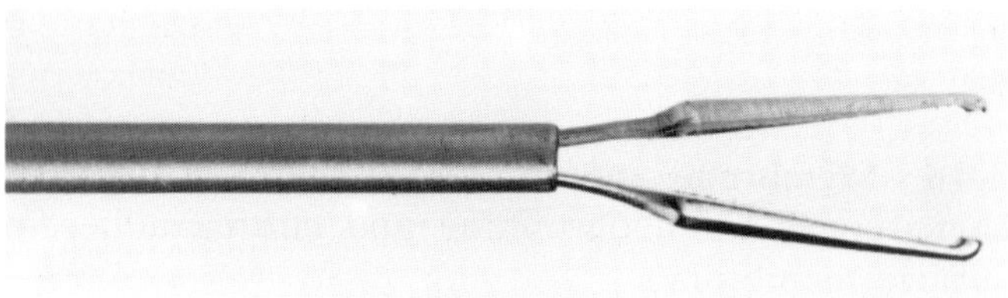

Dorc

3.6a **End-gripping forceps.** The small platform between the blunt tips of the blades is extremely well suited for grasping delicate membranes from the surface of the retina.

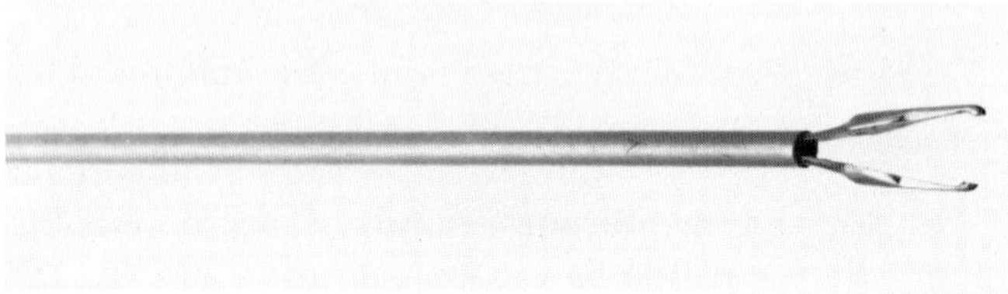

Dorc

3.6b **End-gripping forceps with tapered tips.** The tips of end-gripping forceps are tapered so that membranes between narrow retinal folds can be grasped.

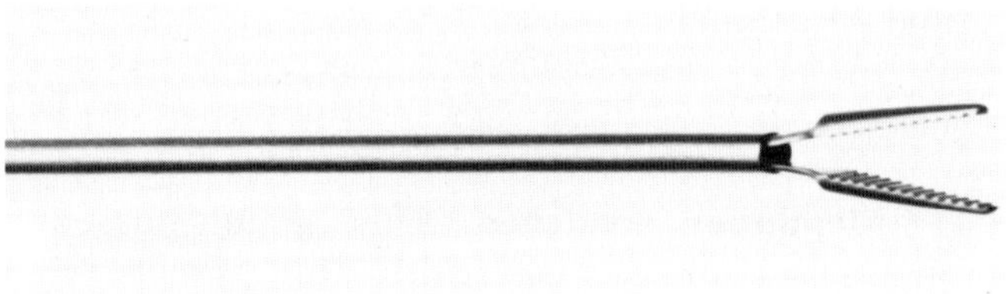

Dorc

3.6c **Forceps with serrated jaws.** The serrated jaws of these forceps are helpful for grasping dense, thick lens capsule, dense membranes, and small foreign bodies.

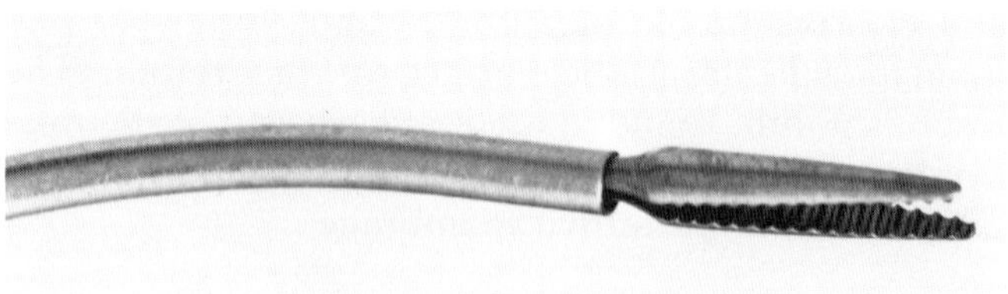

Dorc

3.6d **Curved forceps.** The long, curved shaft and tips of these forceps are suited for reaching through a retinotomy to grasp a subretinal membrane.

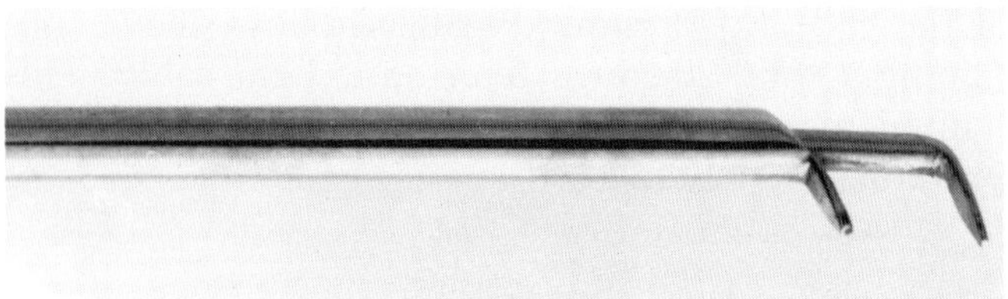

Dorc

3.6e **Side-gripping forceps.** The blades, which close at right angles, can be helpful in peeling membranes from the edge of a buckle.

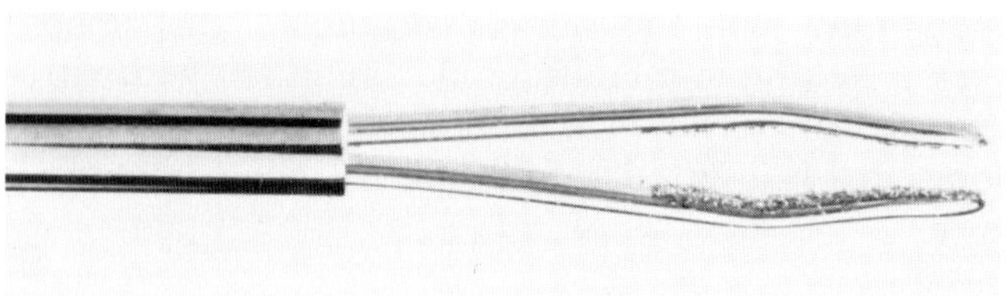

Grieshaber

3.6f **Diamond-coated foreign-body forceps.** These forceps can grasp and hold intraocular foreign bodies of various shapes and composition because of the diamond-chip coating on the internal surfaces of the jaws. A self-closing mechanism holds the foreign body once it is grasped.

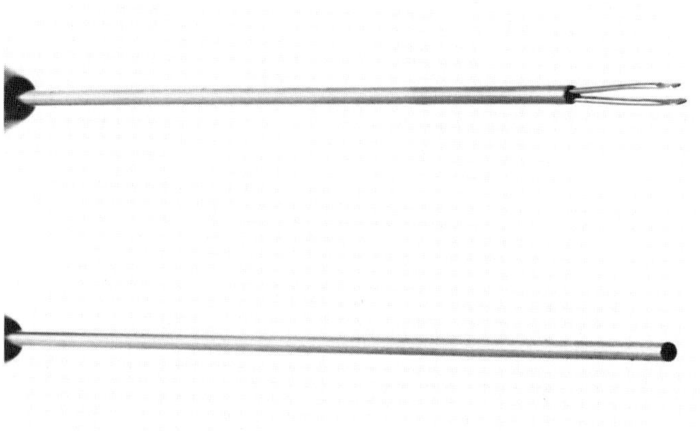

Grieshaber

3.6g **Microsurgical biopsy forceps.** These forceps are designed for the removal of vitreous gel, vitreous membranes, and preretinal membranes. The specimen is grasped between the forceps blades and then partially drawn into the 20-gauge tube by retracting the jaws of the forceps. This protects the specimen from damage and from getting lost while it is passed through the small opening in the pars plana during removal from the eye. Following its removal, the tips of the forceps, together with the specimen, are placed in a glass vial containing a fixative.

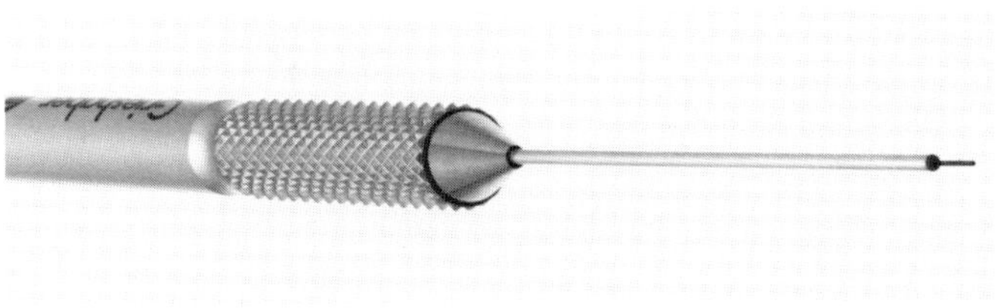

Grieshaber

3.7 **Fiber-optic diathermy tissue manipulator.** This instrument provides illumination, diathermy, and aspiration through a single probe tip. Coaxial bipolar diathermy with a fiber-optic light makes it possible to coagulate vessels. By gently aspirating membranes up to the port, the instrument can be used as a forceps.

When hemorrhage is encountered, thrombin solution can be infused through the probe to irrigate blood away from the site and aid in hemostasis. The tip of the manipulator can then be used to cauterize the bleeding site (4).

Membrane scissors. Scissors are preferable to the vitrectomy probe for cutting membranes that are tough or located close to the retina. Suction required to engage such membranes in the port of a vitrectomy-probe may exert traction on the adjacent retina to produce an iatrogenic retinal break.

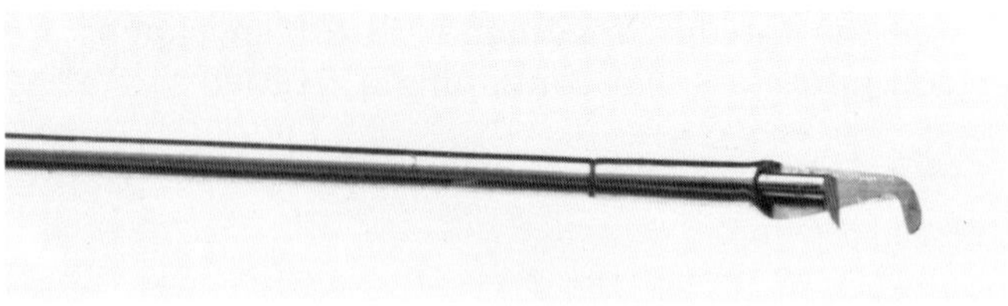

Grieshaber

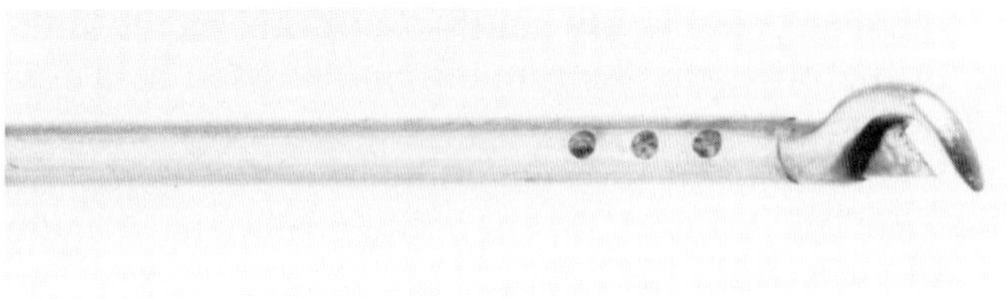

Storz

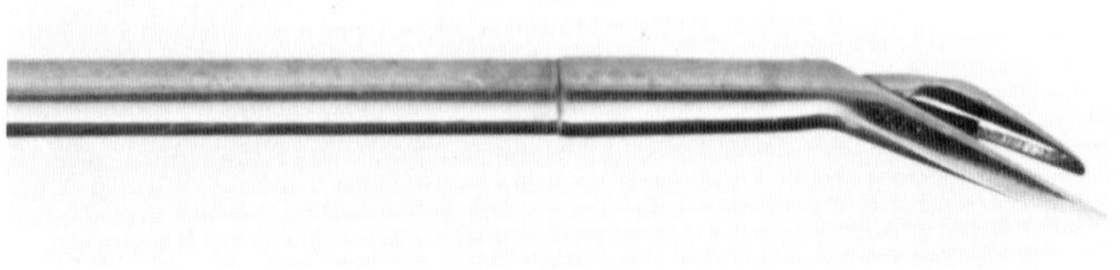

i

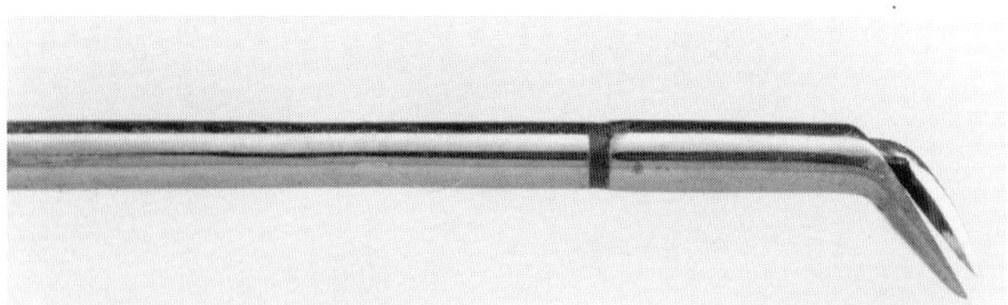

ii

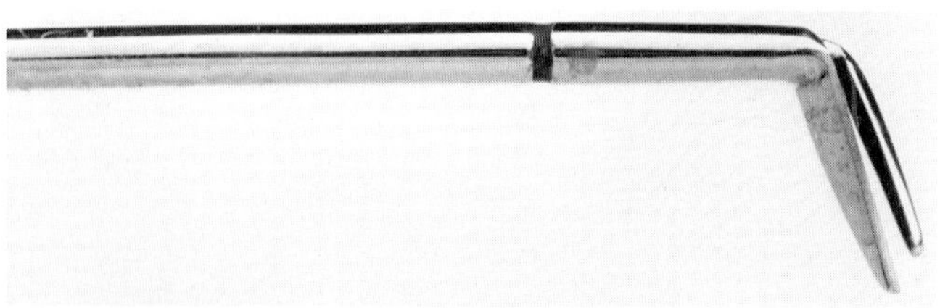

iii

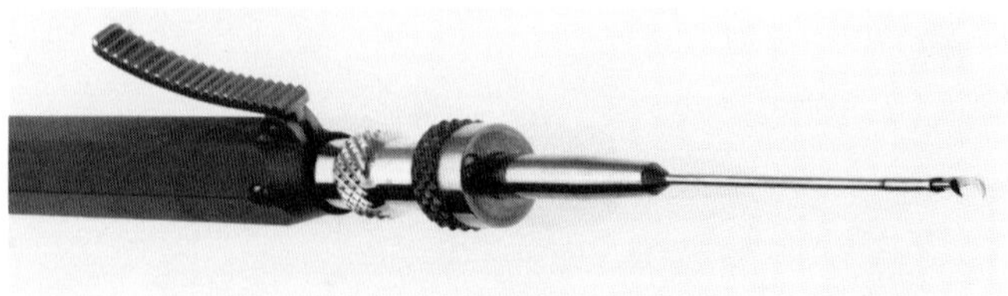

iv

Blunt or sharp-tipped scissor blades at various angulations make it possible to dissect, delaminate, or cut membranes in various locations and planes. Different blade angulations allow the best visualization of the membrane, the scissor blades, and adjacent structures. The blades may be closed manually or by remote control (membrane peeler cutter, dissector cutter).

3.8a **Automated scissors: membrane peeler cutter** (MPC). This vertical-cutting and dissecting instrument has a stationary distal blade (inset) that can be used as a membrane pick, and a proximal blade that moves against the stationary blade to cut the membrane (13). The blades are at right angles for cutting membranes parallel to the retinal surface. The cutter is powered by an electric motor located in the handle and activated by a foot pedal.

3.8b **Automated scissors: dissector cutter.** This vertical-cutting instrument is useful for cutting and dissecting preretinal membranes (22). The smooth, blunt, hook-shaped tip (inset) is designed to isolate and separate the firm adhesion between the preretinal membrane and the retina in diabetic tractional detachments. The guillotine-type blade cuts on an anvil-like chopping block, causing no movement of the instrument and therefore minimal traction to surrounding structures and a reduced risk of retinal perforation. The blade is activated by a foot pedal. The cutting action is powered by compressed air from a console or a compressed air-powered vitrectomy console.

3.8c **Manually operated scissors.** The Sutherland type of scissors have been adapted for vitreoretinal surgery. Blunt or sharp tips with varying angulations offer the versatility necesseary to cut membranes oriented in a variety of planes and locations (7). (i) Angle 25°, blade length 1.7 mm (Stegman). (ii) Angle 55°, blade length 1.7 mm (Tolentino). (iii) Angle 70°, blade length 3.1 mm (Charles). (iv) Vertical-cutting (Machemer). (v) Angle 180° (Freeman).

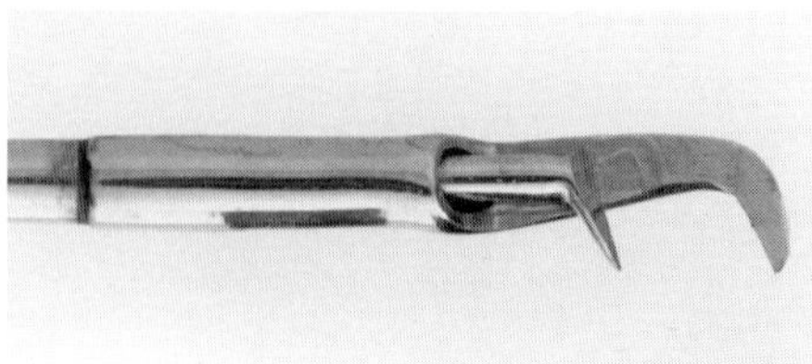

iv

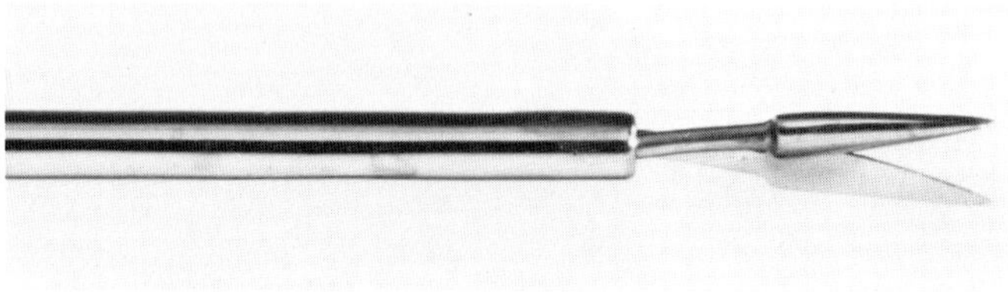

v

Grieshaber iv–v)

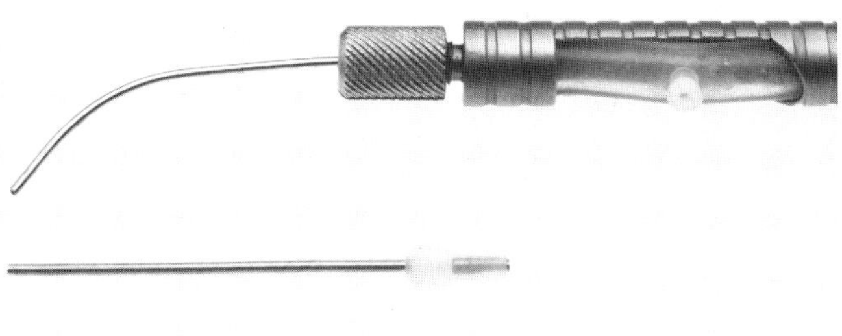

Dorc

3.9a Backflush needle. This needle has the advantage over the flute needle of being able to disengage tissue incarcerated in its tip. Depressing the silicone tubing in which the vent is located closes the vent and forces a jet stream of fluid down and out of the needle, thereby disengaging incarcerated retina, membranes, or blood. This jet stream can be used to stir up blood from the retinal surface, where it can be more safely aspirated. A straight, curved, or hooked needle can be inserted into the handle.

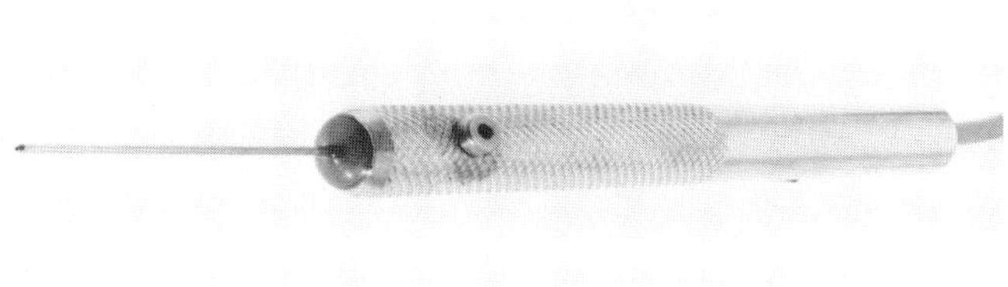

Dorc

3.9b Combined backflush needle and diathermy. This instrument is useful in the presence of profuse intraocular bleeding which obscures the bleeding site so that it cannot be coagulated (5). The backflush capability makes it possible to aspirate blood to permit visualization and simultaneously coagulate the bleeding site without losing time exchanging a diathermy probe for a backflush needle.

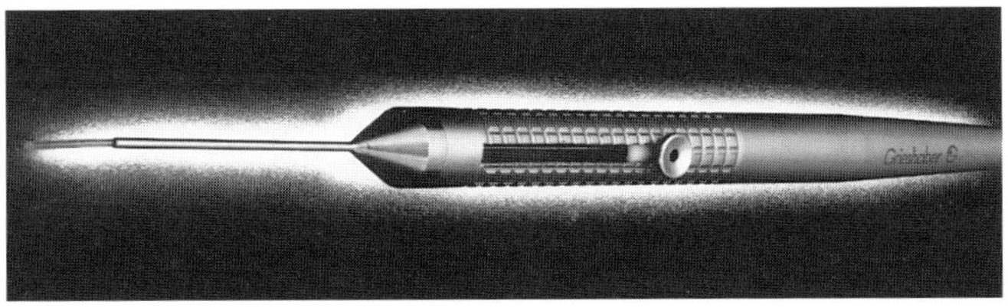

Grieshaber

3.9c Cannulated subretinal fluid aspirator. This extrusion needle makes possible the drainage of subretinal fluid through a peripheral retinal break, and may obviate the need for a retinotomy (5). The instrument is also useful in draining subretinal hemorrhage. A flexible translucent cannula with a 0.6 mm outer diameter and 0.3 mm inner diameter is threaded into the shaft of the 20-gauge stainless steel instrument tube. The cannula fits snugly within the shaft of the tube, preventing egress of fluid from the eye between the cannula and the shaft of the instrument. The cannula is advanced by means of a slide controlled with the index finger. The cannula can be extended 18 mm beyond the blunt end of the 20-gauge instrument. The slide contains a venting hole to allow passive egress of fluid if indicated. The venting hole can be covered by the surgeon's index finger to allow active suction through the central stainless steel tube when connected to the vitrectomy console with the flexible tubing. The instrument tip is positioned near a retinal hole, and then the cannula is advanced into the subretinal space through the retinal hole. The subretinal fluid is aspirated by passive or active linear suction. The cannula is then retracted from the retinal hole after retinal reattachment has been achieved.

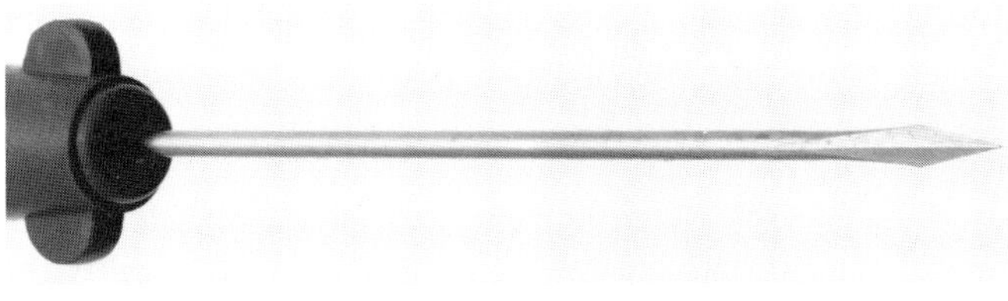

Alcon, Fr. Worth, Tx, USA

3.10 Microvitreal knife (MVR). This knife has a blade 1.4 mm wide that produces an incision that accommodates a 20-gauge instrument snugly.

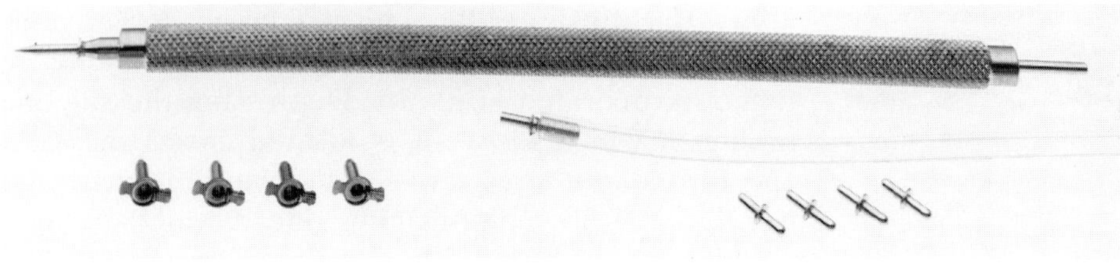

Grieshaber

3.**11a Trochar cannula set.** Microcannulas are used during vitreous surgery to protect the entry site, avoid vitreous base damage, and allow easy exchange of instruments or the infusion line. By using three or four cannulas of equal size, interchangeability of all instruments is achieved. A locking mechanism or an "O" ring seal allows attachment of various infusing lines. The cannulas are inserted into the sclerotomy using a trochar. The cannula opening can be closed with a plug with a locking collar.

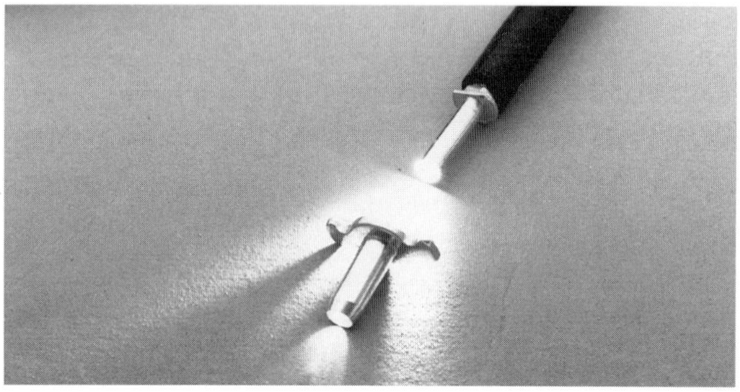

b Light insert. A Grieshaber fiber-optic light insert is used to illuminate the vitreous cavity. It is especially useful in cases requiring bimanual vitreous surgery.

3.**12 Retinal tacks and screws.** The detached retina may be mechanically fixated using retinal tacks or retinal screws.

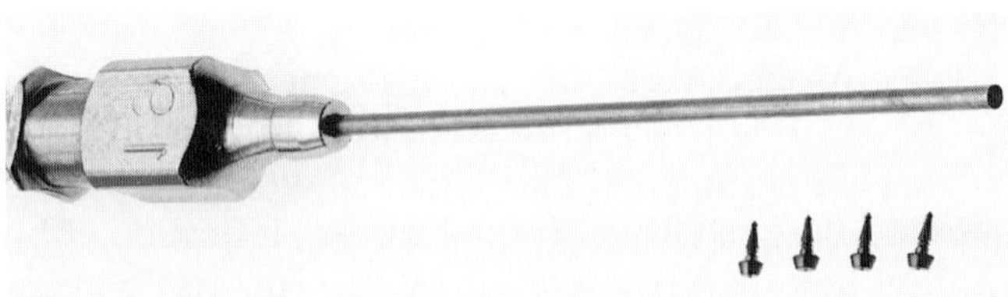

Trek, Milwaukee, WI, USA

a *Retinal tack.* The retinal tack developed by Abrams et al. is composed of the purest form of titanium commercially available (99.448%), machined to a diameter of 1.0 mm and a length of 0.7 or 1.6 mm (1). The tapered conical end allows easy penetration through the sclera, and the grooved shaft becomes enmeshed by the glial cells and choroidal connective tissue.

The tack is inserted with a 1 mm steel cannula machined to accept the tapered head of the tack (inset). The tack is retained by suction in the cannula and released by foot-activated controls. The suction is aborted by equilibration to a preset air infusion pump within the system, so that no suction force is applied to the adjacent retina.

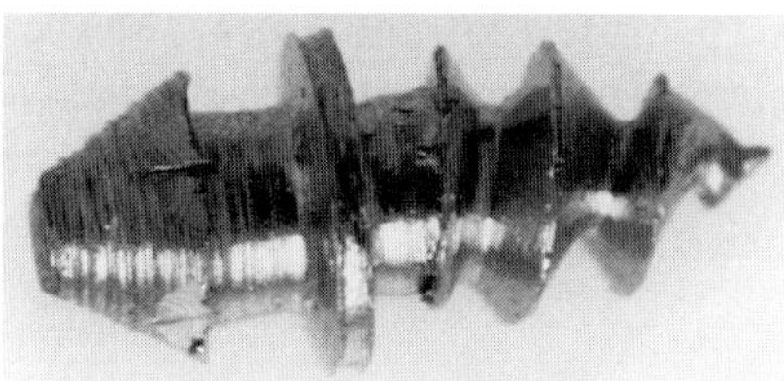

b *Retinal screw.* The tantalum retinal screw designed by Tolentino and Baehr is 2 mm in length. The tapered head of the screw has a maximum diameter of 1.0 mm. The screw design affords a stronger fixation in the sclera and thus reduces the incidence of dislodgement experienced intra- or postoperatively with retinal tacks. The screw is inserted with a forceps-like screwdriver that grasps the screw in the groove distal to its head.

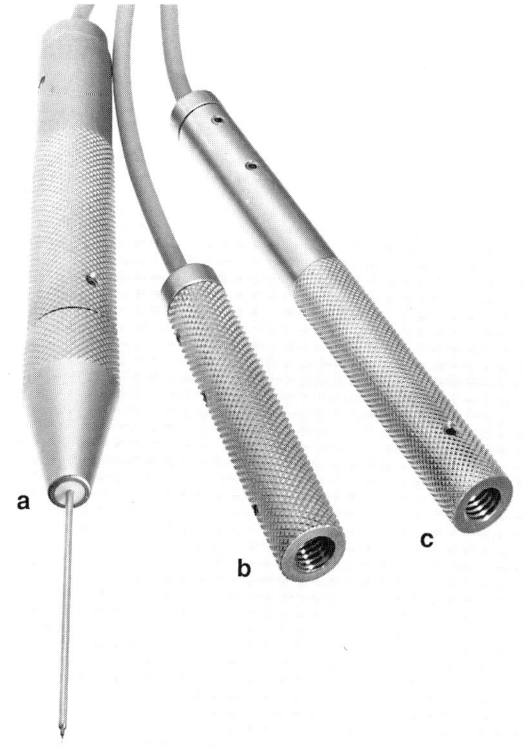

MIRA

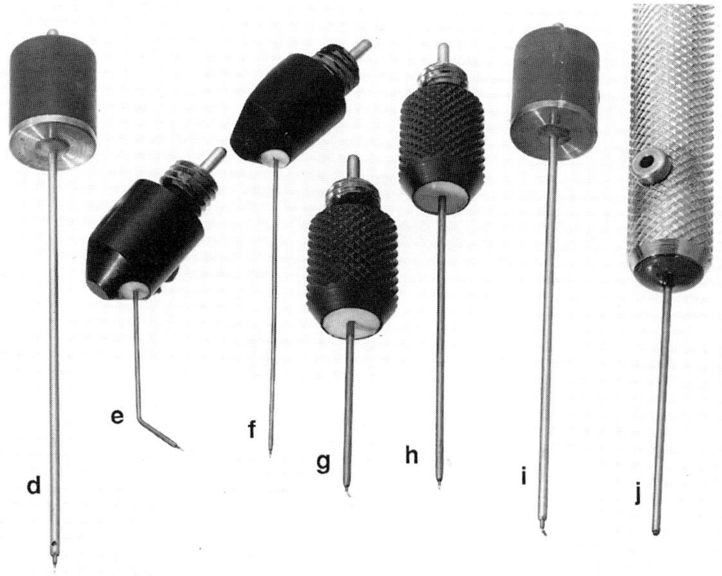

MIRA

3.**13 Endodiathermy probes.** Vitreoretinal surgery demands effective hemostasis, because hemorrhage into the vitreous cavity may obscure the operative field and incite preretinal cellular proliferation postoperatively.

Underwater diathermy probes. Underwater diathermy electrodes are of coaxial design. They have a double insulation, and are shielded to prevent current loss in fluid medium and variation in output through secondary induced currents. Energy is delivered at the tip of the electrode only. This permits the placement of discrete burns that affect only the chosen structure and not the surrounding tissue. The diathermy probe is mounted on a 19-gauge stainless steel tube which is swaged over the diathermy probe. Three lengths of handles (**a**–**c**) and six types of straight and angled electrodes with and without concentric infusion (**d**–**j**) are available. Diathermy is activated by a foot pedal (19).

a Infusion electrode handle with cable, complete with straight coaxial electrode.

b Short electrode handle and cable for use with coaxial electrodes without infusion.

c Long electrode handle and cable for use with coaxial electrodes without infusion.

d Straight coaxial electrode with concentric infusion channel.

e 35° angled coaxial electrode without infusion for use in open-sky procedures.

f Straight coaxial electrode without infusion, designed for use through a sclerotomy in the pars plana.

g Angled anterior chamber coaxial electrode without infusion.

h 20-gauge straight coaxial electrode without infusion.

i Hirose electrode. Right-angled underwater diathermy tip used to scrape the retinal pigment epithelium.

j Aspiration electrode. This electrode is a combination coaxial diathermy and vacuum-cleaner needle. Its purpose is to aspirate loose blood or thin clots from actively bleeding vessels on the retinal surface, and then to coagulate these vessels immediately. The instrument tip is of a 20-gauge size with a small central lumen and a two-layered outer coaxial conductor. The vacuum-cleaning action is controlled by opening or closing a port on the handle with a fingertip, while diathermy application is activated by a foot pedal.

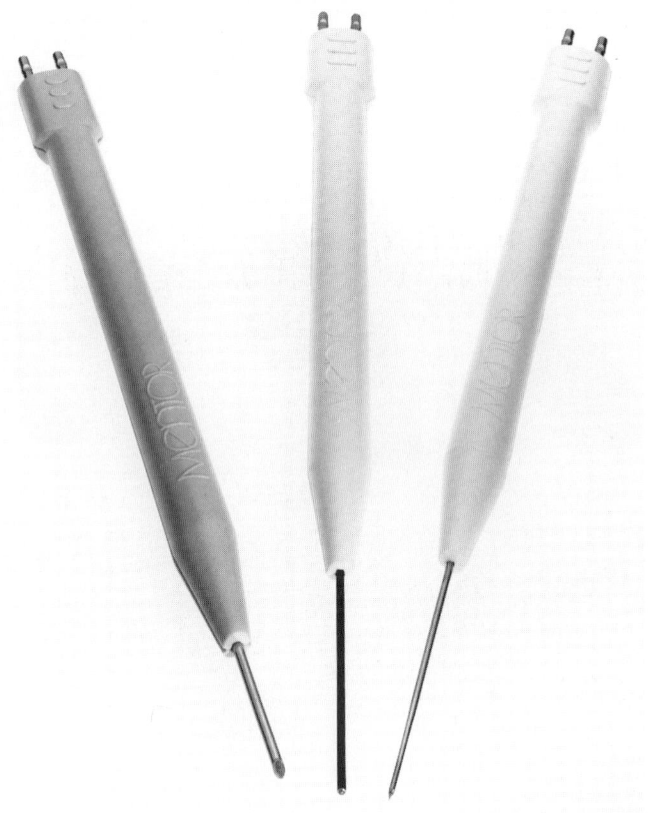

Mentor, Norwell, MA, USA

3.**14** **Endoeraser.** The endoeraser is in reality a modified bipolar coagulating system that combines two electrodes in a single probe. The outer metallic tube serves as one electrode and the inner solid cylinder is the other electrode. Two electric cords connect the terminals of each electrode to a bipolar console which is activated by a pedal. Tissues bridging the outer and inner electrodes at the eraser tip become coagulated when electrical current is activated by the foot pedal. Three tips are available: a beveled tip for use on the external surface of the globe, and 20-gauge flat and tapered tips for intraocular use.

Air pump. A source of continuous supply of sterile air to the vitreous cavity has become an important adjunct of complex vitreoretinal surgery. An air pump with air flow and pressure regulators control the volume and pressure of air flowing into the eye through the infusion line and cannula (3, 6, 11). Various systems are available: the Grieshaber air system for automated fluid-gas exchange, the Aaberg electrically driven air pump, and the simple nonelectric air pump developed by Tolentino, using operating room air supply.

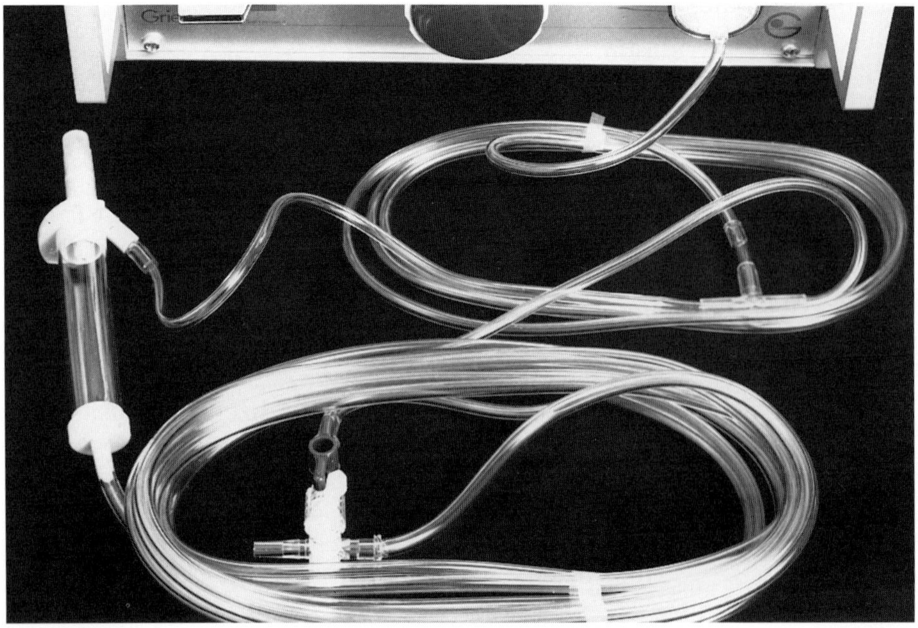

Grieshaber

3.**15** **Global infusion setup.** This setup uses a continuous-infusion air pump to pressurize the infusion fluid bottle and thus allow for more precise control of intraoperative infusion pressure (24). The infusion bottle is placed at the patient's eye level, and air is pumped into the infusion bottle to provide the desired infusion pressure. The infusion pressure can be rapidly changed by adjusting the continuous-infusion air pump, and the appropriate infusion pressure will be displayed digitally. It is possible to switch quickly from fluid air infusion using a stopcock.

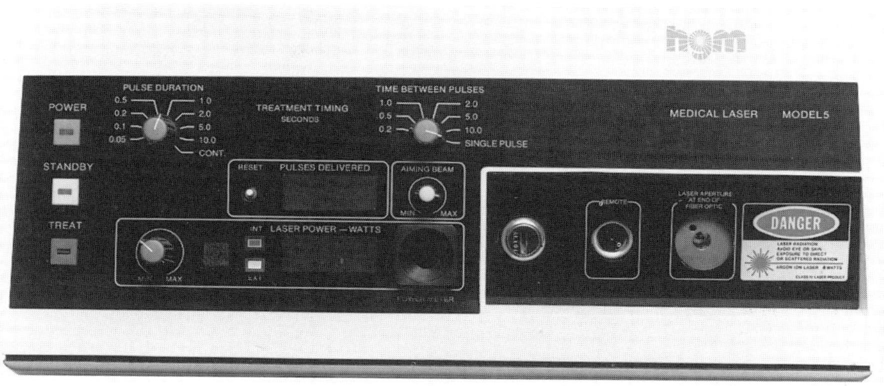

Summit, Great Falls, VA, USA

3.**16a** **Endophotocoagulator.** The endophotocoagulator is an argon laser that operates in the blue-green visible light spectrum. The principal components of the laser energy are at wavelengths of 514 nm (green) and 488 nm (blue). Energy at such wavelengths is strongly absorbed by red pigment. For this reason, argon laser energy is extremely useful in the coagulation of pigmented tissues.

b The operator's eyes are protected from exposure during endophotocoagulation by a safety filter and shutter in the attachment to the operating microscope. The aiming beam is an attenuated laser beam; therefore it has the same spot size as the treating beam. The air-cooling system permits a rapid repetition rate between applications.

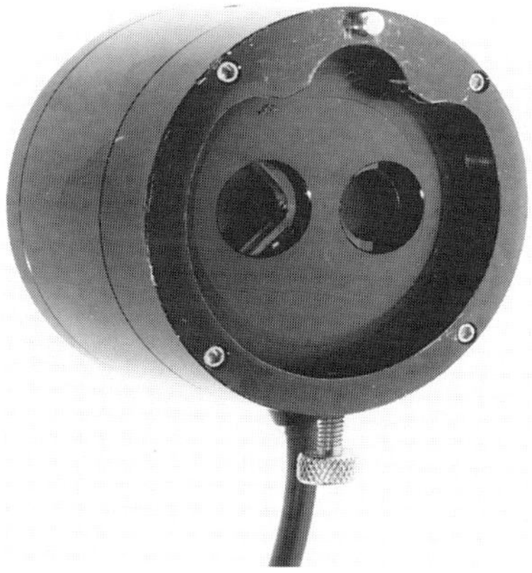

Summit

3.**17** **Endoilluminators.** *Light sources.* Many vitrectomy systems contain a light source for the endoilluminator probe. Different light sources are manufactured by Pilling and by Grieshaber.

a The Pilling light source is fitted with two individually controlled, 150 W lamps. A light signals when a lamp needs replacement, which can be done in a few seconds. The output at the port is nominally 250000 footcandles.

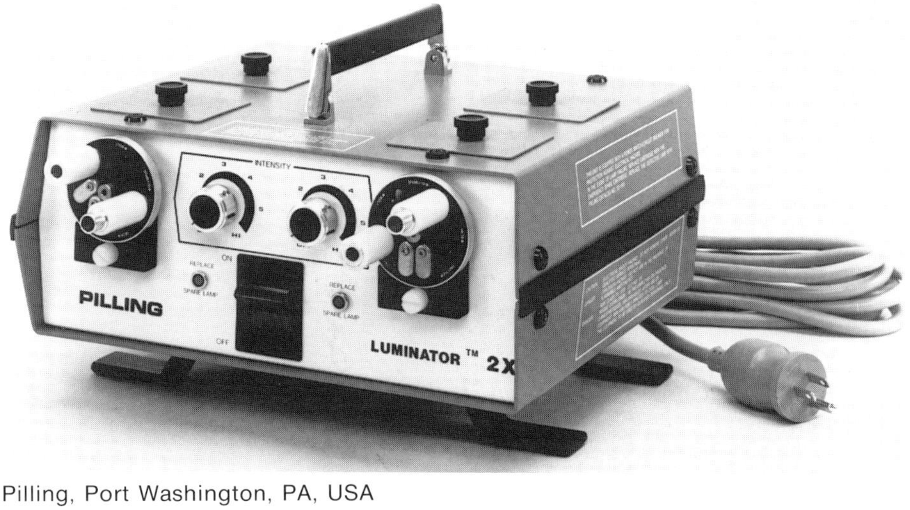

Pilling, Port Washington, PA, USA

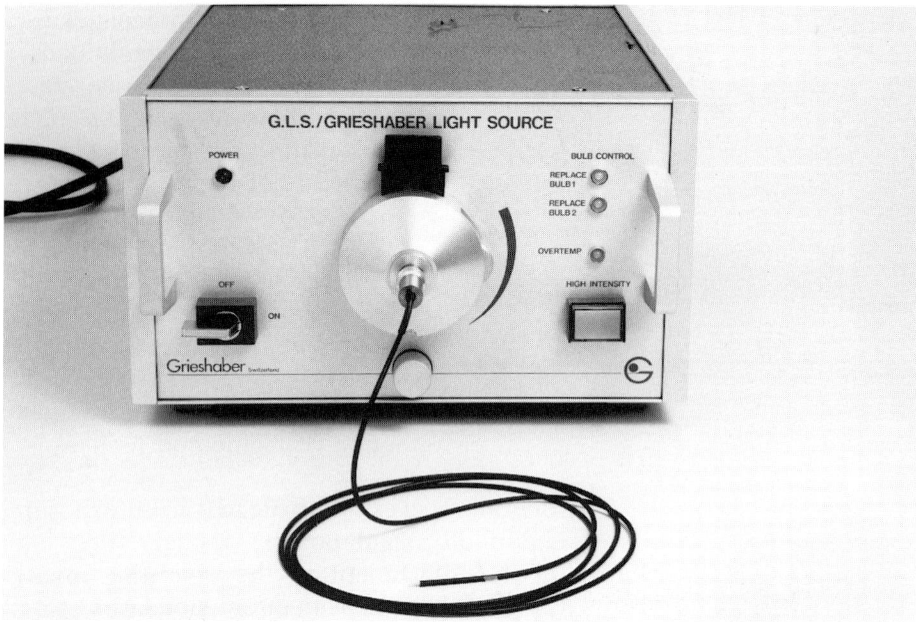

3.**17b** Grieshaber light source. An optical system concentrates halogen light down to the diameter of the fiber optic cable to achieve maximum efficiency. The intensity of the light can be adjusted, and additional filters can be fitted to enhance visualization of vitreous strands. Also pictured (front) is the fiber optic insert for the trochar cannula set.

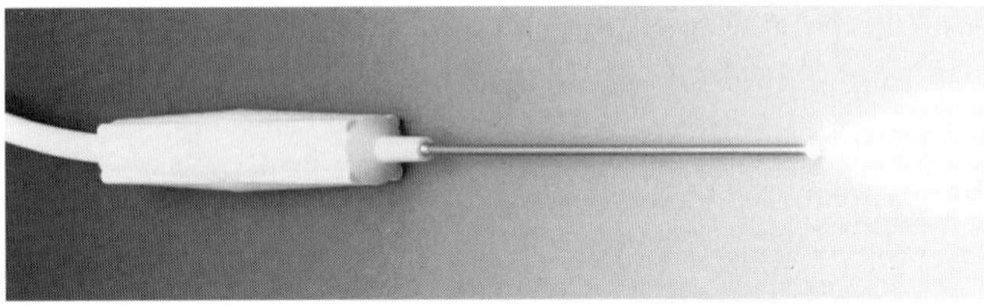

Cooper Vision, Irvine, CA, USA

c Endoilluminator probes. A variety of disposable and nondisposable fiber-optic light probes are available in conjunction with the vitrectomy systems or as separate components. The CooperVision disposable fiber optic illuminator consists of a 20-gauge straight cannula with a tapered tip for ease of insertion. Disposable 20-gauge endoilluminator probes are also made by Storz, Alcon, and Grieshaber.

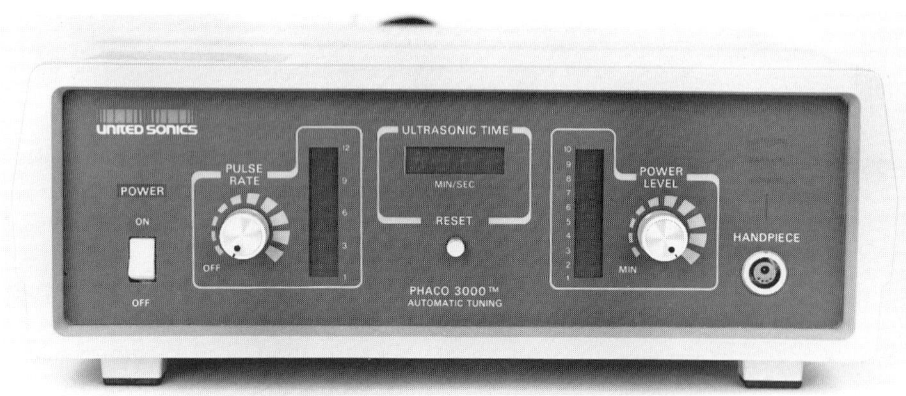

United Sonics, Hauppauge, NY, USA

This unit was specifically designed for ultrasonic extracapsular cataract extractions. It operates at an ultrasonic frequency of approximately 27000 cycles/sec.

The generator converts the normal wall current of 50/60 cycles/sec to this ultrasonic frequency and delivers it to the handpiece, where the electrical signal is converted to mechanical/vibratory motion.

3.**18 Phacoemulsification and phacofragmentation units.**

a The United Sonics Phaco 3000 can be used for either anterior segment phacoemulsification or pars plana phacofragmentation. It features an automatically tuning generator, autoclavable handpieces, variable ultrasonic pulse rate, power control, ultrasonic timer, disposable infusion sleeve and tubing set, and the ability to interconnect to irrigation-aspiration or vitrectomy systems.

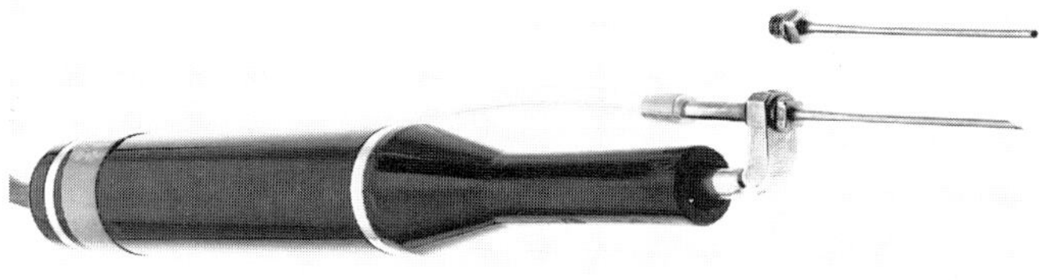

United Sonics

b The titanium needle attached to the handpiece is the final vibrating component, and serves as the ultrasonic aspirating needle. The needles are available in 19 or 20 gauge and in 15°, 30°, 45°, and 60° beveled tips.

Vitrectomy equipment. The various vitrectomy systems have two basic components: a console containing an aspirating and cutting module, and a vitrectomy probe.

The cutting module may be powered by a pneumatic mechanism or an electric motor. Pneumatic-type cutting modules have guillotine cutters. Electric-driven modules have either a guillotine or rotating-type cutter.

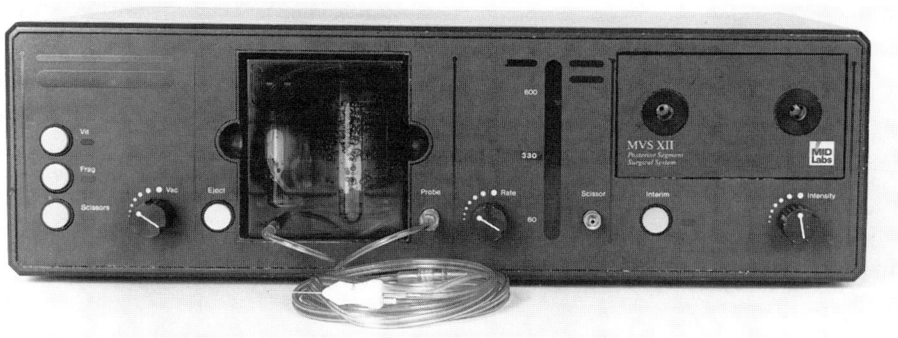

i
Storz

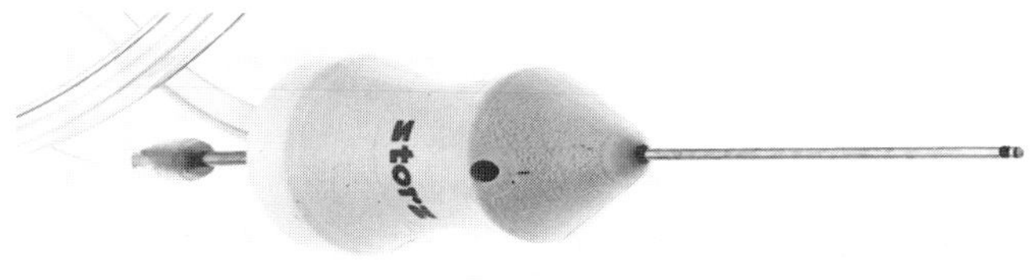

ii
Storz

3.**19a** The MVS System provides four functions including cutting, aspiration, illumination, and infusion. The console (i) is powered both pneumatically and electrically. Power to the probe (ii) is provided by compressed nitrogen or air. The system utilizes a single-use vitreous cutter with a self-sharpening guillotine action and a cutting rate of 300 to 600 cuts per minute. Illumination is provided by a fiberoptic cable inserted into the console. Irrigation is provided by either an infusion cannula or a coaxial irrigation sleeve that fits over the vitrectomy probe. The on-and-off cutting action is controlled by a foot pedal which also controls suction in a linear fashion.

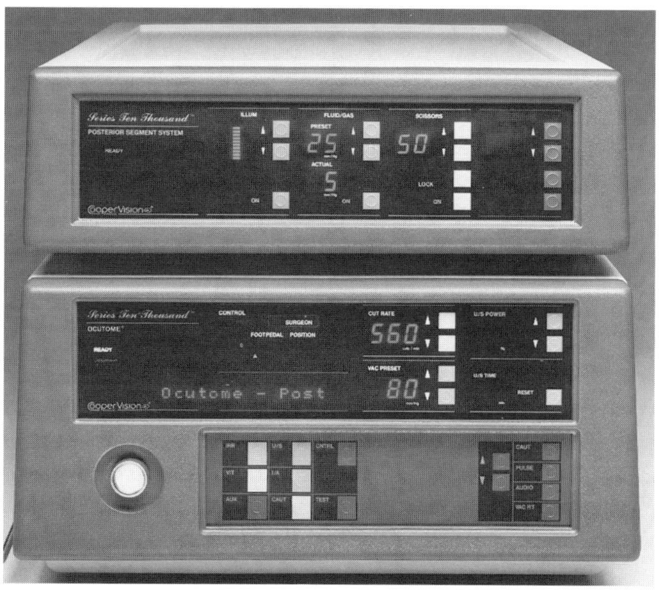

3.**19b** CooperVision Ocutome Vitreoretinal System (Series 10000). This system has the capability for vitrectomy, phakofragmentation, fluid-gas exchange, pneumatic intraocular scissors, and bipolar diathermy. With linear suction, the suction force increases proportionally to depression of the foot pedal. This system has a Micro Reflux feature that automatically backflushes the cutter to release tissue or incarcerated material. This function can be activated instantly by the foot switch.

The disposable and reusable vitrectomy probe has a guillotine cutting action. The single-use Ocutome probe consists of a 20-gauge straight cannula probe. The cutting port is on the side of the cannula 0.0015 mm from the tip. The port size is infinitely variable from 0–1 mm.

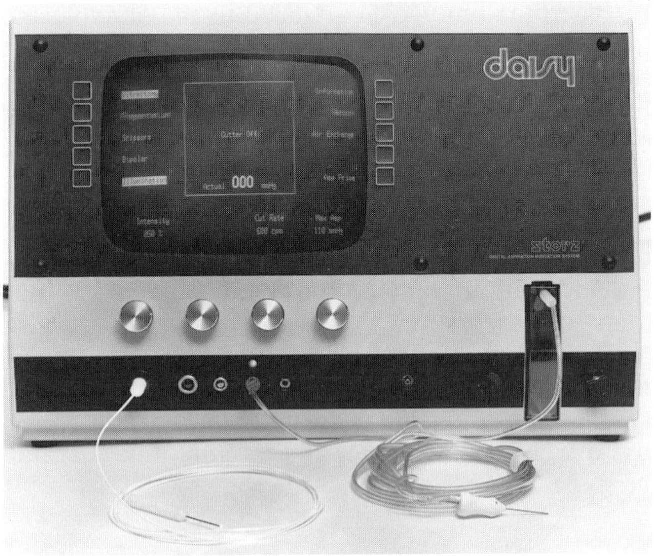

i

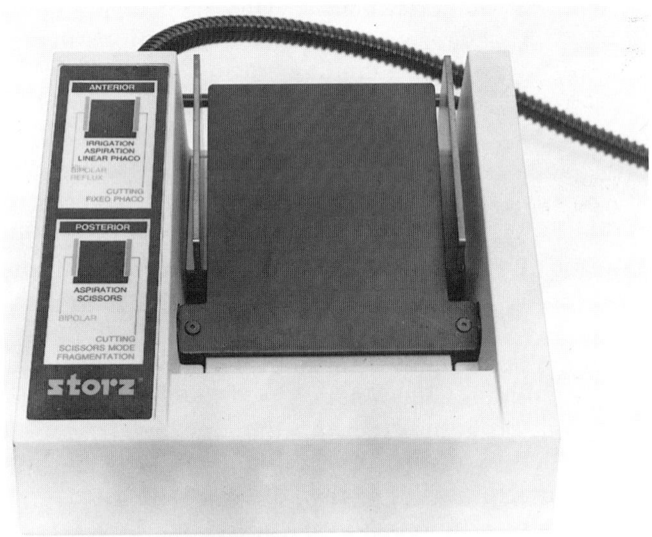

ii

Storz (i and ii)

3.**19 c Digital Aspiration Irrigation System** (DAISY). (i) This system contains a key with electronic information regarding the surgeon's preferred procedures, preferred initial settings, and preferred language for all video displays. Information from the owner's instruction manual is stored, allowing the staff access to this information through use of a videoscreen. This system provides phakofragmentation, phakoemulsification, irrigation-aspiration, microscissors, bipolar diathermy, fiber-optic light source, air exchange, and a disposable vitrectomy probe. The unit is gas and electrically powered. The 20-gauge Microvit Storz 2 probe (front right) cuts with a guillotine action. The endoilluminator probe is also shown (front left).

(ii) The foot pedal controls irrigation, aspiration, and phakoemulsification in anterior segment surgery and diathermy, automated cutting of scissors, fragmentation, and vitrectomy in the posterior segment. The foot switch is controlled fiber-optically, eliminating moisture problems associated with electrical switches.

3.**20 a Ocular connection machine** (OCM). This is a multifunction instrument for both anterior and posterior segment surgery. Designed with a systems engineering analysis of the present operating room environment, the OCM improves surgeon productivity and provides new functions. The Surgeon Interface Module at left contains the display, controls, and surgical tools. This module is used in the sterile field, suspended over the patient by the articulated arm. The cart contains all the support equipment, such as power supplies, pumps, electronics, light sources, etc.

Display, controls, and surgical tools within the sterile field at the Surgeon Interface Module provide the surgeon with total control of the system. A unique handpiece recognition feature automatically changes the system mode upon handpiece pickup. Computer-controlled interconnection of pumps and valves eliminates stopcocks and complex external tubing interconnections and the potential for incorrect connections.

20 a

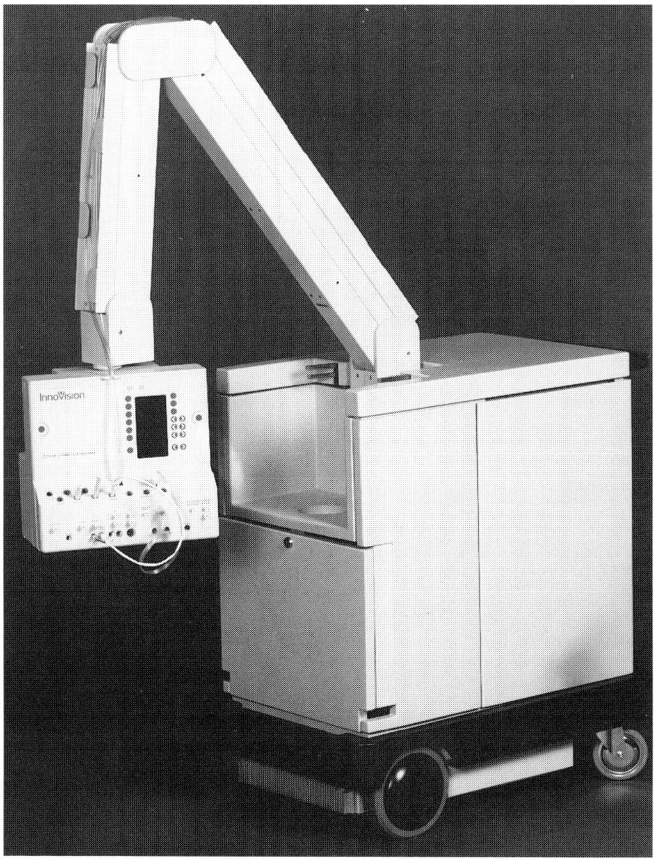

Innovision, Irvine, CA, USA

The OCM consolidates the multiple foot pedals now required into a two foot pedal, surgeon-control system. All primary functions (suction, ultrasound, cutting) are controlled by the primary foot pedal, and all "thermal" functions (1 MHz bipolar cautery, 13.56 MHz unipolar diathermy, and laser) are controlled by a secondary foot pedal. A dual-slope function in the foot pedals allows fine control of a preset first power range, with a second range up to the maximum available power for difficult situations. Immediate increase in intraocular pressure for control of intraocular bleeding or other procedural requirements is also accomplished with one button on the primary foot pedal.

This infusion system is servo-controlled, with infusion pressure monitored at the eye and through automatic feedback control; infusion pressure is changed to compensate for suction or wound leakage to maintain a preset intraocular pressure. The infusate may also be chilled up to 15 °C below room temperature when cooled infusion is preferred. In addition, an irrigating and aspirating lid speculum provides chilled solution for extraocular cooling.

Filtered air and other gases can also be used with the servo infusion control, and are accessed rapidly at the Surgeon Interface Module through a single button. Air-gas mixing is automated, and concentrations can be easily selected.

Suction is controlled by foot pedal through a proportional feedback servo, providing exceptionally fast and precise response. This performance is achieved through short tubing lengths (small controlled volume) and by using digital servo control algorithms.

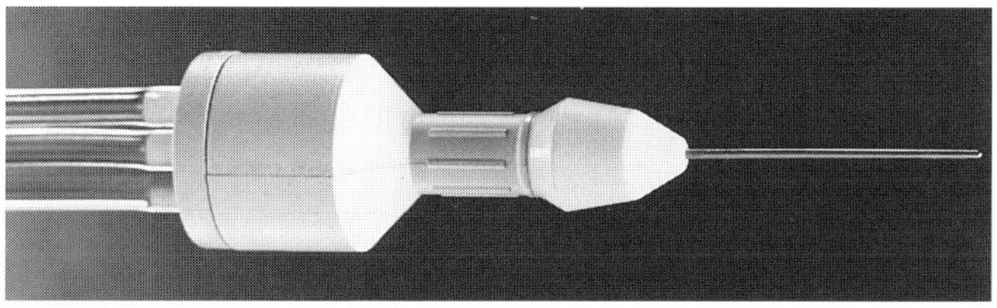

Innovision

3.**20 b** The inertial vitreous cutter uses a revolutionary "snap action" driver design, resulting in higher blade speed and higher cutting frequency. By pneumatically driving the guillotine cutter open as well as closed, the effective cutting power is increased.

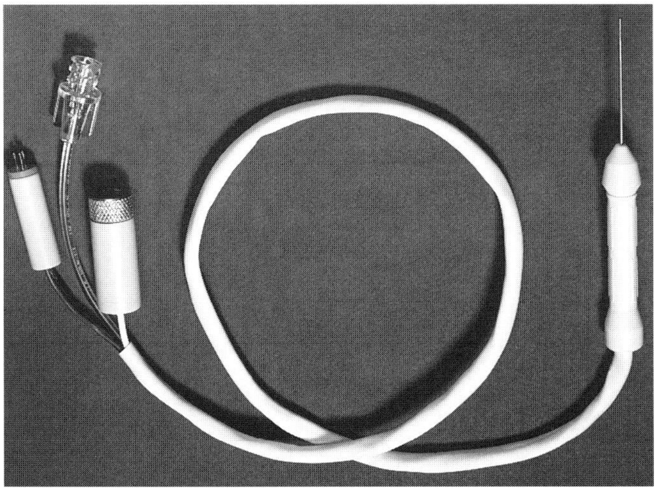

Innovision

3.**20 c** A multiprobe combines illumination, diathermy, and infusion into one 20-gauge needle, an ergonomic unipolar diathermy probe, and high-efficiency, lightweight, ultrasonic handpieces for phakoemulsification and fragmentation.

Instrumentation for Scleral Buckling

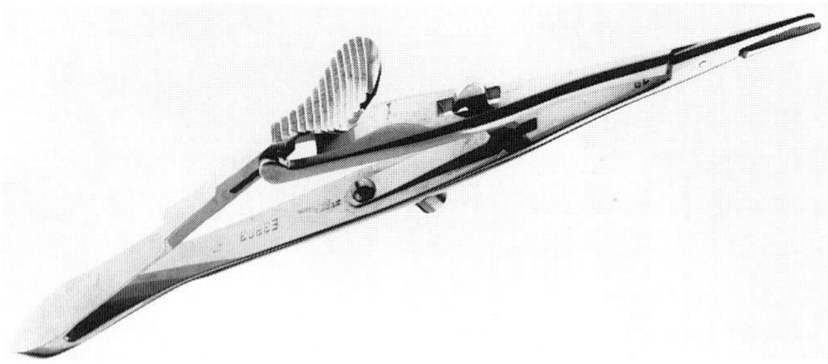

Storz

3.**21** **Kalt Needle holder**

a

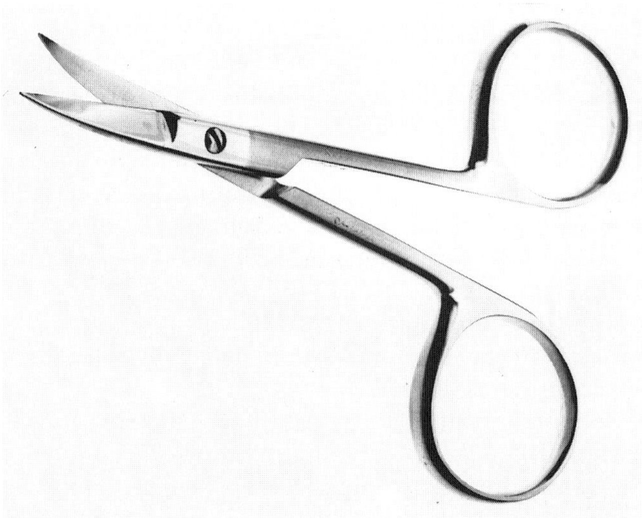

Storz

b

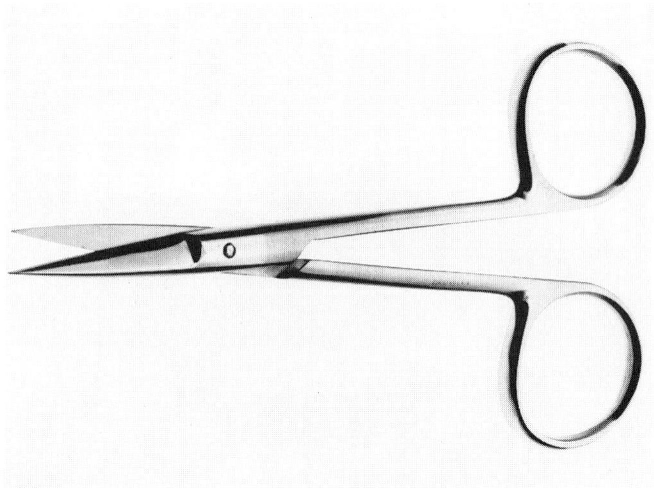

Storz

c

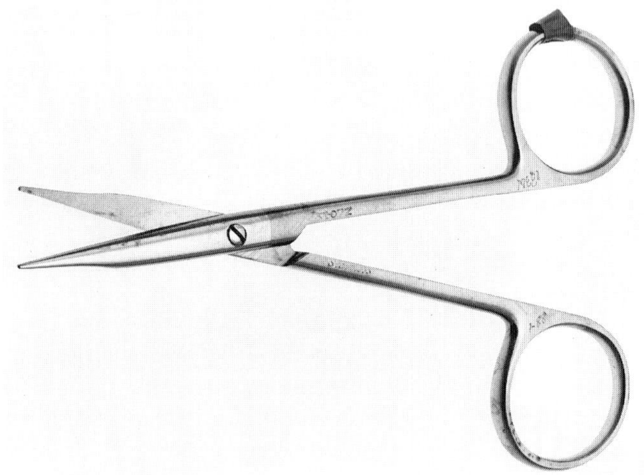

3.**22** **Scissors.** Curved, sharp-pointed to dissect peribulbar tissue (**a**); straight, blunt to cut hydrogel sponge or silicone rubber implants (**b**); straight, sharp-pointed to trim implants and cut sutures (**c**).

a

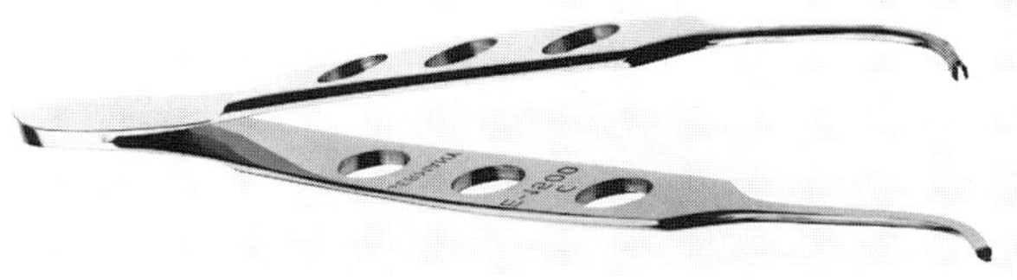

Storz (a–e)

b

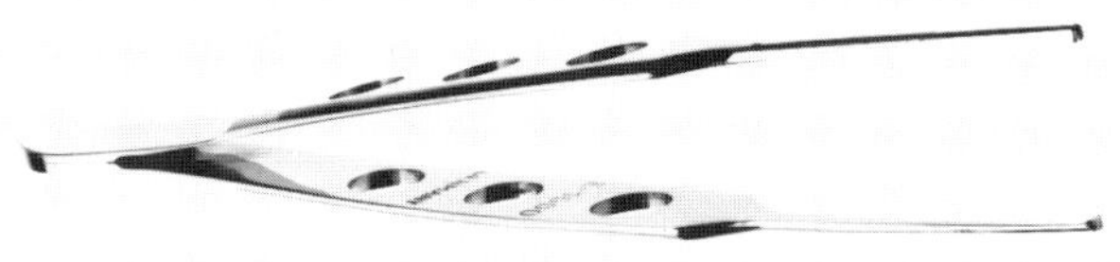

c

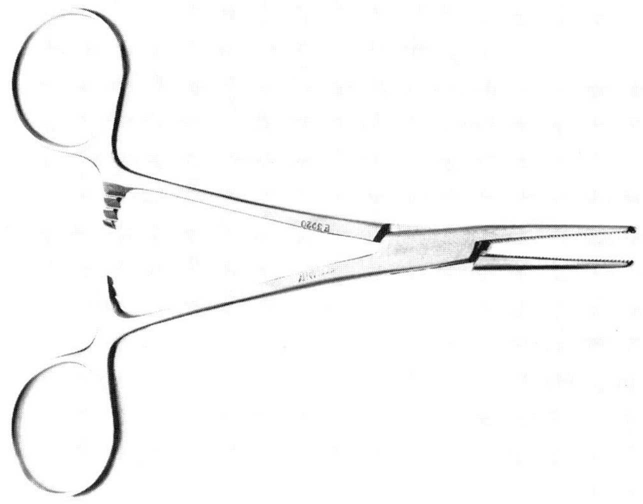

d

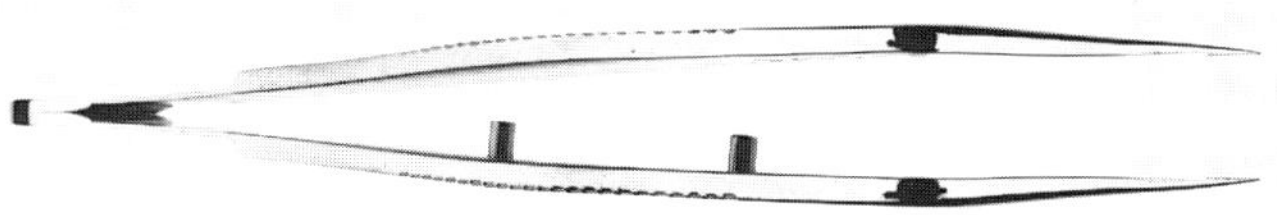

e

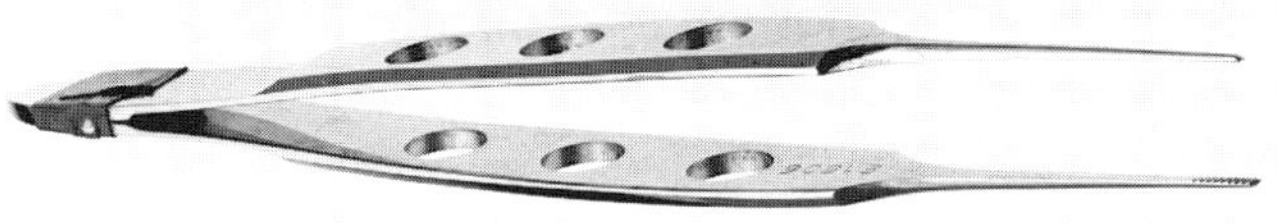

3.**23** **Forceps.** Curved, medium-sized, Bishop-Harmon forceps to grasp soft tissues (**a**); straight, medium-sized, Bishop-Harmon forceps to grasp soft tissues such as sclera and conjunctiva (**b**); straight, fine, mosquito forceps to fixate the lid sutures to the surgical drape (**c**); Elschnig's forceps to grasp the lid to pass traction sutures (**d**); smooth forceps to handle the implant and encircling element (**e**).

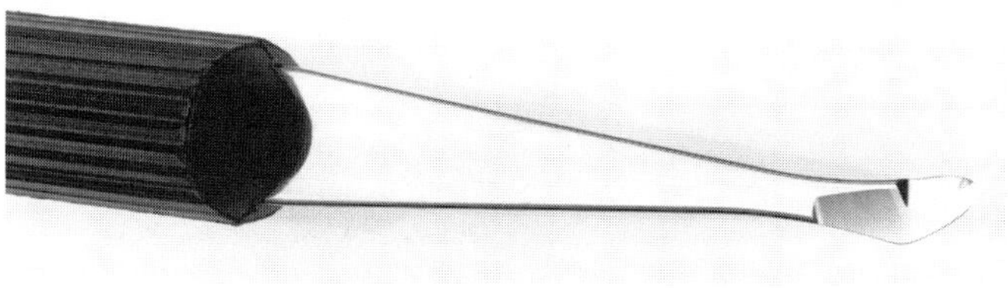

Grieshaber

3.**24** **Scarifier.** A Grieshaber disposable scarifier is used for the lamellar scleral undermining and the sclerotomy for drainage of subretinal fluid.

a

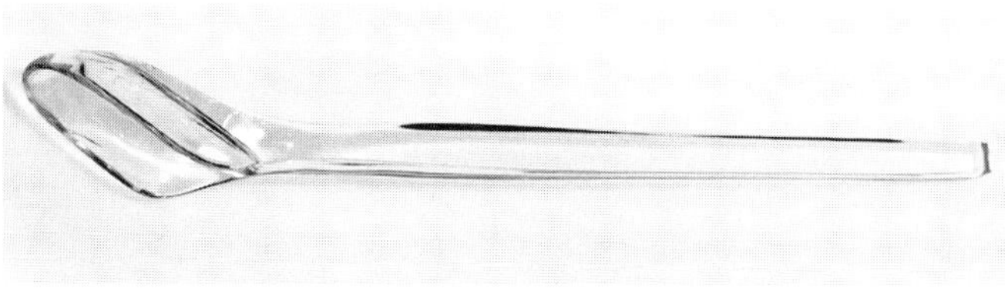

b

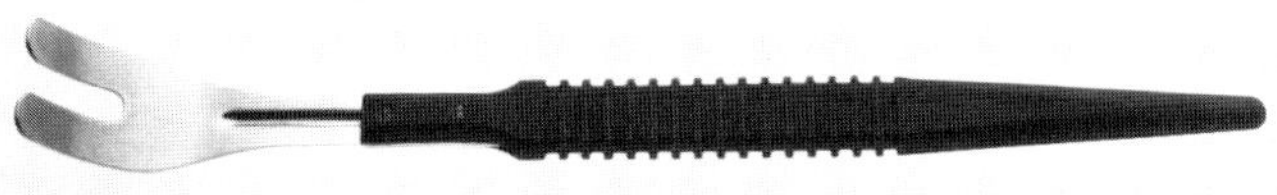

MIRA (a, b)

3.**25** **Retractors.** A plastic Arruga retractor is used during localization of the retinal breaks (**a**); a forked Schepens retractor is used for exposure (**b**).

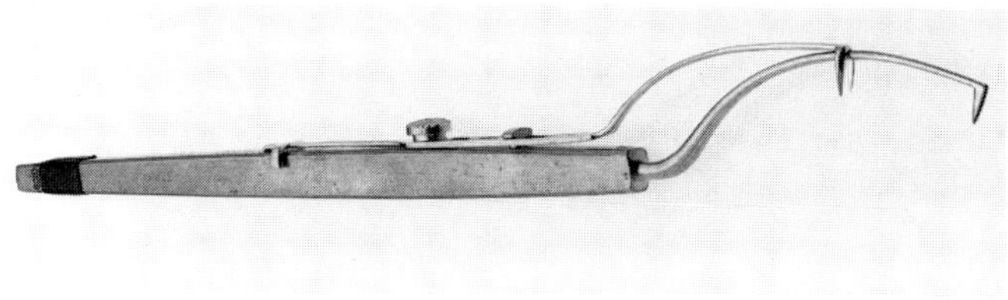

MIRA

3.**26** **Amsler marker.** An Amsler marker is used to measure the distance between the limbus and localizing marks.

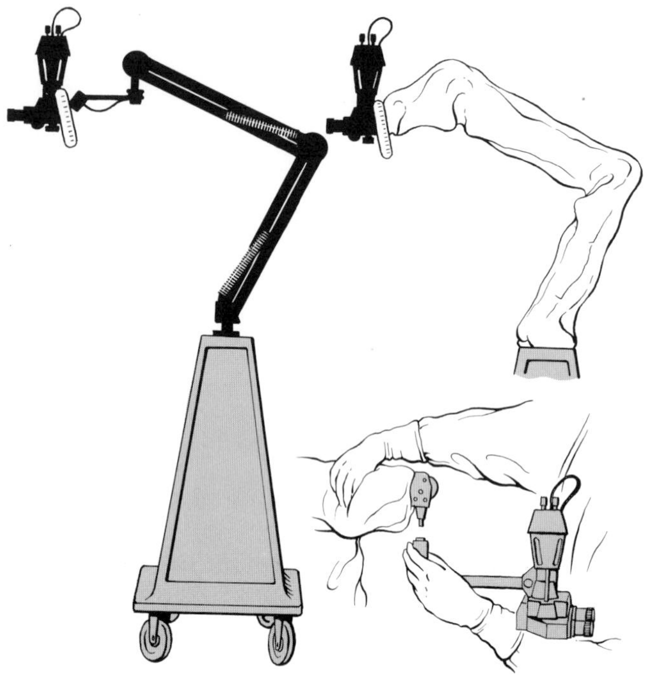

3.**27** **Indirect ophthalmoscopes and condensing lenses.** An ethylene oxide-sterilized, small-pupil ophthalmoscope is mounted on a mobile stand. A second ethylene oxide-sterilized headband-type indirect ophthalmoscope, scleral depressor, fundus drawing sheets, and colored pencil crayons are available for fundus examination under anesthesia. Two ethylene oxide sterilized, aspheric, +20D and +27D condensing lenses are used for ophthalmoscopy.

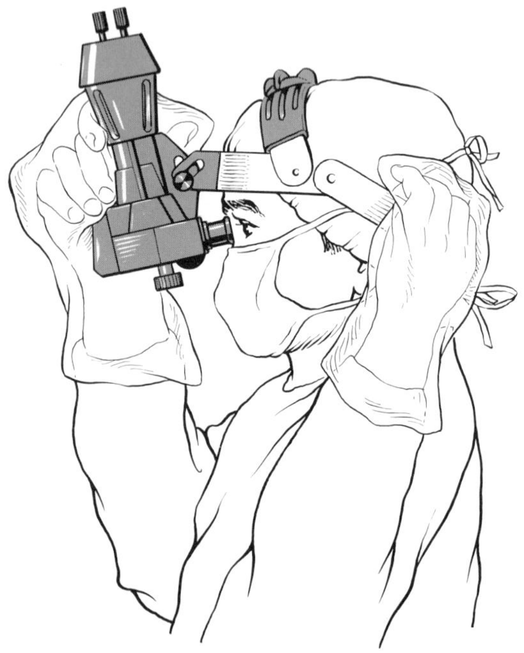

3.**28** An unsterile indirect ophthalmoscope can be handled using sterile plastic bags over the hands.

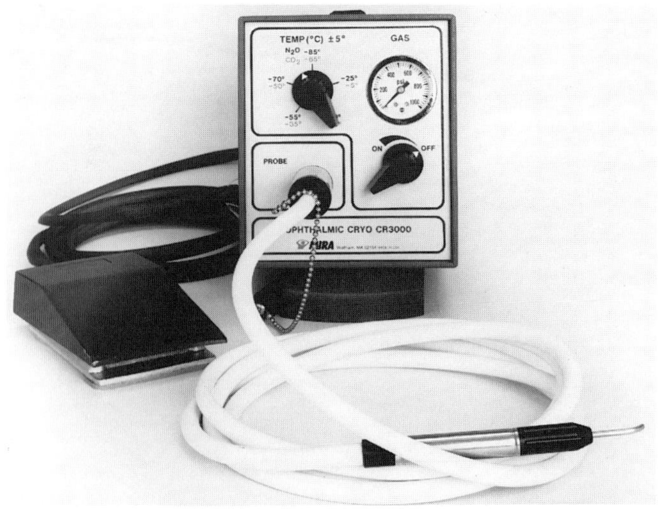

MIRA

3.**29** **Cryogenic console, probe, and pedal.** A cryomachine that uses nitrous oxide or carbon dioxide gas. The probe is designed to freeze only at its tip, in order to reduce unwanted freezing of adjacent tissues. The probe has a rapid freeze-defrost cycle. The probe is designed to evacuate cold gases through the center of the probe shaft to eliminate the need for additional insulation to the probe shaft and handle. This design eliminates the need for silicone boots, and provides the surgeon with greater visibility of the probe tip.

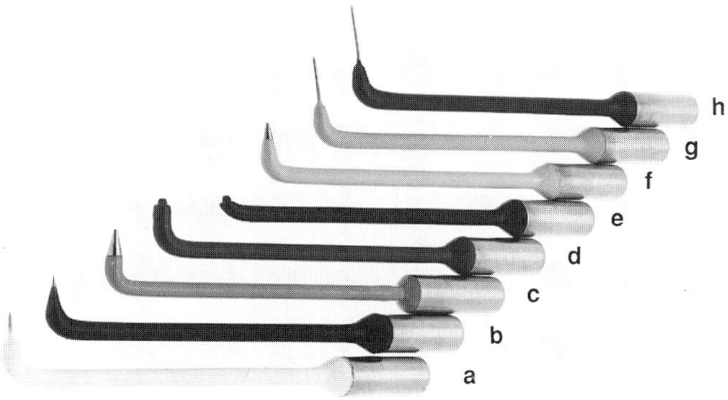

MIRA

3.**30** **Diathermy.** In the transistorized radiofrequency diathermy machine, the radiofrequency current is produced by a crystal-controlled, solid-state amplifier powered by rechargeable nickel-cadmium batteries. A variety of electrodes are available for applying penetrating and non-penetrating diathermy:

a Electrode: white, 2 mm, fine tip. For perforation and release of subretinal fluid.

b Electrode: black. For surface or partially penetrating diathermy.

c Electrode: green. For surface diathermy.

d Electrode: gray. For localization posterior to the equator.

e Electrode: brown. For localization at or anterior to the equator.

f Electrode: aqua, 3 mm, fine tip. For penetrating diathermy and tumor destruction.

g Electrode: pink, 4 mm, fine tip. For penetrating diathermy and tumor destruction.

h Electrode: brown, 5 mm, fine tip. For penetrating diathermy and tumor destruction.

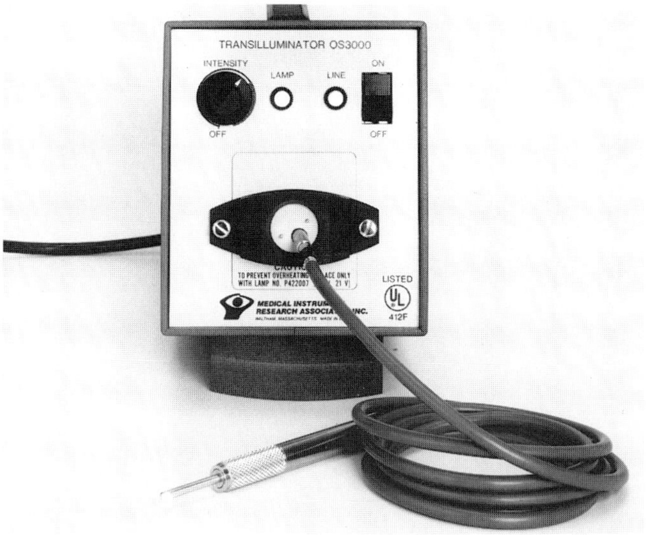

MIRA

3.**31** **Transilluminator.** A hand-held transilluminator with a bright tungsten light source used for transilluminating foreign bodies, choroidal vasculature, the pars plana ciliaris, and the long posterior ciliary arteries and nerves.

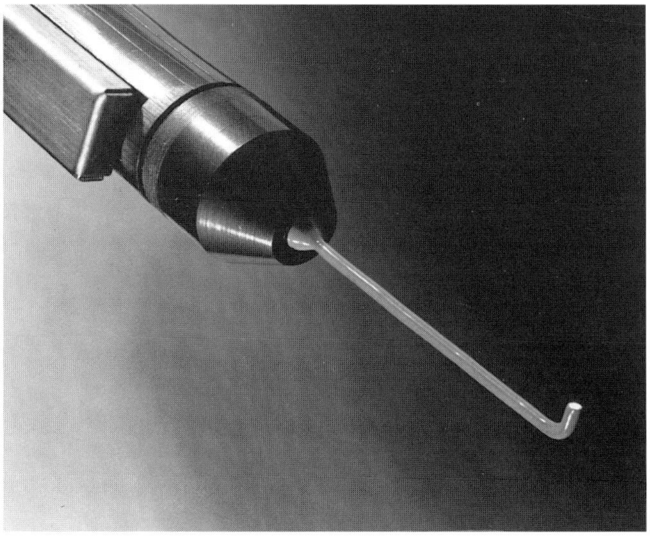

MIRA

3.**32** **Transilluminating electrode.** A transilluminating electrode combines diathermy and transillumination so that a precise localizing mark can be made on the very posterior sclera.

Implants for Scleral Buckling Surgery

Solid silicone rubber implants. Medical-grade soft silicone rubber implants are well tolerated by ocular tissues and do not support bacterial growth (18). These implants are translucent, colorless, and easy to fashion and cut with scissors or a knife. They are sterilized by autoclaving, dry heat, or ethylene oxide gas. The gas is absorbed by the rubber; the sterilized implant must therefore be aerated in its wrapper for 3 days before use.

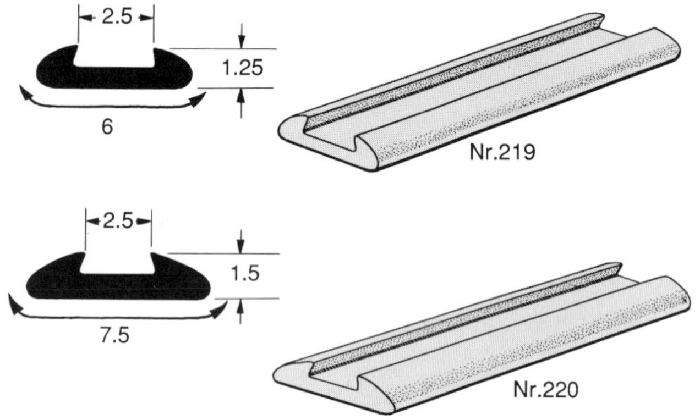

3.**33a** **Straight silicone rubber implants.** Straight silicone implants are available in ungrooved and grooved sections of varying widths and thicknesses.

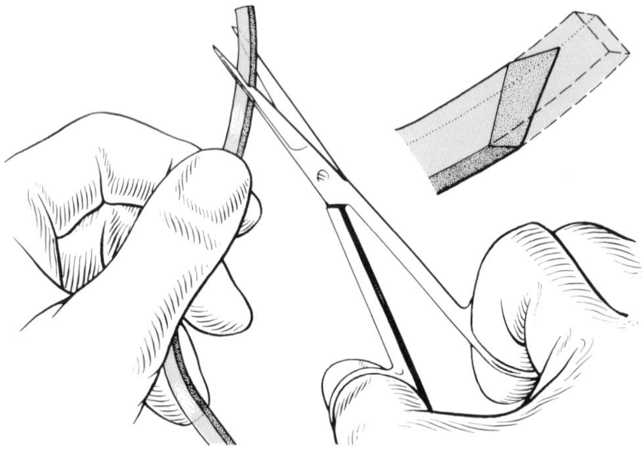

3.**33b** **Encircling element.** An ungrooved strip 2.5 mm wide and 0.6 mm thick is used as a circling element that fits into the groove of the implant. The end of the element is beveled so that it will pass more easily in the groove of the implant.

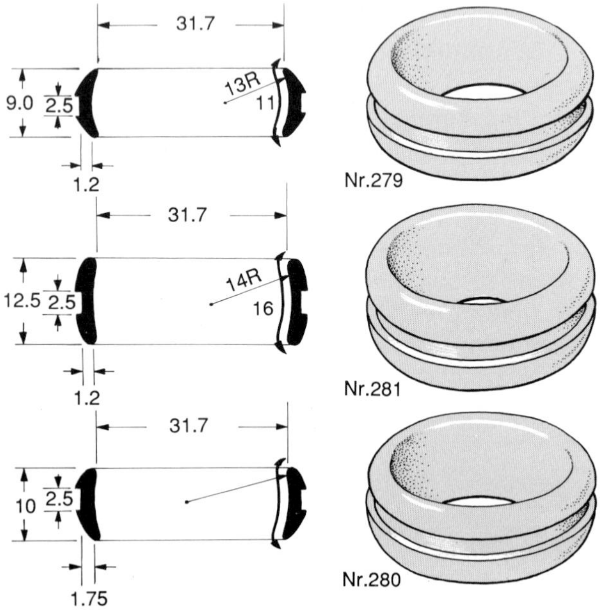

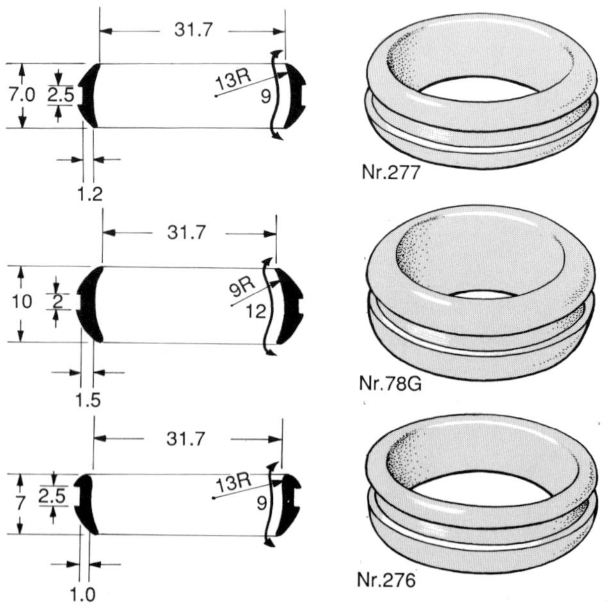

3.**34a, b** **Curved or "tire" implants.** Curved implants are made into tires that have radii of curvature approaching those of the globe. Tires are relatively thin along their margins, which makes them well suited for supporting anterior retinal breaks. There are two types of tires, symmetric and asymmetric, depending on the location of the groove.

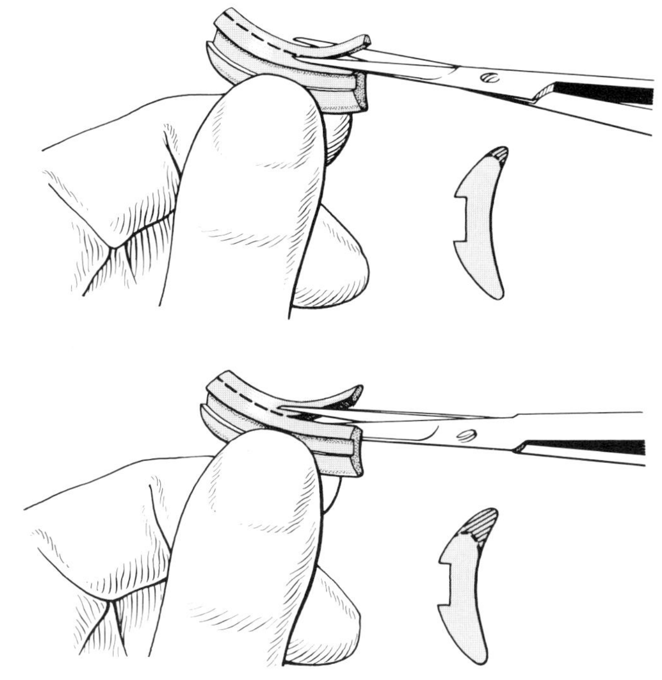

3.**34c** Tire silicone implants can be trimmed with scissors to produce implants of varying lengths and widths.

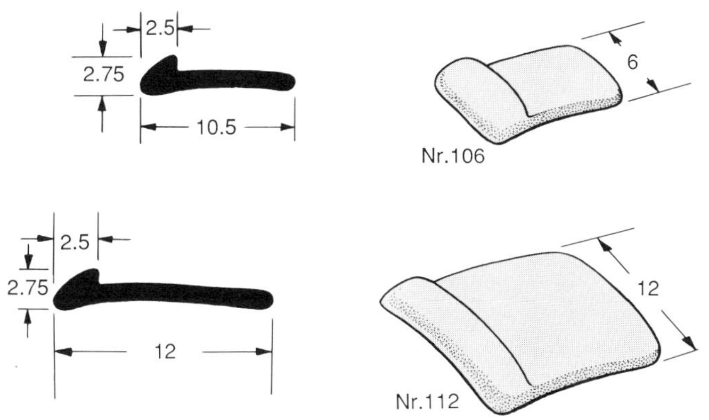

3.**35a** Meridional implants are molded to fit under straight or curved silicone implants to produce an additional buckling effect.

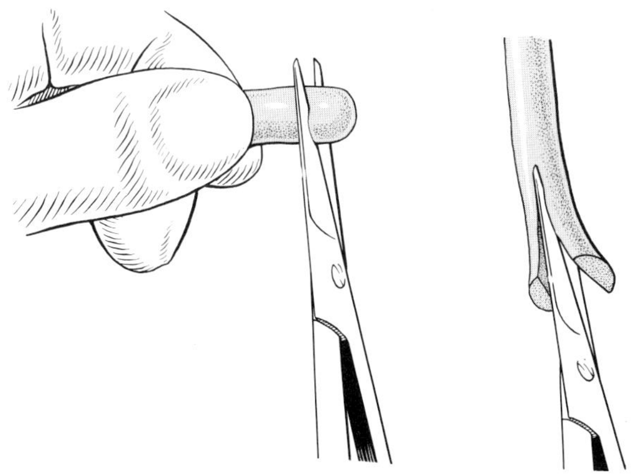

b A meridional implant can also be cut from a sponge implant.

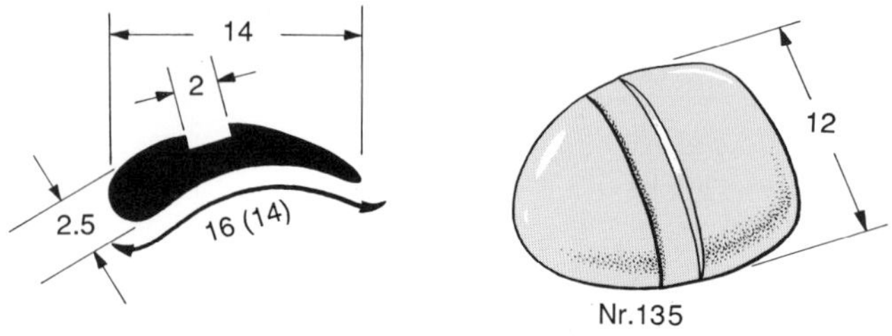

3.36 Wedge implant. A wedge-shaped implant is effective in treating equatorial retinal tears, which have a tendency to fishmouth following the drainage of subretinal fluid (see Chapter 25). The wedge-shaped configuration of the implant with its convex, blunt, rounded tip tends to produce an indentation that counteracts fishmouthing of a retinal break (16).

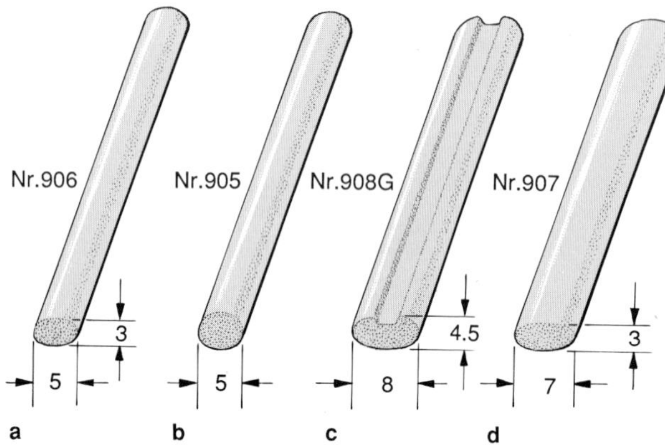

3.37 Hydrophilic acrylate implants. Silicone sponge implants have proved to be very useful in episcleral buckling. A new type of microporous, hydrogel implant is made from methyl acrylate or 2-hydroxyethyl acrylate (23). This material is soft and elastic, properties that help to prevent erosion of the sclera or conjunctiva when the material is implanted intrasclerally or episclerally. Hydrogel differs from silicone sponge in being devoid of dead spaces, which reduces the risk of infection. In addition, when soaked in antibiotic solution, the implant absorbs and retains the antibiotic.

Circular, oval, and grooved hydrogel implants are made in varying sizes (**a**–**d**). Grooved implants are used when an encircling element is desired to produce a more permanent buckling effect. A rod implant can be cut lengthwise to produce a meridional implant with a flat side, which is effective in flattening a radial retinal fold.

References

1. Abrams GW, Williams GA, Neuwirth J, McDonald HR. Clinical results of titanium retinal tacks with pneumatic insertion. Am J Ophthalmol 1986; 102: 13–19.
2. Charles, S. Vitreous microsurgery. 2nd ed. Baltimore; Williams and Wilkins, 1987: 72.
3. Charles S, Wang C. A motorized gas injector for vitreous surgery. Arch Ophthalmol 1981; 99: 1398.
4. Cowan GM. Microinfusion of thrombin solution in vitreous surgery. Am J Ophthalmol 1988; 105: 689–690.
5. Flynn HW, Davis LD, Parel J, Lee WG. Applications of a cannulated extrusion needle during vitreoretinal surgery. Retina 1988; 8: 42–49.
6. Grizzard WS, Slagle C, Gordon S. Infusion of intraocular gas with a pressure-controlled system. Am J Ophthalmol 1979; 88: 1096.
7. Heinze, J. Sutherland rotatable microsurgery instruments. Trans Ophthalmol Soc NZ 1981; 33: 112–115.
8. Ho PC, Mainster MA, Dieckert JP, Tolentino FI. Contact lenses for vitrectomy. Ophthalmology 1984; 91(9S): 88–93.
9. Jabbour NM, Tolentino FI, Hirose T. Vitreoretinal dissection set. Arch Ophthalmol 1986; 104: 1552–1553.
10. Landers MB III, Stefansson E, Wolbarsht ML. The optics of vitreous surgery. Am J Ophthalmol 1981; 91: 611–614.
11. McCuen BW II, Bessler M, Hickingbotham D, Isbey E III. Automated fluid-gas exchange. Am J Ophthalmol 1983; 95: 717.
12. Machemer R, Aaberg TM. Vitrectomy. 2nd ed. New York: Grune and Stratton, 1979: 212.
13. Machemer R, Parel J-M, Hickingbotham D, Nose I. Membrane peeler cutter: automated vitreous scissors and hooked needle. Arch Ophthalmol 1981; 99: 152–153.
14. Parel J-M, Machemer R. Steam-sterilizable fundus contact lenses. Arch Ophthalmol 1981; 99: 151.
15. Peyman GA, Schulman JA. Intravitreal surgery: principles and practice. New York: Appleton-Century Crofts, 1986: 100.
16. Pruett RC. The fishmouth phenomenon, II: wedge scleral buckling. Arch Ophthalmol 1977; 95: 1782–1787.
17. Rice TA, Michels RG, Stark WJ, eds. Operative surgery: ophthalmic surgery. 4th ed. St. Louis: C V Mosby, 1984: 212. (Rob and Smith's operative surgery series.)
18. Schepens CL. Retinal detachment and allied diseases. Philadelphia: W B Saunders, 1983: 334–336.
19. Schepens CL, Delori F, Rogers FJ, Constable IJ. Optimized underwater diathermy for vitreous surgery. Ophthalmic Surg 1975; 6 (4): 82–89.
20. Tolentino FI, Freeman HM. A new lens for closed pars plana vitrectomy. Arch Ophthalmol 1979; 97: 2197–2198.
21. Tolentino FI, Wu G. Diamond-dusted microspatula tips for vitreoretinal surgery. Arch Ophthalmol 1987; 105: 1732–1733.
22. Tolentino FI, Baehr EF, Miyamoto K. New instrument for vitreoretinal membrane surgery. Arch Ophthalmol 1986; 104: 1711–1713.
23. Tolentino FI, Refojo MF, Schepens CL. A hydrophilic acrylate implant for scleral buckling: technique and clinical experience. Retina 1981; 1: 281–286.
24. Witherspoon CD, Morris RE, Goggans WE Jr. Automated regulation of fluid infusion pressure during vitrectomy. Arch Ophthalmol 1986; 104: 1551.
25. Živojnović R. Silicone oil in vitreoretinal surgery. Dordrecht: Nijhoff 1987; 30–33.

4

Liquids, Gases, Visoelastic Substances, and Oils Used in Vitreoretinal Surgery

Infusion Fluids

Two kinds of infusion solutions are used for vitreoretinal surgery: a balanced salt solution enriched with bicarbonate, dextrose, and glutathione (BSS Plus), and Ringer's lactate. BSS Plus is available in a 500 ml bottle; Ringer's lactate, in a 1000 ml plastic bag.

Antibiotics

We routinely add gentamicin (40 μg/ml) to the infusion solution as a prophylaxis against endophthalmitis. To obtain this concentration, 40 mg of gentamicin is added to a 1000 ml bag of Ringer's lactate solution, or 20 mg to a 500 ml bottle of BSS Plus. In cases of known endophthalmitis, 80 mg of gentamicin is mixed with 1000 ml of Ringer's lactate solution, which is infused during vitrectomy after specimens are collected for culture. Clindamycin, 0.06 ml of a 150 mg/ml solution, may be added.

Viscoelastic Substances

Hyaluronic acid or its sodium salt, sodium hyaluronate, is a high-molecular-weight polysaccharide composed of sodium glucuronate and *N*-acetylglucosamine. Sodium hyaluronate is ubiquitously distributed throughout the body tissues and is present in high concentrations in the vitreous, synovial fluid, and umbilical cord, and the dermis of the rooster comb. Sodium hyaluronate functions as a tissue lubricant (19, 21) and a shock-absorbing molecule of the eye and musculoskeletal system (3, 6). In the eye, these molecules not only fill the vitreous, but are also present in the anterior chamber, coating the endothelium (2, 5). The use of sodium hyaluronate as a viscosurgical tool or vitreous injection does not, therefore, constitute the use of a foreign material (4). The unique physical properties of sodium hyaluronate solutions – their lubricating property, viscoelasticity, transparency, and cushioning effect – make them a useful adjunct in vitreoretinal surgery.

Sodium hyaluronate can be used to improve visualization through a cornea which has marked wrinkling of Descemet's membrane (see Chapter 9). It is helpful in protecting the corneal endothelium in eyes in which an intraocular lens must be removed. Sodium hyaluronate can be used in the hydraulic dissection of preretinal membranes (see Chapter 25) and in the dissection of iris that has been flattened against the endothelium by a bubble of gas or air in an aphakic eye. After release of subretinal fluid, air can be injected into the vitreous cavity and then exchanged with sodium hyaluronate to tamponade the retina.

A transient postoperative increase in intraocular pressure has been observed following the use of sodium hyaluronate in the anterior segment. A mild inflammatory response may occur postoperatively in the anterior and posterior segments (8, 18).

Intraocular Gases

The injection of perfluorcarbon gases into the vitreous cavity can be a useful adjunct in the management of certain retinal detachments (9, 15–17). The insolubility of perfluorocarbon gases limits their ability to cross the blood-aqueous barrier and thus to leave the eye. This property results in a prolonged tamponading effect to the retina postoperatively, during the formation of the chorioretinal adhesion. The half-life of 1 ml of pure perfluoropropane (C_3F_8) is 35 days, and the gas is absent in 70 days. The insolubility of perfluorocarbon gases increases their expansile properties. Long-acting gases expand in the vitreous because tissue gases, particularly nitrogen, enter the bubble from the surrounding fluid. This expansion is clinically important because it may result in increased intraocular pressure, closure of the ophthalmic artery, or closure of the filtration angle. A pure bubble of C_3F_8 injected into the eye will expand to 4 times the injected bubble volume; a bubble of SF_6 will expand to 2.6 times the injected volume. Expansion of the gas can be reduced during vitreoretinal surgery under general anesthesia by shutting off the nitrous oxide at least 15 minutes before C_3F_8 is injected into the eye. Experimentally, the nonexpansile concentration of C_3F_8 is 14% and 86% air; the nonexpansile concentration of SF_6 is 20% SF_6 and 80% air. To tamponade an inferior retinal tear, it is necessary to maintain at least a 50% fill of the vitreous cavity volume with gas. With anteriorly-located inferior retinal breaks, a 90–100% filling of the vitreous cavity is desirable. If an eye is filled with a mixture containing 14% C_3F_8, a complete gas fill can be expected for several days, and a 50% fill can be maintained without a repeat injection for 3 weeks. If a 90–100% fill is required, one or two additional fluid-gas exchanges with C_3F_8 are required to maintain an adequate fill for 2–3 weeks (W. S. Stern, personal communication).

Potential complications. In addition to the potential risk of acute ocular hypertension due to expansion of the gas, prolonged contact of gas with the corneal endothelium may produce corneal edema or a bullous keratopathy in extreme cases. Prolonged contact of gas with the lens may produce posterior subcapsular cataract (9).

Management following gas or air injection. If a complete gas-fluid exchange is done using a nonexpansile gas, patients are instructed to maintain the prone position for at least 8 hours each day for one week postoperatively. Prone positioning will reduce the chance of secondary lenticular changes and closure of the filtration angle. Elevated intraocular pressure can usually be controlled with topical 0.5% timolol and acetazolamide. Patients are followed at weekly intervals and then biweekly until the bubble is absorbed. Air travel should be avoided until the gas is absorbed (12).

Perfluorocarbon gases may be used to provide an intermediate duration of tamponade between the shorter duration of sulfur hexafluoride gas or air and the permanent vitreous substitutes, such as fluorosilicone or silicone oil.

Silicone Oil

Medical-grade silicone oil is used to provide prolonged postoperative tamponade for complex retinal detachments because it is a transparent, viscid liquid. It is quite inert chemically, highly water-repellent, and has a high surface tension. Its low specific gravity (0.972) gives it tamponading properties. Viscosities of 1000 to 10,000 centistokes are used. Silicone oil produces cataractous changes when in contact with the lens, keratopathy, and glaucoma. Controversy exists as to whether it is toxic to the retina (1, 7, 8, 11, 13, 14, 20).

Fluorosilicone oil (polymethyl-3,3,3-trifluroropropylsiloxane) is chemically modified silicone oil. Fluorosilicone oil has a higher specific gravity and better thermal stability than silicone oil. The high specific gravity causes the oil to sink posteriorly in the vitreous cavity to tamponade the pigment epithelium against the retina. This tamponade effect is most beneficial with inferior retinal detachments or retinal breaks in the posterior pole. The posterior location of the fluorosilicone oil tends to produce less keratopathy than silicone oil, which may float into the anterior chamber when the patient is supine or in the sitting position (10). Fluorosilicone oil with a viscosity of 1000 centistokes is used. It is injected through a 19-gauge needle over the optic disc in an air-filled eye, and the vitreous cavity is filled to the level of the iris plane.

References

1. Alexandridis E, Daniel H. Results of silicone oil injection into the vitreous. Dev Ophthalmol 1981; 2: 24–27.
2. Balazs EA. Molecular morphology of the vitreous body. In: Smelser GK, ed. The structure of the eye. New York: Academic Press, 1961: 293–310.
3. Balazs EA. Viscoelastic properties of hyaluronic acid and biological lubrication. (Symposium: prognosis for arthritis: rheumatology research today and prospects for tomorrow. Ann Arbor, Michigan). Univ Mich med Ctr J 1968 (suppl): 255–259.
4. Balazs EA. Viscosurgery: features of a true viscosurgical tool and its role in ophthalmic surgery. In: Miller D, Stegman R, eds. Treatment of anterior segment trauma. Montreal; Medicopea, 1986: 121–127.
5. Balazs EA, Armand G. Glycosaminoglycans and proteoglycans of ocular tissues. In. Varmas R, ed. Glycosaminoglycans and proteoglycans in physiological and pathological processes of body systems. Basel: Karger, 1983: 480–499.
6. Balazs EA, Gibbs DA. The rheological properties and biological function of hyaluronic acid. In: Balazs EA, ed. Chemistry and molecular biology of the intercellular matrix. New York: Academic Press, 1970: 1251–1254.
7. Cox MS, Trese MT, Murphy PL. Silicone oil for advanced proliferative vitreoretinopathy. Ophthalmology 1986; 93: 646–650.
8. Chan C, Okun E. The question of ocular tolerance to intravitreal liquid silicone: a long-term analysis. Ophthalmology 1986; 93: 651–660.
9. Chang S, Coleman DJ, Lincoff H, et al. Perfluoropropane gas in the management of proliferative vitreoretinopathy. Am J Ophthalmol 1984; 98: 180–188.
10. Chung H, Acosta J, Refojo MF, Tolentino FI. Use of high-density fluorosilicone oil in open-sky vitrectomy. Retina 1987; 7: 180–182.
11. Cockerham WD, Schepens CL, Freeman HM. Silicone injection in retinal detachment. Arch Ophthalmol 1970; 83: 704–712.
12. Dieckert JP, O'Connor PS, Schacklett DE, et al. Air travel and intraocular gas. Ophthalmology 1986; 93: 642–645.
13. Grey RHB, Leaver PK. Results of silicone oil injection in massive preretinal retraction. Trans Ophthalmol Soc UK 1977; 97: 238–241.
14. Leaver PK, Grey RHB, Garner A. Silicone oil injection in the treatment of massive preretinal retraction, II: late complications in 93 eyes. Br J Ophthalmol 1979; 63; 361–367.
15. Lincoff H, Coleman J, Kreissig I, et al. The perfluorocarbon gases in the treatment of retinal detachment. Ophthalmology 1983; 90: 546–551.
16. Lincoff A, Lincoff H, Iwamoto T, et al. Perfluoro-*n*-butane: a gas for a maximum duration retinal tamponade. Arch Ophthalmol 1983; 101: 460–462.
17. Lincoff H, Mardirossian J, Lincoff A, et al. Intravitreal longevity of three perfluorocarbon gases. Arch Ophthalmol 1980; 98: 1610–1611.
18. Pruett RC, Schepens CL, Swann DA. Hyaluronic acid vitreous substitute: a six-year clinical evaluation. Arch Ophthalmol 1979; 97: 2325–2330.
19. Radin EL, Paul IL, Swann DA, Schottstaedt ES. Lubrication of synovial membrane. Ann Rheum Dis 1971; 30: 322.
20. Sugar SH, Okamura ID. Ocular findings six years after intravitreal silicone injection. Arch Ophthalmol 1976; 94: 612–615.
21. Swann DA, Radin EL, Nazimiec M, Weisser PA, Curran N, Lewinnek G. Role of hyaluronic acid in joint lubrication. Ann Rheum Dis 1974; 33: 318.

5

Operating Room Layout and Preoperative Preparation

Operating Room Layout

Vitreoretinal surgery requires numerous pieces of equipment and many personnel. Efficient use of the limited space that is available is mandatory (1).

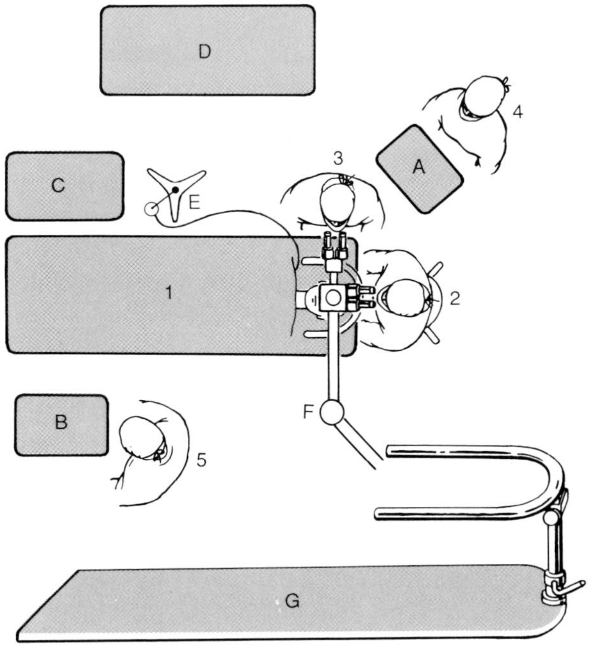

5.**1** **Recommended layout.** Numbers indicate personnel: 1 patient; 2 surgeon; 3 assistant; 4 scrub nurse or instrument technician; 5 anesthesiologist.

Letters indicate equipment: A Mayo tray for vitreoretinal instruments; B anesthesia machine; C portable stand with shelves for vitrectomy machine, gas pump, diathermy, and other auxiliary equipment; D instrument table; E pole for infusion bottle; F floor- or ceiling-mounted microscope; G arm rest.

The layout illustrated is for the right eye. For surgery on the left eye, the elements on the right and the left sides are interchanged.

The operating table is controlled electrically and lowered or elevated by remote switches. The patient is anesthetized on the table. The Chan arm rest is adjusted to the level of the patient's ears.

For vitrectomy, the surgeon sits at the head of the operating table and the assistant at the patient's temporal side. The scrub nurse and the Mayo tray with the instruments are located between the surgeon and the assistant. This arrangement allows the nurse to pass the instruments efficiently to both the surgeon and the assistant. The locations of the vitrectomy console, auxiliary equipment, and infusion bottle make it possible to run sterile electrical cords, tubings, and other cords connected to the surgeon's instruments on the sterile field.

For scleral buckling, the layout is basically the same as for vitrectomy, except that the microscope and the Chan arm rest are omitted. An indirect ophthalmoscope stand is located in one corner of the room and moved beside the table when needed. The Mayo instrument tray is placed across the middle portion of the table.

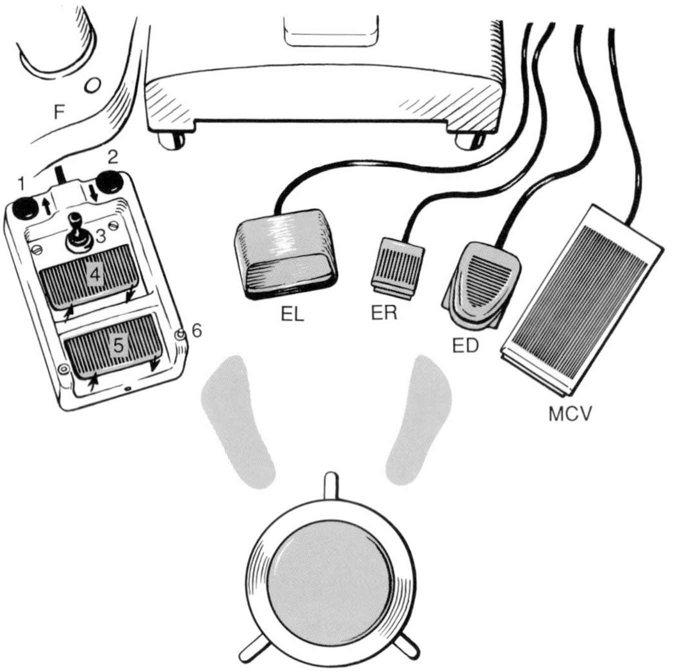

5.2 **Layout of foot pedals.** Most of the equipment used in vitreoretinal surgery is activated by remote-control pedals located on the floor beneath the head of the operating table. The pedal for the vitrector and the operating microscope are located near the corners of the table because they are used most frequently. The infrequently used pedals are located between the microscope pedal (far left) and microvit pedal (MCV): EL, endolaser; ER, endoeraser; ED, endodiathermy.

The surgeon should master the location of switches on the microscope pedal:
1 and 2, gross up-and-down focusing;
3, x-y movement control;
4, fine up-and-down focusing;
5, zoom control;
6, OFF/ON switch for the microscope light.

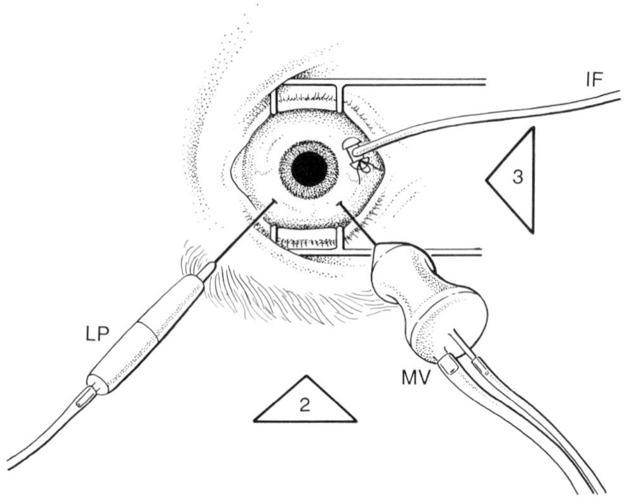

5.3 **Sitting arrangements.** The 12 o'clock position, which is at the top of the patient's head, offers the most convenient location for the surgeon to sit during routine vitrectomy. In this position, there is adequate leg room to allow the surgeon to operate the multiple foot pedals that control the instruments. In addition, this position permits the surgeon to use the two upper quadrants for instrument entry and the lower temporal quadrant for the infusion cannula. The active instruments can reach most of the vitreous cavity through the upper quadrants. Furthermore, the lower temporal quadrant is available for the infusion cannula (IF), a location in which the cannula interferes least with the rotation of the globe against the lids.
2, surgeon;
3, assistant;
LP, light pipe;
MV, vitrectomy probe.

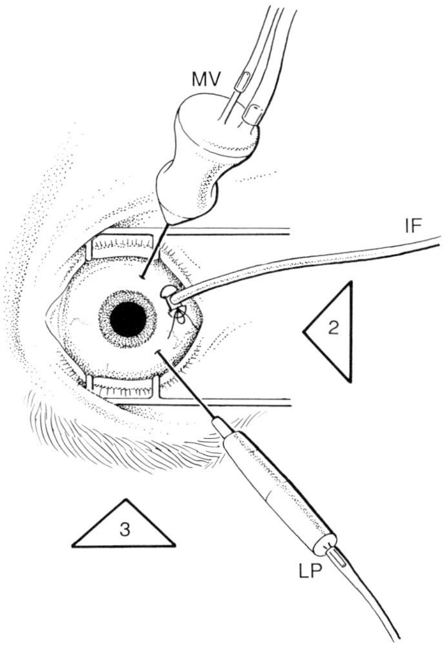

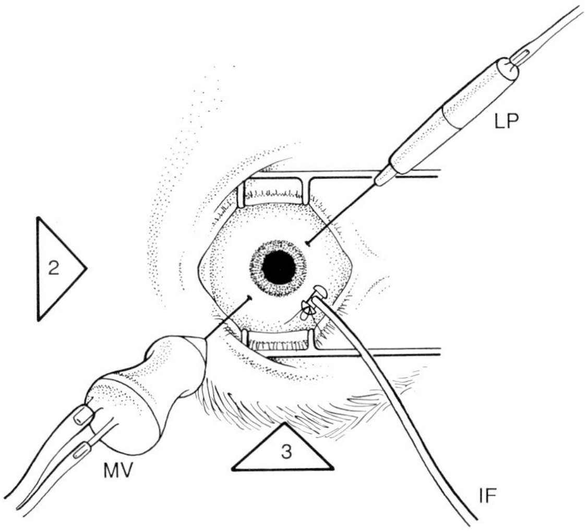

5.**4** Occasionally, the surgeon located at 12 o'clock cannot reach vitreoretinal membranes, and the surgeon, 2, and assistant, 3, must exchange positions. In such cases, the routine setup is changed. The patient is placed with his or her head at the foot of the operating table, providing more leg room for the surgeon sitting on the temporal side of the patient. The infusion cannula (IF) may be located along the border of the lateral rectus muscle; the upper and lower temporal quadrants may be used for the active instruments.

5.**5** Access to the upper temporal quadrant of the vitreous may be difficult from the surgeon's 12 o'clock or temporal location. If vitreoretinal pathology must be operated in this quadrant, the surgeon, 2, may have to be located at the nasal side of the eye. The infusion cannula is located in the upper temporal quadrant. The active instrument may be inserted in the upper nasal or lower temporal quadrant to reach the pathology in the upper temporal quadrant.

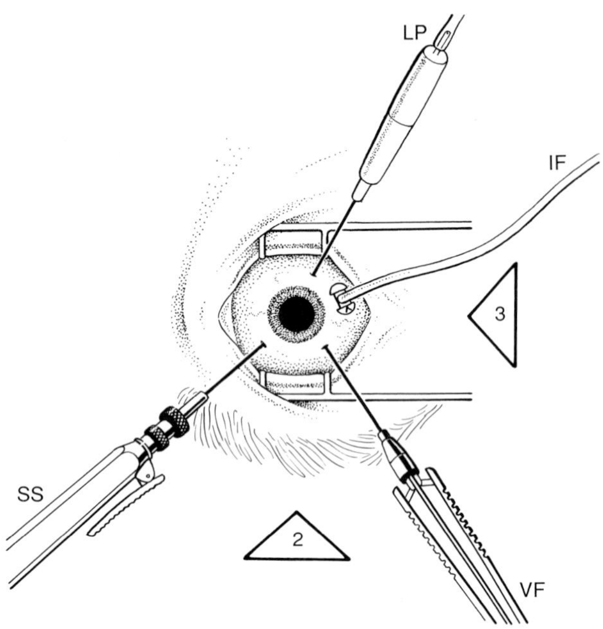

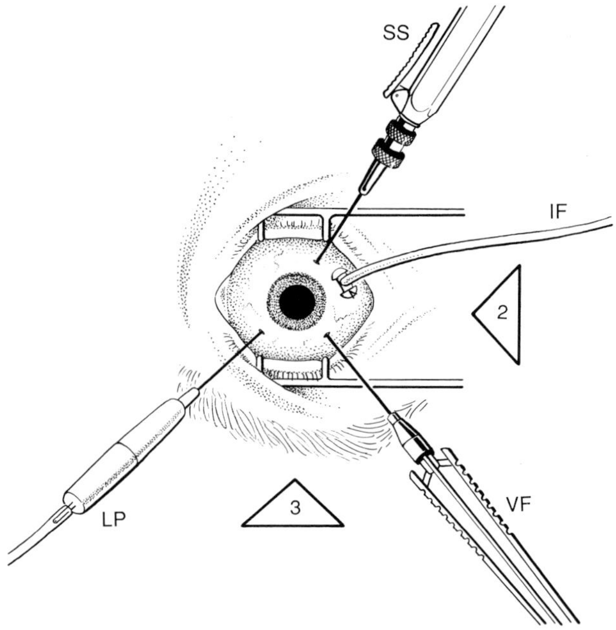

5.**6** Two active instruments, Sutherland scissors (SS) and vitreous forceps (VF), may be required for bimanual dissection of vitreoretinal membranes. These are held by the surgeon, 2. A fourth slcerotomy is required for introduction of a light pipe held by an assistant, 3, or of a cannula holding a fiber-optic illuminator. A modification of this approach is the use of four-port cannulas anchored in four quadrants, allowing the infusion to be fitted in all ports and three functional elements to be in the vitreous cavity simultaneously.

5.**7** With a four-port approach, the surgeon, 2, handles the Sutherland scissors (SS) and vitreous forceps (VF), and can change position from 12 o'clock to the patient's temporal side. The microscope and operating table setup are modified accordingly. The assistant holds and directs the light pipe to the operative field, or an indwelling fiber-optic light is used.

The skin over the lids and around the eye is scrubbed thoroughly with surgical soap solution in a circular pattern that includes the nose, cheek, forehead, and preauricular region. The scrubbed area is swabbed with surgical prep solution containing 70% isopropanol and 0.01% D and C red dye no. 39 (1, 3).

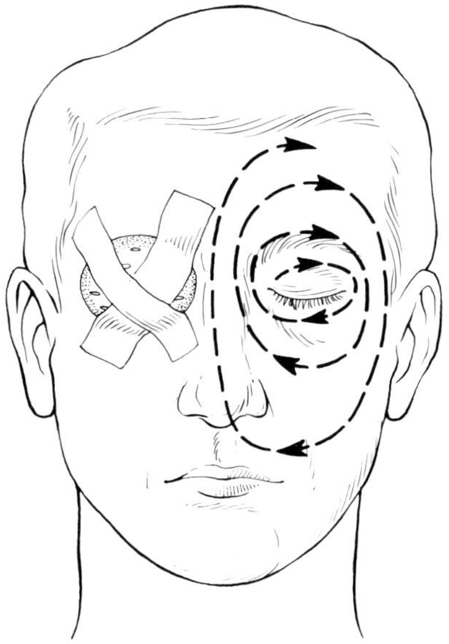

Preoperative Preparation

5.**8** The preoperative preparation of patients for retinal or vitreous surgery is identical. The patient is instructed to wash his or her face thoroughly with soap and water the night before surgery and the morning of surgery. Eyelashes are clipped with scissors the night before surgery. Gentamicin eye drops are instilled three times at 15-minute intervals the night before surgery and again the morning of surgery.

The morning of surgery, the pupil is dilated with 1% cyclopentolate hydrochloride and 2.5% phenylephrine hydrochloride instilled three times at 15-minute intervals. In addition, a 0.1% antiprostaglandin drop, which promotes sustained intraoperative pupillary dilation, is instilled four times at 30-minute intervals.

Operating Room Preparation. Pupillary dilation is routinely checked, and additional mydriatic solutions are instilled as needed. The fellow eye is protected with a Fox shield. A culture is taken from the cul-de-sac of the conjunctiva. Topical 0.5% proparacaine hydrochloride solution is instilled when the patient is to have retrobulbar anesthesia, and omitted when general anesthesia is being given. A 10% solution of Argyrol is instilled in the conjunctival cul-de-sac to coagulate mucus. This is supplemented with 5% povidone-iodine solution for antisepsis.

Draping procedure. A. *Scleral buckling.* Drapes for a scleral buckling operation include separate sterile drapes for the head and body. The head drape consists of two sheets. The patient's head is lifted so that the bottom sheet can be placed under it. Then the top sheet is wrapped around the head and face. A plastic eye drape is placed over the head and chest, centering the hole of the sheet on the operated eye. A body drape is placed over the patient with the hole of the drape centered on the eye. The body drape is anchored to the side of the table with towel clips.

B. *Vitrectomy.* Patients requiring both vitrectomy and scleral buckle are draped in a similar fashion, to that described for A, with the addition of a plastic sheet placed over the patient's head and under the table head to catch dripping irrigating fluids (2).

For a "routine" vitrectomy, the use of an arm rest facilitates draping. Three layers of drapes are placed: a plastic drape as first layer, a body drape as second layer, and a plastic drape as third layer. The drapes are pushed between the patient's head and the arm rest to form a well to catch the dripping irrigating fluids that are sucked out through a catheter connected to a suction pump.

References

1. Charles S. Vitreous microsurgery. 2nd ed. Baltimore: Williams and Wilkins, 1987: 40–41.
2. Machemer R, Aaberg TM. Vitrectomy. 2nd ed. New York: Grune and Stratton, 1979: 33–35.
3. Schepens CL. Retinal detachment and allied diseases. Philadelphia: W B Saunders, 1983: 385–388.

6

Basic Vitrectomy: Preparation of Sclerotomies

Preparing Sclerotomy Sites

A lid speculum, preferably a heavy-duty Barraquer wire speculum, is inserted between the lids. If scleral buckling is to be performed, a traction suture is placed in both the upper and lower lids, using 4-0 black silk.

6.1 **Peritomy.** If scleral buckling is planned, a 360° peritomy is carried out. If only vitrectomy is contemplated, peritomy is performed in the quadrants requiring sclerotomies. In eyes that have had previous retinal detachment surgery, the conjunctival incision follows the line of the previous peritomy. In eyes with a functional filtering bleb, the conjunctival incision should extend posterior to the bleb.

Peritomy is done using curved, sharp-pointed iris scissors and fine-toothed Bishop-Harmon forceps. The peritomy is made slightly posterior to the limbus so that a 2 mm rim of conjunctiva is left to facilitate conjunctival closure.

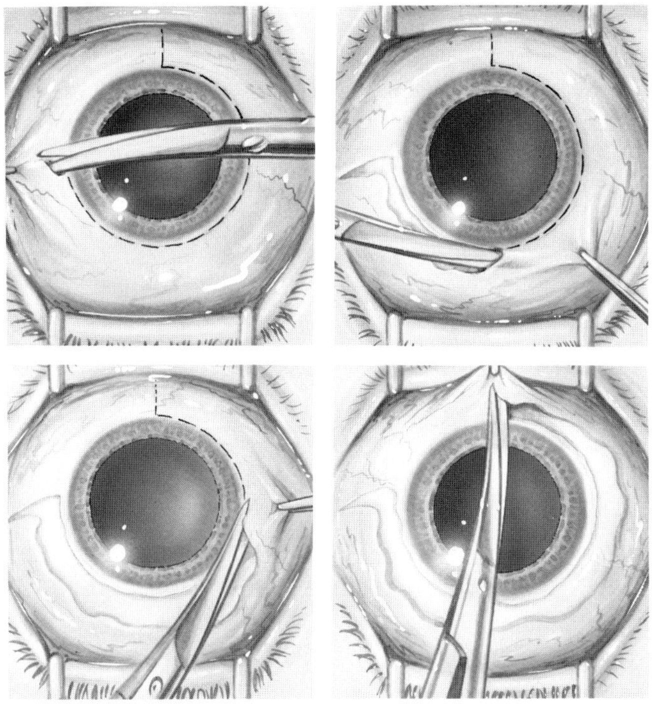
a b c d

a The conjunctiva is grasped with the forceps, lifted up, and opened with the scissors.
b, c The opening is extended along the limbus, undermining the conjunctiva and splitting Tenon's fascia with the tip of the scissors.

d In eyes requiring a 360° peritomy, an 8 mm relaxing radial conjunctival incision is made slightly above or below each horizontal meridian. If peritomy involves three quadrants, a relaxing conjunctival incision is made at each extreme end of the peritomy.

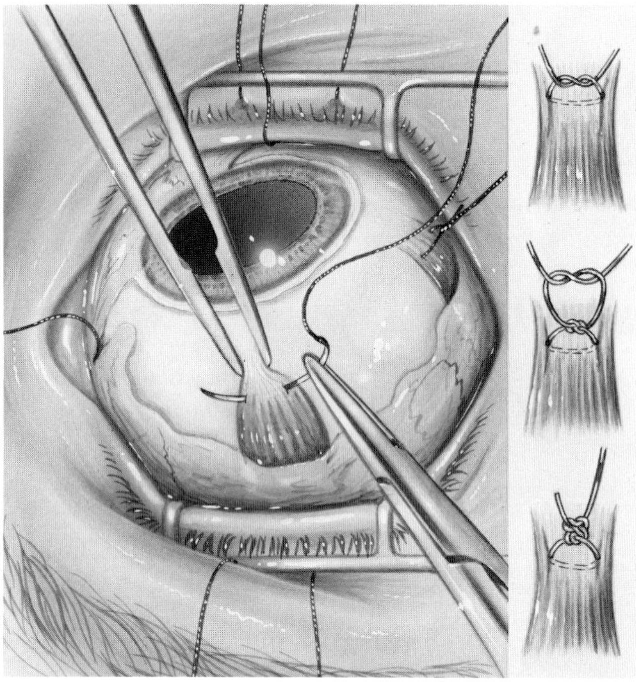

6.2 Placement of traction sutures. If scleral buckling is included in the surgical plan, 4-0 silk traction sutures may be placed through or under the tendons of the rectus muscles. The suture through the tendon is tied loosely with a square knot, leaving a loose loop to facilitate suture cutting at the end of surgery.

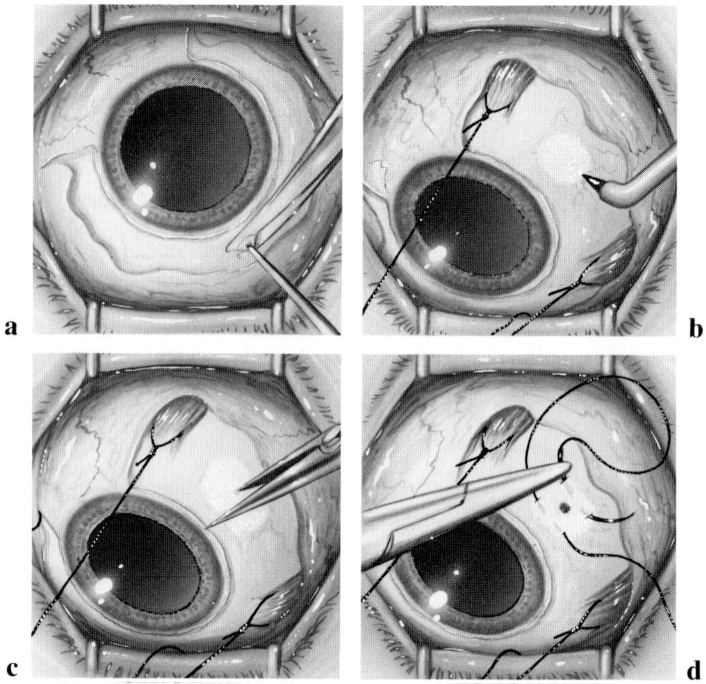

6.3 Sclerotomy for infusion cannula. The most practical location for the infusion cannula is the lower temporal quadrant along the inferior border of the lateral rectus muscle, because when the globe is moved, the cannula does not impinge on the nose or the lower lid margin or lid speculum (1).

a Episcleral tissue over the slcerotomy site is meticulously excised with scissors or scraped with a scarifier.

b Episcleral vessels in the area intended for the sclerotomy are coagulated with diathermy or eraser. Excessive diathermy should be avoided to prevent scleral necrosis. Pinpoint applications of diathermy to blood vessels is recommended to minimize damage ot the sclera.

c While visualizing with the operating microscope, the sclerotomy site is measured 3.5 mm from the limbus, using a caliper, and marked with a gentian violet pen.

d The first bite of the 6-0 polyglactin scleral suture is placed in front of the 3.5 mm mark, and the second bite behind it.

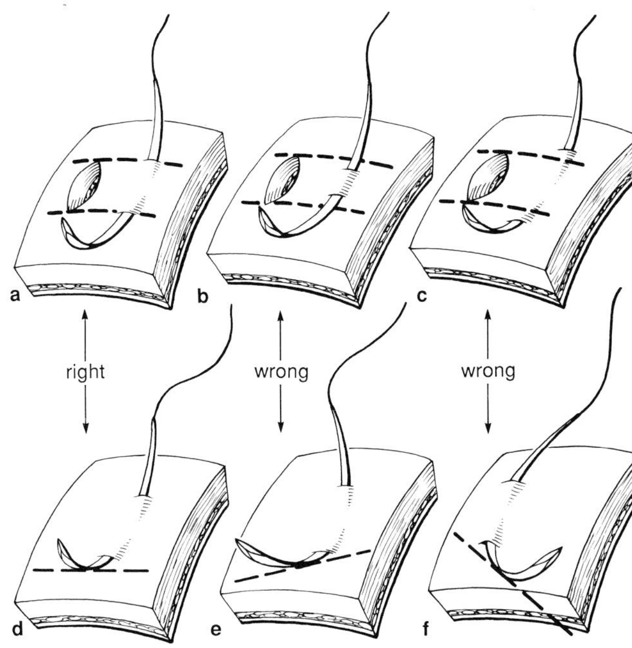

6.**4** We prefer a 6-0 polyglactin suture with a spatula needle to anchor the infusion cannula. The scleral bite for the anchor suture must be of adequate depth and length to make the cannula secure and stable.

a Its depth should be half the scleral thickness, and its length should be approximately the same as that of the sclerotomy.

b A short and shallow suture bite may cause the suture to cut through the sclera.

c On the other hand, an excessively long scleral bite would make it difficult to secure the suture loop on the shoulder of the cannula.

d Passage of the needle parallel to the surface of the sclera may prevent the suture from cutting through the sclera.

e, f A tilt of the spatula needle to either side will cause a shallow scleral tract which results in a weak anchoring suture.

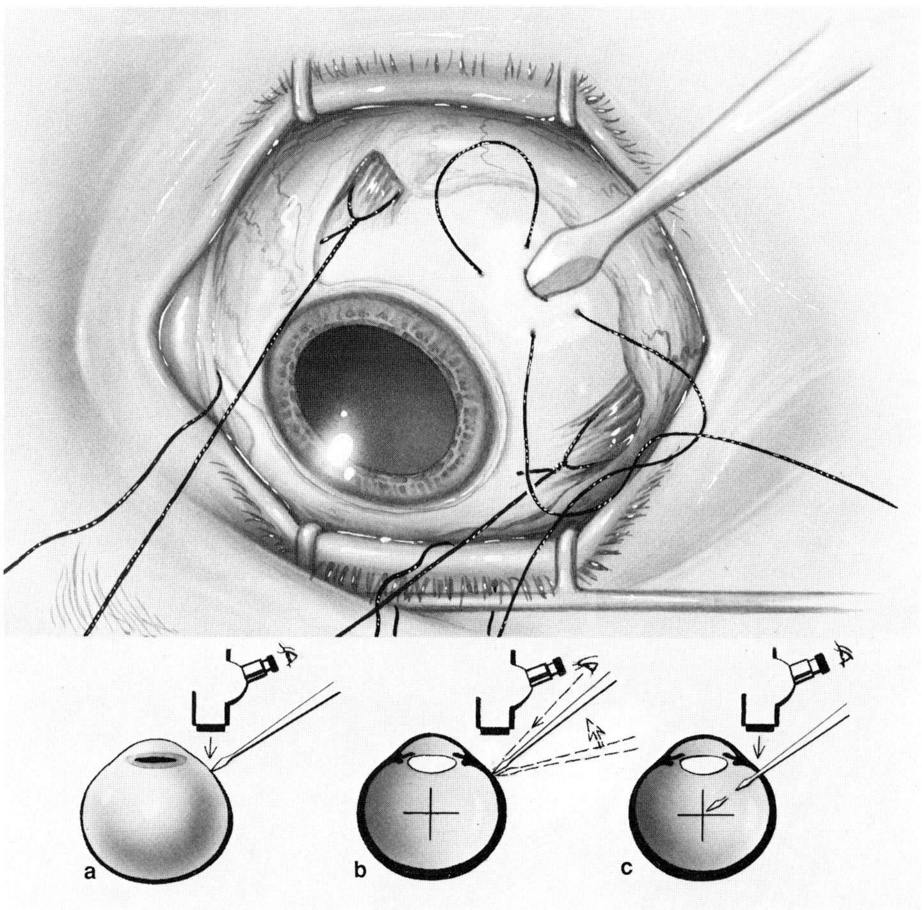

6.**5a** While viewing with the operating microscope, the tip of a microvitreoretinal (MVR) blade is rested on the gentian violet mark on the sclera.

b The surgeon's view is directed away from the microscope to the knife, which is inclined so that its point is directed toward the enter of the vitreous cavity.

c The surgeon's view is directed back to the microscope. The MVR knife is carefully passed through the pars plana, vitreous base, and anterior vitreous, then withdrawn slowly from the eye.

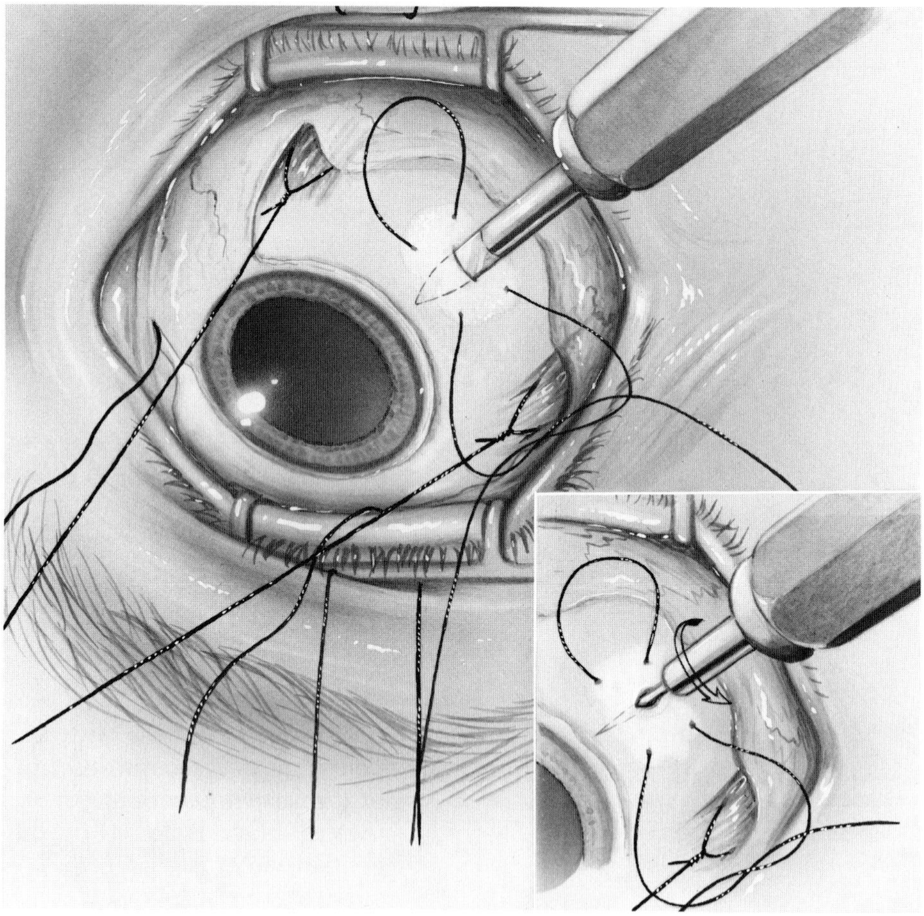

6.**6** The slit-like sclerotomy is enlarged with a stiletto which is rotated 180°, facilitating insertion of a cannula.

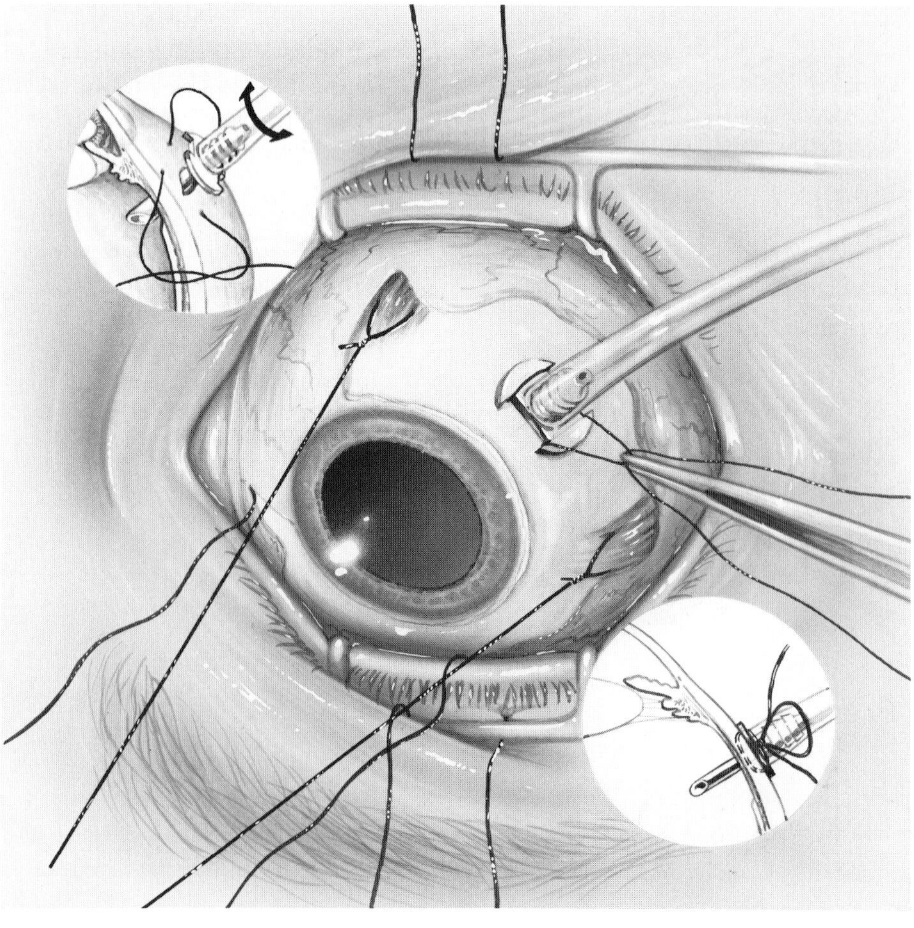

6.**7** A cannula with a 4 mm shaft is inserted through the sclerotomy in a rotating manner, while its tubing is held between the thumb and index finger. One suture loop is placed on the shoulder of the cannula while the opposite loop is pulled up. Then the other loop is tied with a slip knot over the opposite shoulder.

With aphakic and pseudophakic eyes, the cannula is pushed toward the anterior vitreous and the tip inspected under the microscope to check that it has entered the vitreous cavity. In phakic eyes, the tip is examined with the indirect opththalmoscope while the cannula is depressed toward the center of the vitreous cavity.

The infusion line is opened. The intraocular pressure is regulated by adjusting the height of the infusion bottle or the pressure in the air pump.

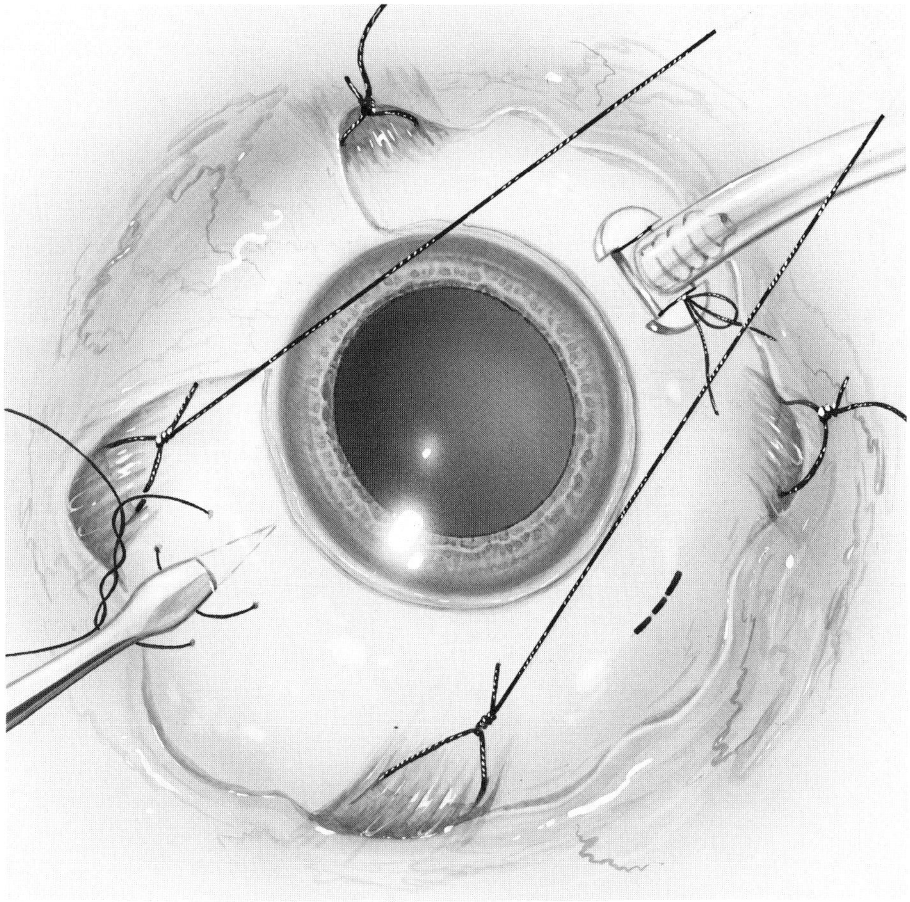

6.**8** Sclerotomy for insertion of the light pipe and vitrectomy probe is made in the same manner as that for the infusion cannula. It is located 3.5 mm from the limbus in the 9:30 and 2:30 o'clock meridians.

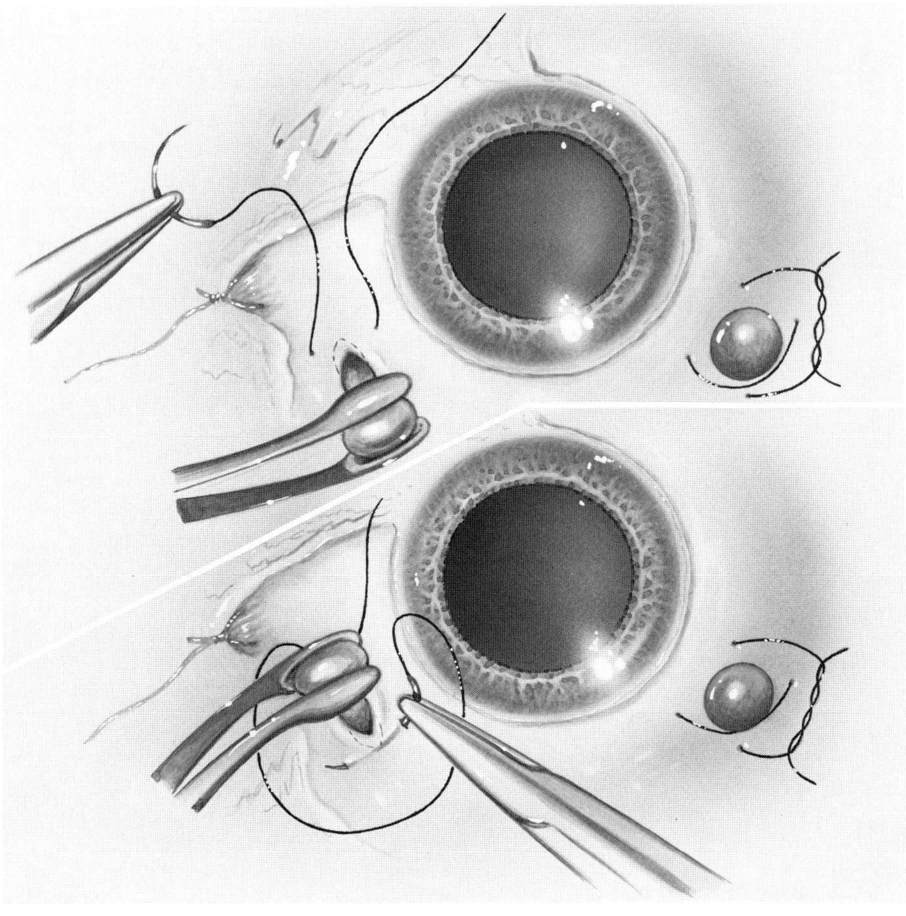

6.**9** Scleral plugs are placed in the sclerotomies to prevent vitreous prolapse. Running sclerotomy sutures of 8-0 polyglactin may be placed while the plug is in position. These sutures keep the sclerotomies tight around the intraocular instruments, preventing hypotony and leakage of air during air-fluid exchange and endolaser. To facilitate suture placement, the plug is held with the forceps and moved to one side to expose the end of the sclerotomy.

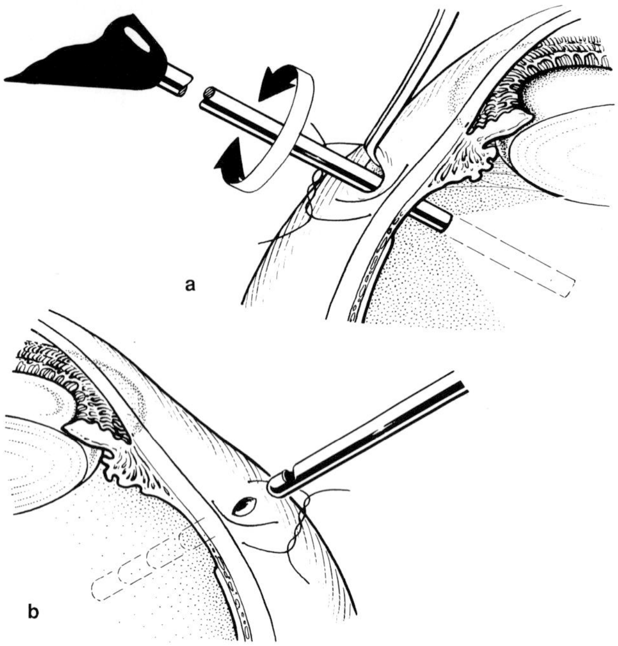

Introducing and Switching Instruments

6.**10 a** Insertion of a flat-tipped instrument, such as the endoilluminator, through a sclerotomy requires a special technique. The anterior or posterior lip of the sclerotomy is held with the colibri forceps. The cylindrical shaft of the endoilluminator is tilted along the length of the sclerotomy so that the tip of the pipe enters the opening at a 45° angle. This angulation allows the shoulder of the tip to gain partial entry and enlarge the opening. The shaft is gradually moved 90° as the entire tip gains entry to the opening. With a rotating motion, the instrument is pushed gradually into the vitreous cavity. The tip is inspected with the microscope to ensure that no tissue is being pushed in front of it.

b Introduction of a vitrectomy probe is less difficult, because it has a conical tip that enters and slides more easily through the sclerotomy, choroid, and vitreous base.

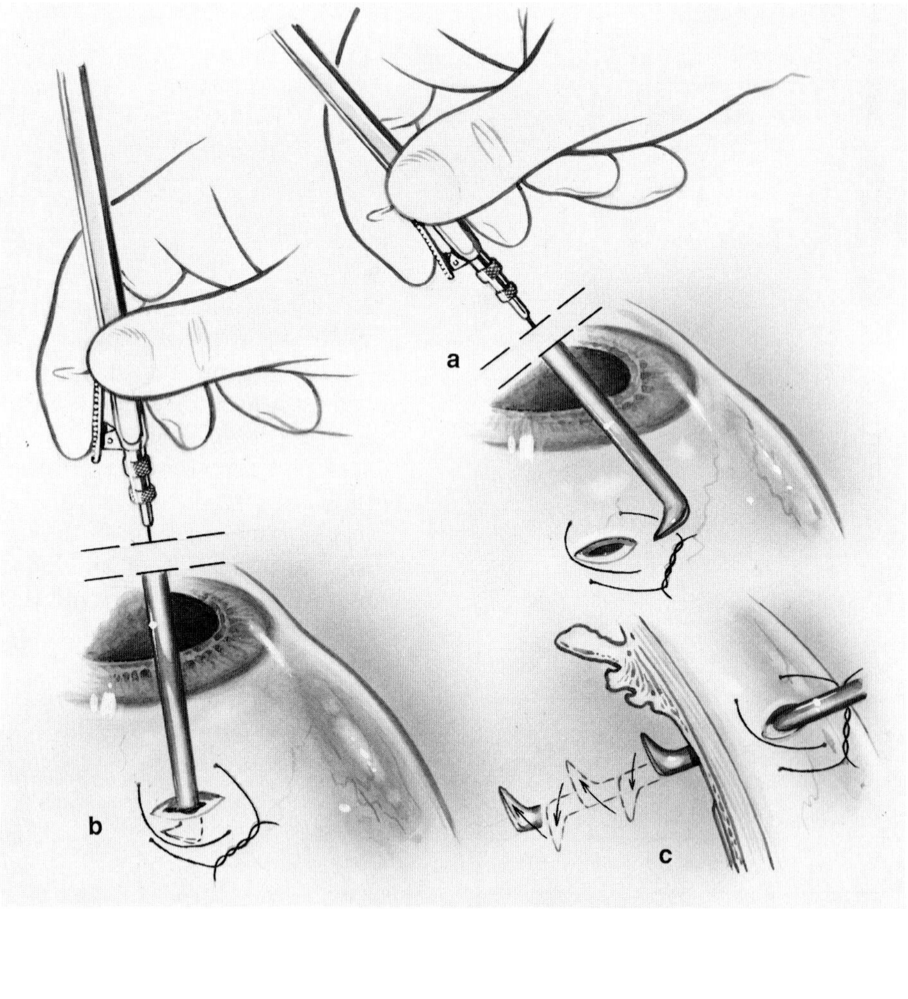

6.**11** Angled-tip instruments such as Sutherland scissors and angled spatulas require special maneuvers for safe introduction into the vitreous cavity.

a Scissor blades are closed during insertion.

b As a rule, the angled tip of the instrument enters the opening at a right angle to the scleral surface, making it necessary to incline the handle. After entry, the tip of the blade is oriented toward the anterior vitreous.

c Once the tip has reached the vitreous base, the instrument is rotated partially from one side to the other to prevent vitreous fibers or membranes along its track from being pushed forward by the blades.

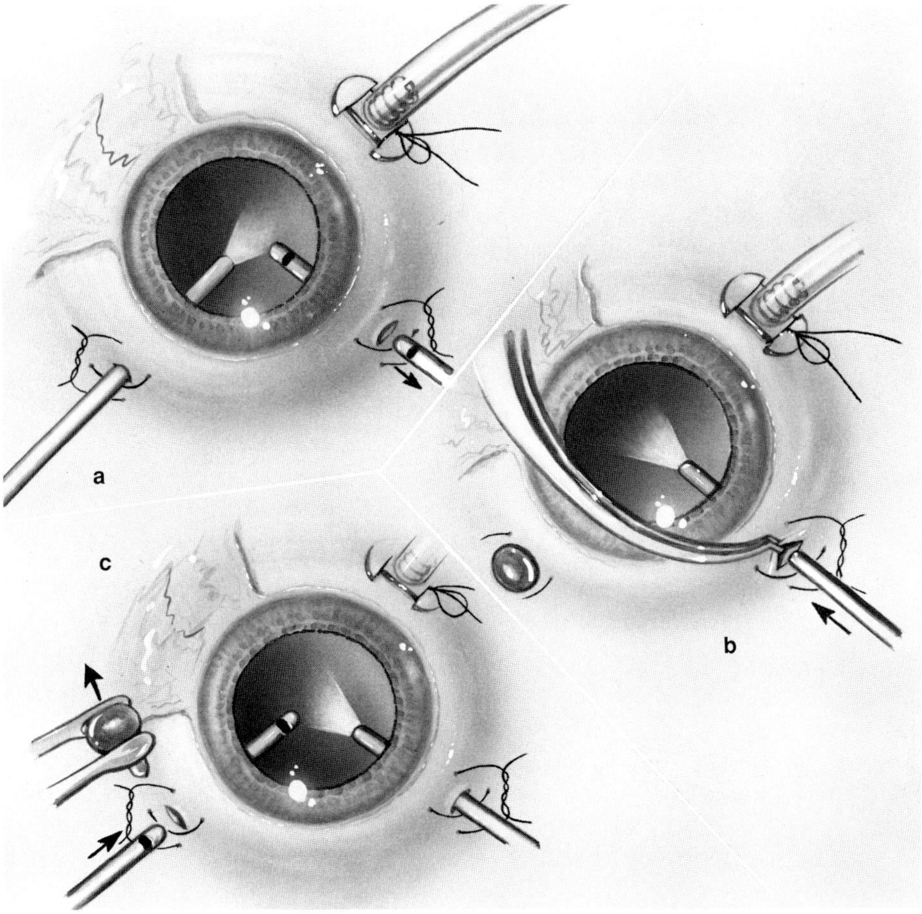

6.**12** During the course of vitreoretinal surgery, it may be necessary to switch the instruments from the left to the right hand, and vice versa, to provide better access to certain regions of the vitreous cavity. The infusion bottle is lowered to decrease the intraocular pressure and prevent vitreous prolapse.
a The instrument held in the dominant hand is removed first; the sclerotomy is closed with a plug. The instrument in the non-dominant hand is now withdrawn and the sclerotomy is closed immediately with a plug.
b The instrument swap is now carried out. The instrument from the other side is introduced after removing the plug.
c The swap is completed with removal of the plug and insertion of the other instrument into the vitreous.

References

1. Charles S. Vitreous microsurgery. 2nd ed. Baltimore: Williams and Wilkins, 1987: 68–69.

7

Basic Vitrectomy: Removal of Opaque Vitreous

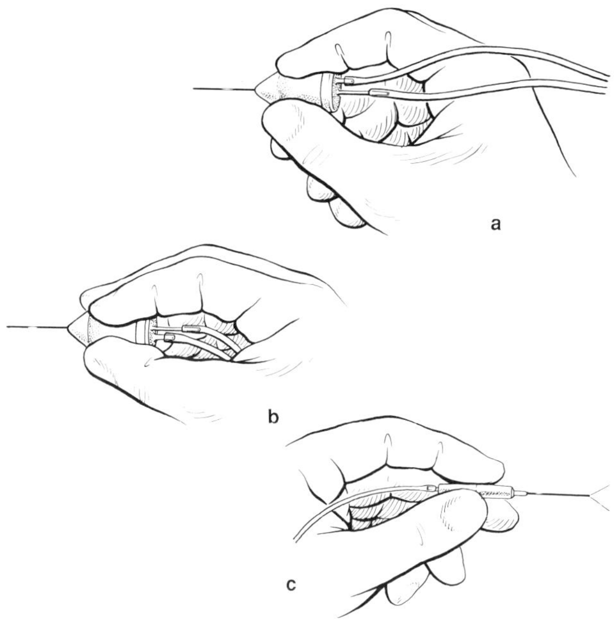

7.**1a** To remove opaque vitreous, the most natural way of holding the vitrectomy probe is the way one holds a pencil, i.e. overhand between the thumb, index, and middle fingers.

b Instruments with a short but large-diameter handle may be held underhand, using the thumb, index, and middle fingers.

c In both instances, movement of the instrument can originate from the fingers or the wrist, or both. The narrow handle of the endoilluminator is held overhand.

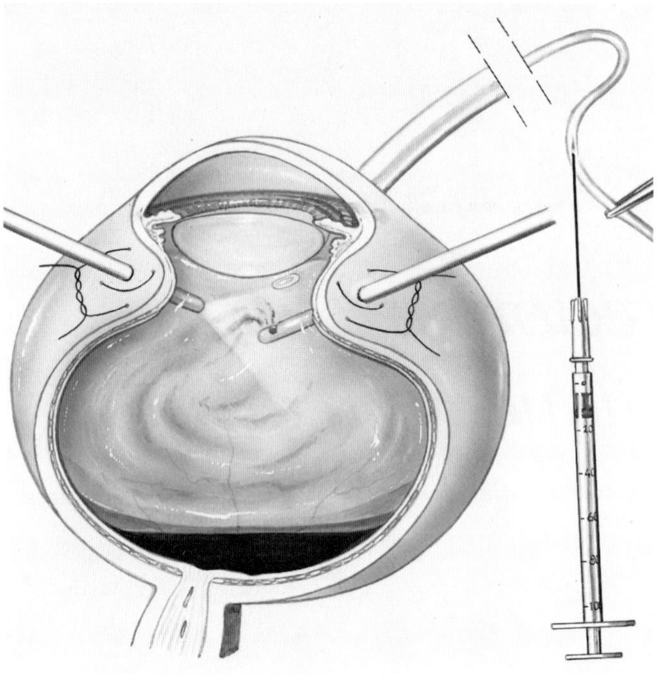

7.**2** Every effort should be made in eyes with diabetic retinopathy to preserve a clear, crystalline lens (1, 2, 3, 7). The posterior surface of the crystalline lens sometimes becomes difficult to differentiate from the adjacent, opaque, anterior vitreous gel in cases of longstanding vitreous hemorrhage. Use of a tuberculin syringe to inject a small bubble of sterile air through the infusion tubing may help overcome this difficulty. The air bubble rises to settle against the back surface of the lens, delineating it from the underlying opacities. An excessively large air bubble can be aspirated with the vitrectomy probe.

Although coaxial light from the microscope may be adequate to visualize the anterior vitreous, direct and indirect illumination from the light pipe provides better visualization.

A vitrectomy lens is not necessary during anterior vitrectomy.

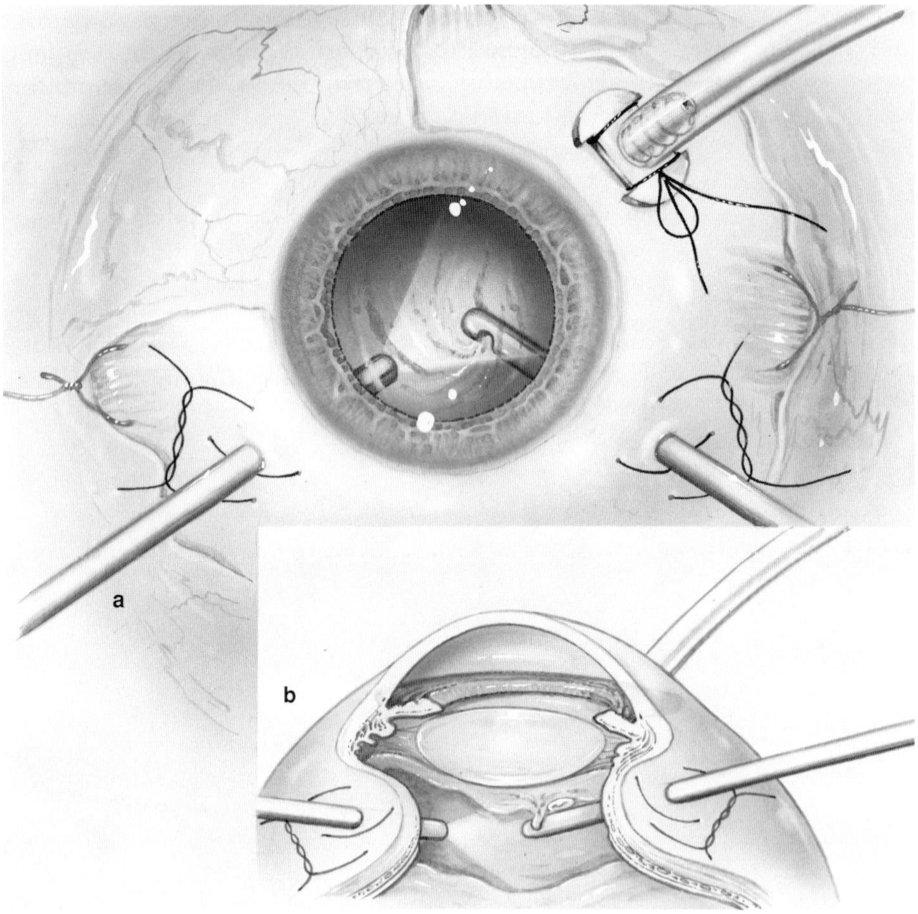

7.**3** The vitreous gel behind the posterior capsule may be opaque, as in cases of amyloidosis or massive vitreous hemorrhage. Removal of this gel requires special techniques to avoid damage to the lens. Visualization of this opaque vitreous may be enhanced by indirect endoillumination, utilizing light reflected from vitreous opacities from behind.

Once a central cavity has been created in the opaque vitreous, visibility may improve so that vitrectomy of retrolental opacities can be done more safely. The microscope magnification is increased to improve visualization of the posterior surface of the lens. The port of the vitrectomy probe is brought close to the anterior vitreous layer and turned sidewise, facing 90° from the lens surface (**a**). The cutting speed of the blade is increased, but suction is set at a low level.

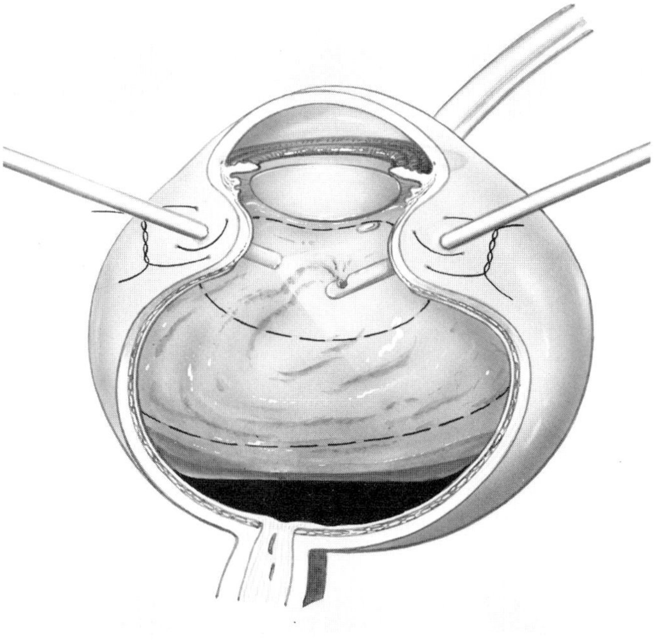

7.**4** As soon as the retrolental region has been cleared of opacities, removal of opaque vitreous proceeds posteriorly (broken line). The gel is engaged with the cutting port, aspirated with moderate suction, and cut at low cutting frequency.

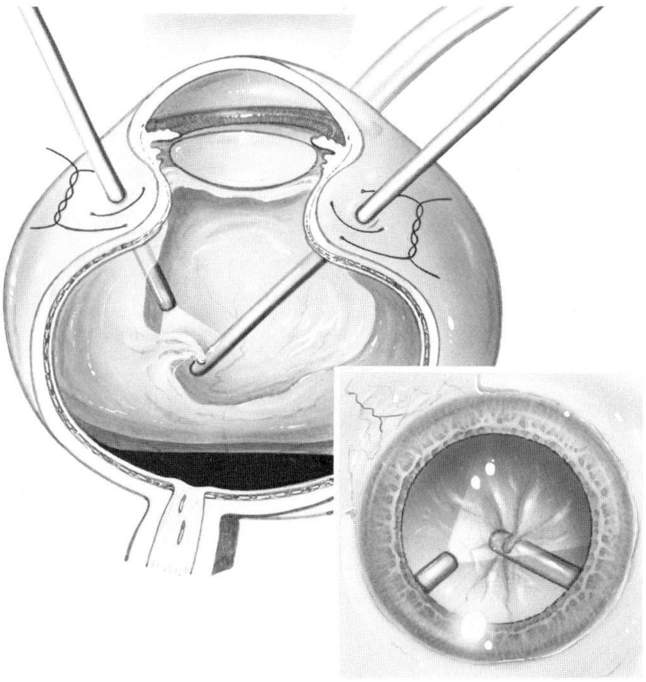

7.**6** When vitrectomy approaches the retina, the cutting port is turned to face anteriorly (inset) to avoid premature penetration of the cortical vitreous, which would allow sughyaloid blood to disperse and obscure the entire vitreous cavity.

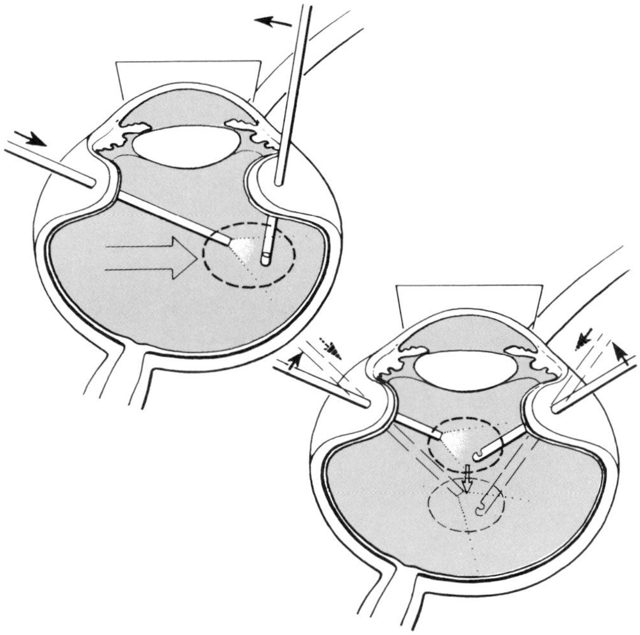

7.**5** If vitrectomy moves toward the middle and posterior vitreous, use of a vitrectomy lens is mandatory. With a vitrectomy lens on the cornea, the images of objects in the vitreous appear smaller as the field of view increases. The tips of the two instruments in the vitreous should move in tandem with the endoilluminator, which is used like a flashlight to illuminate the active instrument (vitrectomy probe, endodiathermy probe, or forceps). To move the location of the operative field (area inside broken line) from one side or plane the vitreous to another, it is necessary to coordinate the microscope focusing, x-y movement, and changes in the position of the instruments. The sclerotomies serve as the fulcrum for these movements (arrows) of the shafts of the instruments (5).

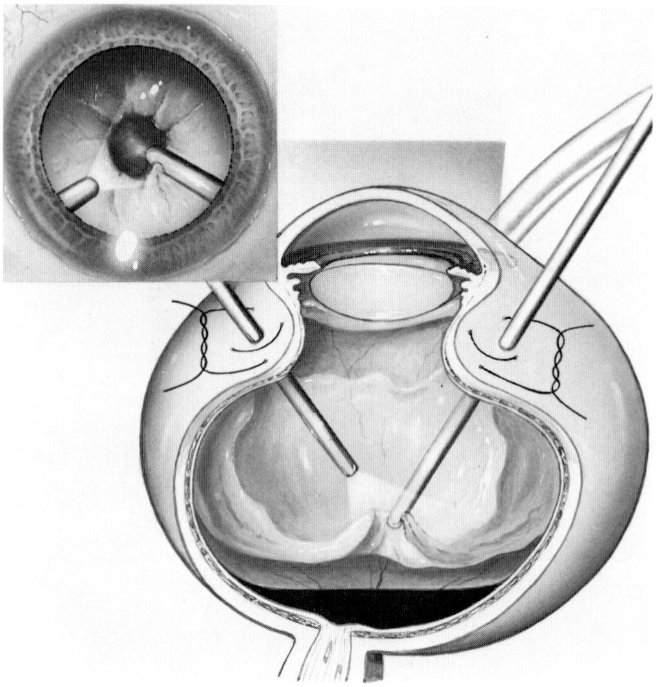

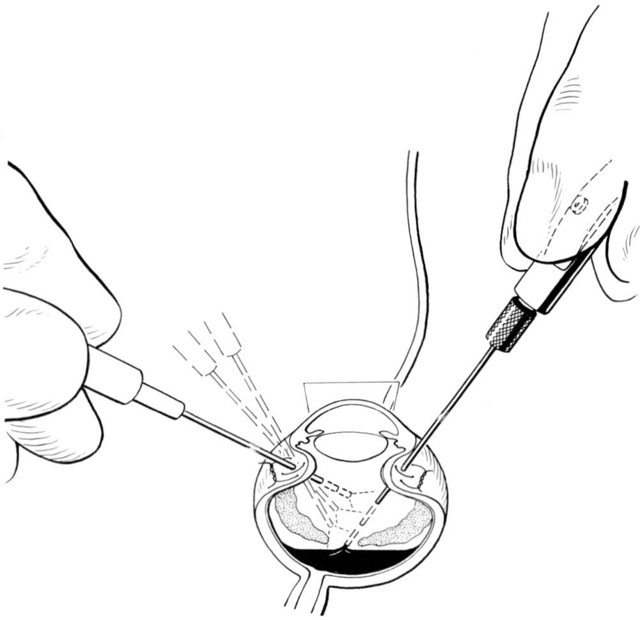

7.7 Before proceeding with vitrectomy of the posterior vitreous, the surgeon reviews the preoperative ultrasonographic findings so that the locations of elevated retina can be avoided until the latter part of the procedure. Vitrectomy proceeds over attached retina, removing posterior opacities until retinal details can be visualized.

The state of the posterior vitreous cortex, subhyaloid space, and retina is surveyed. In case of complete posterior vitreous detachment with a large accumulation of degenerated red blood cells in the subhyaloid space, a small hole the size of the optic disc is created in the posterior cortical layer.

7.**8** After the infusion bottle is lowered to decrease intraocular pressure and prevent vitreous prolapse, the vitrectomy probe is withdrawn and an extrusion needle is substituted (8). During insertion, the vent is closed with the thumb or index finger. With the endoilluminator moving in tandem, the tip of the needle is carefully introduced into the subhyaloid space through the opening in the posterior vitreous cortex.

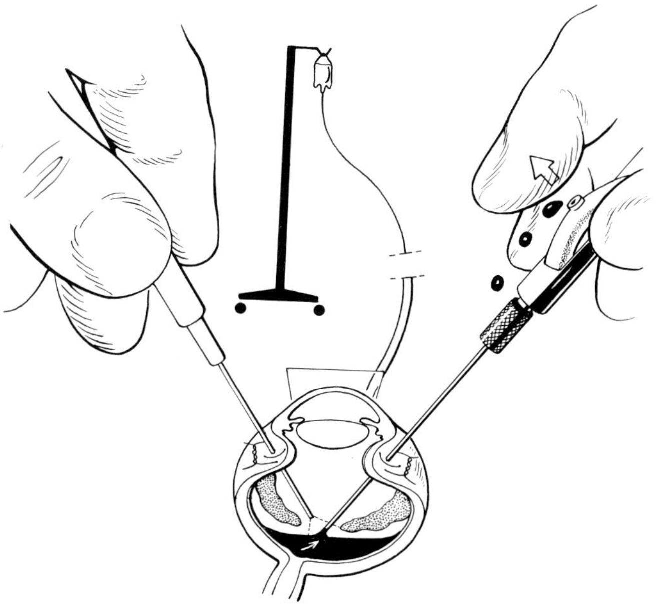

7.**9** Once the tip of the extrusion needle has reached the surface of the blood, the finger is removed from the vent. When the vent is uncovered, fluid and dispersed blood will flow out of the eye, because of the pressure gradient between the vitreous cavity at the needle tip and the lower atmospheric pressure at the vent. Elevation of the infusion bottle increases the evacuation rate of fluid from the vitreous cavity.

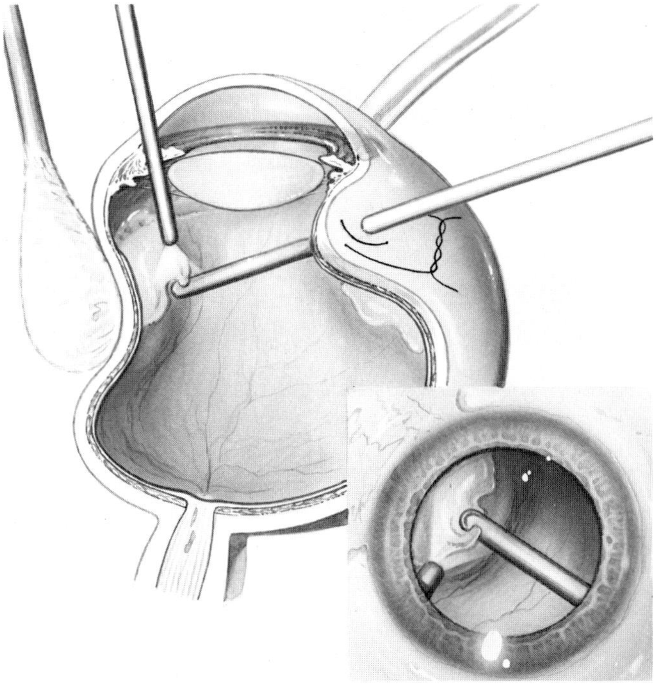

7.**11** As soon as the vitreous cavity has been cleared of opacities, the surgeon inspects the entire fundus, including the periphery. In eyes with longstanding, massive vitreous hemorrhage, the vitreous base is usually opaque and loaded with degenerated red blood cells that may become dispersed into the vitreous cavity postoperatively. To avoid this, vitrectomy is directed to the vitreous base. The assistant applies a scleral depressor or a cotton swab in the area of the opaque vitreous base, pushing it toward the axial region and making it more safely accessible to vitrectomy. The light pipe and vitrectomy probe are brought close to the opaque gel, which is removed carefully. The cutting frequency of the probe is increased, and suction is set at a low level to minimize traction ot the peripheral retina. Vitrectomy should stop when visibility of the surgical field is no longer optimal.

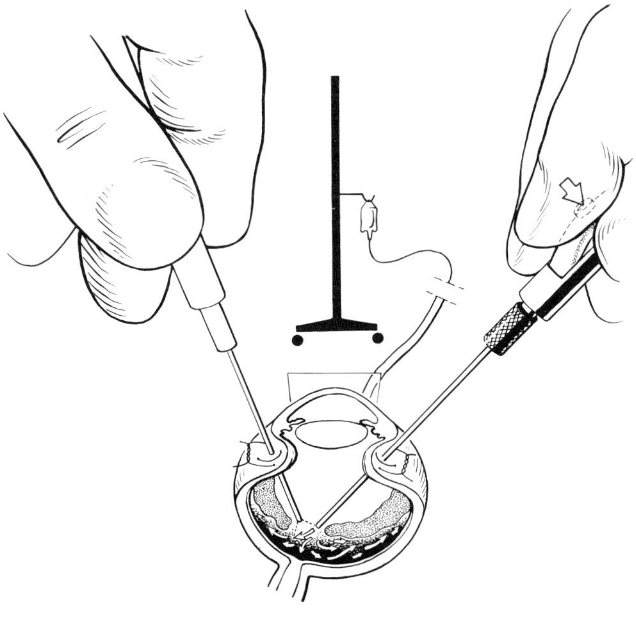

7.**10** Degenerated red blood cells may behave like thick sediment on the retinal surface (4, 6). These cells are usually resistant to evacuation unless they are agitated mechanically. Sediment-like blood is stirred up by squeezing the silicone tubing with a finger over the vent. This forces fluid in a jet stream out of the needle into the layered blood, dispersing it into the vitreous cavity, where it can be evacuated. During this maneuver, the intraocular pressure is decreased by lowering the infusion bottle.

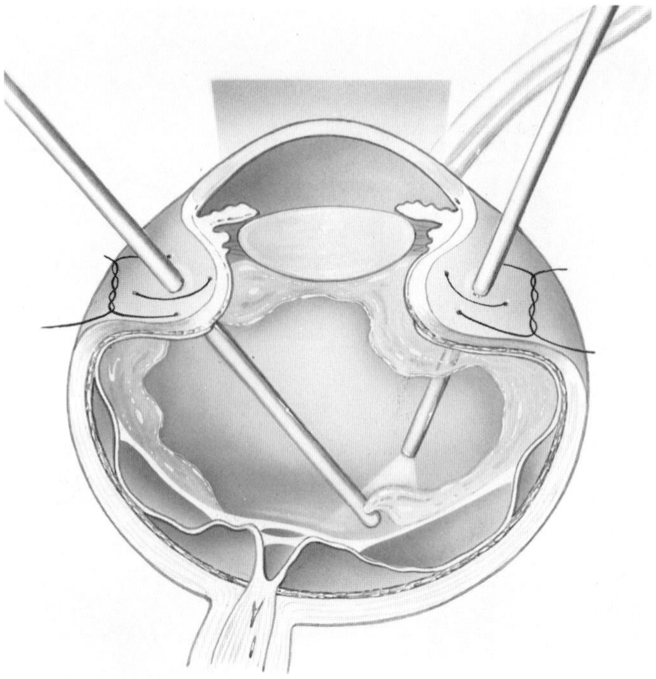

7.**12** Opaque vitreous may be associated with retinal detachment, whether or not a retinal elevation is evident by ultrasonography. Posterior vitrectomy should proceed with great caution, first removing vitreous in areas least likely to have retinal detachment, and reserving areas of suspected detachment for last. As soon as the fundus becomes visible, it is surveyed with the light pipe to determine vitreoretinal adhesions, traction membranes, preretinal membranes, fibrovascular membranes, or retinal breaks. The procedures for handling these vitreoretinal findings are described in later chapters. In preparation for these procedures, the vitreous gel lining the inner surface of traction membranes is removed with the vitrectomy probe. Removal of gel facilitates dissection and segmentation of membranes. As a general principle, the cutting port of the probe should be positioned 180° from the membrane or retinal surface from which the gel is being removed. During this somewhat risky procedure, the infusion pressure should be reduced, the vitrectomy probe cutting speed increased, and its suction pressure decreased.

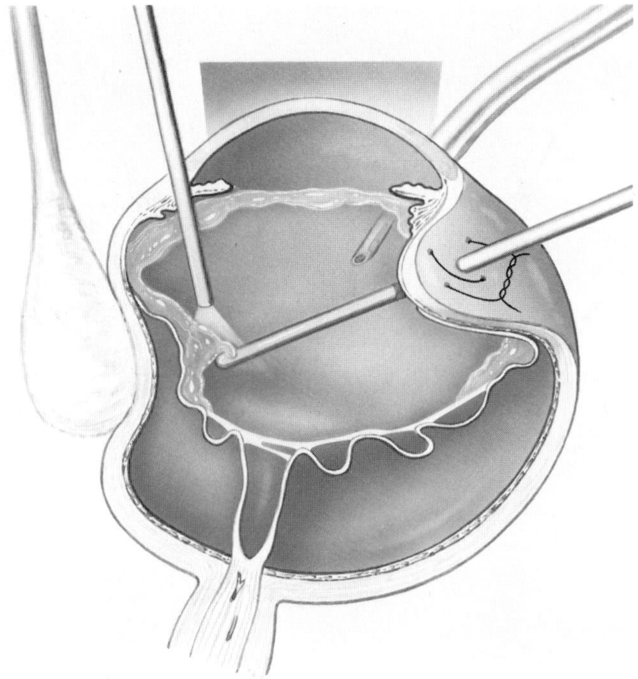

7.**13** Vitrectomy in the peripheral vitreous overlying detached retina requires an optimum view of the vitrectomy field. Scleral depression of the peripheral retina improves the binocular and stereoscopic view of the peripheral vitreous, and enhances safe vitreous removal. The same precautions as those described in Figure 7.**11** regarding cutting speed, suction, cutting port position, and infusion pressure are observed. When visibility deteriorates, vitrectomy should be terminated in that region.

References

1. Blankenship GW. The lens influence on diabetic vitrectomy results: report of a prospective randomized study. Arch Ophthalmol 1980; 98: 2196–2198.
2. Blankenship G, Cortez R, Machemer R. The lens and pars plana vitrectomy for diabetic retinopathy complications. Arch Ophthalmol 1979; 97: 1263–1267.
3. Blankenship GW, Stirpe M, Gonvers M, Binder S. Basic and advanced vitreous surgery. Padua: Liviana, 1986: 255–258.
4. Landers MB III. Removal of blood from the retinal surface in pars plana vitrectomy. Am J Ophthalmol 1978; 86: 427-429.
5. Machemer R, Aaberg TM. Vitrectomy. 2nd ed. New York: Grune and Stratton, 1979: 57–65.
6. Michels RG. Vitreous surgery. St. Louis: C V Mosby, 1980: 161–172.
7. Rice TA, Michels RG, Maguire MG, Rice EF. The effect of lensectomy on the incidence of iris neovascularization and neovascular glaucoma after vitrectomy for diabetic retinopathy. Am J Ophthalmol 1983; 95: 1–11.
8. Živojnović R, Vijfvinkel GJ. A modified flute needle. Am J Ophthalmol 1983; 96: 548–549.

8

Basic Vitrectomy: Closure of Sclerotomy and Conjunctiva

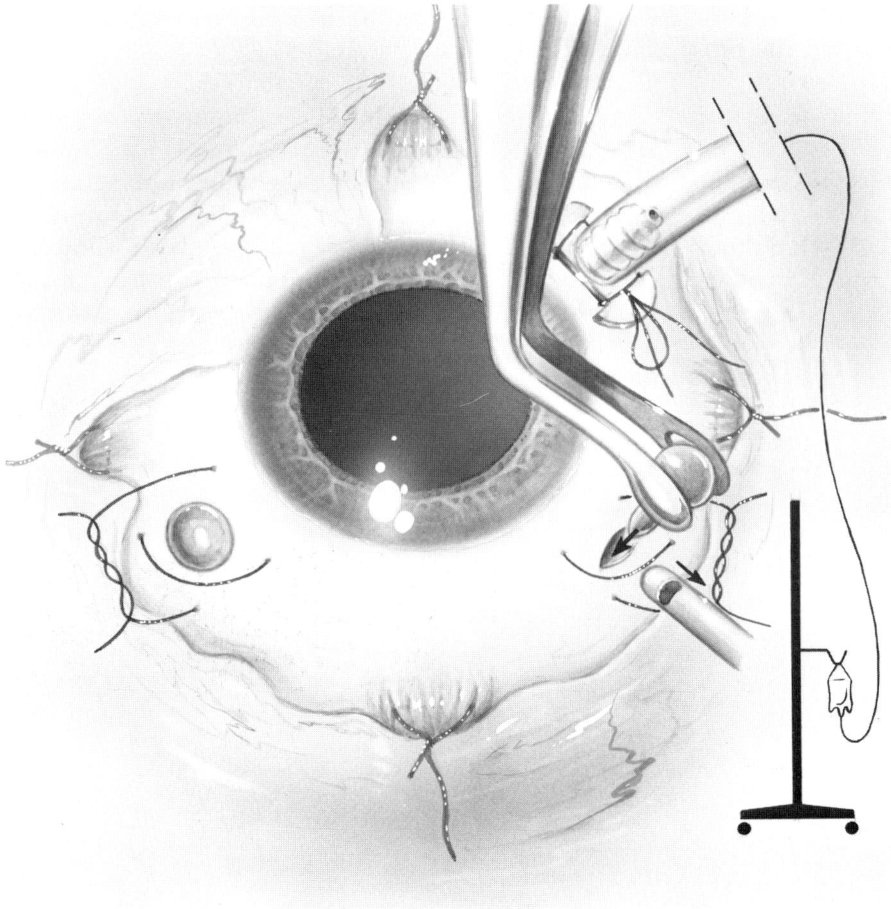

8.**1** Before withdrawing the instruments from the vitreous cavity, the fundus is inspected thoroughly for retinal pathology. The port of the vitrectomy probe is inspected to make sure that no vitreous is incarcerated that may be dragged when the probe is withdrawn. The infusion bottle is lowered to reduce intraocular pressure and lessen the tendency toward vitreous prolapse through the sclerotomy. As a rule, the active instrument is the first to be withdrawn.

The instrument tip is observed constantly through the microscope until it disappears from view in the periphery. The sclerotomies are covered immediately by plugs which are inserted with a plug forceps. The preplaced sutures are tied and closed.

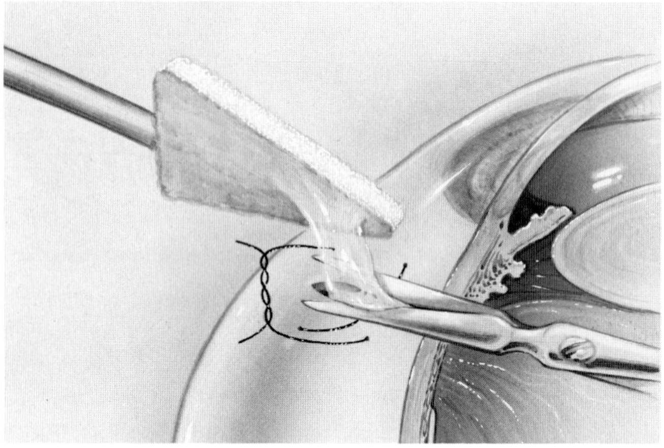

8.2 If vitreous has prolapsed through the sclerotomy, the infusion pressure is reduced, and the prolapsed vitreous is excised with Vannas scissors.

Excision of prolapsed vitreous is done using the operating microscope. A dry cellulose sponge is applied to the sclerotomy to pick up vitreous strands, which are pulled away from the sclera and cut with scissors. This procedure is repeated until all strands have been cut.

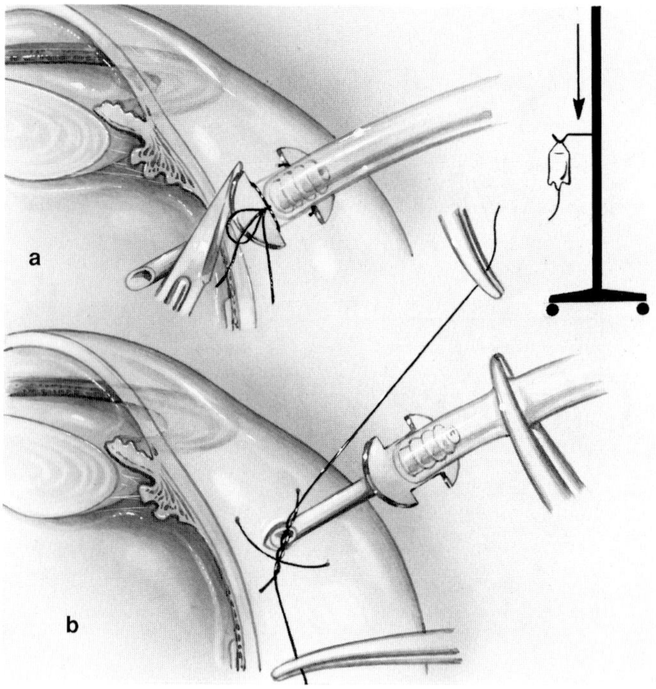

8.4 A temporary suture is used to anchor the infusion cannula during vitrectomy.

a During removal of the cannula, the anchor suture is cut under the shoulder of the cannula with a sharp knife; then the sclerotomy is closed with an 8-0 nylon suture in a figure-of-eight fashion while the cannula is in the eye.

b One of us (H.M.F.) uses the preplaced suture to close the sclerotomy. Pulling on the arms of this suture as the assistant slowly withdraws the cannula prevents loss of vitreous gel. An additional 8-0 nylon suture is placed across the sclerotomy.

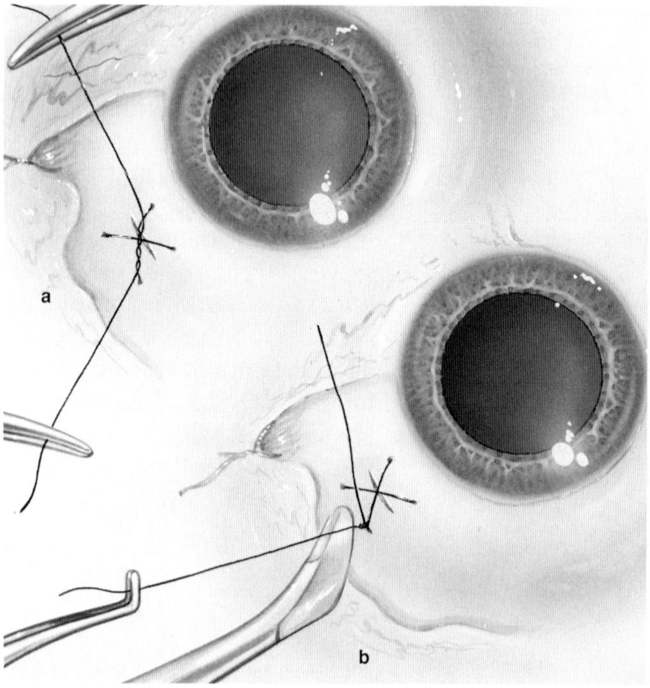

8.3**a** The sclerotomy suture is pulled up tight with two tying forceps and tied with a square knot so that the sclerotomy is closed in a figure-of-eight fashion.

b If the sclerotomy has become enlarged inadvertently, interrupted sutures may be added. The suture ends are trimmed to the knot with a knife or Vannas scissors.

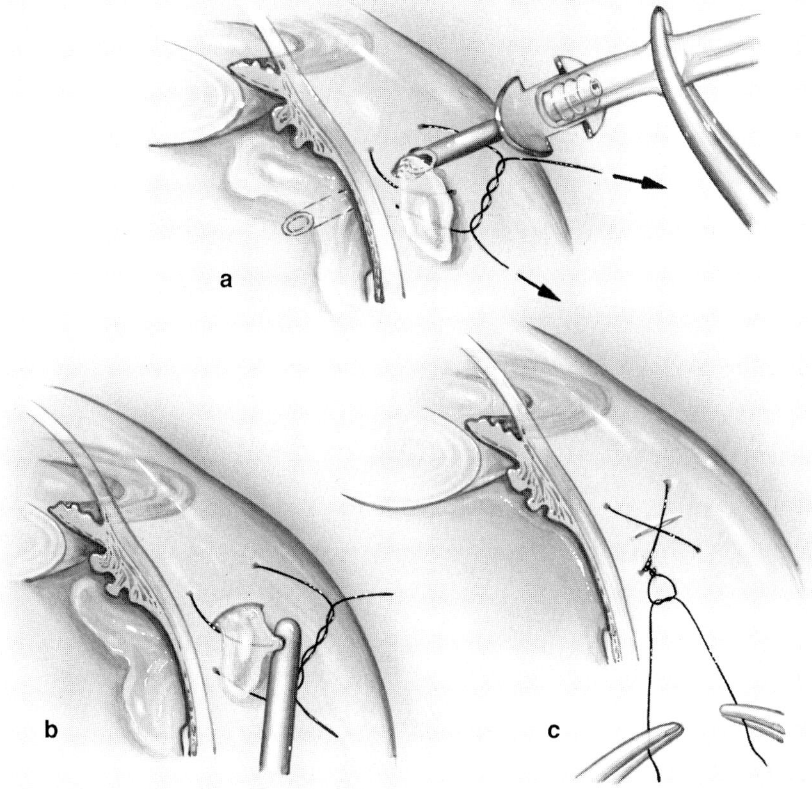

8.5a Vitreous prolapse may occur when the infusion pressure is not reduced prior to the removal of the cannula. Vitreous incarcerated in the sclerotomy will prevent proper closure and healing of the sclerotomy; it must therefore be meticulously excised.
b The prolapsed vitreous may be removed using the vitrectomy probe. The port of the probe is passed around the edge of the sclerotomy to engage prolapsing vitreous gel. Then the probe tip is inserted in the sclerotomy to aspirate and cut the incarcerated vitreous.
c The preplaced suture is pulled up tightly and closed with a square knot, and the excess suture is trimmed close to the knot with the scissors or knife.

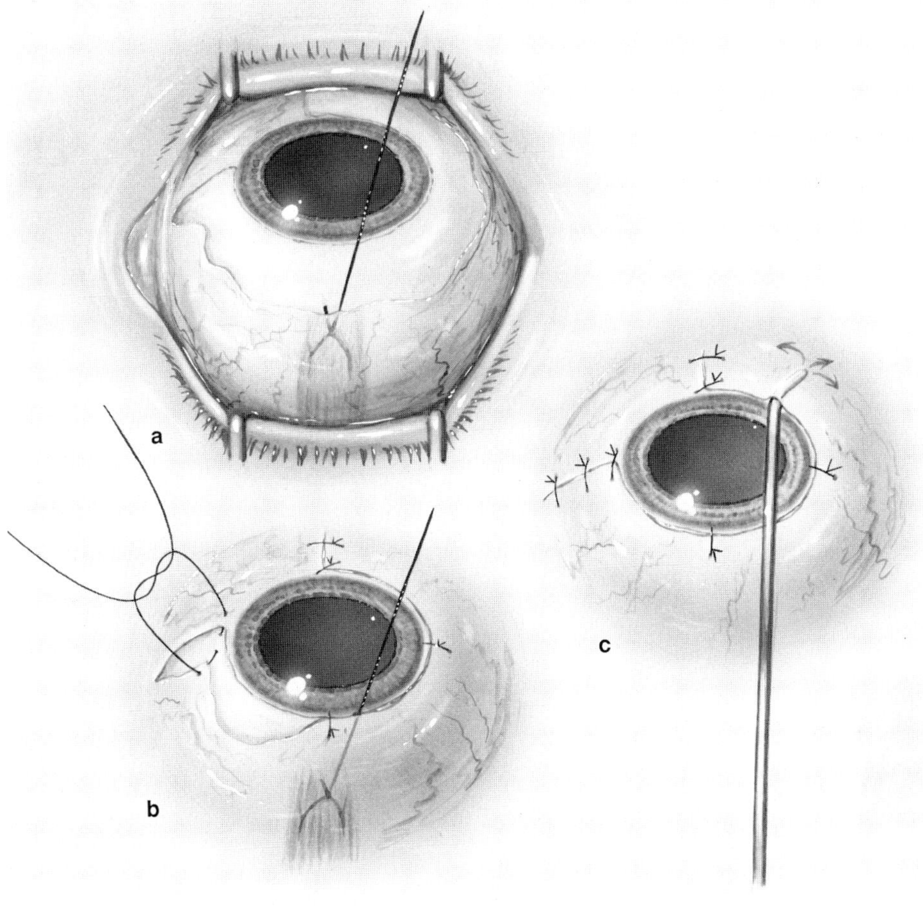

8.6a While the globe is stabilized with the superior rectus traction suture, the posterior edge of the conjunctival peritomy is pulled back to the limbus.
b The corners of the relaxing incision are approximated and sutured with 8-0 polyglactin.
c Additional interrupted sutures are placed to achieve tight conjunctical closure. Antibiotics are injected under Tenon's capsule after obtaining a culture.

9

Basic Vitrectomy: Prevention and Management of Complications

Intraoperative Corneal Haze

Corneal haze hinders vitreous and fundus visibility, and can compromise the results of vitrectomy. It is likely to occur in the eyes of patients with diabetes, or of elderly patients with a history of multiple intraocular procedures. Corneal haze may be due to epithelial, stromal, or endothelial edema. Stromal and endothelial edema are usually caused by damage to the endothelium.

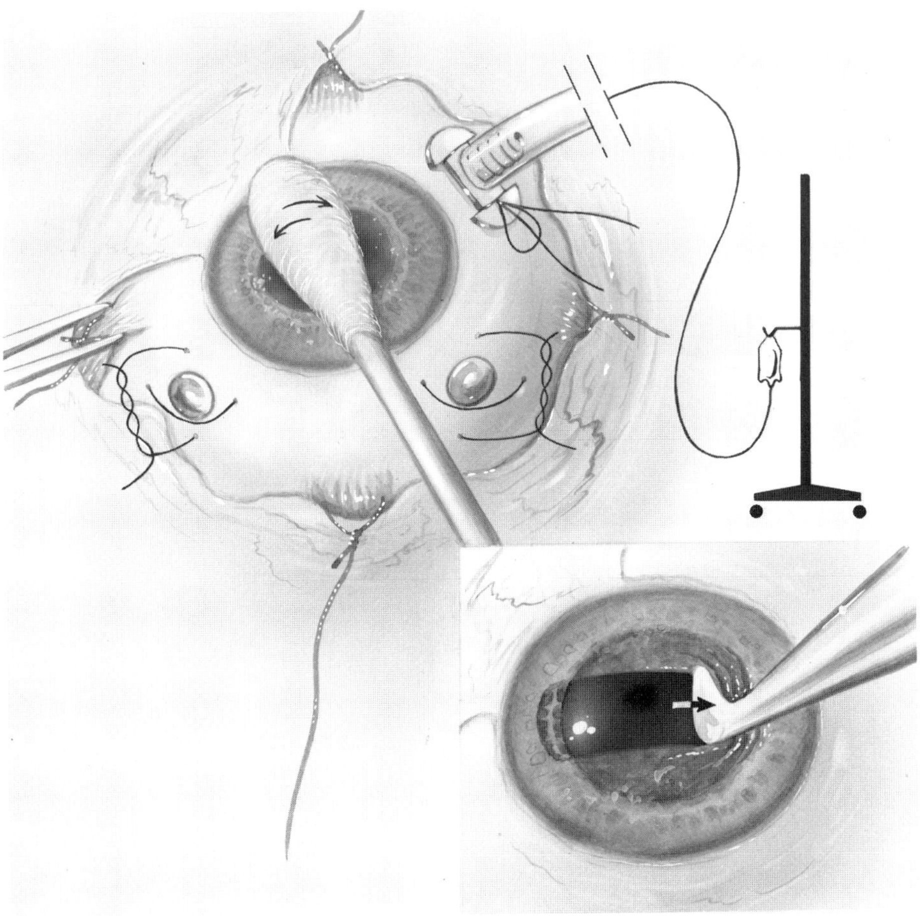

9.**1** Elevated intraocular pressure can cause epithelial and stromal edema in a cornea with marginally healthy endothelium. If the cornea becomes hazy, the height of the infusion bottle should be checked immediately and lowered if indicated. Epithelial edema causing a persistently hazy cornea may be cleared by rolling a dry cotton swab back and forth over the cornea with firm pressure.

Inset: If the above measures fail, the corneal epithelium is removed using a scarifier. The procedure requires gentle scraping of the epithelium with the dull heel of the knife.

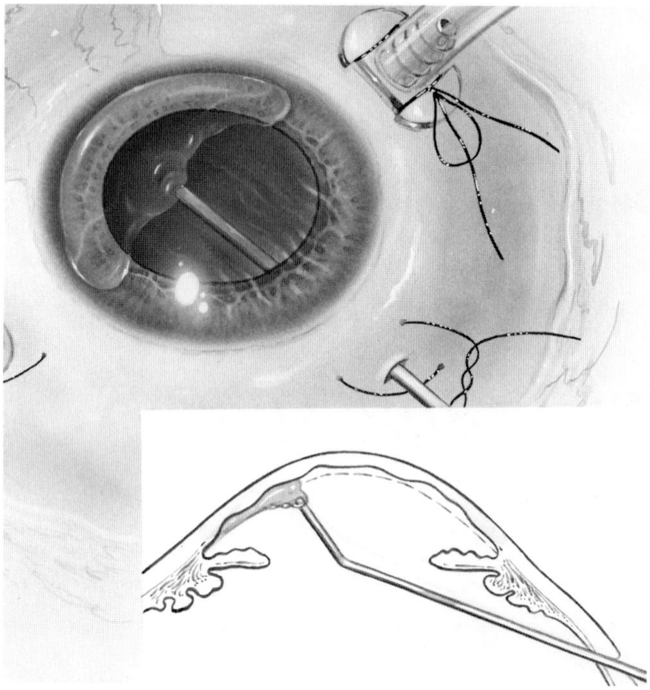

9.**2** Prolonged vitrectomy in aphakic or pseudophakic eyes may produce edema of the corneal stroma and wrinkling of Descemet's membrane. During air-fluid exchange, these wrinkles produce light reflections that interfere with visualization of the fundus. Sodium hyaluronate 1% injected between the endothelium and the air interface reduces these reflections and results in improved visualization.

In an aphakic gas-filled eye, sodium hyaluronate is injected from a tuberculin syringe through a curved, blunt, 30-gauge cannula. One sclerotomy is closed with a plug to maintain intraocular pressure at 20–25 mmHg. The needle is passed into the anterior chamber through the other sclerotomy. A small amount of sodium hyaluronate is injected to form a tiny globule at the cannula tip. The globule is applied to the endothelium, and then sodium hyaluronate is injected in a thin film over the entire endothelial surface.

In pseudophakic patients, the injection of sodium hyaluronate requires the removal of aqueous fluid, which is usually trapped in the the anterior chamber, using a 30-gauge needle. The fluid is replaced with sodium hyaluronate solution.

Complications Involving the Sclerotomy

Complications involving the peripheral retina are likely to be associated with the sclerotomy, insertion of instruments, and placement of an infusion cannula (3, 6, 7, 9). Prevention of these complications is easier and simpler than their management.

Meticulous measurement of the sclerotomy sites under microscope observation should be a routine procedure to avoid peripheral retinal damage during incision and insertion of instruments. It should be remembered that the eyes of children and hyperopic eyes have an anteriorly located ora serrata. The sclerotomy sites in these eyes should therefore be located 3.0 mm from the limbus.

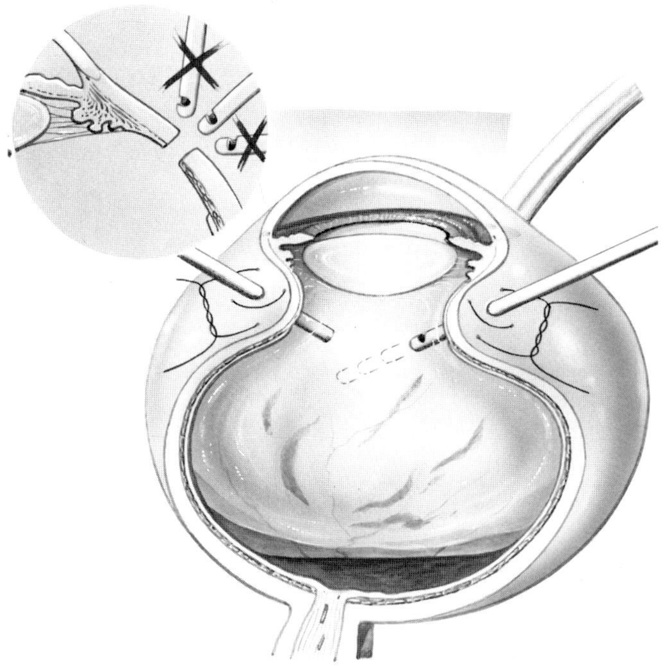

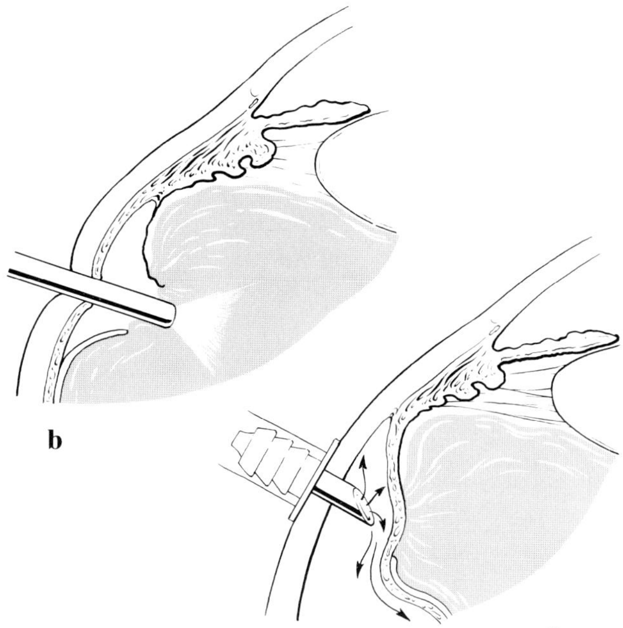

b

c

9.**3a** An understanding of the basic mechanics of inserting instruments through the sclerotomy may avoid dire peripheral retinal complications. *Inset:* To prevent traumatizing the choroid and vitreous base, the tip of the instrument is inserted perpendicularly to the scleral surface along the track of the MVR blade incision. Any resistance encountered during insertion should be considered abnormal, an indication of a problem, and a warning to stop the insertion. The sclerotomy knife may be reinserted to enlarge the scleral and choroidal incision. The instrument tips should be inspected as soon as they come into view in the peripheral vitreous before they are introduced more deeply. A tip that is pushing a tissue in front of it is withdrawn. The sclerotomy site is closed with a plug, and indirect ophthalmoscopy is performed to determine if an iatrogenic retinal dialysis has been produced and requires endolaser, cryoapplications, or scleral buckling.

9.**3b** Instruments such as the light pipe, the endolaser probe, and the endoeraser electrode, have flat tips that prevent resistance-free insertion into the vitreous. Insertion of such instruments is difficult and risky in a hypotonic eye that becomes distorted, causing distortion of the sclerotomy track. Insertion in a soft eye may produce a retinal break (**b**), vitreous base avulsion and hemorrhage of the choroidal detachment. To prevent these complications, the eye should be firmed up with an injection or infusion of balanced salt solution before the introduction of blunt instruments into the vitreous cavity.

c A choroidal detachment that develops during the early stages of vitrectomy should immediately alert the surgeon to a complication involving the infusion cannula. A cannula that fails to penetrate the vitreous cavity and lies in the subchoroidal space may result in a massive choroidal detachment. This may occur when a short cannula is used in an eye with thickened, edematous sclera, or an eye in which a detachment of the pars plana ciliaris and ora serrata has not been detected. This complication is prevented by the use of a 4 or 6 mm infusion cannula and routine inspection of the cannula tip before opening the infusion line. Management requires relocation of the infusion cannula and drainage of the suprachoroidal fluid through a scleral incision in the area of choroidal detachment. With the new infusion line open and eye pressure lowered by readjusting the bottle height, suprachoroidal fluid is completely drained. The procedure for choroidal tap is described in Chapter 22.

9.4

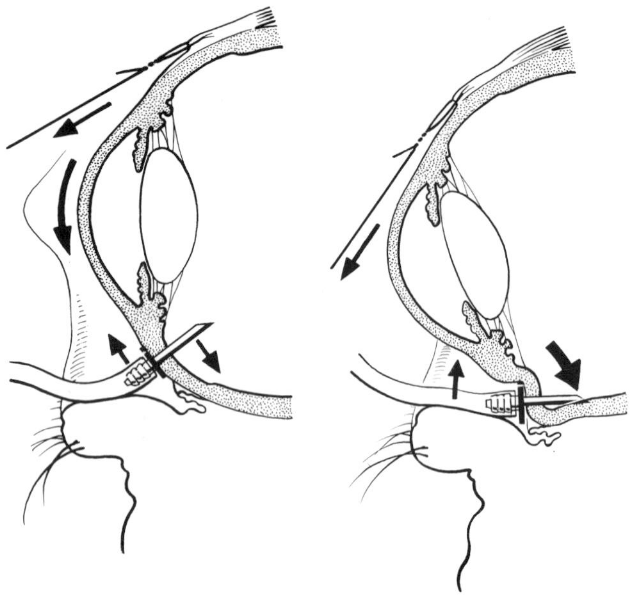

a b

9.5

a

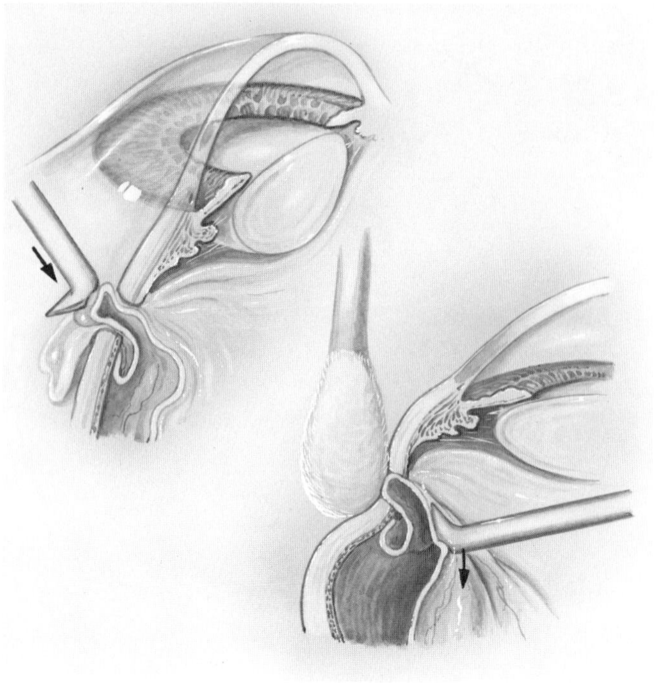

b

9.4 A long infusion cannula located closer to the vertical than the horizontal meridian may damage the peripheral retina in an eye with a tight palpebral fissure.

a When the eye is rotated inferiorly, the outer element of the cannula may be forced against the lower lid or lid speculum.

b This causes the cannula tip to come into contact with the peripheral retina, and is likely to happen when the eye is soft.

To avoid this complication, the infusion cannula is located closer to the horizontal meridian in eyes with a narrow palpebral fissure. In addition, the infusion pressure should be increased slightly when vitrectomy is performed in the periphery of the lower quadrants. The eye is rotated inferiorly as the surgeon attempts to gain a better view of the periphery of the vitreous cavity. When the eye is rotated downward, the infusion cannula or tubing may be compressed against the lid margin or speculum, resulting in a lowering of the intraocular pressure, which is compensated by raising the infusion bottle.

If an iatrogenic break been produced, it is treated with cryoapplications or endolaser, and supported with a meridional scleral buckle if it is large.

9.5 **Prolapse of retina and vitreous in sclerotomy.** Prolapse of retinal and vitreous tissue through a sclerotomy is a serious, but fortunately infrequent, complication of vitrectomy. Bullous retinal detachment, excessive infusion pressure, and an open sclerotomy may lead to this complication. Multiple, fixed retinal folds converging in the peripheral retina near a sclerotomy site indicate the occurrence of this complication (10:888).

There are two approaches in managing this problem: the external approach utilizes a blunt spatula to reposition the retina; the internal approach uses a curved vitreous spatula to dissect and release the incarcerated retina from the sclerotomy.

a With the external approach, the eye is made hypotonic by lowering the height of the infusion bottle to reduce the intraocular pressure to atmospheric level. The edge of the sclerotomy is held with colibri forceps. The spatula tip is inserted between the sclera and the incarcerated retina, which is pushed back into the vitreous cavity with the flat surface of the spatula. An alternative is to use the vitrectomy probe rather than a spatula. The infusion pressure is increased, and the sclerotomy is closed securely with 8–0 polyglactin suture. The area of incarceration is inspected with indirect ophthalmoscopy and scleral depression. If incarceration is still present, the internal approach is carried out.

b With the internal approach, coaxial illumination of the operating microscope is used to aid in inserting the vitrectomy probe and bringing it near the incarceration. The surgeon's other hand depresses the sclerotomy with a cotton swab. The infusion pressure is reduced to allow more scleral depression of the incarcerated retina into the anterior and axial regions of the vitreous. Vitrectomy is carried out around the incarcerated retina to isolate the incarcerated vitreous from the vitreous base. The vitrectomy probe is replaced with a curved vitreous spatula which is used to tease and release the retina (arrow) from the sclerotomy.

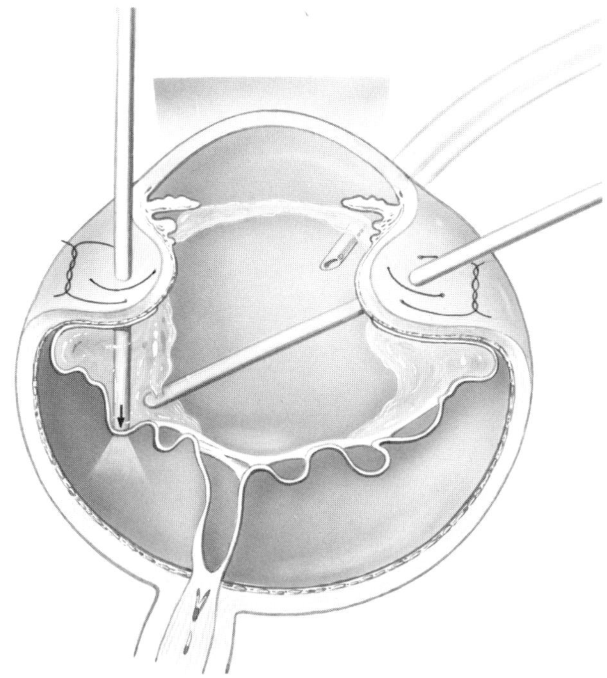

b

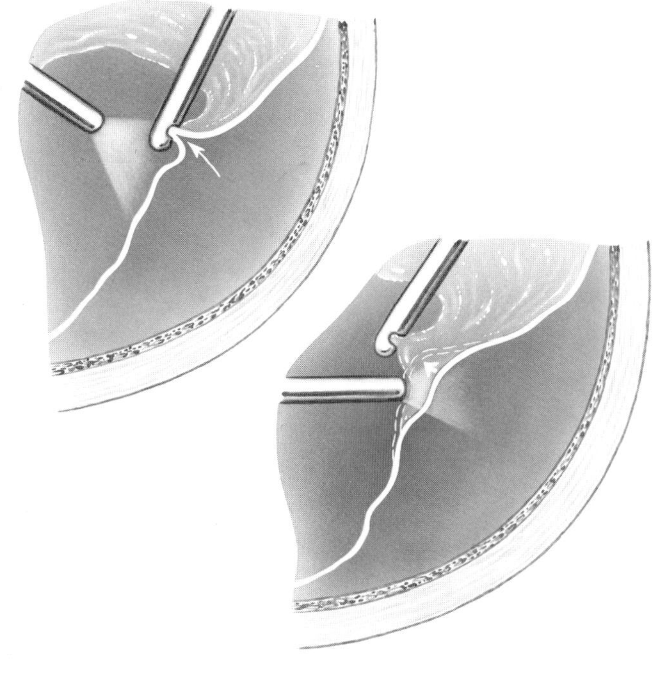

c

9.**6a** **Vitreous adherent to the retina.** When vitreous gel remaining adherent to the retina is trimmed with the vitrectomy probe, the risk of cutting the retina is high. To avoid this complication, the front surface of the light pipe is held near the retina to prevent it from being accidentally aspirated into the vitrectomy probe during vitrectomy.

9.**6b, c** Extraordinary precautions should be observed in vitrectomy in eyes with no posterior vitreous detachment and a mobile, ballooning retinal detachment, because the retina can easily become sucked into the port of the probe. In addition to using the light pipe as a shield to hold back the retina, the port of the probe is directed away from the retina. The level of suction is reduced, and the cutting speed of the probe is increased so that the cutting port is open only briefly.

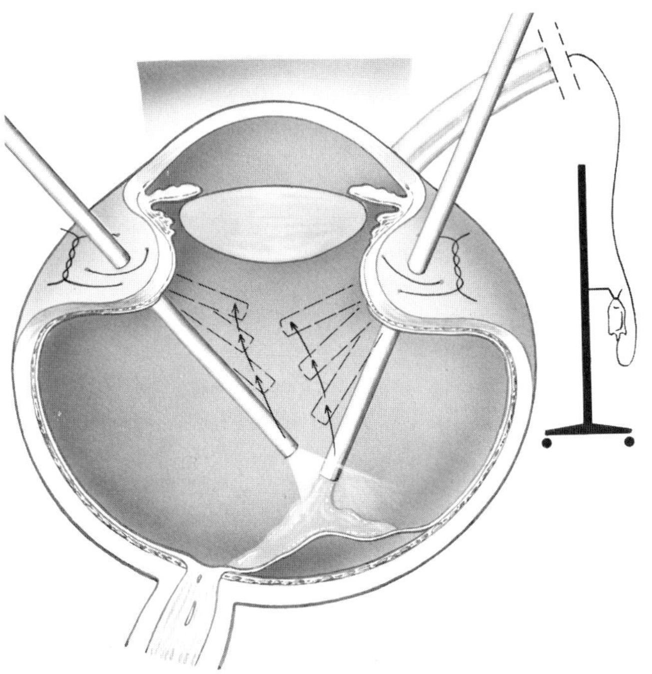

9.**7** Vitreous gel or blood clot that is firmly adherent to the retina may become inadvertently caught in the lumen of the extrusion needle when vitreous fluid is vented out of the eye. If the incarceration of vitreous or clot is not recognized, a retinal tear may develop when the needle tip is moved away from the retina (arrows on right). When the extrusion needle is moved within the vitreous cavity, the vent should be covered with the finger so that vitreous or clot adherent to the retina cannot surge into the needle tip. In this way, tears in the retina can be avoided.

9.8

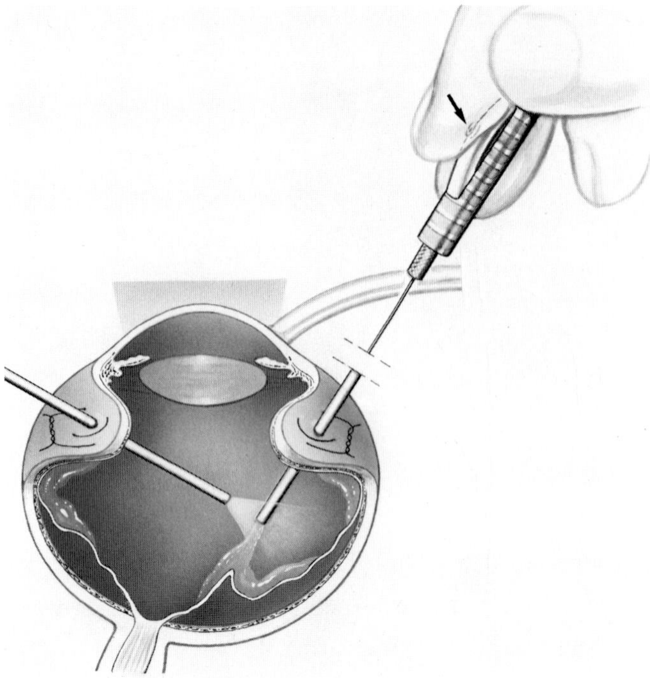

9.10

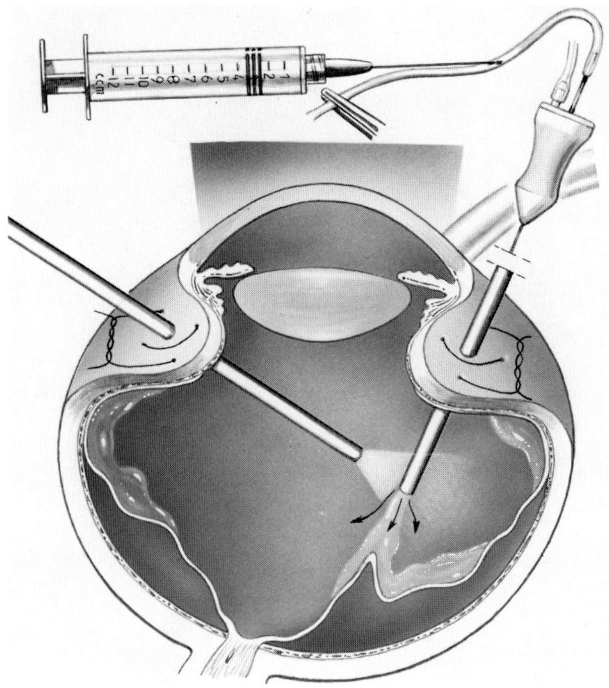

9.9

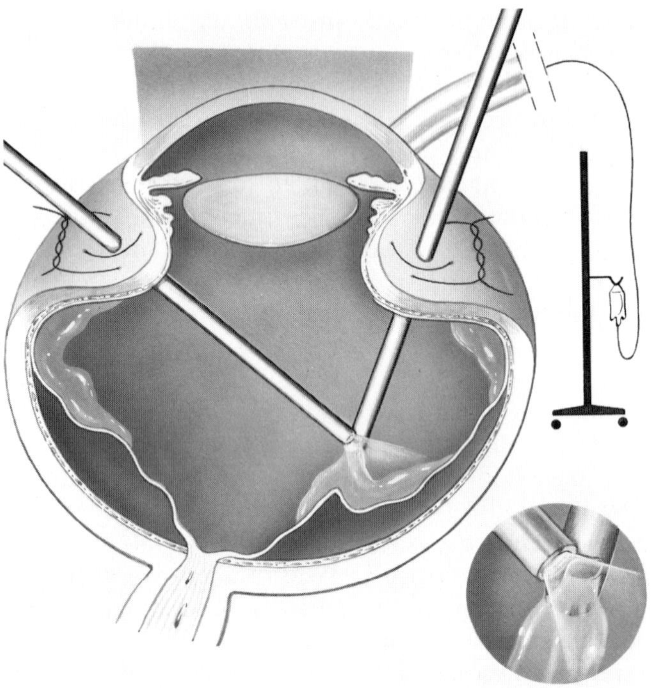

9.**8** The backflush mechanism in extrusion needles allows release of vitreous gel caught in the needle tip (13). When the silicone tubing in the shaft of the instrument is squeezed with the index finger, fluid is forced out of the needle, releasing incarcerated tissue.

9.**9** Some vitrectomy probes do not have a machine-operated reverse-flow mechanism. If the vitrectomy probe fails to cut vitreous, vitreous may become incarcerated in the cutting port. If this vitreous is attached to the retina, a retinal break may develop when the probe is moved. If it is noted that vitreous gel is incarcerated in the vitrectomy probe, the probe is held stationary.

Inset: The light pipe is rubbed against the sharp edge of the port, cutting the gel into shreds, thus releasing it from the probe. The vitrectomy probe is replaced and discarded, because vitreous incarceration may have been due to a defective cutting action.

9.**10** If the technique described in Figure 9.**9** is unsuccessful, the infusion bottle is lowered to reduce the infusion pressure. The evacuation line of the vitrectomy probe is clamped near the probe. Balanced salt solution is injected into the infusion line to expel the gel caught in the vitrectomy probe. As balanced salt solution is injected through a 25–gauge needle into the evacuation line between the clamp and the eye, incarcerated vitreous is expelled from the probe.

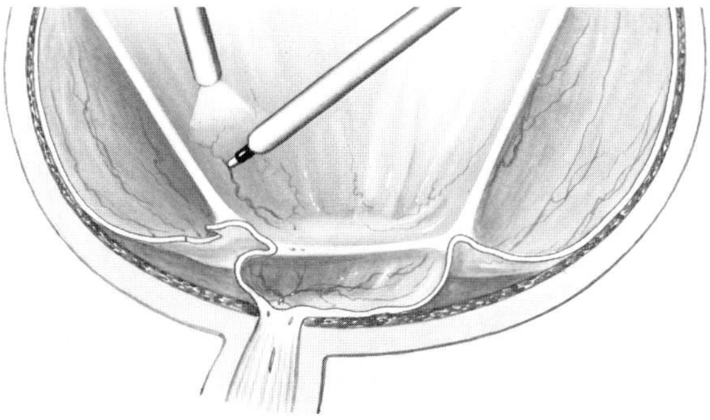

9.**11 a** **Bleeding from fibrovascular membranes** may obscure the surgical field during vitrectomy and preclude successful completion of the procedure. As a routine, all blood vessels lying on membranes to be cut are treated with light endodiathermy to produce minimal contraction of the membrane. Excess diathermy can produce membrane contraction which may cause a retinal break if the retina is atrophic. Light diathermy is applied along the length of the blood vessels. A faint white reaction indicates the ideal endpoint of diathermy coagulation.

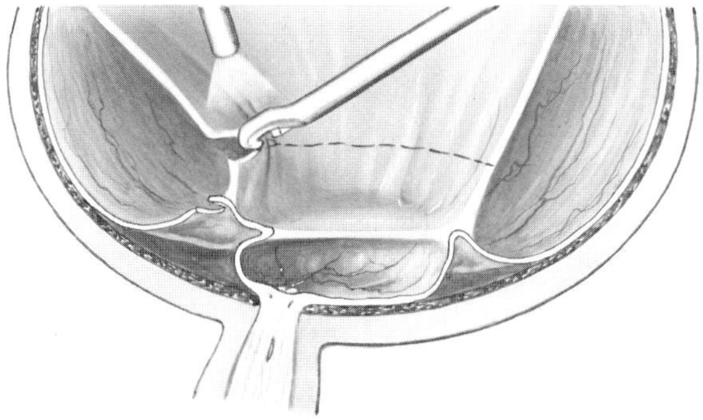

b Vitreous membrane traction may result in thinning and atrophy of the retina where the membrane is attached. This atrophic retina is prone to develop iatrogenic retinal breaks if excessive traction is exerted on the membrane. To be cut by a vitrectomy probe, the membrane must be suctioned into the cutting port. Less traction is exerted when the membrane is cut with scissors.

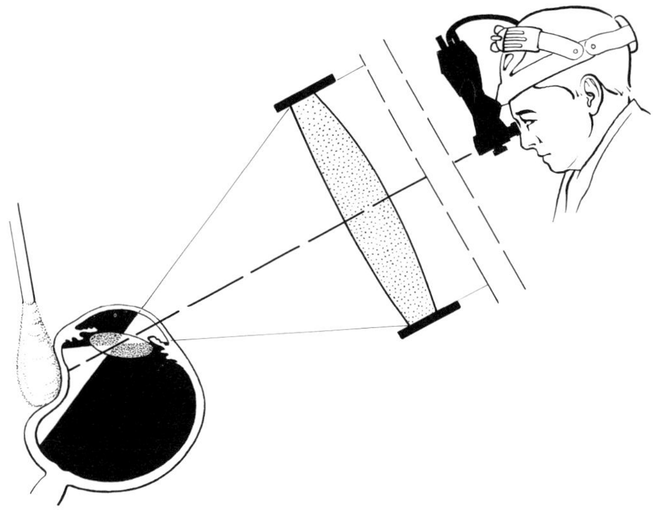

9.**12** Since the peripheral retina is usually difficult to visualize with the microscope, it is routinely checked with indirect ophthalmoscopy and scleral depression for iatrogenic retinal breaks when vitrectomy has been performed in the periphery of the vitreous cavity (4, 5, 8). A cotton swab is used as a scleral depressor.

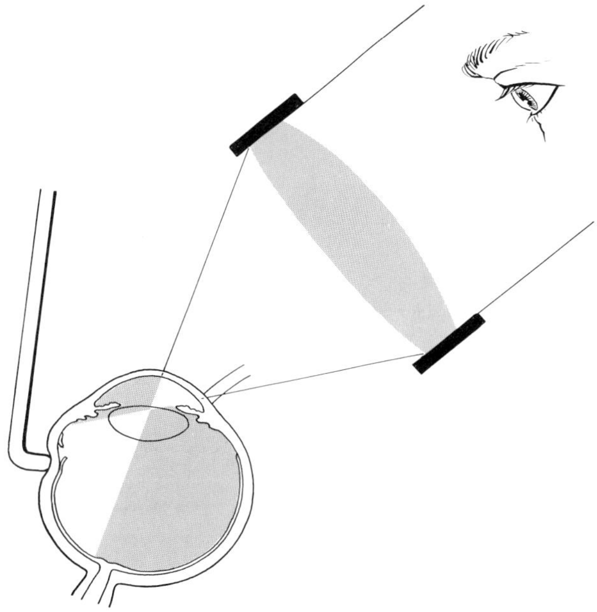

9.**13** **Iatrogenic retinal breaks** in the extreme retinal periphery near the ora serrata are very difficult to reach with the endolaser probe. They are best treated with cryoretinopexy under indirect ophthalmoscopic control.

9.**14**

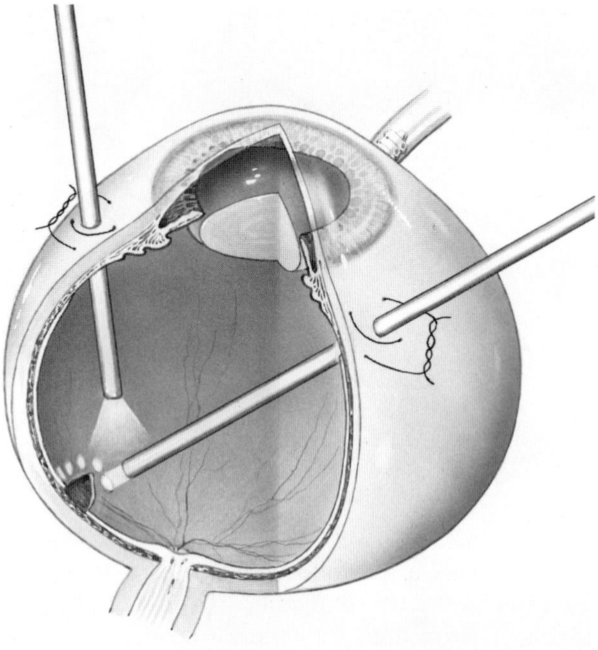

9.1

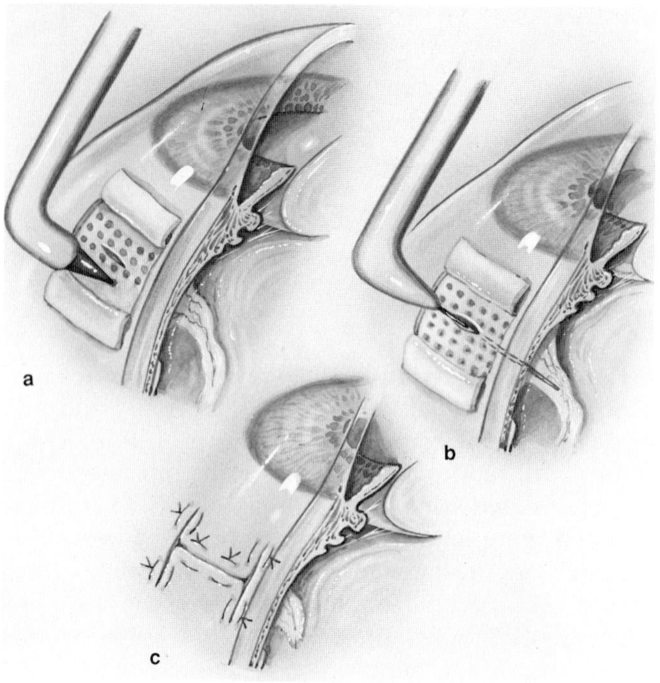

9.**15**

a

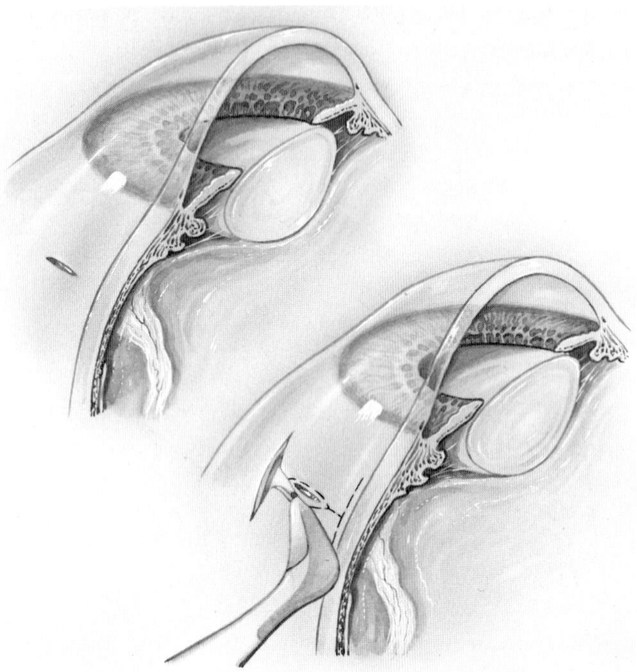

b

9.**14** Iatrogenic retinal breaks in attached posterior retina are surrounded by two or three rows of endolaser applications. Development of a retinal detachment around the breaks negates endolaser applications; retinal breaks in attached retina are therefore treated immediately.

Breaks in detached posterior retina are treated after internal drainage of subretinal fluid and air-fluid exchange. To facilitate identification of the retinal break after fluid-air exchange, endodiathermy is applied around the break to form a white circle of coagulated retina.

9.**15** **Fibrovascular proliferation through the sclerotomy. a** The sclerotomy may be the site of fibrovascular proliferation (11, 12). Proliferation through a sclerotomy seems to occur preferentially in eyes with poor circulation, such as in advanced diabetes or following multiple operations. Spontaneous bleeding at the site of proliferation may cause recurrent mild or massive vitreous hemorrhage. In cases with mild hemorrhage, diagnosis can be made with indirect ophthalmoscopy and scleral depression. The fibrovascular growth is usually covered by red, clotted blood. In cases with massive hemorrhage, a trail of hemorrhagic debris originating from the sclerotomy site may be observed with ultrasonography.

b A scleral groove is made parallel to the limbus with a scarifier, passing along each side of the sclerotomy. The groove is extended 3 mm beyond each end of the sclerotomy. A meridional incision is made at both ends of the scleral groove. Anterior and posterior scleral flaps are raised on each side of the sclerotomy to create a 5–6 mm scleral bed.

9.**16a** Using a sharp conical electrode, diathermy is applied to the dissected scleral bed, and the sclerotomy site is surrounded with heavier applications. Acetazolamide 500 mg is given intravenously to decrease intraocular pressure, which may become elevated as a result of scleral shrinkage caused by diathermy.

b The sclerotomy is treated with a fine, 3 mm penetrating diathermy. Multiple heavy applications are made along the entire length of the sclerotomy, making certain that the electrode has penetrated the vitreous cavity.

c The scleral flaps are closed over the treated scleral bed with interrupted 8–0 polyglactin sutures.

a

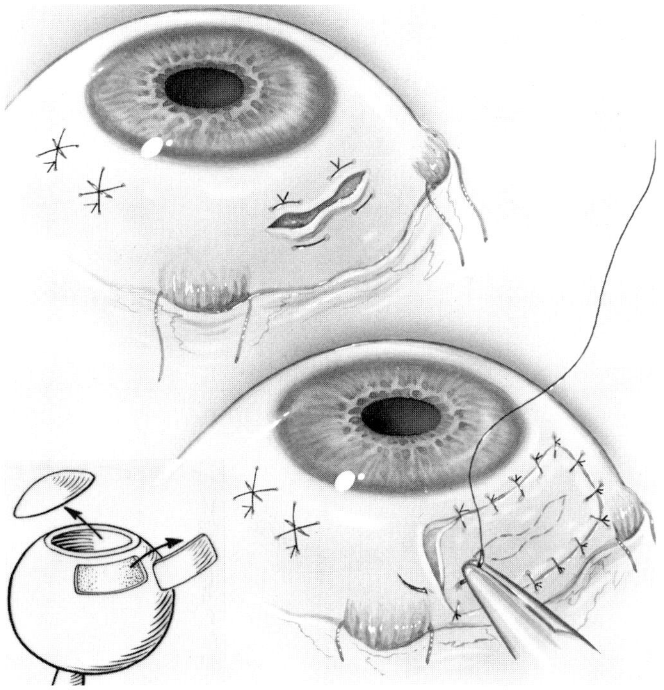

b

9.**17** **Necrotic sclerotomy site.** **a** The sclerotomy site may become necrotic as a result of previous cryoapplications, or diathermy, or faulty closure. Small- to moderate-size defects may be closed with mattress sutures of 6–0 polyglactin or nylon.

b Extensive areas of scleral necrosis are covered with a scleral graft. The area to be grafted is marked with a gentian violet pen. The border of the area should be at least 3 mm from the necrotic margin. Donor sclera is cut to fit the outlined area and then sutured to the globe using multiple 9–0 polyglactin interrupted sutures. Tenon's fascia and conjunctiva are sutured to the limbus in separate layers. Further vitreoretinal surgery is delayed 4–6 weeks.

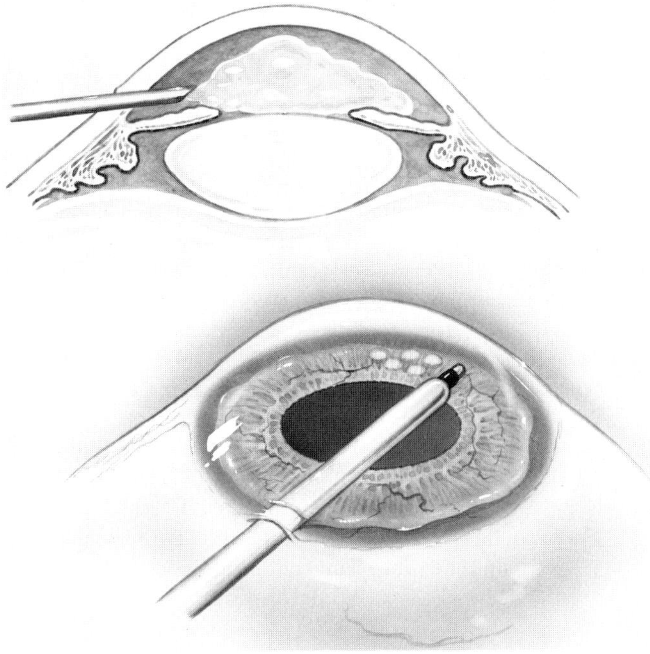

9.**18** **Rubeosis irides.** Extensive rubeosis irides may develop following any intraocular surgery in eyes with diabetic retinopathy, central retinal vein occlusion, or ocular ischemia associated with carotid artery disease (1, 2, 4, 10:886). To minimize complications of recurrent hyphema and neovascular glaucoma in these eyes, panphotocoagulation is added intraoperatively following vitrectomy. Panretinal ablation with cryoapplications may be done when endolaser applications in the peripheral retina are not feasible.

New-formed iris blood vessels that bleed recurrently are treated with diathermy coagulation. Photocoagulation is not effective in these eyes because of hyphema. Blood is irrigated from the anterior chamber with a 20-gauge needle introduced through the limbus and attached to BSS Plus infusion tubing. The vitrectomy probe is introduced through a separate limbal incision to aspirate the anterior chamber blood. Sodium hyaluronate 1% is injected to fill the anterior chamber, to prevent its collapse and impede further hemorrhaging. The endodiathermy electrode is introduced into the anterior chamber and applied to all new iris vessels to close them completely. This procedure is a heroic effort to save any residual vision in these near-hopeless cases.

References

1. Blankenship GW. Lens influence on iris neovascularization and glaucoma. In: Blankenship GW, Stirpe M, Gonvers M, Binder S, eds. Basic and advanced vitreous surgery. Padua: Liviana, 1986: 255–258.
2. Blankenship G, Cortez R, Machemer R. The lens and pars plana vitrectomy for diabetic retinopathy complications. Arch Ophthalmol 1979; 97: 1263–1267.
3. Buettner H, Machemer R. Histopathologic findings in human eyes after pars plana vitrectomy and lensectomy. Arch Ophthalmol 1977; 95: 2029–2033.
4. Charles S. Vitreous microsurgery. 2nd ed. Baltimore: Williams and Wilkins, 1987: 127–128.
5. Ghartey KN, Tolentino FI, Freeman HM, et al. Closed vitreous surgery, XVII: results and complications of pars plana vitrectomy. Arch Ophthalmol 1980; 98: 1248–1252.
6. Kreiger AE. Complications in closed vitrectomy. In: Freeman HM, Hirose T, Schepens CL, eds. Vitreous surgery and advances in fundus diagnosis and treatment. New York: Appleton-Century-Crofts, 1977: 355–364.
7. Michels RG. Complications of vitreous surgery. In: Blankenship GW, Stirpe M, Gonvers M, Binder S, eds. Basic and advanced vitreous surgery. Padua: Liviana, 1986: 347–351.
8. Peyman GA, Schulman JA. Intravitreal surgery: principles and practice. New York: Appleton-Century-Crofts, 1986: 395–400.
9. Pulhorn G, Teichmann KD, Teichmann I. Intraocular fibrous proliferation as a incisional complication in pars plana vitrectomy. Am J Ophthalmol 1977; 83: 810–814.
10. Schepens CL. Retinal detachment and allied diseases. Philadelphia: W. B. Saunders, 1983.
11. Tardif YM, Schepens CL. Closed vitreous surgery, XV: fibrovascular ingrowth from the pars plana sclerotomy. Arch Ophthalmol 1977; 95: 235-239.
12. Tardif YM, Schepens CL, Tolentino FI. Vitreous surgery, XIV: complications from sclerotomy in 89 consecutive cases. Arch Ophthalmol 1977; 95: 229–234.
13. Živojnović R, Vijfvinkel GJ. A modified flute needle. Am J Ophthalmol 1983; 96: 548-549.

10

Ancillary Vitreoretinal Surgical Techniques

This chapter describes procedures that are common to all vitreoretinal surgical techniques.

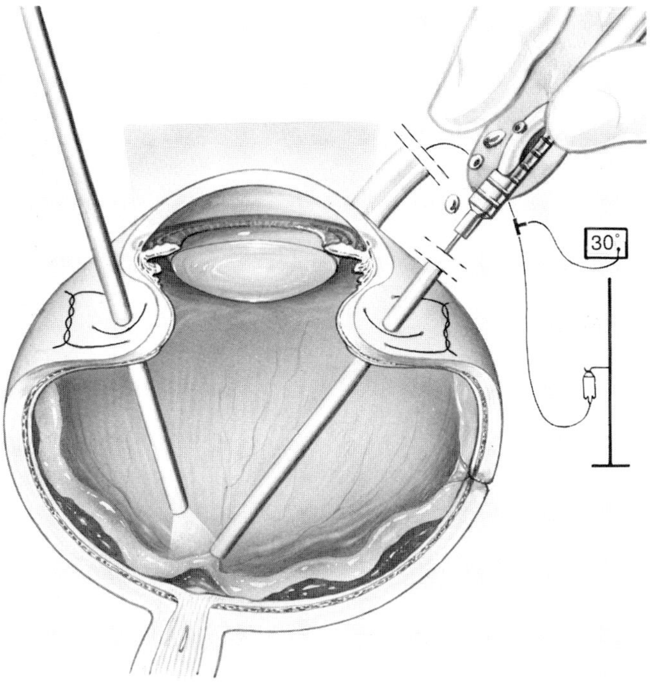

Stripping of the Cortical Vitreous

10.**1a** In young patients who have suffered perforating injury to the posterior segment of the eye, the vitreous cortex becomes a liability, because proliferative tissue within it can cause tractional retinal detachment. During vitrectomy for such cases, stripping of vitreous cortex may be undertaken if fundus visibility is optimal. Stripping of the vitreous cortex may also be indicated in cases of proliferative diabetic retinopathy with subhyaloid vitreous hemorrhage.

The stripping procedure follows a core vitrectomy to clear vitreous opacities. The extrusion needle, with its vent closed by the surgeon's finger, is inserted into the cavity. Liquid vitreous is washed out by venting the extrusion needle to the atmosphere. If the cortex has not partially separated, its separation is started near the optic disc. The cortex is sucked into the tip of the extrusion neddle, which is pulled up to separate the cortex from the retina. To increase the suction force on the tip, the vent is left open and the infusion pressure is increased. While the cortex is pulled away from the disc and then toward the periphery, the retina under it is observed very closely. If the retina appears to be under traction, the pulling procedure is discontinued.

1b

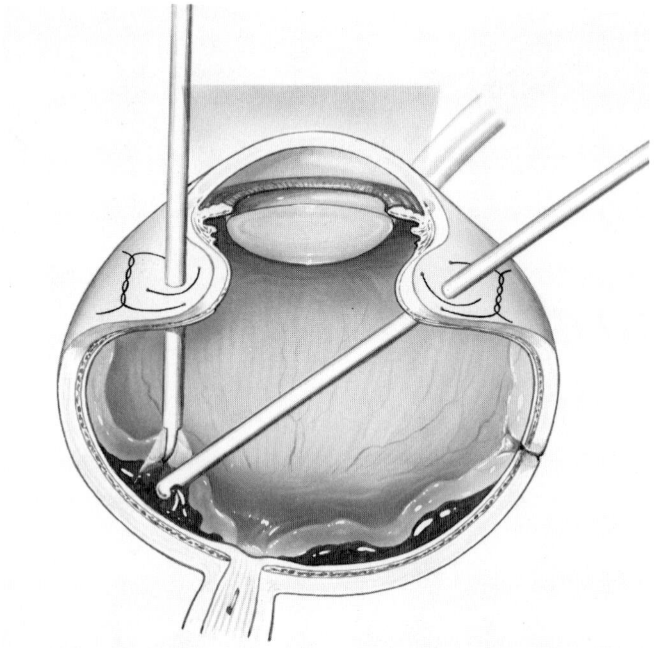

1d

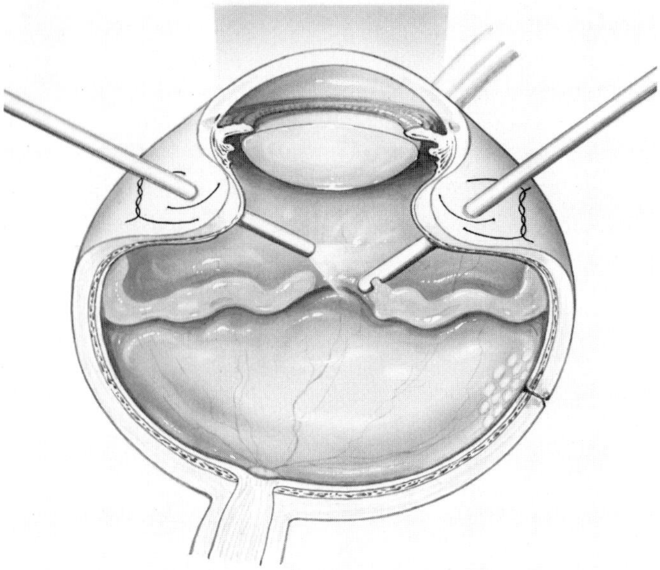

1c

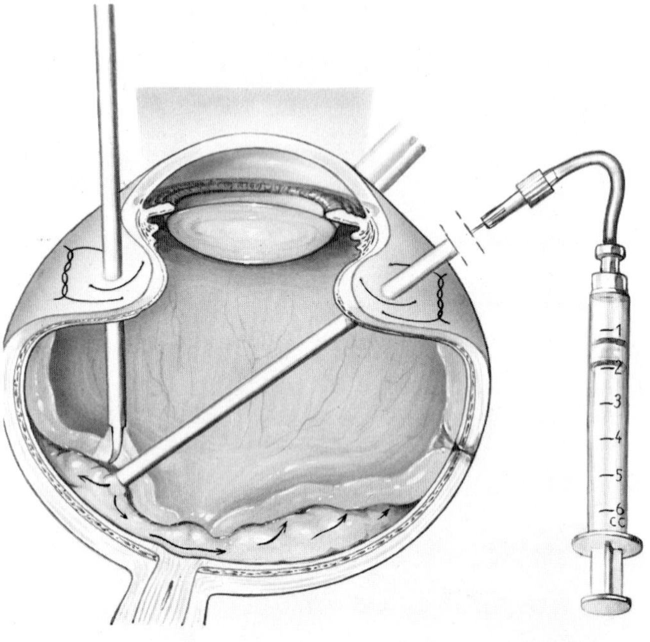

1e

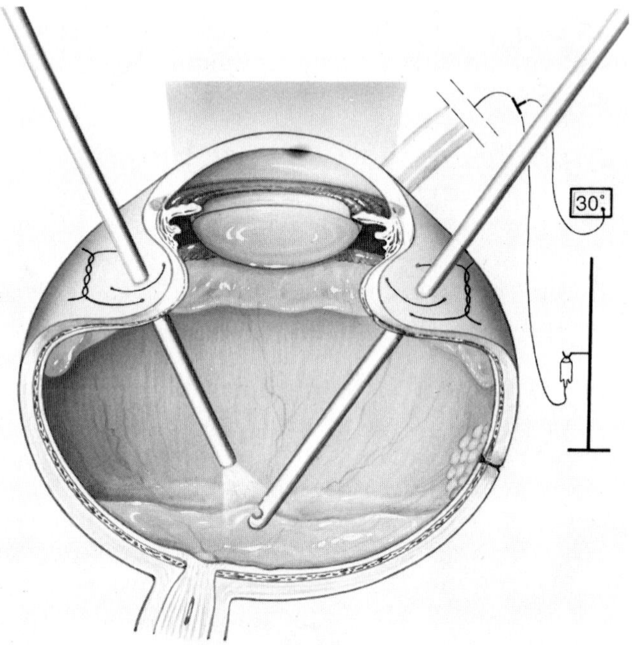

10.**1b** Subhyaloid blood, between the cortex and the retina, facilitates stripping vitreous cortex from the retina (24:91–96, 27:225–226). A small hole is created in the cortex overlying the maximum accumulation of blood. Blood is aspirated through the hole to identify the outer surface of the cortical layer. Before further stripping, all subhyaloid blood is evacuated with an extrusion needle. The layer of cortical vitreous is lifted with an illuminating pick and a vitrectomy probe.

10.**1c** An alternative technique for separating the cortex from the retina utilizes sodium hyaluronate as a hydraulic dissector. After subhyaloid blood is removed through the hole in the cortex, sodium hyaluronate 1% is injected slowly into the subhyaloid space with a blunt, 20-gauge needle attached to a 6 ml syringe. This viscous material behaves like a hydraulic wedge that splits the cortex from the retina.

10.**1d** The separated vitreous cortex usually retracts anteriorly, and is removed with the vitrectomy probe. Three or four rows of endolaser are applied around any traumatic retinal breaks.

10.**1e** If sodium hyaluronate was used, the infusion pressure is increased and the sodium hyaluronate is washed out from the vitreous cavity with the vitrectomy probe.

Endodiathermy

Use of a tissue-coagulating probe to control bleeding from retinal and vitreous blood vessels is mandatory in modern vitreoretinal surgery (26:163, 27:227, 30). A number of endodiathermy probes are commercially available (see Chapter 3). In addition, bipolar diathermy, which uses low-frequency diathermy, can function through any two intraocular instruments or one intraocular and one extraocular instrument. Unshielded wires or clips connect the diathermy machine to the instruments (5).

10.**2a** Before an endodiathermy probe is introduced into the eye, it is tested on wet episcleral blood vessels under microscope magnification. To prevent adhesion of coagulated tissue to the probe, it is dipped in silicone oil, which forms a coating around it.

2a

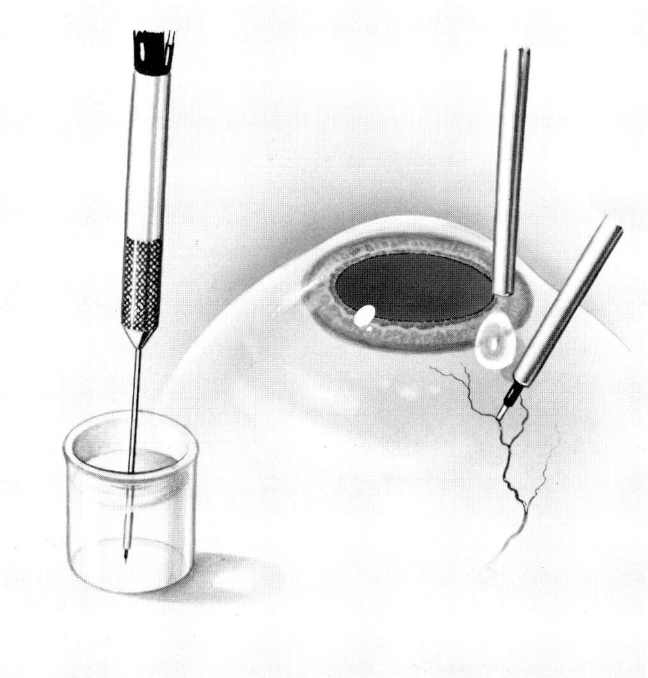

2b

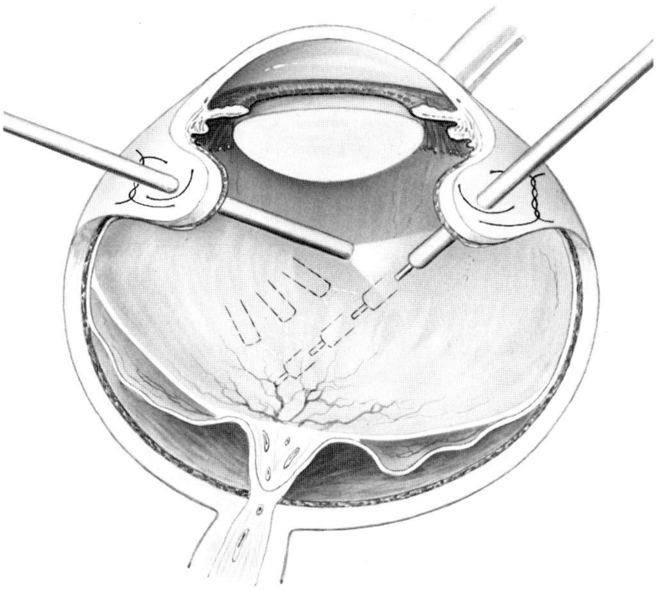

2c

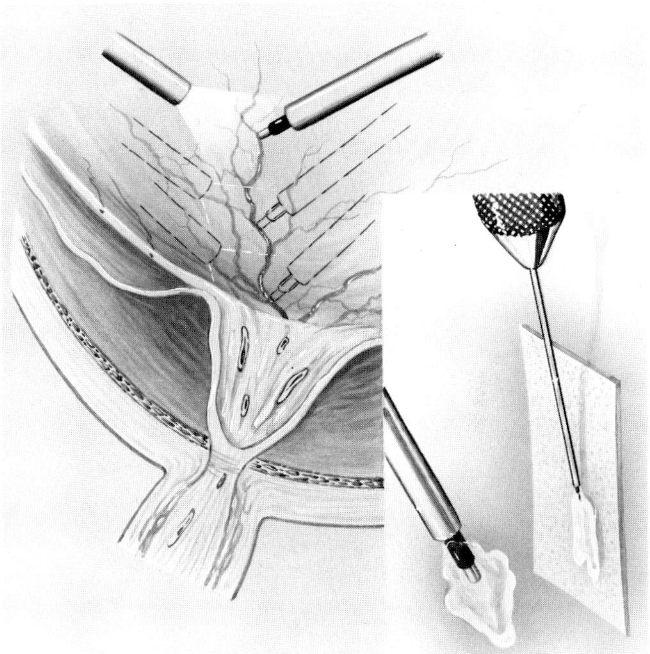

10.**2b** The endodiathermy probe is inserted into the eye and brought to the operative field simultaneously with the light pipe.

10.**2c** The diathermy probe is applied in a systematic manner from small to large vessels to prevent abrupt hemodynamic changes causing spontaneous rupture of delicate-walled vessels. The electrode is applied directly to the abnormal blood vessel, using a low energy level, and watching for the endpoint, which is a slight whitening of the blood column. Excessive coagulation should be avoided, to prevent protein adhesion to the endodiathermy tip and shrinkage of the fibrovascular membrane. *Inset:* Protein coagulum is removed from the tip with the micro-wipe instrument sponge.

Endophotocoagulation

This has the advantage over endocryopexy and endodiathermy that it does not require contact with the retina. There is therefore less chance of creating a retinal break or of chorioretinal bleeding, provided that the power levels of the photocoagulating source are not excessive. The retina should be in contact with the retinal pigment epithelium to allow energy absorption of the photocoagulating beam. If the retina is detached, drainage of subretinal fluid and air-fluid exchange must precede endophotocoagulation. A more rapid firing time, better imaging in gas, and a greater distance between the probe tip and the retina make argon laser a preferable source of energy to xenon arc light.

A solenoid-operated filter attached to the microscope and connected to the foot switch of the endophotocoagulator is activated during laser applications to protect the operator's eye. Activation of the probe causes the filter to swing in front of the observation axis of the microscope before each coagulation. The intensity of the burn is regulated by adjusting the power setting, exposure time, and distance of the probe from the retina.

The indications for endophotocoagulation are for coagulation of neovascular tissues to prevent bleeding, closure of retinal breaks or retinotomies, walling-off of retinectomies, or panphotocoagulation after vitrectomy in the treatment of rubeosis iridis. Endophotocoagulation may be applied to iris neovascularization, or to the ciliary processes, to decrease intraocular pressure.

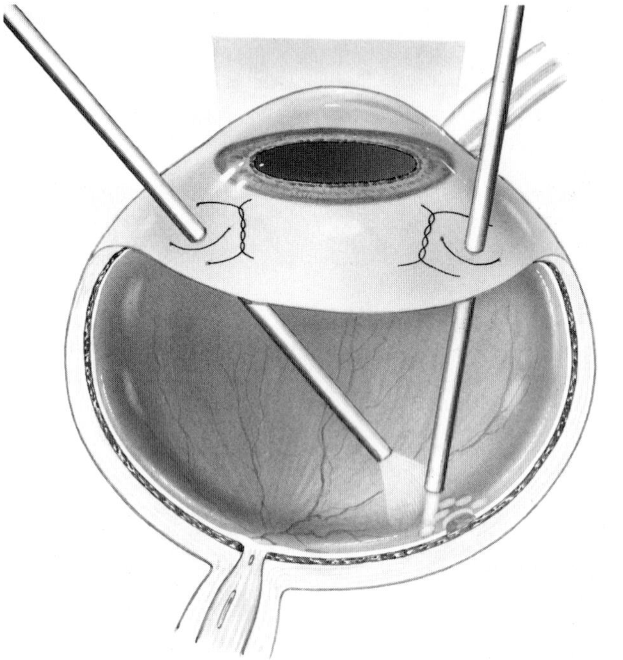

10.**3** After the endoilluminator and the endolaser probe have been introduced into the eye, the console is switched to treatment mode, with initial settings at 200 mW and 400 milliseconds. The probe tip is held 5–8 mm from the retina. With the light probe illuminating the retinal break, a few laser applications are made around it. The energy and time settings are then adjusted until a yellowwhite reaction is obtained. This reaction can be increased or decreased in size by holding the probe closer to or farther from the retina.

One of us (H. M. F.) usually uses a setting of 500 mW and a "manual" exposure time.

4a

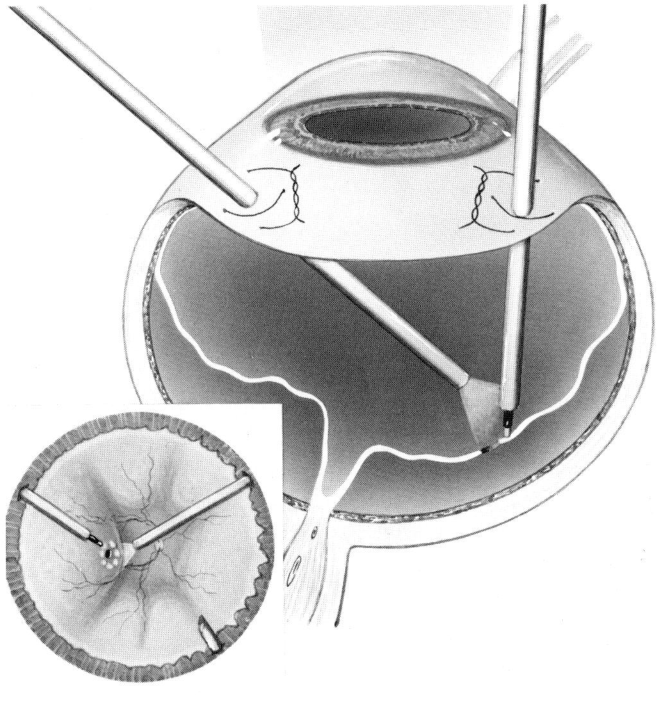

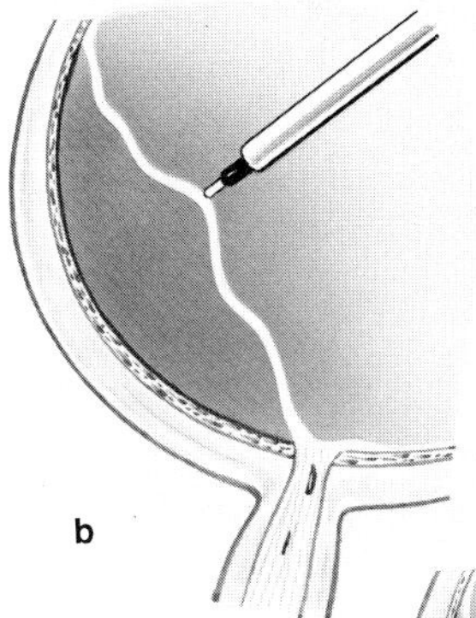

b

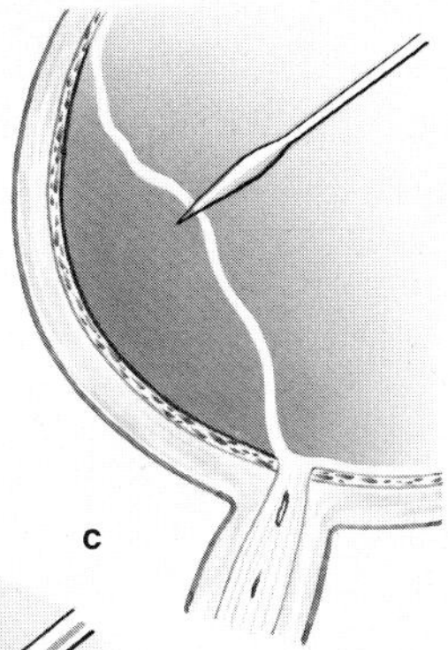

c

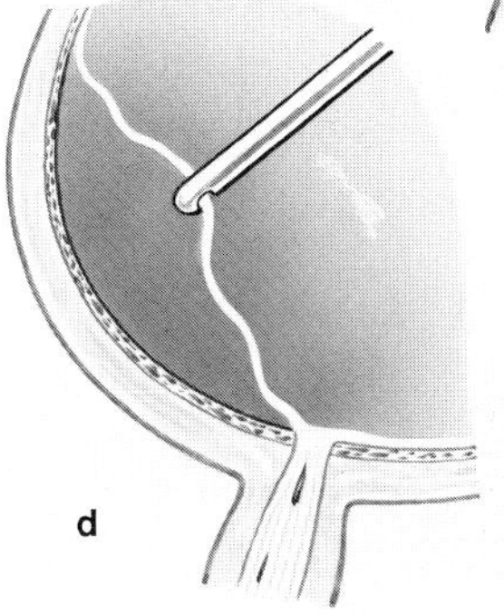

d

Internal Drainage of Subretinal Fluid

This is used in cases that require fluid-air or air-gas exchange combined with endolaser applications. Subretinal fluid may be drained internally through a preexisting retinal break or through a retinotomy (3:89–91, 7).

10.**4a** Subretinal fluid drainage through a preexisting retinal break is begun by surrounding the retinal break with white diathermy marks (inset). These marks assist in identifying the retinal break at the time of air-fluid exchange when visibility is not optimal through the air bubble.

Subretinal fluid can be drained through a peripheral retinal break using a cannulated subretinal aspirator (8). The instrument tip is positioned near a retinal break, and the cannula is advanced into the subretinal space through the retinal break. The subretinal fluid is aspirated by passive or active linear suction. The cannula is then retracted from the retinal break after retinal reattachment has been achieved.

10.**4b** When a retinal break cannot be visualized or is unsuitable for drainage of subretinal fluid, a retinotomy is made. The upper nasal quadrant in eyes with total retinal detachment is a good site for the retinotomy, because this quadrant can be tamponaded effectively with gas or silicone oil, which floats superiorly when the patient's head is erect. The lower nasal quadrant close to the 9 or 3 o'clock meridian is the preferred site in detachment involving the lower quadrants, because effective tamponade to this area is feasible when the patient lies on the side opposite the involved eye. In addition, the nasal quadrants are preferable to avoid such complications as subretinal neovascularization, or tissue proliferation that might extend to involve the macula.

The first step is the application of endodiathermy using a moderate level of coagulating energy at the site of retinotomy.

c The coagulated retina is perforated with the tip of the endodiathermy probe or incised with an MVR blade.

d If the incision in the retina does not gape, one of us (F. I. T.) rounds and enlarges its edge with the vitrectomy probe.

4e

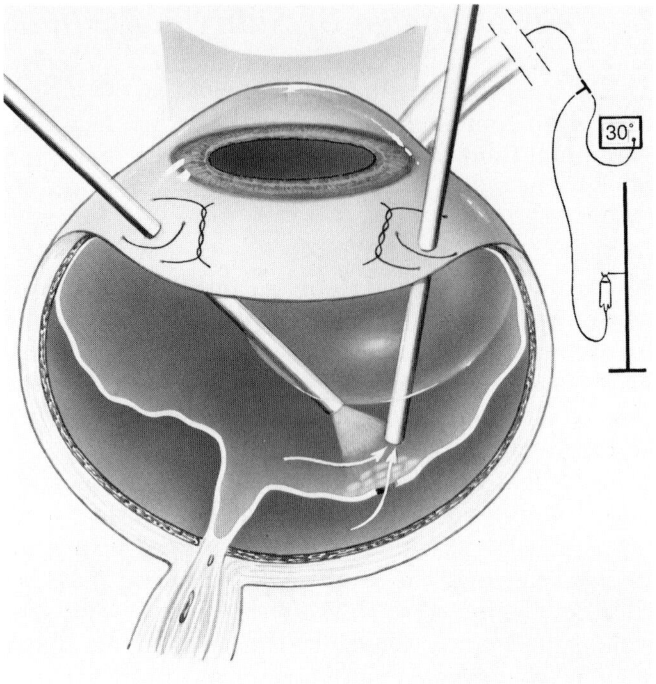

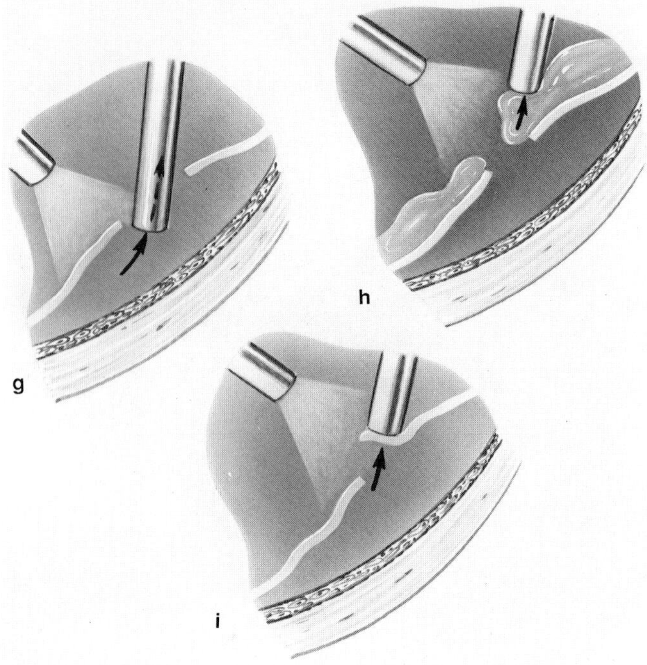

4f

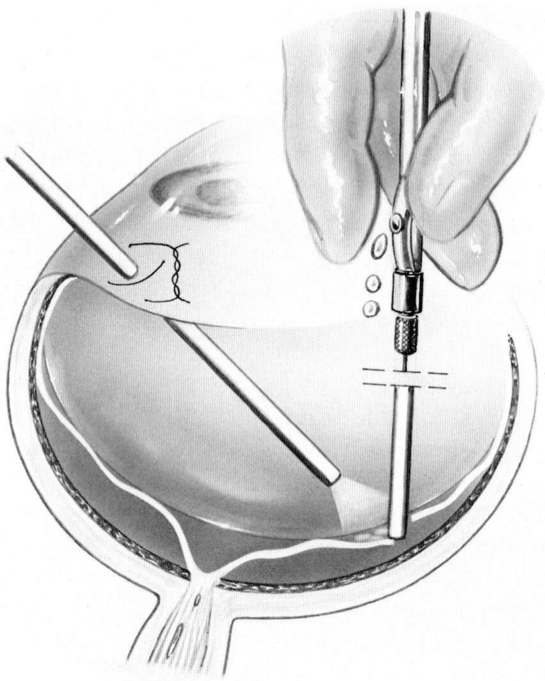

10.**4e** Subretinal fluid drainage is carried out in conjunction with fluid-air exchange (2, 4, 11, 15, 17, 19, 21, 24:96–99, 26:167–171, 27:228–229). The vent of the extrusion needle is closed with the index finger, and its tip and the endoilluminator are positioned near the retinotomy. A Landers' lens is placed on the cornea of phakic eyes, and the microscope magnification is increased to visualize the retinotomy. In aphakic eyes, a regular planoconcave vitrectomy lens may be used for fundus visualization under air. With the air pump set at 30 mmHg, the vitreous is infused with sterile air. The finger is lifted to vent vitreous fluid through the extrusion needle.

10.**4f** When the air bubble covers the retinotomy, the tip of the extrusion needle is inserted into the retinotomy, then vented until the subretinal space is evacuated (35). The eye is positioned so that the area of the retinotomy is the lowest point in the eye, allowing subretinal fluid to gravitate under the hole.

10.**4g** The tip of the extrusion needle should be located within the retinotomy. If the preexisting retinal break is small, the tip of the extrusion needle should be placed over the break. To decrease the incidence of subretinal neovascularization, an effort is made to avoid trauma to the pigment epithelium or to Bruch's membrane by the tip of the extrusion needle.

h, i Failure to drain the subretinal space completely may be explained by residual vitreous cortex, viscoelastic material, blood (**h**), or a retinal flap (**i**) obstructing the opening of the extrusion needle. This problem can be corrected by clearing the tissue from the needle by covering the vent, then relocating the needle tip.

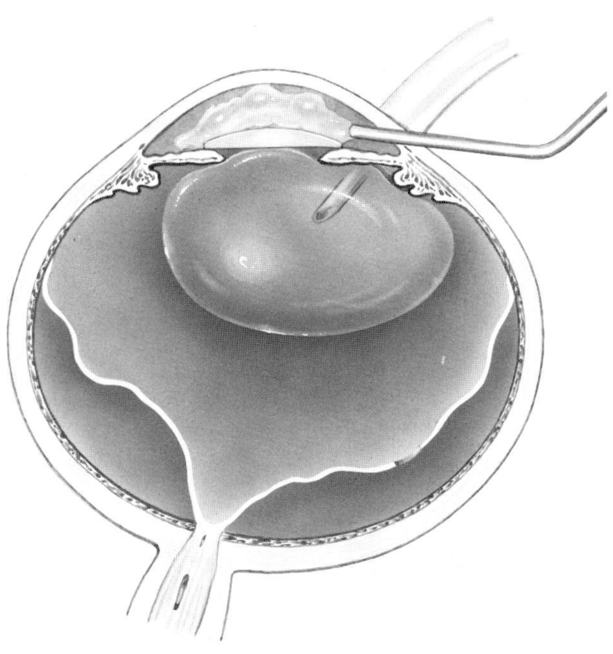

10.**4j** Fluid-air exchange in pseudophakic eyes with an anterior chamber intraocular lens is risky, because air can migrate to the anterior chamber and hamper fundus visualization. To prevent this, sodium hyaluronate is injected to fill the anterior chamber (18).

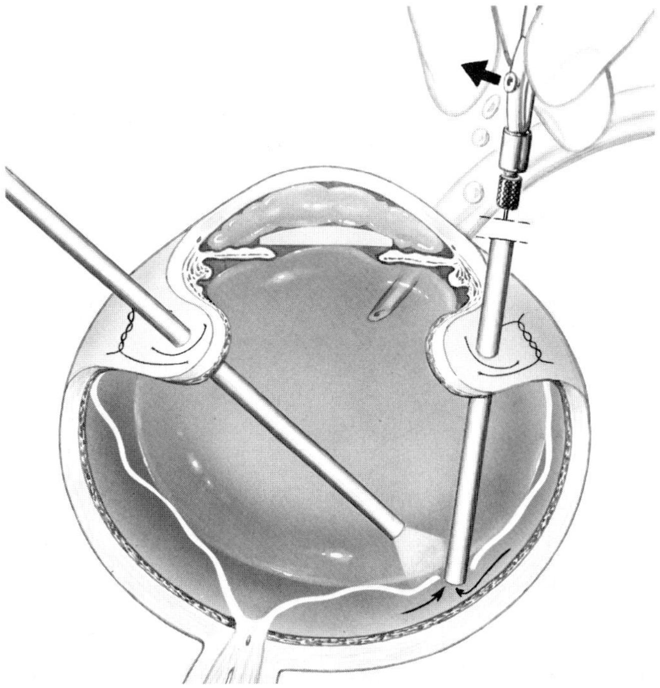

10.**4k** The extrusion needle tip is introduced into the retinotomy to complete the fluid-air exchange. The instrument tip is positioned near a retinal hole, and the tip of the cannula is advanced into the subretinal space through the retinal hole. The subretinal fluid is aspirated repeatedly until it appears to have been evacuated completely.

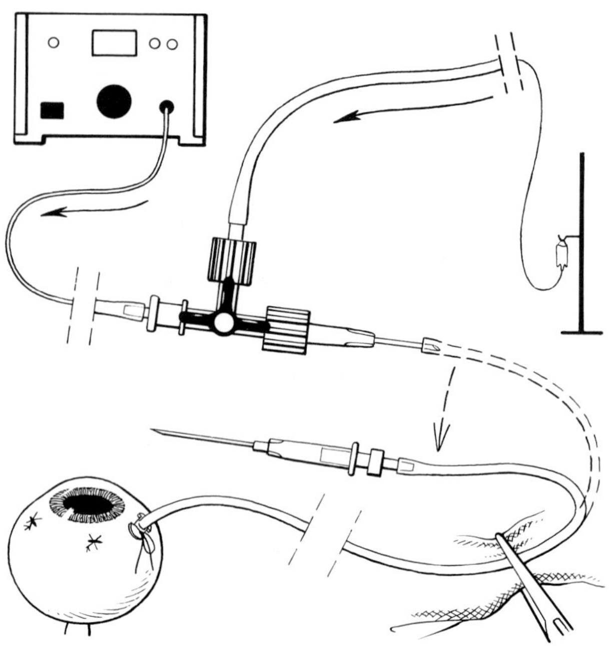

Air-Gas Exchange

10.**5a** Prior to closure of the conjunctiva, air in the vitreous cavity is exchanged for long-acting gas, usually perfluorocarbon (12). The infusion line, which is connected through a stopcock to the infusion solution and air pump (upper arrows), is closed by clamping it to the drape a few inches from the eye (lower right). The proximal end of the infusion line is detached from the three-way stopcock (dashed central arrow), and a 25-gauge needle is attached using a plastic female adaptor. The relatively small bore of the 25-gauge needle will prevent sudden hypotony when the clamp is opened during injection of gas into the eye.

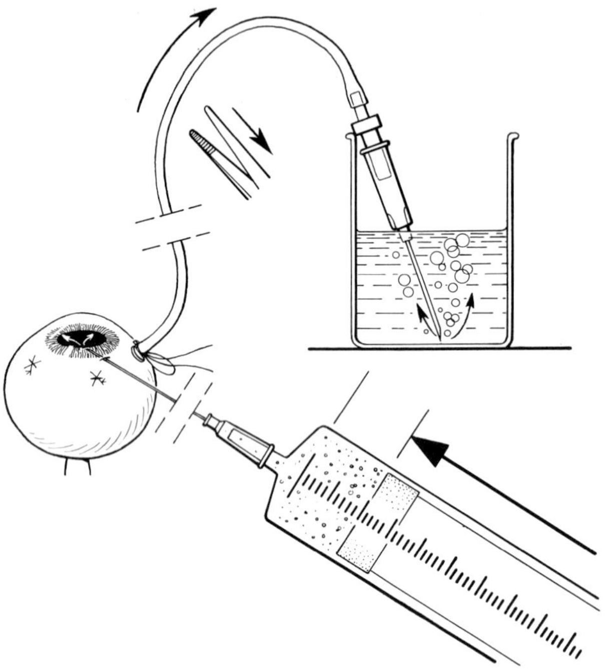

10.**5b** A 20% mixture of perfluorocarbon gas and air is injected through a 30-gauge needle on a 50 ml syringe. The needle is inserted through the limbus in aphakic eyes (left), and through the preexisting superior temporal sclerotomy in phakic eyes. After removing the clamp from the infusion line (top), 40 ml of the gas mixture is lavaged through the vitreous cavity over a period of 2 minutes. Bubbles in the fluid in the glass beaker indicate a continuous lavage of gas through the vitreous cavity.

An alternative method utilizes the infusion cannula tubing which is connected to replace vitreous air, which is vented through a 27-gauge needle inserted in one of the sclerotomies.

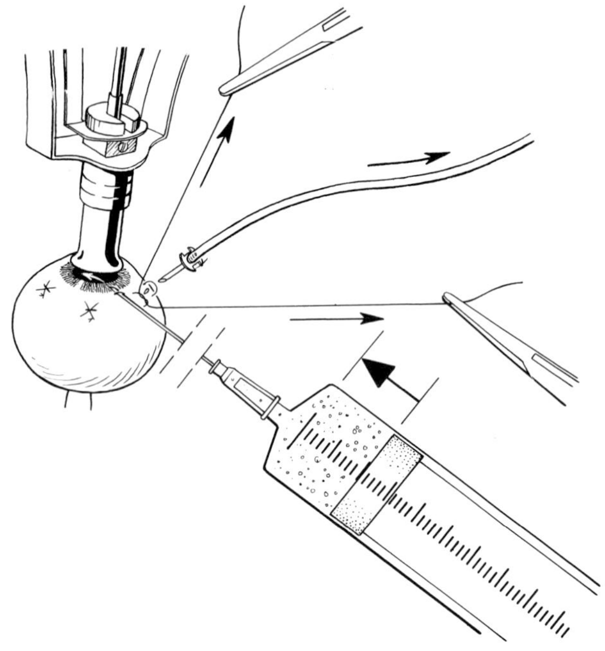

10.**5c** With 10 ml of the mixture of gas and air remaining in the syringe, the sutures surrounding the sclerotomy for the infusion cannula are tightened (arrows), and the cannula is removed (arrow, upper right). Additional gas is injected (arrow, lower right) if tonometry indicates low intraocular pressure.

Outpatient Fluid-Gas Exchange

A postoperative fluid-gas exchange may be used to remove persistent vitreous hemorrhage, or to prolong tamponade of the retina after surgery for retinal detachment. Removal of vitreous hemorrhage after vitrectomy permits visualization and photocoagulation, if indicated (1). It is desirable in some cases of retinal detachment with residual preretinal traction to perform a postoperative outpatient fluid-gas exchange to provide an extensive tamponade with gas for at least 2–3 weeks.

Because outpatient fluid-gas exchange is an intraocular procedure, it carries the risk of hyphema, ocular hypertension, flat chamber, and endophthalmitis. To minimize and deal promptly with these potential complications, we perform the procedure in an ambulatory operating room rather than at the slit lamp in an examining room. The skin around the eye is scrubbed with a povidone-iodine solution. A preoperative culture is taken from the conjunctival cul-de-sac.

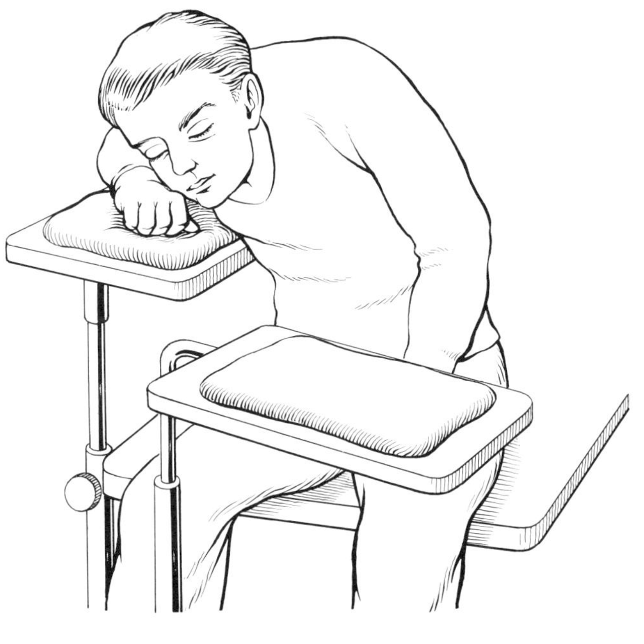

10.**6a** The patient is placed with the chin resting on a closed fist and supported on a Mayo stand.

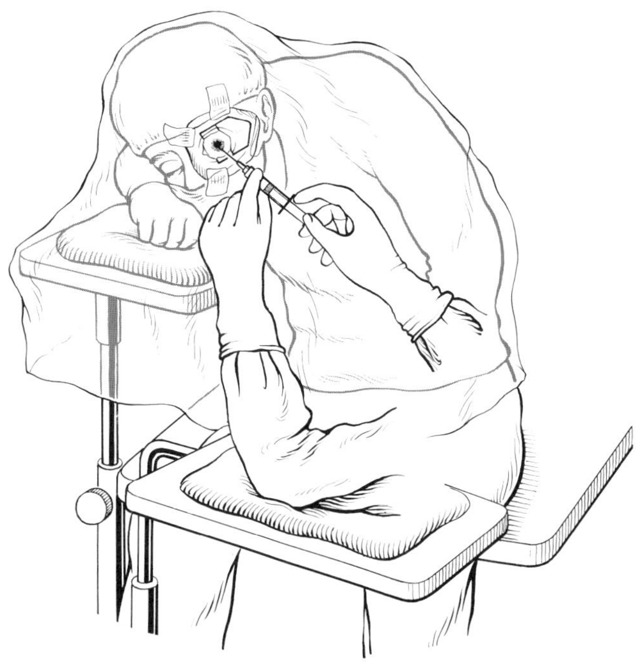

10.**6b** A small plastic drape is applied to the periorbital region. The gowned and gloved surgeon sits on a adjustable stool with his or her elbow supported on a Mayo stand. Topical 4% cocaine is applied at the limbus at the selected injection site. To steady the globe, the conjunctiva is grasped with toothed Bishop-Harmon forceps. 3 ml of a mixture of 20% perfluoropropane gas and air is drawn into a 6 ml syringe and attached to a short 27-gauge needle. In aphakic eyes, the needle is inserted parallel to the iris into the anterior chamber. In phakic or pseudophakic eyes, the needle is inserted through the pars plana.

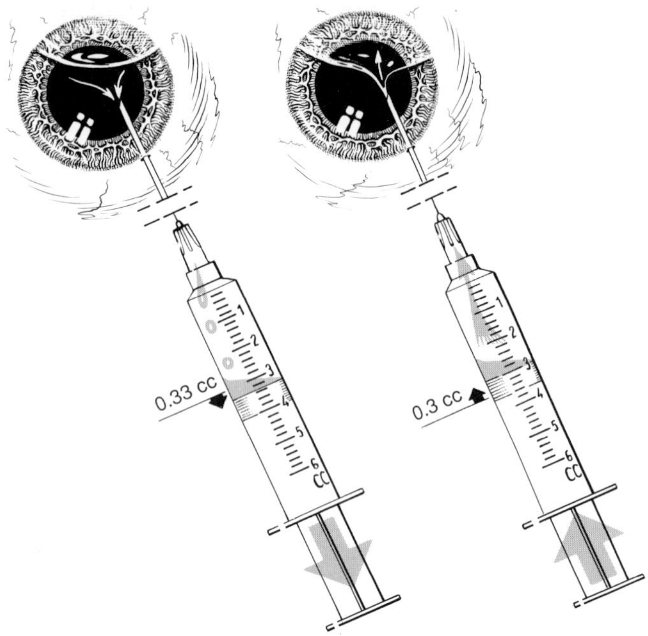

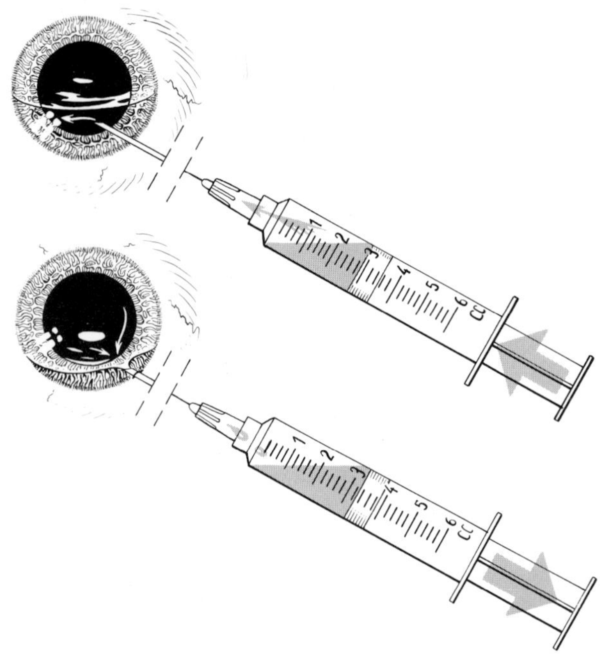

10.**6c** Small amounts of fluid are aspirated and exchanged for an equal volume of gas until most of the intraocular fluid is removed. The syringe is depressed so that fluid that is aspirated will trickle down the barrel to accumulate below the 3 cc of gas mixture (left). The plunger of the syringe is slightly withdrawn (large arrow) until 0.3 cc of intraocular fluid is aspirated (small arrow); then an equal volume of gas is injected. If the eye was slightly hypotonous prior to the procedure, 0.4 cc or more of gas is injected.

10.**6e** As the gas bubble becomes larger, the tip of the needle is withdrawn slightly and directed below the level of the bubble (below). Additional fluid is exchanged for gas until the gas bubble fills the pupil (top).

After the gas-fluid exchange, the paracentesis site is inspected for leakage, intraocular pressure is measured, and the ophthalmic artery is examined to be sure it is patent.

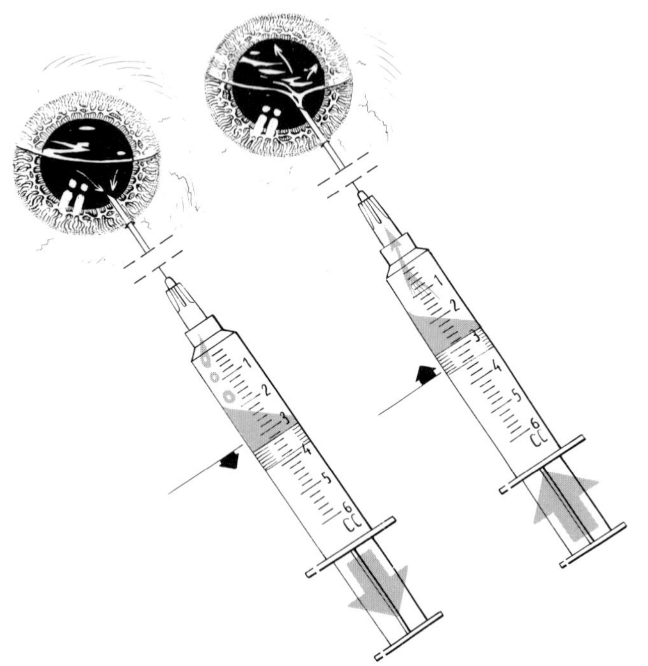

10.**6d** The tip of the needle is directed below the meniscus of the gas bubble (left); then another 0.3 ml of fluid is aspirated and replaced with an equal volume of gas (right).

Relaxing Retinotomy

In eyes in which scleral buckling, vitrectomy, membrane peeling or segmentation, and gas injection have failed to reattach the retina, relaxing retinotomy can be attempted as a last resort in an effort to relieve intractable retinal traction (25). Relaxing retinotomy may be helpful in cases of retinal incarceration associated with penetrating ocular injuries. Penetrating injuries of the posterior segment with choroidal and subretinal hemorrhage may produce a retinal detachment associated with extensive subretinal membranes that prevent retinal reattachment. A circumferential retinotomy makes possible the exposure and removal of extensive subretinal membranes. In severe cases of anterior PVR, the peripheral retina may be dragged so far anteriorly that it becomes adherent to the posterior surface of the iris or pupillary margin in an iridoretinal adhesion (10, 28). If efforts to separate this adhesion with a membrane spatula are unsuccessful, retinotomy is performed along the pupillary margin. In cases of anterior PVR in which severe preretinal organization and very adherent membranes cannot be peeled by bimanual dissection, retinotomy is performed slightly posterior and parallel to the vitreous base and extended over the circumference of unrelieved traction (see Chapter 25). It should be repeated that relaxing retinotomy should be attempted only as a last resort.

a

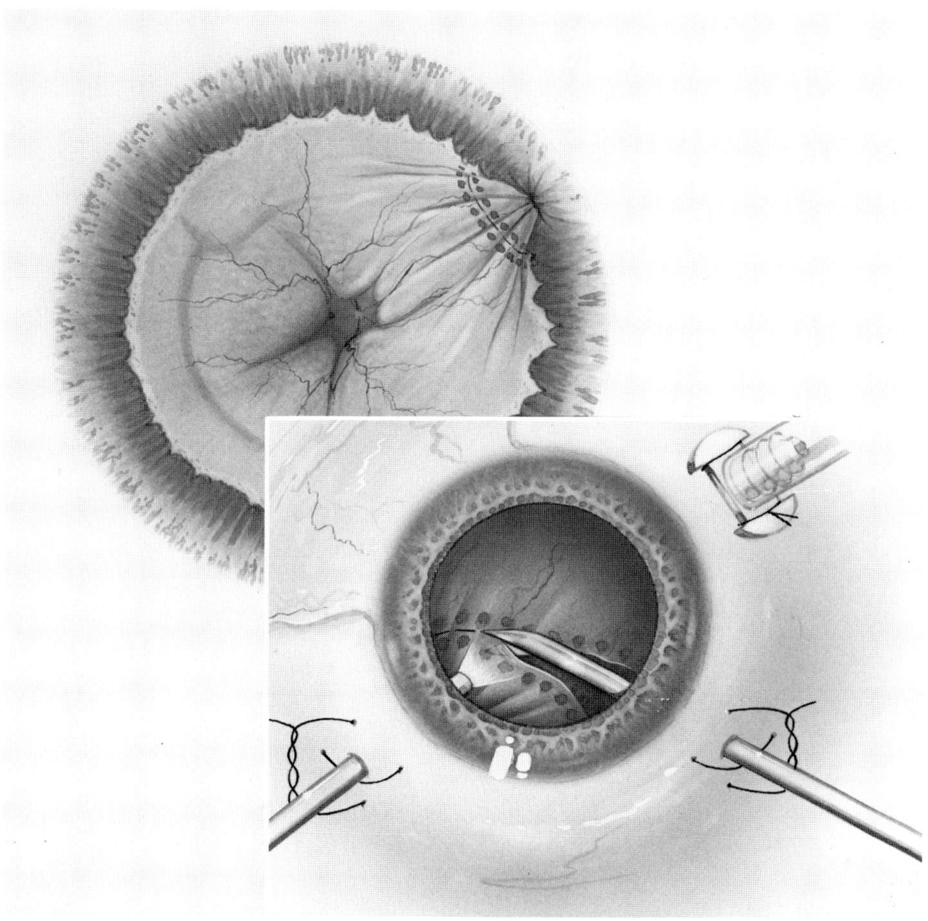

b

10.7 a This fundus drawing illustrates the right eye of a patient who had three unsuccessful vitreoretinal operations complicated by incarceration of vitreous and retina in a superior nasal sclerotomy. A lensectomy was necessary for optimum visualization of the anteriorly located pathology. Vitrectomy was extended anteriorly to include the vitreous base in the quadrant of the incarceration. Diathermy was applied along both sides of the proposed retinotomy.

b A superior nasal relaxing retinotomy may be carried out with the surgeon sitting at the patient's head or, alternatively, at the patient's temporal side. Because the curvature of the 25° Sutherland scissors follows the direction of the curvature of the retinotomy, these scissors are used in combination with other Sutherland scissors with different angles of inclination of the blades with the shaft. Scleral depression and a 15° prism vitrectomy lens help to enhance the view of the fundus periphery. The incarcerated retina and vitreous are amputated, releasing the retina and leaving a napkin-like retinal stalk at the incarceration site.

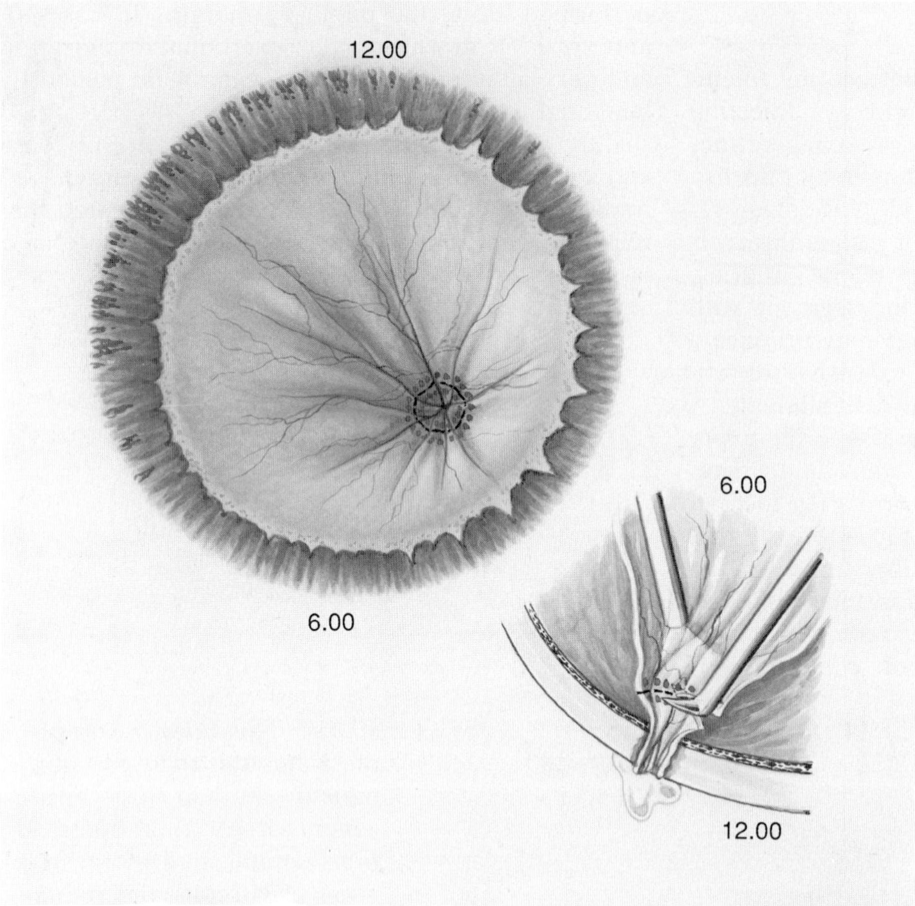

10.**7c** This fundus sketch illustrates total retinal detachment with retina and vitreous incarcerated in a scleral wound. The incarcerated tissue is organized and contracted, dragging the retina inferiorly so that the optic disc is not visible. The site of the relaxing retinotomy is indicated by the broken line. One row of endodiathermy applications is made on each side of the intended retinotomy.

Inset: Sutherland scissors being used for the retinotomy, which amputates the incarcerated retina from its scleral attachment.

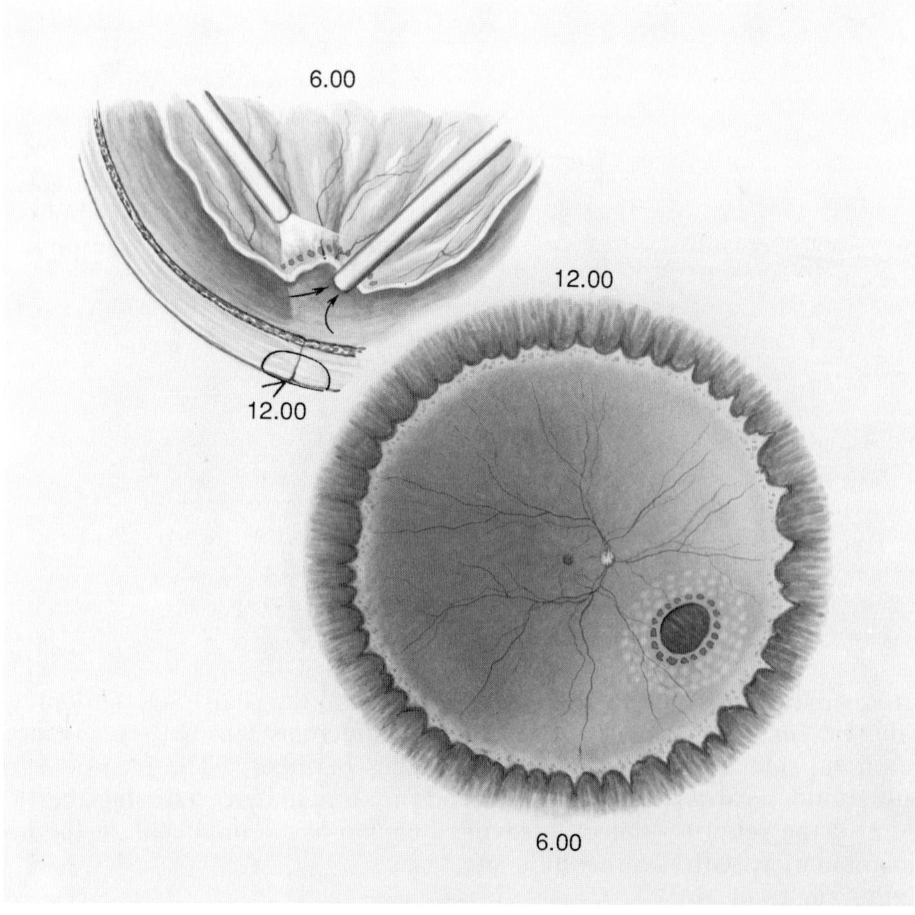

10.**7d** *Inset:* After preretinal membranes are removed, the tip of the extrusion needle is introduced into the retinotomy for drainage of subretinal fluid and fluid-air exchange.

Three rows of endolaser are applied around the retinotomy. Prior to closure of the conjunctiva, air is replaced with a mixture of 20% perfluorocarbon gas and air.

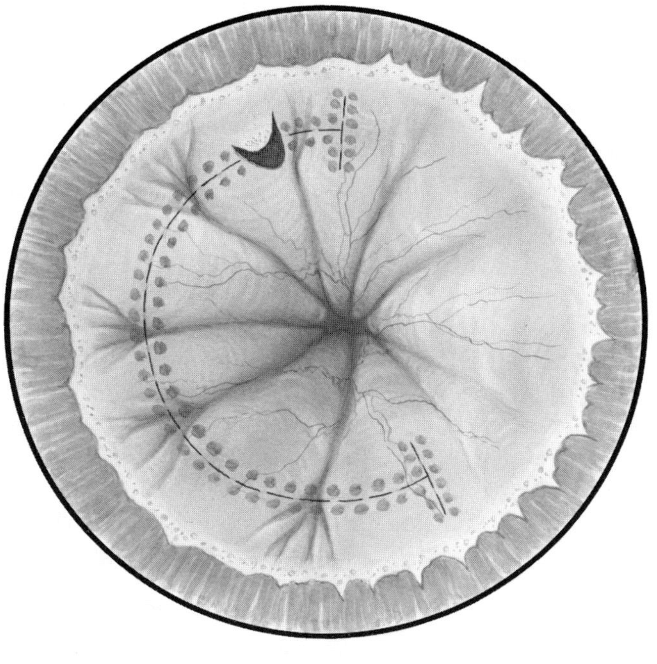

10.7e Despite several fluid-air exchanges, a thorough vitrectomy involving the vitreous base, sectioning of an anterior membrane, meticulous membrane peeling, as well as a high and broad scleral buckle, the temporal retina failed to flatten in this case. A relaxing retinotomy was therefore performed. The extent of retinal incision, from 5 to 12 o'clock, was outlined with two rows of endodiathermy. The circumferential retinotomy was made to extend one clock hour beyond the organized retina. A radial retinotomy was made, extending anteriorly and posteriorly from both ends of the circumferential retinal incision.

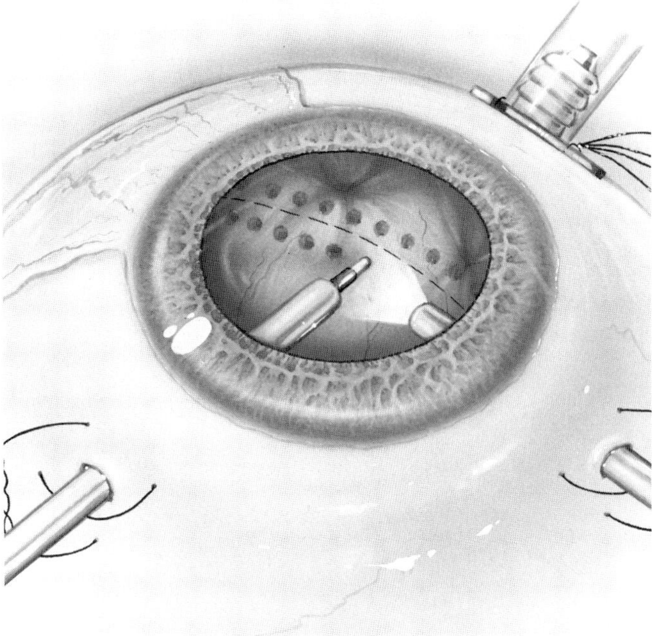

10.7f The illustration shows the inferior temporal fundus of the right eye as seen by the surgeon, seated at the patient's head. Endodiathermy is applied to the retina along the line of the intended retinotomy (broken line). Retinal blood vessels crossing the incision line are coagulated to prevent bleeding. The automated vitreous dissector cutter is used to perform the retinotomy.

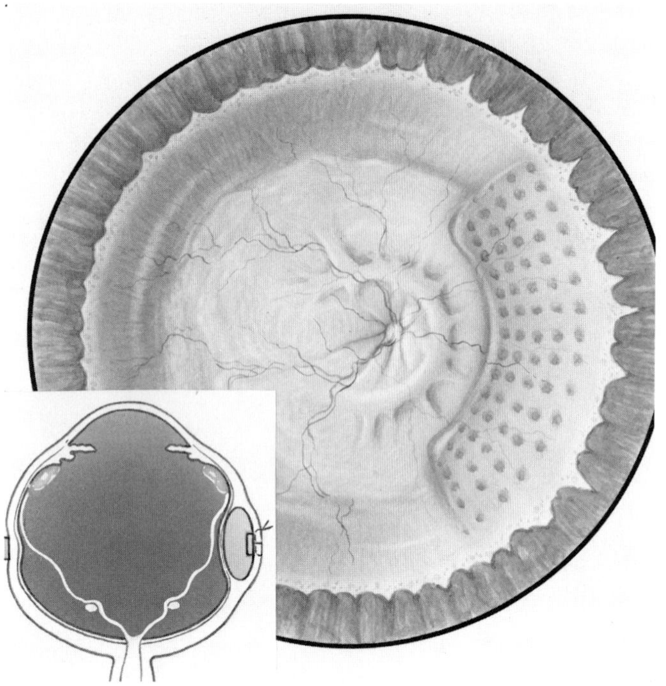

Retinotomy for Subretinal Organization

10.**8a** Subretinal membranes are seldom removed unless they prevent retinal reattachment. They may form a circular band under the posterior retina, producing a funnel-shaped retinal detachment with a napkin-ring configuration.

Inset: the cord-like subretinal membrane may be adherent to the back surface of the retina. Although uncommon, this napkin-ring subretinal membrane usually develops following penetrating trauma or recurrent retinal detachment complicated by subretinal or choroidal hemorrhage. In such cases, the retina remains detached, even though the retinal breaks have been closed and the preretinal membranes removed.

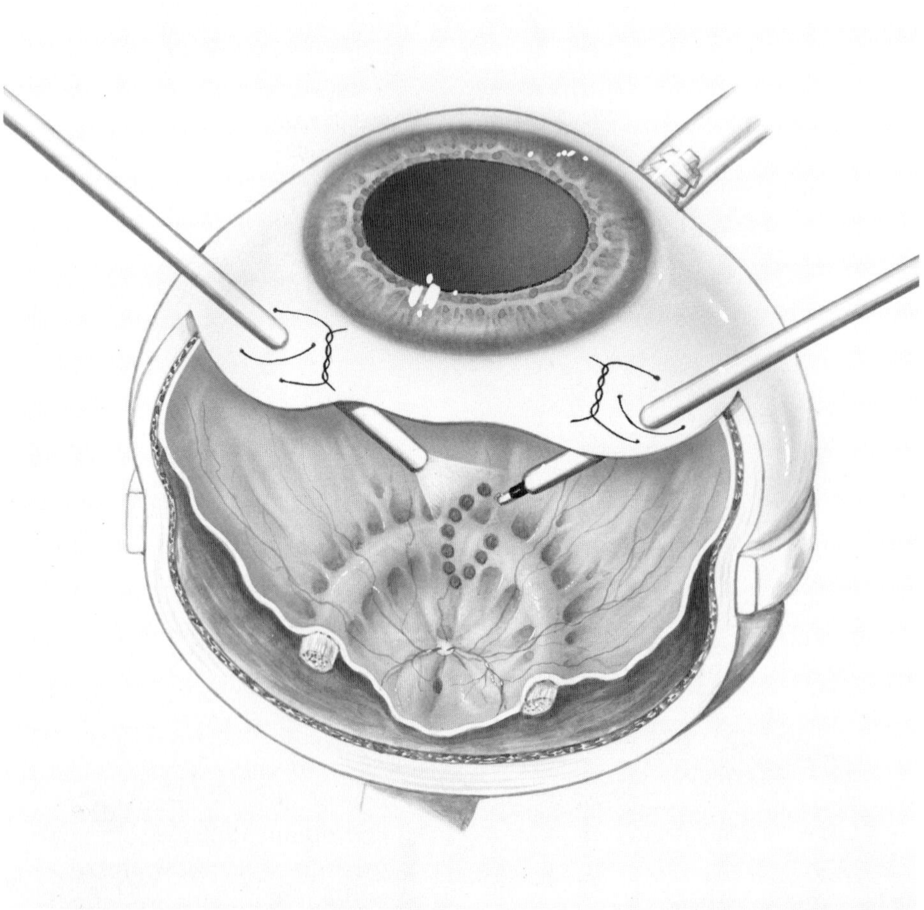

10.**8b** Subretinal bands may be exposed by a retinotomy (23). The site selected for a radial retinotomy is an area devoid of vessels where the membrane is maximally elevated and has numerous branches that can be reached with forceps or scissors through the retinotomy. Endodiathermy is applied around the proposed retinotomy site, using a low energy setting and prolonged duration of application.

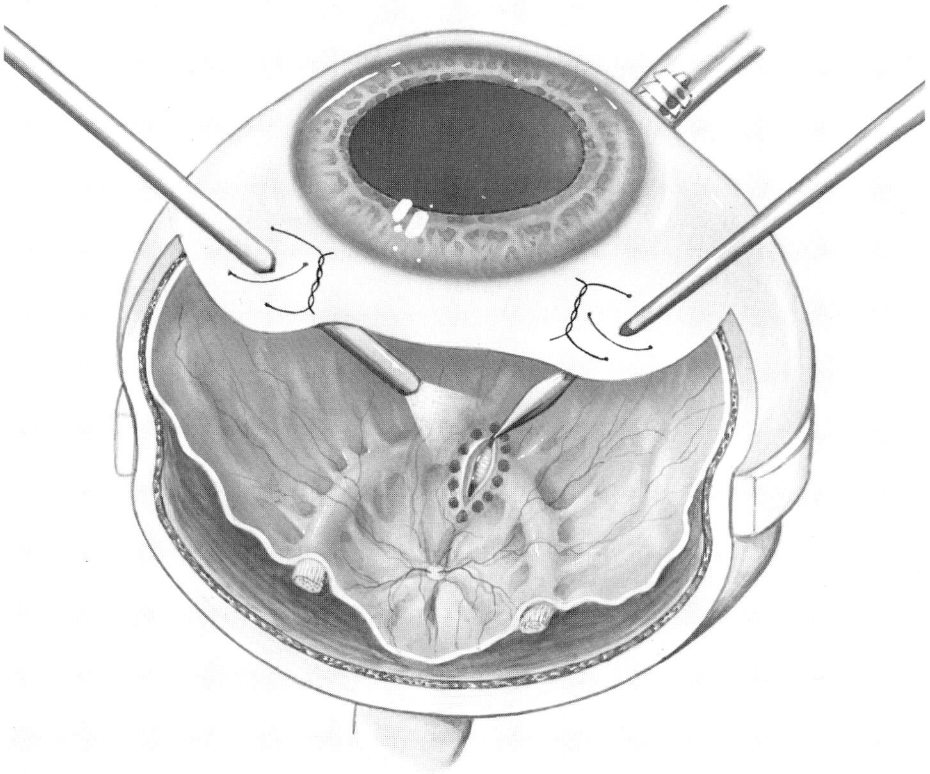

10.**8c** Retinotomy is made with an MVR knife inserted through the diathermized retina. The incision is enlarged to expose the width of the membrane.

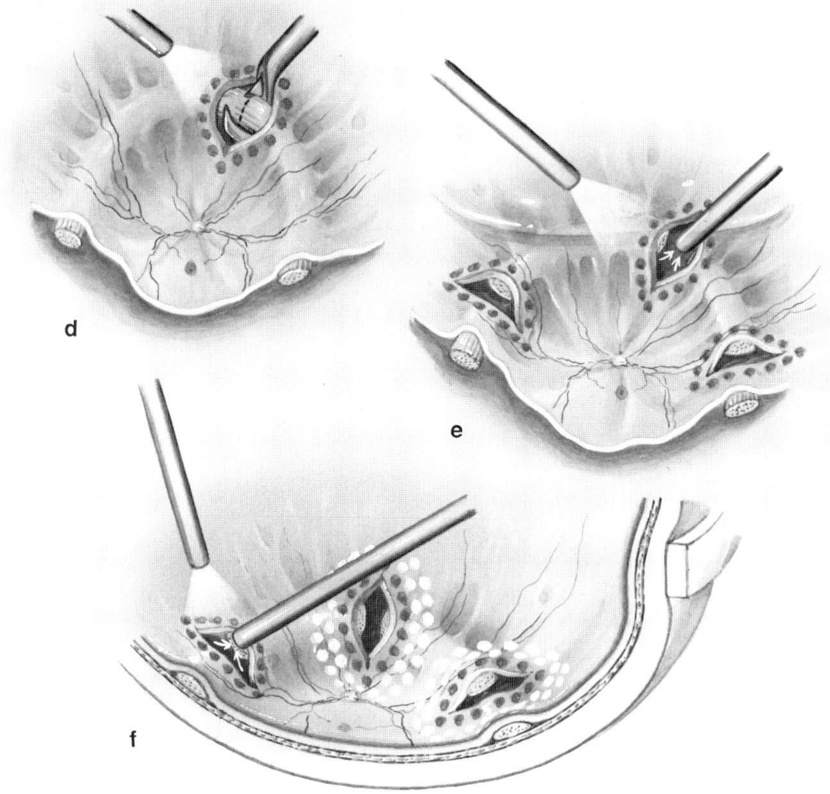

d

e

f

10.**8d** A membrane spatula is inserted into the subretinal space to separate the membrane from the back surface of the retina. This maneuver is carried out as distally as possible on both sides of the retinotomy. The membrane exposed by the retinotomy is cut with vertical-cutting scissors.

e Tough leathery subretinal membranes are best cut with the guillotine cutting blade of the automated vitreous dissector scissors. Some membranes may have firm and broad adhesions that cannot be separated from the posterior retinal surface. Therefore, multiple radial retinotomies are made overlying the membrane. Fluid-air exchange is done after each retinotomy to determine whether the subretinal membrane has been adequately divided to allow retinal reattachment.

f When the detached retina has been flattened against the pigment epithelium as a result of internal drainage of subretinal fluid (left), the retinotomies are surrounded by endolaser (center and right).

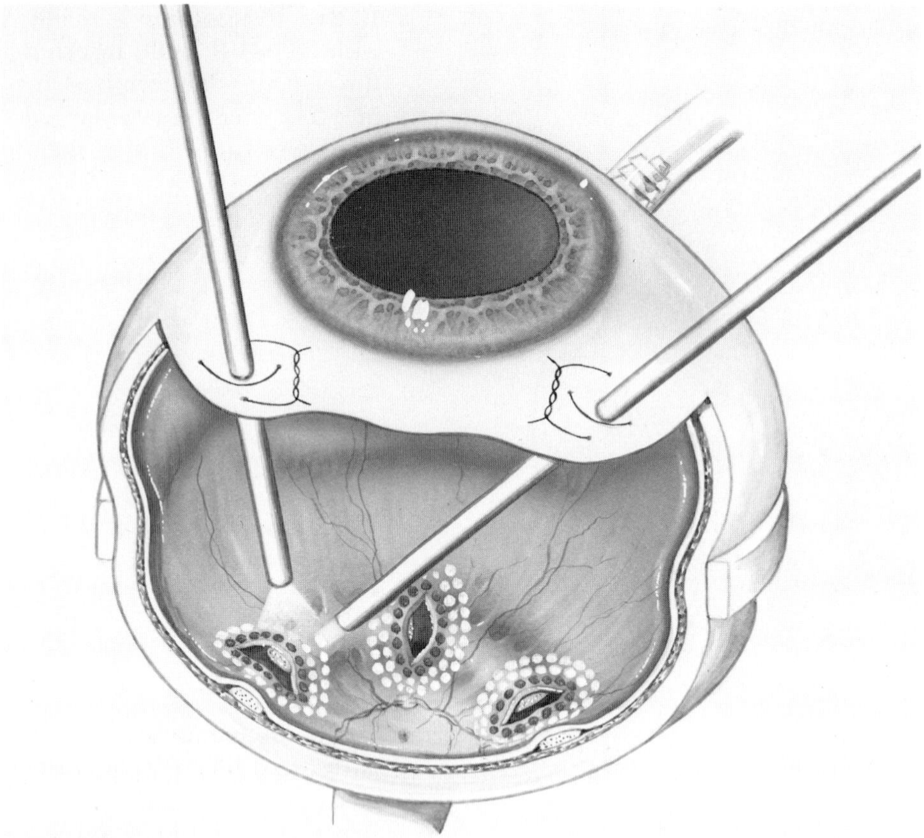

10.**8g** Additional rows of endolaser are placed around the retinotomies. The procedure is completed with the replacement of air by a 20% mixture of perfluoropropane gas (C_3F_8) and air. When multiple breaks have been produced in the posterior retina, postoperative prone positioning of the patient's head is important. Because the retinotomies are located below the horizontal meridian of the fundus, it is important that the gas bubble occupy at least 70% of the vitreous cavity for a period of two weeks during the formation of the endolaser chorioretinal adhesion. It may be necessary to perform a postoperative fluid-gas exchange with C_3F_8 to maintain a sufficiently large gas bubble for that period.

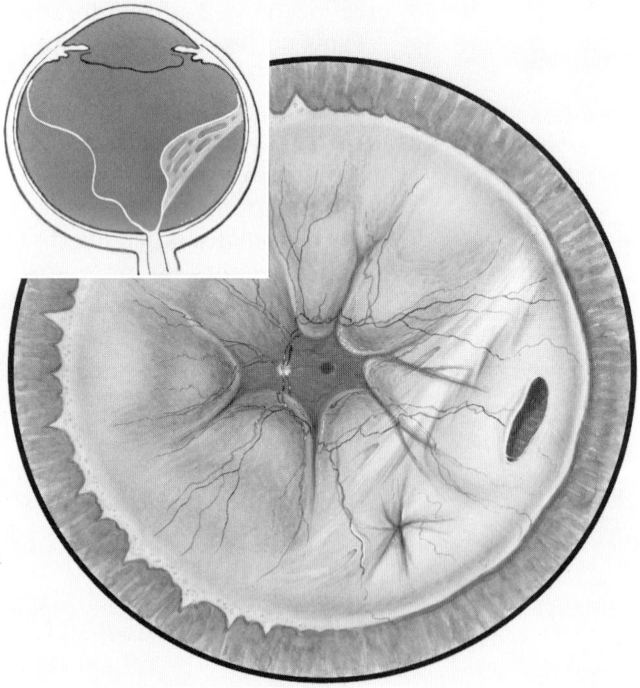

10.**8h Retinotomy for extensive subretinal membranes.** Penetrating injuries of the posterior segment with subretinal and choroidal hemorrhage may produce a traumatic retinal detachment associated with extensive subretinal membranes that prevent retinal reattachment.
Inset: an extensive subretinal membrane with a Swiss cheese-like appearance extends posteriorly from the site of a corneoscleral laceration.

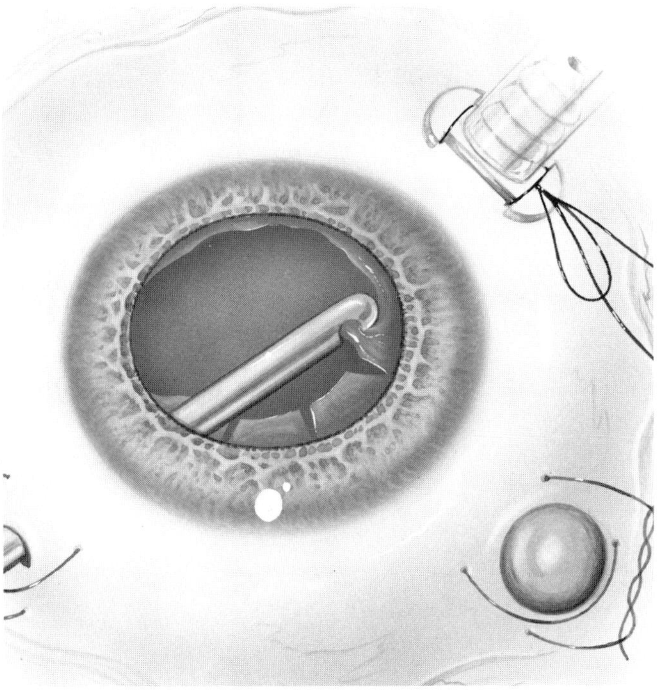

10.8i **Removal of capsular remnants of the traumatic cataract** that interfere with visualization of the region of the vitreous base. Using vitreous scissors, radial cuts are made in the thick capsular remnant so that it can be engaged and removed with the vitrectomy instrument.

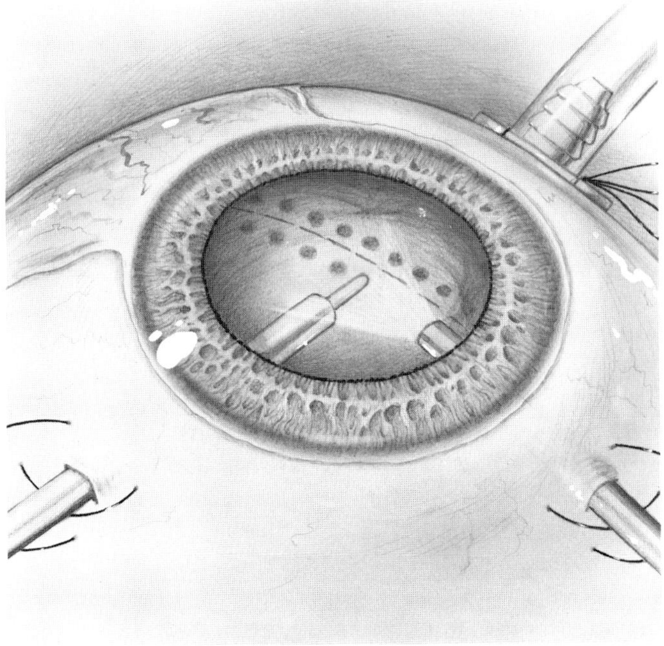

10.8j A double row of endodiathermy applications are made in the intended path of the retinotomy.

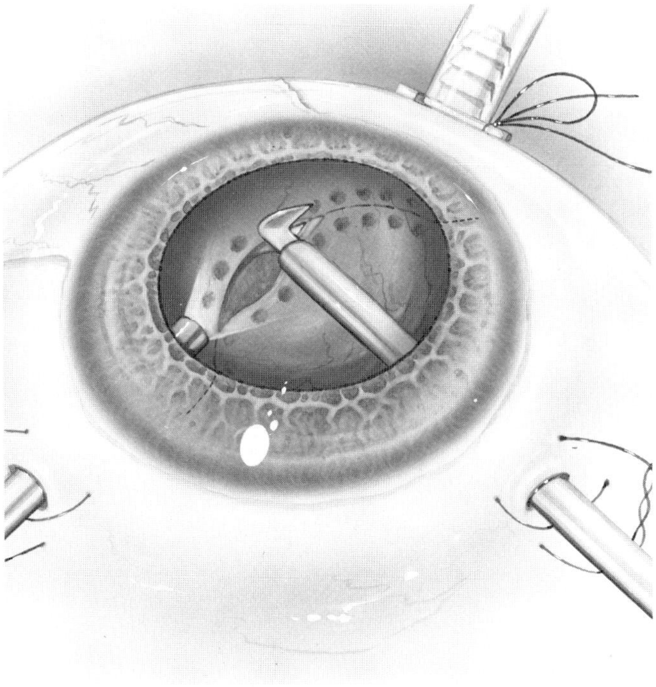

10.8k The retinotomy is extended inferonasally using scissors with blades at right angles to the shaft.

8l

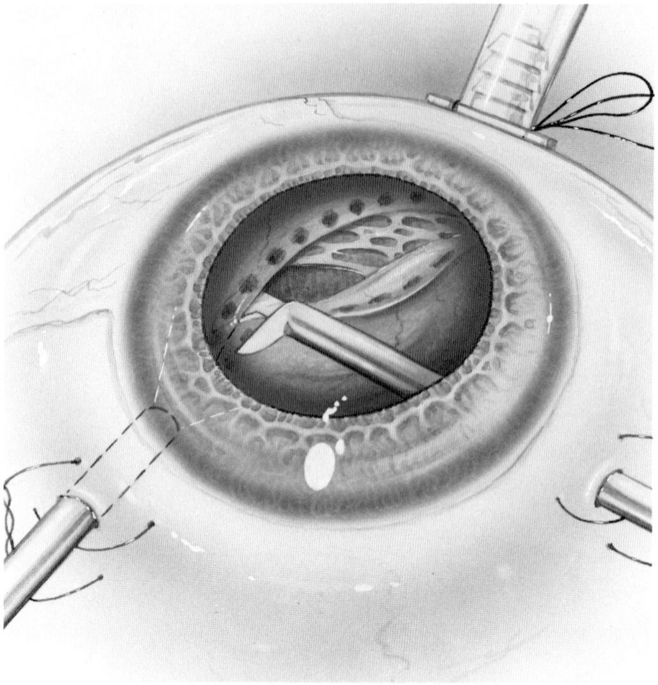

8n

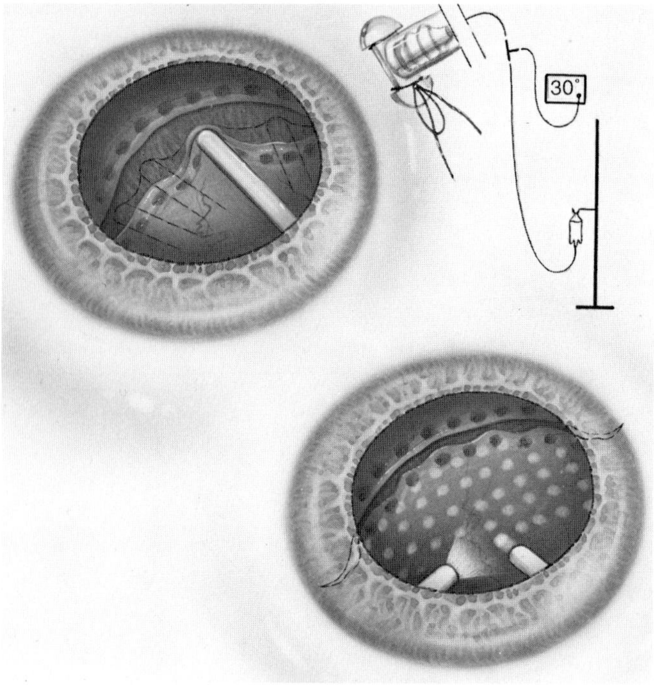

8m

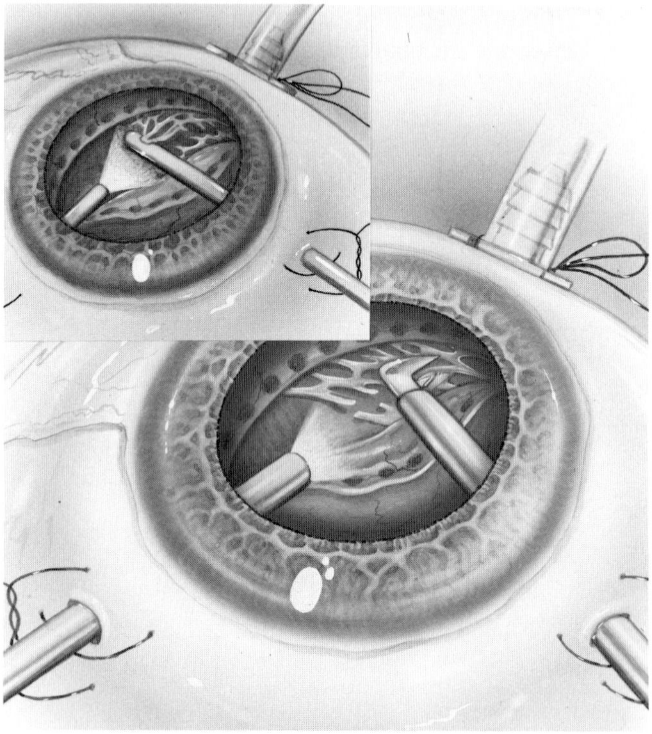

10.**8l** With the blades of the scissors directed in the opposite direction, the retinotomy is extended inferotemporally. The posterior flap of the giant retinotomy becomes inverted to expose the subretinal membrane which may have numerous oval-shaped holes, giving it a Swiss cheese-like appearance.

10.**8m** The attachment of the subretinal membrane to the outer surface of the sensory retina is severed with scissors, and the membrane is then removed using a vitrectomy instrument (inset). After a giant retinotomy has been made, the posterior flap is inverted over the optic disc so that the back surface of the retina can be examined for subretinal organization. Using a bimanual technique, with the flap steadied by a spatula or peeler, membranes on the back surface of the flap are removed with forceps. Using the backflush needle, pigment debris is removed from the subretinal space.

10.**8n** Fluid-air exchange is performed to tamponade the posterior retinal flap against the pigment epithelium. The posterior edge of the giant retinotomy is dragged as far anteriorly as possible using the backflush needle.

Endolaser is applied in five rows along the posterior edge of the giant retinotomy and in four rows around the remaining circumference of the fundus periphery. A 20% mixture of perfluoropropane gas with air is exchanged for the air prior to closure of the conjunctiva.

Retinectomy

Penetrating injuries involving the region of the vitreous base may cause the peripheral retina to become thickened, opaque, and organized into a mass of fixed retinal folds because of intra-, pre-, and subretinal organization. When efforts to peel membranes from both surfaces of the retina are unsuccessful, retinectomy is performed with the vitrectomy probe (9, 16, 34:84–94). To avoid excising an excessive amount of viable retinal tissue, the slowest possible cutting speed and low suction pressure are used. In cases where the retina is markedly thickened and cut with difficulty with the vitrectomy probe, retinal tissue is removed using a bimanual technique, with forceps holding the tissue which is excised with scissors. The retina is reattached as described in Chapter 23.

Bimanual Vitreoretinal Surgery

Preretinal membranes may be so adherent that attempts to peel them produce iatrogenic retinal breaks. Traction by the anterior membrane in anterior PVR causes the peripheral retina to become stretched, thin, and atrophic (13). This atrophic retina is very prone to develop retinal breaks during peeling of peripheral preretinal membranes. A bimanual technique is used in eyes with atrophic peripheral retina to reduce the incidence of iatrogenic retinal breaks. While peeling or sectioning membranes using the bimanual technique, the membrane is held with forceps in the surgeon's nondominant hand while membranes are separated from the retina with a spatula or membrane peeler held in the dominant hand (34:97–98). Holding the membrane reduces excessive tractional movements during attempts to peel it, and decreases the incidence of iatrogenic retinal breaks.

In addition, during retinectomy of severe intraretinal and periretinal organization of the posterior edge of a giant retinal break, it is helpful to hold the flap steady while amputating or peeling tissue from both surfaces of the retinal flap.

In vitrectomy involving the vitreous base, scleral depression can be more precise and safer when it is performed by the surgeon rather than the assistant. A long-handled scleral depressor is held in the surgeon's nondominant hand, and the vitrectomy probe is held in the dominant hand. Providing the pupil is well dilated and the media clear, it is possible to illuminate the peripheral retina with coaxial illumination from the operating microscope. Bimanual posterior dissection requires a fiber-optic illuminator introduced into the vitreous cavity through a cannula in the pars plana, an endoilluminator introduced by the assistant through a fourth sclerotomy, or forceps or picks with a fiber-optic sleeve.

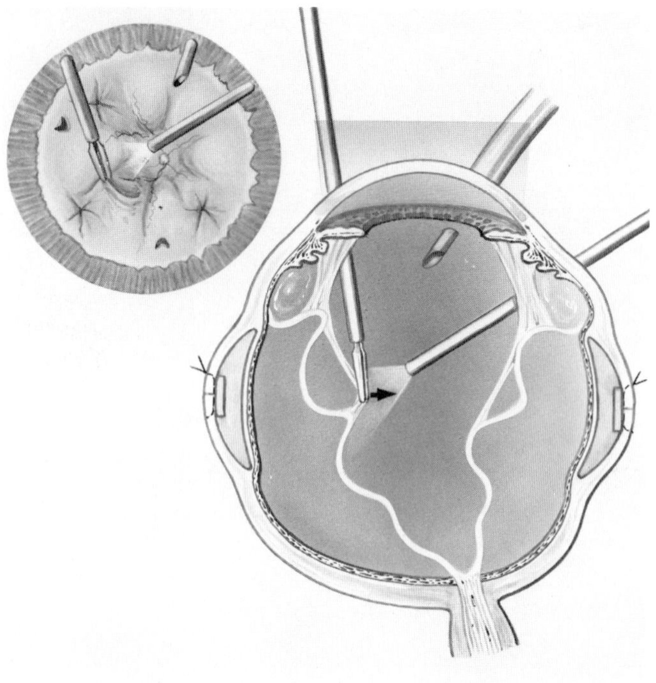

Silicone and Fluorosilicone Oil Injection

10.**9a** Silicone oil injection is reserved for complex cases of retinal detachment with severe proliferative vitreoretinopathy (6, 14, 20, 22, 31) as indicated in the inset. The oil should be injected only after the detached retina has been completely relieved of surface traction membranes. Fluorosilicone or silicone oil is removed 4–6 months after injection because of the postoperative complications of keratopathy, cataract formation, and glaucoma (29, 34:127–138).

The large illustration shows a surface membrane being grasped with end-gripping forceps, drawing it first toward the midline.

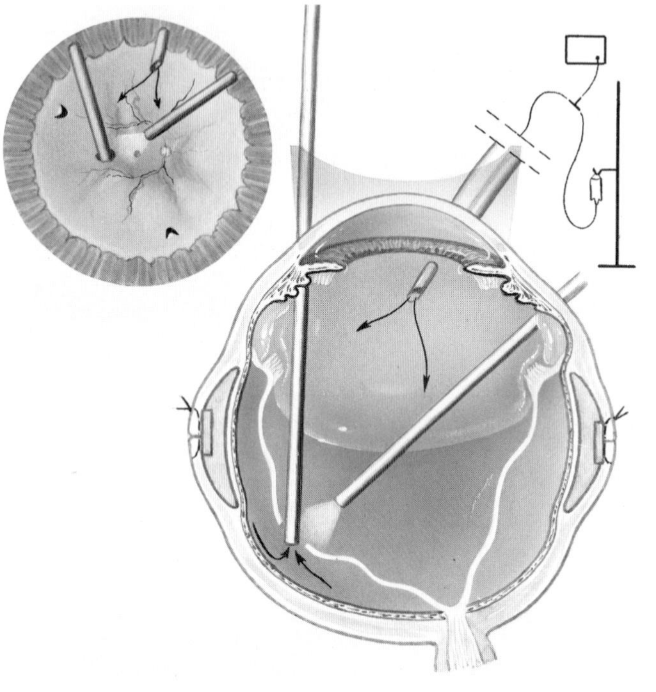

10.**9b** A preexisting scleral buckle is left in place if it is felt that it extends far enough posteriorly to encompass the retinal breaks. If retinal breaks are located so far anteriorly that they cannot be used for internal drainage of subretinal fluid, a retinotomy is made between the equator and the posterior retina. Fluid air exchange is performed at the completion of the intraocular dissection. Internal drainage of subretinal fluid combined with fluid-air exchange is a useful test to determine whether traction on the retina has been relieved. Charles has termed this pneumohydraulic reattachment of the retina "air-traction test" (3:91–92). If the retina remains elevated following fluid-air exchange, further preretinal dissection or sectioning of subretinal bands should be performed. Membrane dissection may be done under air or after refilling the vitreous cavity with infusion fluid.

If retinal breaks continue to remain open after additonal membrane peeling and pneumatic reattachment with air, a revision of the scleral buckling should be attempted to close these retinal breaks; otherwise, silicone oil will tend to pass subretinally. If revision of the buckle fails to close the retinal breaks and relieve residual retinal traction, a relaxing retinotomy is performed.

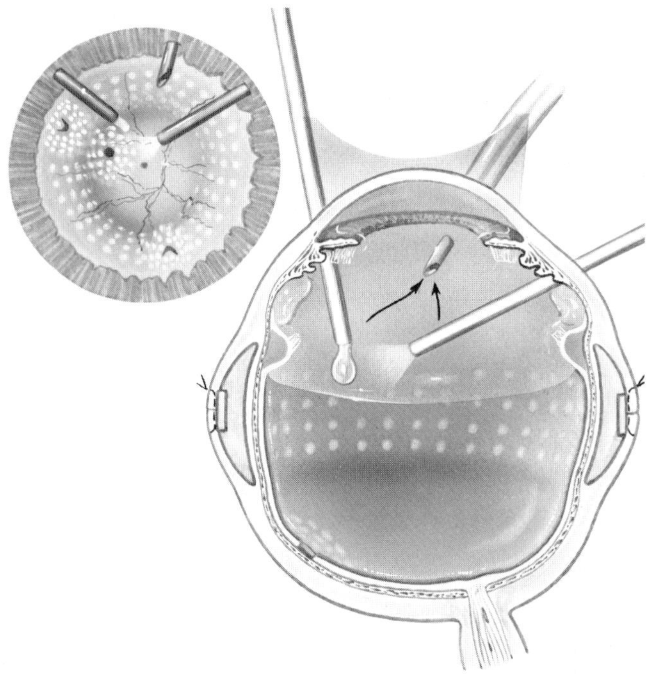

10.9c The inset shows endolaser photocoagulation applied around retinal breaks and the peripheral fundus prior to silicone oil injection. Several rows of laser photocoagulation have been applied over the buckle and the indentation produced by the encircling element.

Silicone oil of 1000 centistokes viscosity is injected into the air-filled vitreous cavity using a 19-gauge blunt needle attached to a mechanical injection pump or a 20-gauge intravenous catheter connected to a 6 ml Luer-Lok syringe. The cannula tubing is disconnected from the three-way stopcock and attached to a 20 ml syringe. As the oil is injected, air in the vitreous cavity is released into the syringe. The oil is injected to the level of the pupil. An inferior peripheral sector iridectomy is made with the vitrectomy probe prior to air-fluid exchange, to prevent silicone oil from causing pupillary block glaucoma. The sclerotomies are closed in the usual manner.

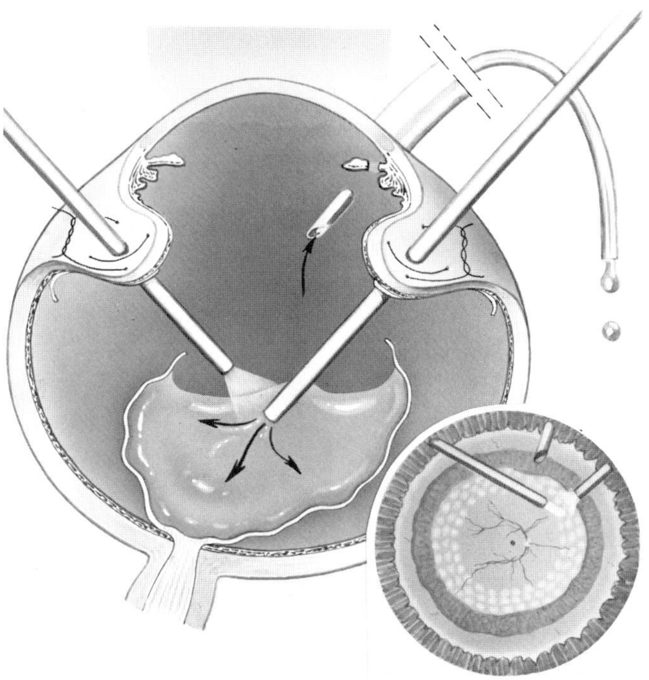

10.9d Fluorosilicone oil has a specific gravity of 1.28 and sinks posteriorly in the fluid-filled vitreous cavity (33). This facilitates the reattachment of extensive giant retinal tears.

After the removal of preretinal membranes, the oil is injected directly inside the folded retina near the optic disc.

When the retina has been reattached, endolaser is applied in four rows along the edge of the giant tear, as shown in the inset.

Nd:YAG Laser Photodisruption

The Nd:YAG laser may be used to disrupt pupillary or thin cyclitic membranes that hinder biomicroscopic or ophthalmoscopic preoperative assessment of the posterior segment. In some circumstances, vitreous membranes causing isolated peripheral retinal traction or traction to the macula can be lysed by photodisruption (32). In very rare instances, vitreous opacities producing disabling visual symptoms may be considered for treatment with this modality.

10.**10** **Pupillary Membranes.** The membrane is examined with the slit lamp microscope for tension lines, which are preferred sites of photodisruption.
a The procedure requires no topical anesthesia. The slit beam of the Nd:YAG laser is directed at an angle to the microscope axis, to reduce glare from the membrane. Single- or multiple-burst applications at energy levels determined by trial are made to create multiple holes. Blood vessels within the membrane should be pretreated with argon laser photocoagulation to minimize bleeding after application of the Nd:YAG laser.
b The membranes between the holes are photodisrupted to interconnect the holes and create a large, single pupillary opening.
c, d To prevent pitting of the anterior surface of the intraocular lens, the focusing beam of the Nd:YAG laser is placed slightly behind the membrane.

10.**11** **Tractional Bands.** Traction bands or membranes can be sectioned effectively with the Nd:YAG laser. The multiple-burst mode can be effective in disrupting thick bands.

There is always a risk of producing a retinal break or vitreous hemorrhage during this procedure. To prevent development of a retinal tear, areas of retina at which the membrane is attached can be surrounded with three rows of argon laser treatment 4 weeks before the treatment with the Nd:YAG laser is attempted. Vascularized membranes are also treated first with argon laser and later sectioned with Nd:YAG laser.

Procedure. Contraction of the equatorial membrane has produced a retinal elevation where it is attached to the retina. Using a Peyman 18 mm or 25 mm contact lens, the single mode is used to minimize tension on the membrane upon impact of the YAG laser beam. The narrowest portion of the membrane is chosen as the site of sectioning. In addition, the edge and not the center of the membrane is always cut, chipping across the membrane with series of applications until the entire width of the membrane has been divided. The retina is carefully inspected after the membrane has been cut to check for retinal breaks.

10.

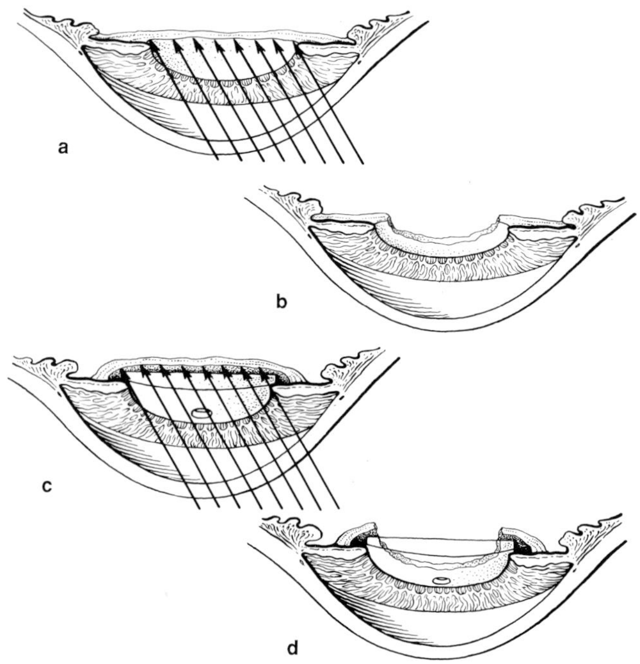

10.

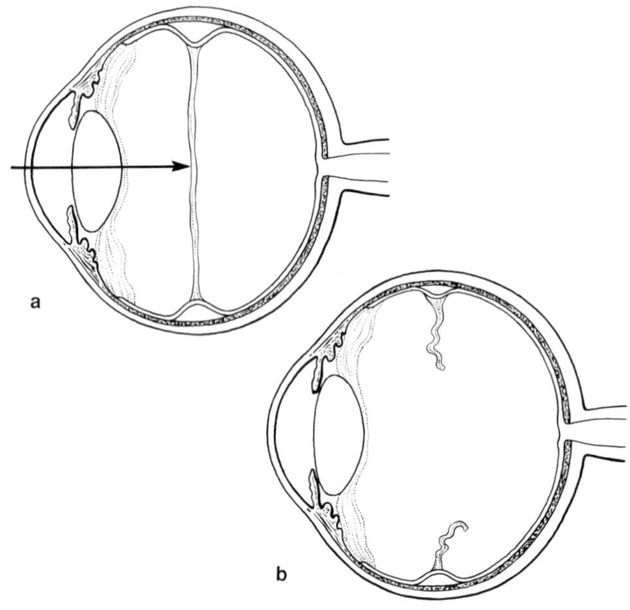

Vitreous floaters occurring after a posterior vitreous detachment are actually glial or fibrous opacities that are adherent to the surface of detached posterior cortex. Surgical or Nd:YAG laser removal is very rarely indicated unless the floaters cause permanent visual loss and disabling visual symptoms that interfere with the patient's ability to function normally. The anterior two-thirds of the vitreous cavity is considered a zone of safety for photodisrupting vitreous opacities. Vitreous floaters within the posterior third of the vitreous cavity or at 6 mm to the retina are a contraindication for Nd:YAG laser photodisruption, because at this location there is considerable risk of creating a retinal hole.

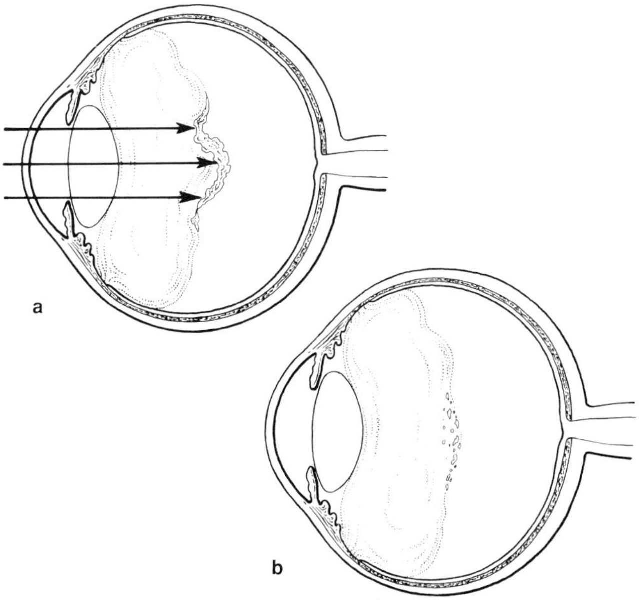

a

b

10.**12** A vitreous floater located in the anterior vitreous can be photodisrupted without using a posterior segment contact lens. Photodisruption of a floater located in the mid-vitreous requires a Peyman YAG laser contact lens. The cornea is anesthetized topically with 0.5% proparacaine hydrochloride. The Nd:YAG laser settings are determined by trial applications. The energy setting is increased step-by-step to reach a level that results in minimal photodisruption of the tissue.

a To stabilize the floater to be disrupted, the patient is instructed to fixate an object with the fellow eye. The YAG laser is focused on the posterior surface of the thickest portion of the floater, and it is photodisrupted in a piecemeal fashion.

b At the end of the procedure, the opacity has been broken into tiny fragments.

The fundus should be checked with indirect ophthalmoscopy and scleral depression. It must be emphasized that this procedure is attempted in very rare instances, and only when the visual symptoms are disabling.

References

1. Blankenship GW. Management of postvitrectomy diabetic vitreous hemorrhage. In: Blankenship GW, Stirpe M, Gonvers M, Binder S, eds. Basic and advanced vitreous surgery. Padua: Liviana, 1986: 295–300.
2. Brucker AJ, Hoffman ME, Navyas JH, et al. New instrumentation for fluid-air exchange. Retina 1983; 3:135.
3. Charles S. Vitreous microsurgery. 2nd. ed. Baltimore: Williams and Wilkins, 1987: 89–91.
4. Charles S, Wang C. A motorized gas injector for vitreous surgery. Arch Ophthalmol 1981; 99:1398.
5. Charles S, White J, Dennison C, Eichenbaum D. Bimanual bipolar intraocular diathermy. Am J Ophthalmol 1976; 81:101–102.
6. Cox MS, Trese MT, Murphy PL. Silicone oil for advanced proliferative vitreoretinopathy. Ophthalmology 1986; 93:646–650.
7. Doft BH. Intentional retinotomy for internal drainage of subretinal fluid. Arch Ophthalmol 1986; 104:807.
8. Flynn HW, Blumenkranz MS, Parel JM, et al. Cannulated suretinal fluid aspirator for vitreoretinal surgery. Am J Ophthalmol 1987; 103:106–108.
9. Freeman HM. Curent management of giant retinal breaks and fellow eyes. In: Glaser, BM, and Michels, RG, eds. Retina Vol. III, Surgical Retina, Mosby, St. Louis, 1989; 431–448.
10. Freeman HM. Surgery of the retina and vitreous. In Jaffe NS, ed. Atlas of ophthalmic surgery. New York: Gower (in press).
11. Freeman HM. Surgery of the retina and vitreous. In Jaffe NS, ed. Atlas of ophthalmic surgery. New York: Gower (in press).
12. Freeman HM, Johnson MR. Current management of giant retinal breaks and fellow eyes. In: Spaeth GL, Katz LJ, eds. Current therapy in ophthalmic surgery. Philadelphia: Decker 1989; 256–263.
13. Freeman HM, Elner SG, Tolentino FI, Schepens CL, Elner VM, Albert DM. Anterior proliferative vitreoretinopathy, part 1: clinical findings and management. In: Freeman HM, Tolentino FI, eds. Proliferative vitreoretinopathy (PVR). New York: Springer, 1988: 22–33.
14. Gonvers M. Temporary silicone oil tamponade in the management of retinal detachment with proliferative vitreoretinopathy. Am J Ophthalmol 1985; 100: 239–245.
15. Grizzard WS, Slagle C, Gordon S. Infusion of intraocular gas with a pressure-controlled system. Am J Ophthalmol 1979; 88:1096.
16. Haut J, Larricart P, Flamand M. Indications of limited retinectomies in the treatment of retinal detachment and its prevention. Int Ophthalmol 1982; 5:118.
17. Hueneke RL, Aaberg TM. Instrumentation for continuous fluid-air exchange during vitreous surgery. Am J Ophthalmol 1983; 96–547.
18. Landers MB. Sodium hyaluronate (Healon) as an aid to internal fluid-gas exchange. Am J Ophthalmol 1982; 94:557–559.
19. Landers MB III, Robinson KR, Olsen JR. Fluid/gas exchange in vitreous surgery. In: Blankenship GW, Stirpe M, Gonvers M, Binder S, eds. Basic and advanced vitreous surgery. Padua: Liviana, 1986: 357–368.
20. Lean JS, Leaver PK, Cooling RJ, McLeod D. Management of complex retinal detachment by vitrectomy and fluid silicone exchange. Trans Ophthalmol Soc UK 1982; 102:203–205.
21. McCuen BW II, Bessler M, Hickingbotham D, et al. Automated fluid-gas exchange. Am J Ophthalmol 1983; 95:717.
22. McCuen B, de Juan E, Machemer R. Silicone oil in vitreoretinal surgery, part I: surgical techniques. Retina 1985; 5:189–197.
23. Machemer R. Surgical approaches to subretinal strands. Am J Opthalmol 1980: 90:81–85.
24. Machemer R, Aaberg TM. Vitrectomy. 2nd ed. New York: Grune and Stratton, 1979.
25. Machemer R, McCuen BW, de Juan E. Relaxing retinotomies and retinectomies. Am J Ophthalmol 1986, 102:7–12.
26. Peyman GA, Schulman JA. Intravitreal surgery: principles and practice. New York: Appleton-Century-Crofts, 1986.
27. Rice TA, Michels RG, Stark WJ, eds. Operative surgery: ophthalmic surgery. 27. Stoneham, MA: Butterworth, 1984. (Rob and Smith's operative surgery series.)
28. Ryan SJ. The pathophysiology of proliferative vitreoretinopathy in its management. Am J Ophthalmol 1985; 100:188–193.
29. Silicone Study Group. Proliferative vitreoretinopathy. Am J Ophthalmol 1985; 99:593–595.
30. Schepens CL. Retinal detachment and allied diseases. Philadelphia: W B Saunders, 1983: 796–801.
31. Scott JD. The treatment of massive vitreous retraction by the separation of pre-retinal membranes using liquid silicone. Mod Probl Ophthalmol 1975; 15:285.
32. Steinert RF, Puliafito CA. Nd–YAG laser in ophthalmology: principles and clinical applications of photodisruption. Philadelphia: W B Saunders, 1985: 72–94.
33. Tolentino FI, Cajita VN, Chung H, Acosta J, Freeman HM, Refojo MF. High-density fluorosilicone oil in vitreous surgery. In: Freeman HM, Tolentino FI, eds. Proliferative vitreoretinopathy (PVR). New York: Springer, 1988: 177-181.
34. Živojnović R. Silicone oil in vitreoretinal surgery. Dordrecht: Nijhoff, 1987.
35. Živojnović R, Vijfvinkel GJ. A modified flute needle. Am J Ophthalmol 1983; 96:548.

11

Impaired Visualization of Posterior Segment: Preoperative and Intraoperative Miosis; Updrawn Pupil

Preoperative and Intraoperative Miosis

Miosis may exist preoperatively as a result of diabetic iridopathy, long-standing miotic therapy for glaucoma, or posterior synechiae. It can occur intraoperatively when the eye becomes hypotonic, or an instrument inadvertently touches the iris sphincter.

There are several ways of handling a miotic pupil. Phenylephrine 10% and cyclopentolate hydrochloride 1% are a strong mydriatic combination and produce wide pupillary dilation. The use of Ocufen, an antiprostaglandin drug, enhances pupillary dilation and sustains it intraoperatively in most cases. Ocufen 0.03% is instilled four times at 30-minute intervals prior to surgery. In aphakic and pseudophakic eyes, pupillary dilation may be obtained intraoperatively using 1:5000 epinephrine hydrochloride with no preservative in the infusion solution, or 0.1 ml of a 1:1000 solution injected into the anterior chamber (2).

Updrawn Pupil

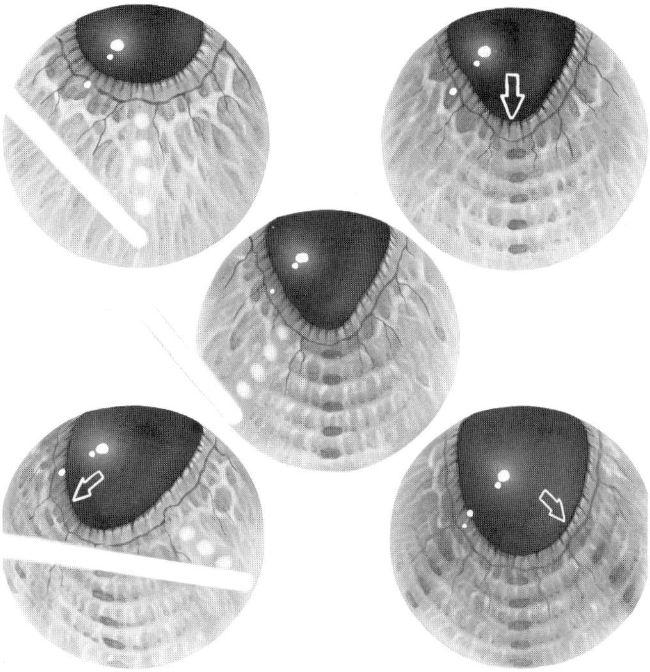

11.1a Updrawn pupil hindering ophthalmoscopy.

Upper left: using a spot size of 200 μm and an argon laser power setting of 0.5–0.6 W in dark irides and 0.75–0.8 W in blue irides, laser applications are made in a radial fashion from the pupillary margin to the peripheral iris (2).

Upper right: radial laser burns cause radial shrinkage of iris collagen fibers to change an updrawn pupil to a U-shaped one (arrow).

Center: an additional radial row of laser burns is applied from the pupillary margin to the peripheral iris.

Lower left: the additional row of laser burns tends to increase the pupillary diameter in the direction of the arrow.

Lower right: another radial row of laser burns (arrow) rounds out the pupil.

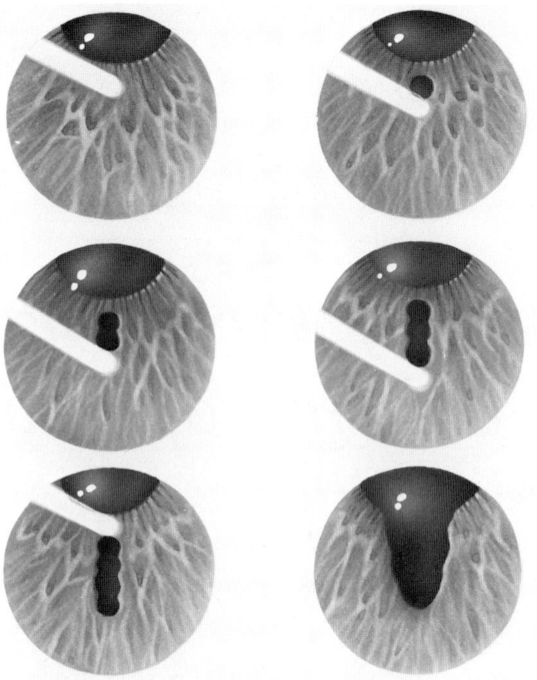

11.1b Nd:YAG laser sphincterotomy.

Upper left: using a setting of 6–10 mJ, applications of Nd:YAG laser are begun away from the iris sphincter, to reduce the risk of hemorrhage early in the procedure (1).

Upper right, center left, center right: confluent applications are added in a radial direction.

Lower left: the sphincter is cut last so that bleeding is minimized for as long as possible.

Lower right: following cutting of the sphincter, a spacious pupillary opening may be obtained. Pressure on the globe with a contact lens or finger for a few minutes may stop bleeding from the iris; if not, subsequent treatment sessions must be carried out.

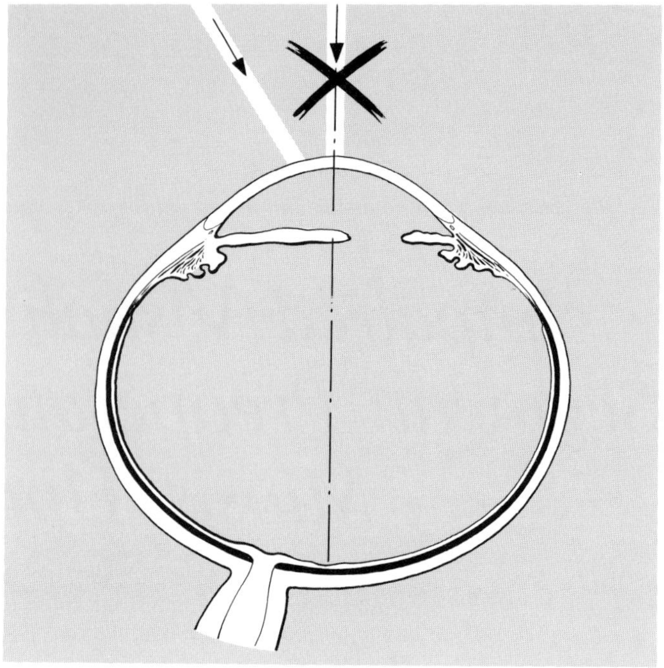

11.1c Care must be taken to apply the laser at an angle that avoids the posterior pole of the fundus, so that if the iris is perforated, the beam will not fall on the macula.

2a

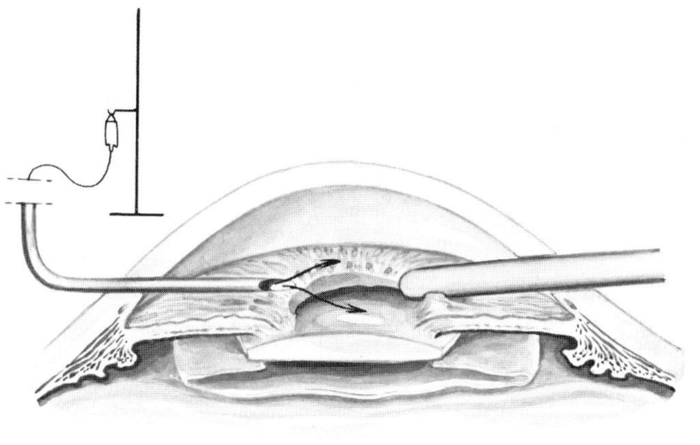

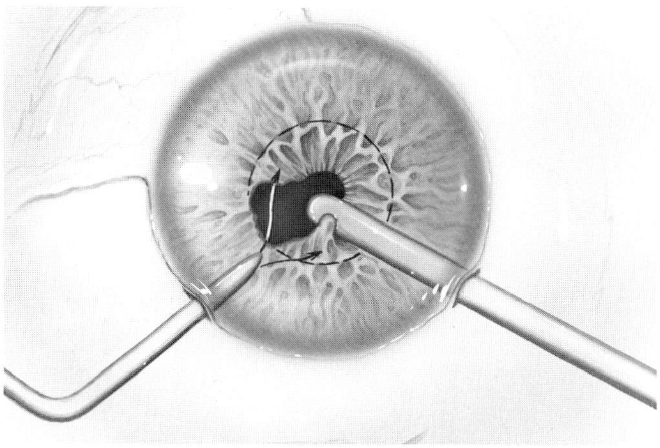

2b

11.**2a** A small pupil in a pseudophakic eye with a posterior chamber intraocular lens may be caused by posterior synechiae. This complication may develop as a result of iridocyclitis, endophthalmitis, or rubeosis iridis. Since experience has shown that Nd:YAG laser coreoplasty is inadequate when extensive posterior synechiae are present, we perform coreoplasty with the vitrectomy probe.

The anterior chamber is infused with BSS Plus using a 25-gauge bent needle inserted through the limbus. The vitrectomy probe is introduced into the anterior chamber through the limbus, 180° from the infusion needle. Epinephrine hydrochloride (1:1000) 0.3 ml is added to 500 ml of the BSS Plus infusion fluid to control bleeding from the iris. A small iridectomy is made between the peripheral and pupillary iris using the vitrectomy probe at a low level of suction. When a full thickness of iris is engaged in the cutting port, the iris is lifted slightly and cut. Sodium hyaluronate 1% is injected under the iris through the iridectomy to separate the iris from the lens. Synechiae at the pupillary margin are broken with a round wire spatula that is swept between the lens and iris. The iridectomy is enlarged toward the pupil and around it until the desired pupillary opening has been accomplished.

11.**2b** The pupillary opening is enlarged with the vitrectomy probe by nibbling the iris margin until the desired pupil size is attained. Sodium hyaluronate is removed from the anterior chamber by aspiration with the vitrectomy probe and continuous irrigation with BSS Plus. Opacities on the anterior surface of the intraocular lens are scraped gently with a flat spatula and aspirated with the vitrectomy probe. After withdrawal of the instruments from the eye, limbal incisions are closed securely with 9–0 nylon sutures.

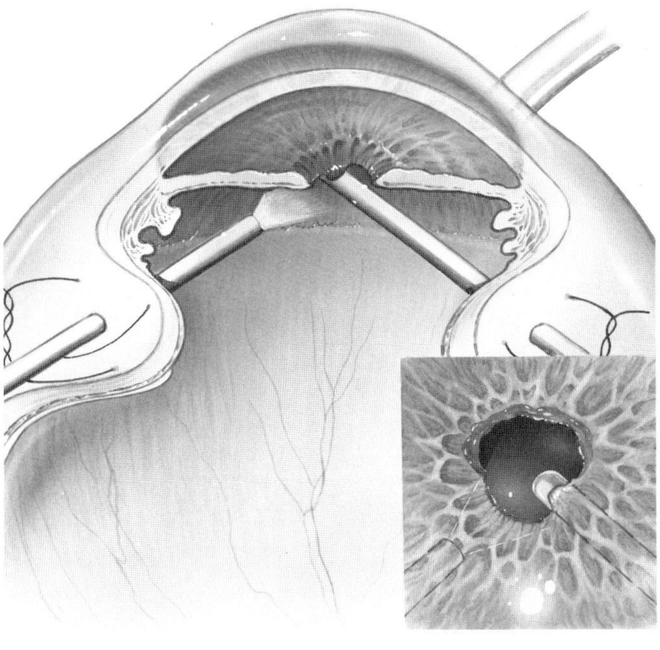

11.**3** In aphakic eyes, enlargement of the pupil is carried out using a vitrectomy probe inserted through the pars plana. Iris tissue at the pupillary margin is removed at low suction level and high cutting speed, which removes small bites.

4

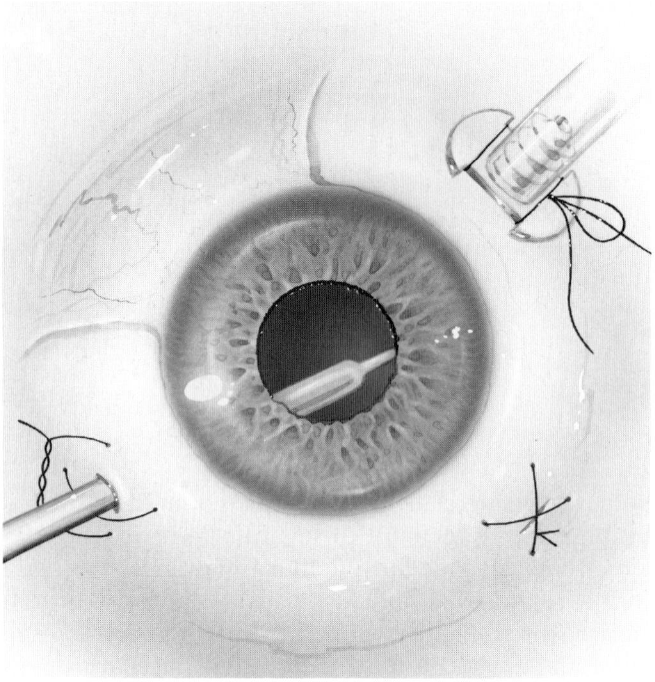

11.**4** The vitrectomy probe produces a circular but scalloped pupil. Application of light endodiathermy to the pupillary margin converts it to a circle. Vitrectomy for vitreous hemorrhage or posterior retinal pathology requires only a moderately enlarged pupil; a large pupil is necessary if vitreous surgery is contemplated in the fundus periphery or the region of the vitreous base.

11.**5a** Permanent enlargement of the pupil may be objectionable to some patients for cosmetic reasons. In addition, removal of iris tissue may produce postoperative hyphema and a marked inflammatory response in the anterior chamber, resulting in the formation of a pupillary membrane. An intact pupil may facilitate future intraocular lens implantation. Temporary enlargement of the pupil may be obtained with sutures exerting traction on the pupillary margin. The procedure requires a special needle with a long straight shaft and sharp point, and a 10–0 polypropylene suture. Limbal incisions are made with a Wheeler knife in oblique meridians of the eye. Sodium hyaluronate is injected into the anterior chamber. The needle and its suture are passed across the anterior chamber through the limbal incisions. The suture is cut, leaving long ends outside the anterior chamber.

b Using an MVR blade, pars plana incisions are made 3.5 mm from the limbus, in the same meridians as the suture. A Sinsky hook is inserted through the sclerotomy to reach the pupil, the suture is hooked through the pupil, pulled out of the eye, cut with a long end, and tied temporarily. The same steps are followed in pulling the suture out from the anterior chamber in the opposite quadrant.

5a

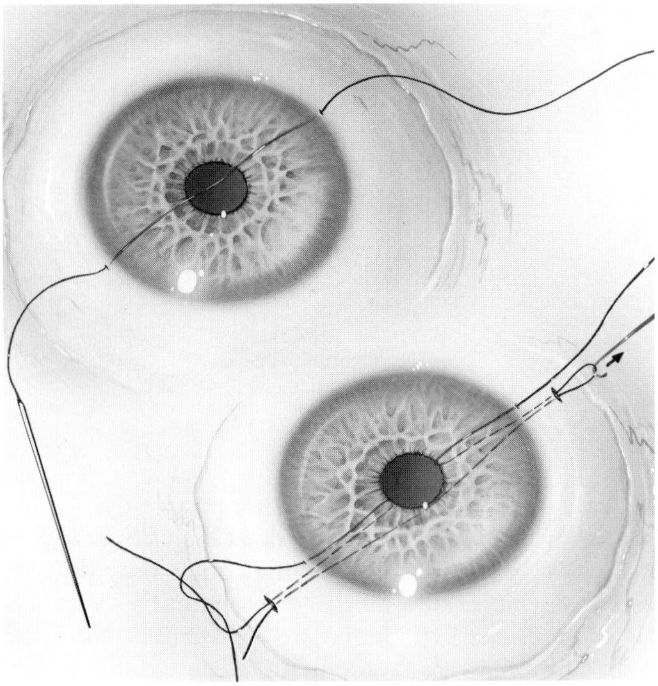

5b

5c

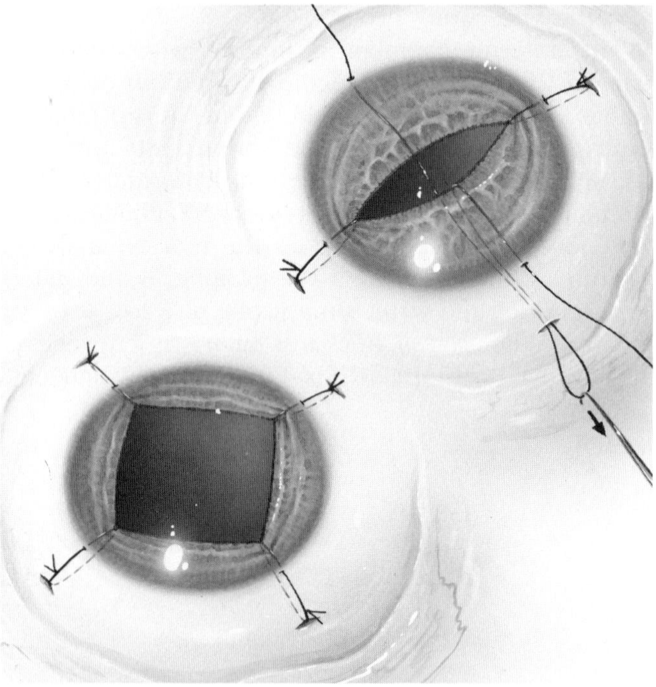

5d

11.**5c** The arms of the suture in each quadrant are tied snugly to create an obliquely elongated pupil.
d The same steps are followed for the other oblique meridians to form a temporarily enlarged, square pupil.

References

1. Eckardt C. Pupillary stretching: a new procedure in vitreous surgery. Retina 1985; 5:235–238.
2. Schepens CL. Retinal detachment and allied diseases. Philadelphia: WB Saunders, 1983; 971–972.

12

Impaired Visualization of Posterior Segment: Pupillary Membranes in Aphakic Eyes; Miosis and Pupillary Membranes in Pseudophakic Eyes

Pupillary Membranes in Aphakic Eyes

Pupillary membranes may hinder visualization of the vitreous and fundus during vitreoretinal surgery. The membranes are often associated with penetrating injury to the eye, previous intraocular surgery, intraocular inflammation, or intraocular lens implantation (4–6).

If the pupillary membrane cannot be photodisrupted by the Nd: YAG laser, it may be approached surgically through the limbus or pars plana, depending on the type of surgery planned in the posterior ocular segment. The limbal approach is suitable for cases requiring scleral buckling only. The pars plana approach is used when the pathology of the posterior segment requires vitrectomy with or without scleral buckling. There are some exceptions: the limbal approach may be used initially for removing the pupillary membrane if a high detachment of the peripheral retina including the ora serrata is suspected. When the pupillary space has been cleared and the peripheral vitreous and retina are visible, a sclerotomy can be more safely made through the pars plana. Variations of the technique and alternative steps are offered if one technique or step fails.

a

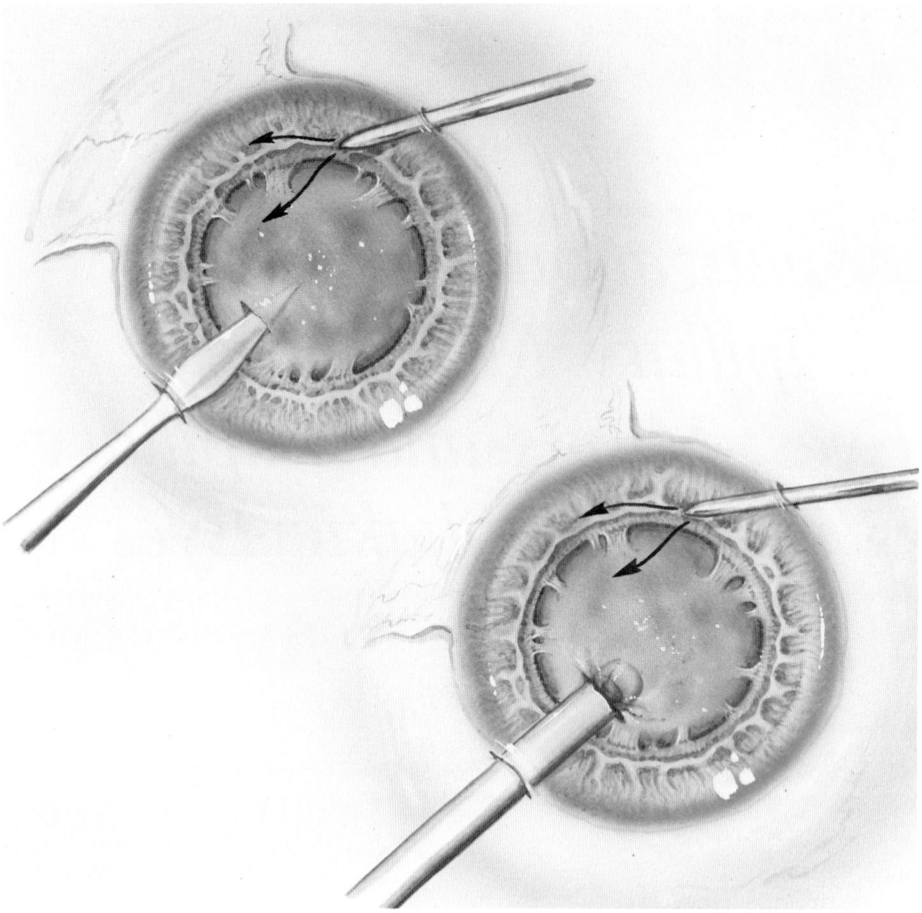

b

12.**1** Anterior chamber infusion is used to keep the anterior chamber formed.

a Using an MVR knife, an incision is made in the membrane.

b The vitrectomy probe is inserted into the anterior chamber and into the incision in the membrane, which is nibbled away until the pupillary area is clear (2: 294–303).

Limited anterior vitrectomy is performed. The limbal incision is closed with a 9–0 polypropylene suture. The infusion needle is removed and the incision sutured. The surgeon proceeds with the planned scleral buckling.

a

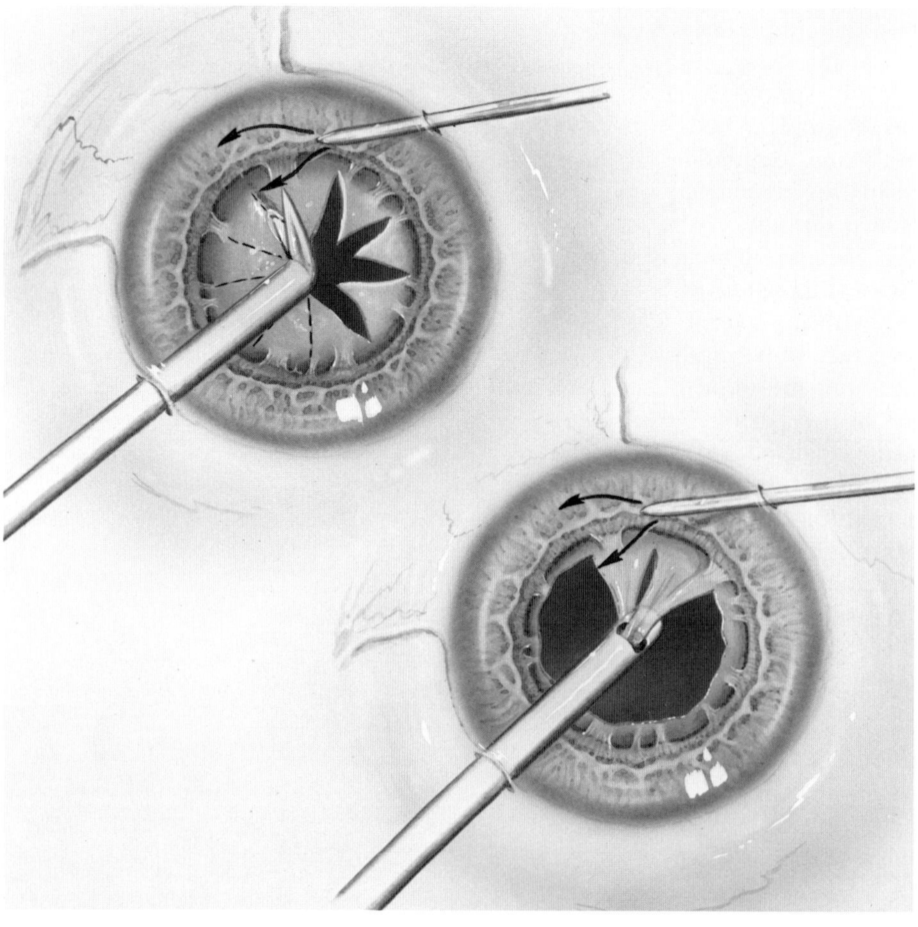

b

12.**2** Thick, rigid pupillary membranes cannot be cut effectively with the vitrectomy probe, because they cannot be molded and aspirated into its cutting port.

a An incision is made in the center of the membrane using an MVR knife. Using 60° angulated Sutherland scissors, the membrane is cut into small thin wedges that can be aspirated into the probe. One blade of the scissors is inserted through the incision in the center of the membrane, and radial cuts are made extending to the margin of the pupil. The infusion needle and scissors are interchanged so that all areas of the membrane can be reached and cut.

b The scissors are replaced with the vitrectomy probe, which is used to trim the pie-shaped segments and to clear the pupillary space. The cutting frequency setting is low, the suction and infusion settings are high.

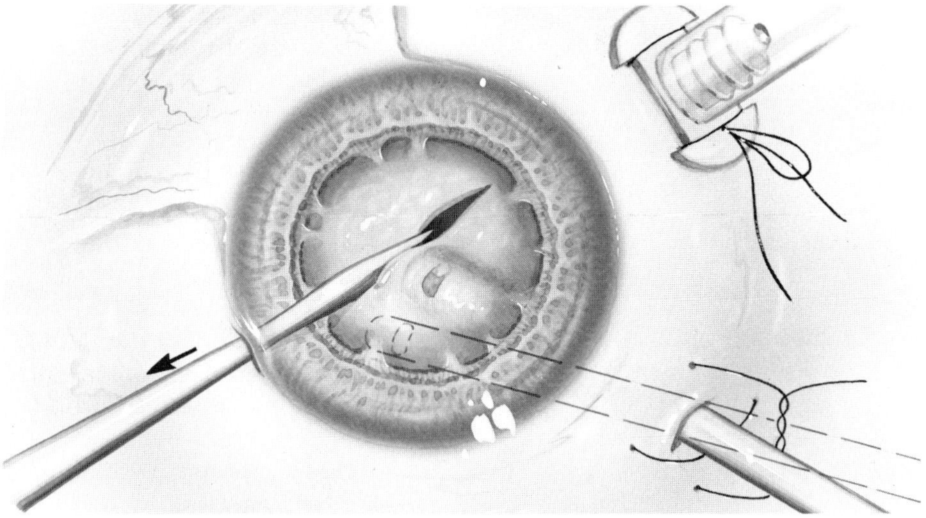

12.**3a** Counterpressure with a vitrectomy probe may be helpful if difficulty is encountered in trying to penetrate a thick pupillary membrane (2: 296). In this illustration, a pars plana infusion cannula has been inserted, since vitrectomy is necessary.

A pars plana sclerotomy is made with an MVR blade to allow introduction of a vitrectomy probe behind the pupillary membrane. The MVR blade is introduced into the anterior chamber through the limbus. To cut the membrane effectively, the membrane is pushed gently forward by the vitrectomy probe from behind, increasing tension on the membrane while slicing it near the probe tip. The probe is moved in the direction of the slicing action.

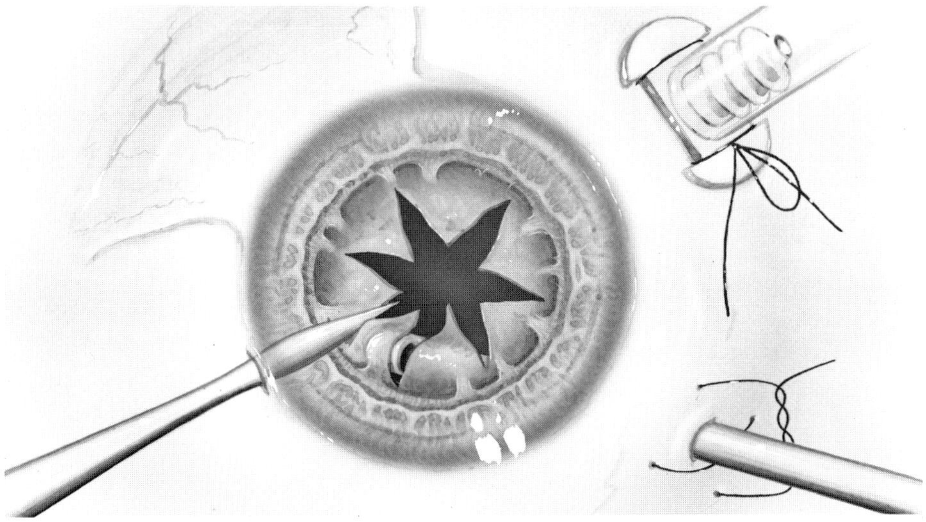

12.**3b** The slicing action with the knife is continued until the pieces of sectioned membrane are sufficiently small to be aspirated into the cutting port of the probe (3). The fundus is checked after the pupil has been cleared.

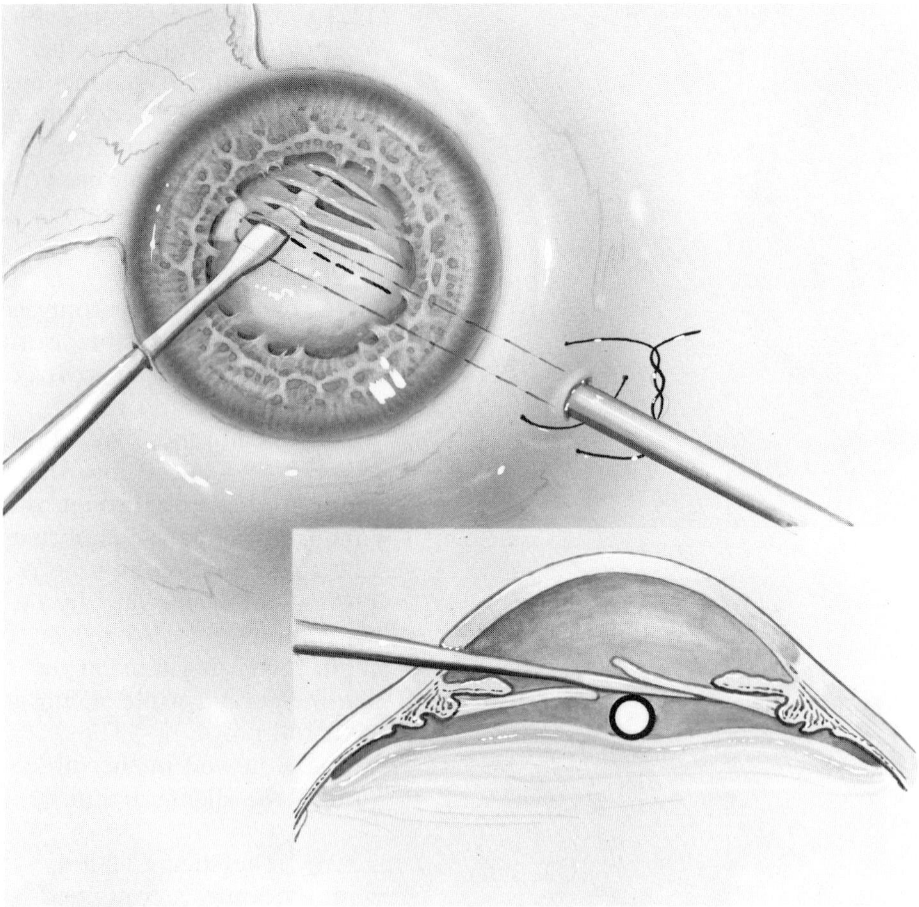

12.**3c** Some pupillary membranes are so tough that they cannot be cut into small pieces with scissors. In such cases, an MVR knife is inserted through the limbus into the anterior chamber to slice the tough membrane into narrow parallel strips. Sodium hyaluronate 1% is injected to maintain the depth of the anterior chamber. The light pipe is inserted through one of the pars plana sclerotomies in the upper quadrant to illuminate the pupillary area and to support the membrane as the knife slices it (inset). Multiple slices are made, converting the membrane into parallel strips. These strips are cut across on one end along the pupillary margin, allowing their free end to be removed with the vitrectomy probe.

If there is no need for a vitrectomy, an infusion needle is inserted into the anterior chamber through the limbal incision for the knife. The light pipe is replaced with the vitrectomy probe, which aspirates and removes the membrane strips.

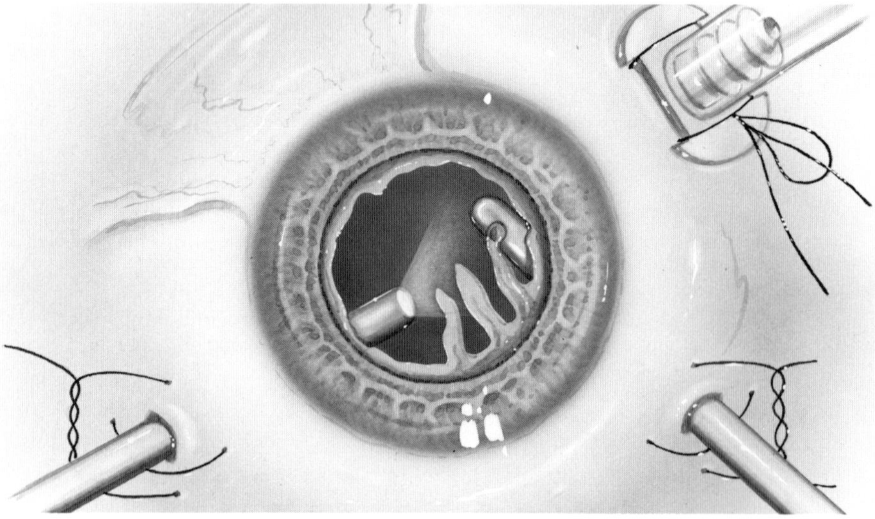

12.**3d** If an aphakic eye with a tough pupillary membrane requires a vitrectomy, the procedure described in Figure 12.**4** is followed. The limbal opening is closed with 9–0 polypropylene suture. Sclerotomies for the infusion cannula and a second instrument are prepared. The membrane which has been sliced into strips is removed with the vitrectomy probe inserted through the sclerotomy in the pars plana.

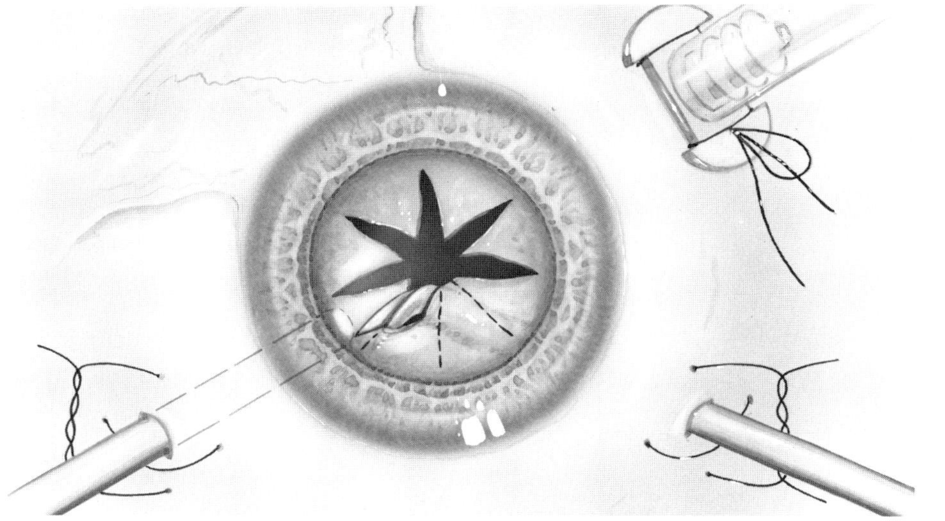

Miosis and Pupillary Membranes in Pseudophakic Eyes

12.**4** In cases in which the pupillary membrane is associated with posterior segment pathology that requires vitrectomy, the membrane is removed using a pars plana approach. The light pipe is introduced into the vitreous to retroilluminate the pupillary membrane. Sutherland scissors are inserted into the anterior vitreous and pupillary area; one blade is made to penetrate the membrane from behind, and the membrane is cut into multiple radial strips. Sutherland scissors with different blade angles may be needed to reach all the meridians effectively. The scissors are replaced with a vitrectomy probe, which is used to remove the strips.

a

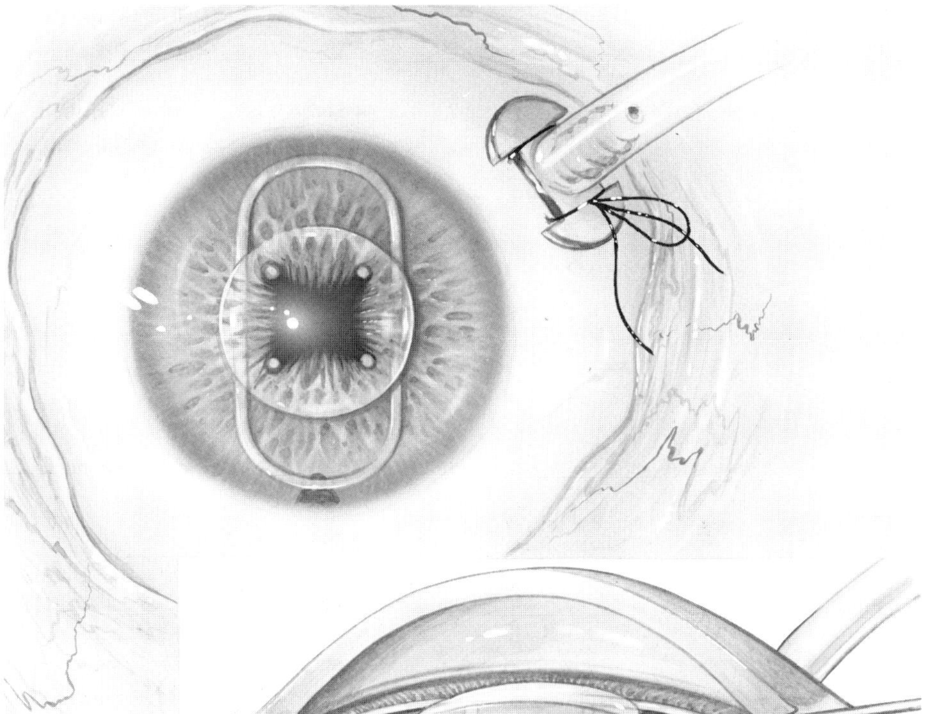

b

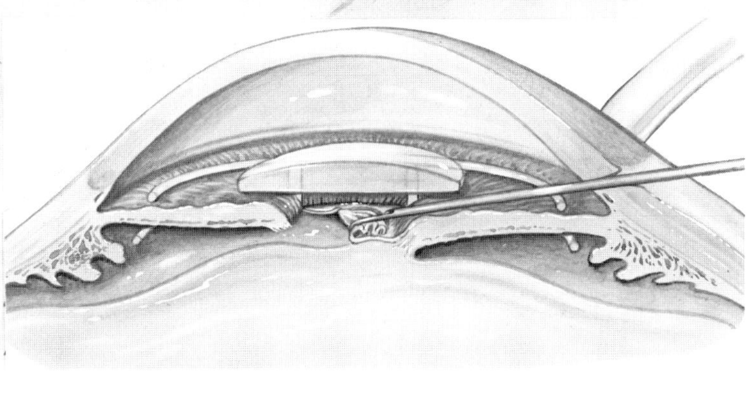

12.**5a** Although iris-fixed lenses are no longer implanted, eyes in which these lenses were implanted may develop posterior segment problems requiring vitreous or retinal surgery. Visualization of the fundus may be impaired by a small pupil or by pupillary membranes in eyes with anterior chamber lenses. If vitrectomy is not planned or is doubtful, a limbal approach is used. If vitrectomy is contemplated, as in this case, the pars plana approach is employed; an infusion cannula is therefore inserted as shown.

b Sodium hyaluronate 1% is injected into the anterior chamber in front of the lens to prevent contact between cornea and lens. A 25-gauge needle with a bent, sharp end is used to perform a capsulotomy (1: 263–267). A discission of the pupillary membrane is made using a bent 25-gauge needle inserted through a limbal incision. The needle is passed beneath the lens to engage the membrane near the opposite pupillary margin. A pupillary opening is created toward the limbal incision.

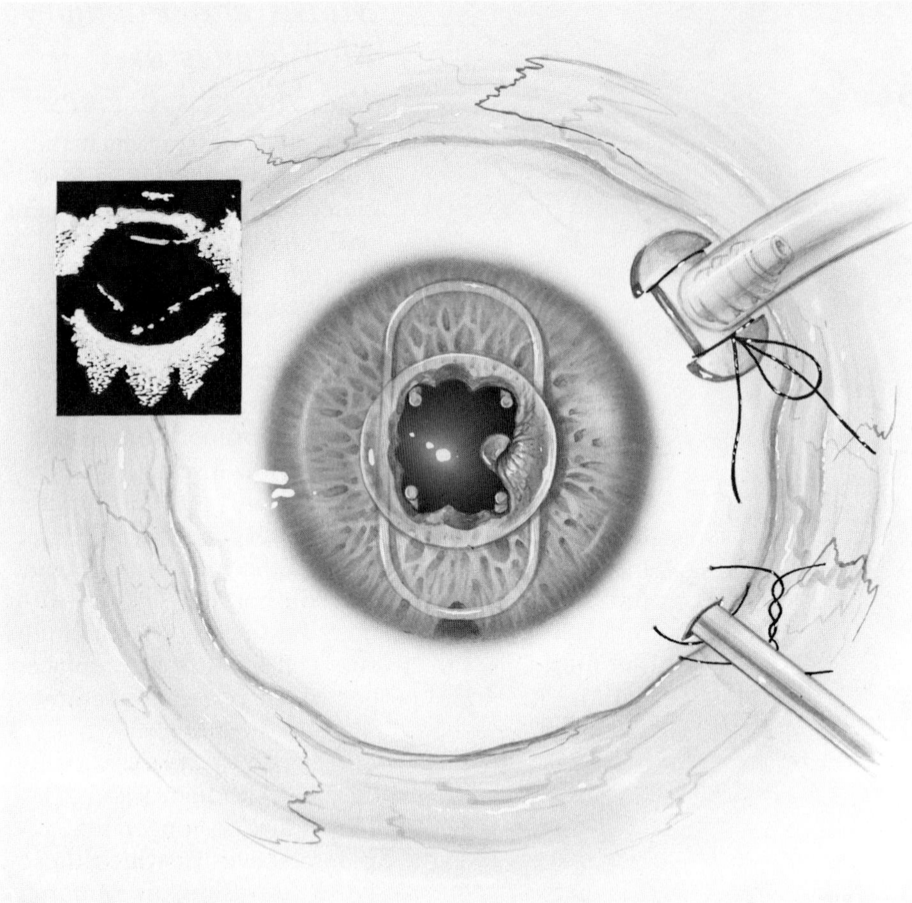

12.**5c** The pupil is enlarged with a vitrectomy probe inserted through a sclerotomy in the pars plana. At high cutting frequency, low suction level, and moderate infusion pressure, the margin of the pupil is trimmed with the vitrectomy probe, without producing a large pupil through which the lens can dislocate posteriorly.

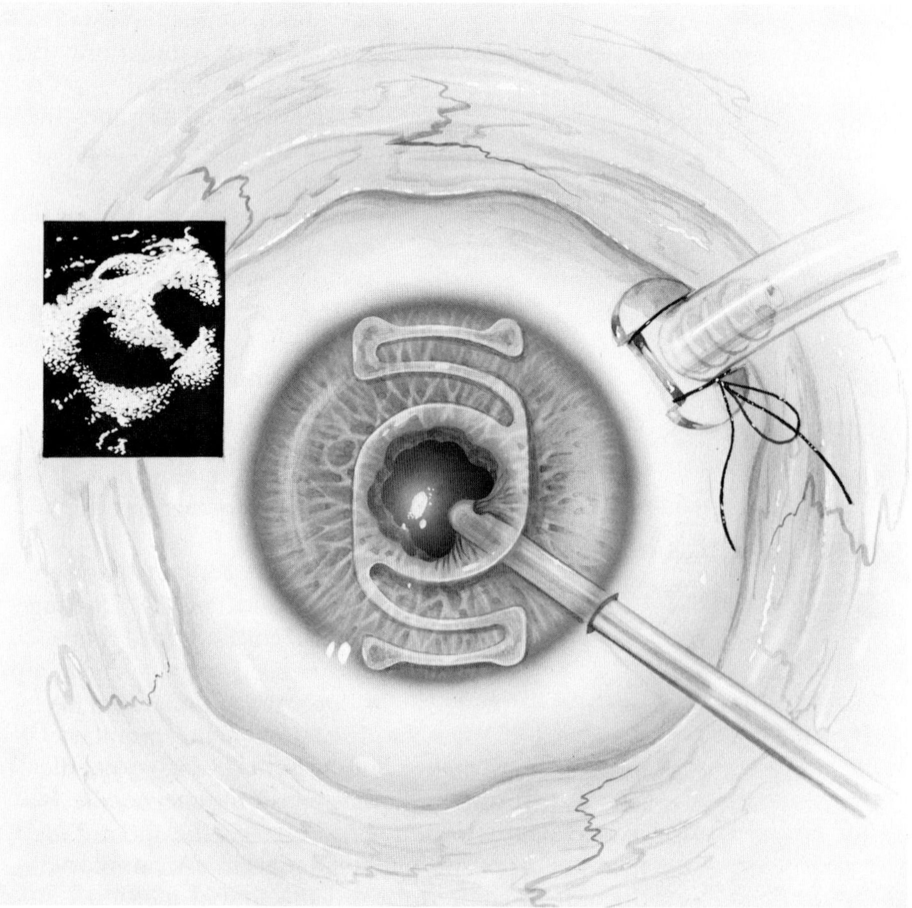

12.**6** An anterior chamber lens in an eye with an opaque pupillary membrane and posterior synechiae which prevent visualization of retinal breaks in a retinal detachment. *Inset:* ultrasonography indicates that the inferior temporal ora serrata and pars plana are not highly detached; therefore, an infusion cannula is placed in that quadrant. Sodium hyaluronate 1% is injected through a limbal incision to maintain the depth of the anterior chamber.

The vitrectomy probe is inserted through the limbal incision and introduced between the intraocular lens and iris. Using a high cutting frequency and low suction, tissue is removed along the iris margin to enlarge the pupil to a size no larger than the optical portion of the lens. An incision is made in the capsule to permit penetration of the vitrectomy probe. With the cutting port facing anteriorly, the central portion of the capsule is removed.

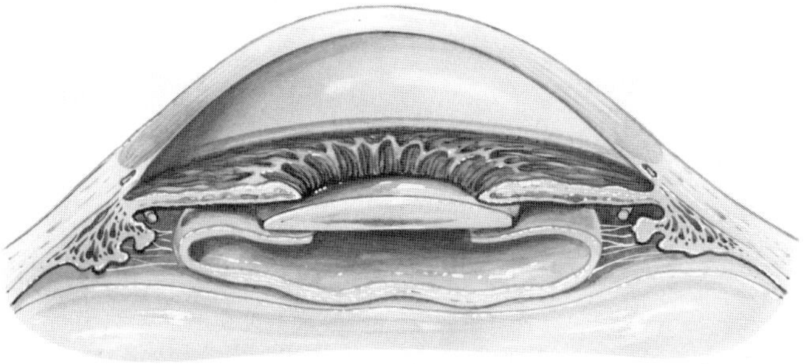

12.**7a** In an eye with a posterior chamber lens, opacification of the posterior capsule may prevent visualization of the fundus (1: 257–262). If the capsule is so thickened that a capsulotomy cannot be made with the Nd:YAG laser, an intraocular procedure is necessary for removal of the capsule.

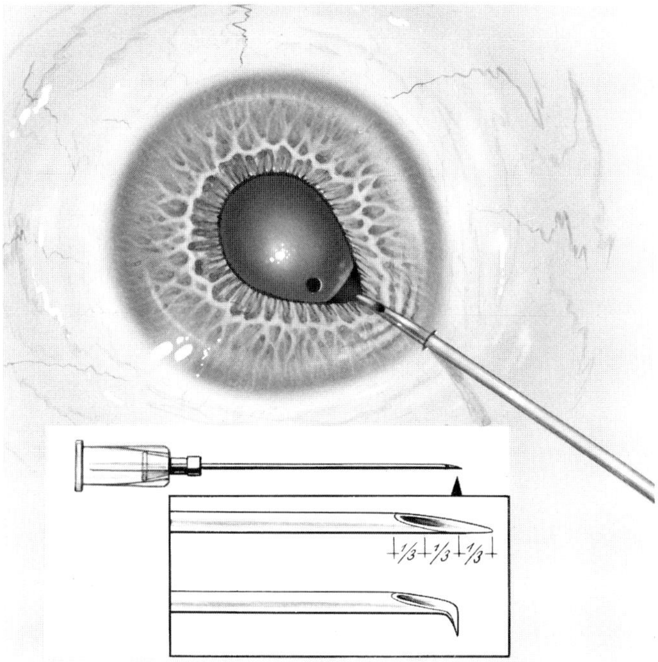

12.**7b** *Inset:* a 25-gauge needle is bent 90° at two-thirds of the distance along its bevelled edge, and attached to an infusion bottle containing balanced saline solution.

A limbal incision is made through which the needle is inserted and used to retract the iris to expose the edge of the intraocular lens.

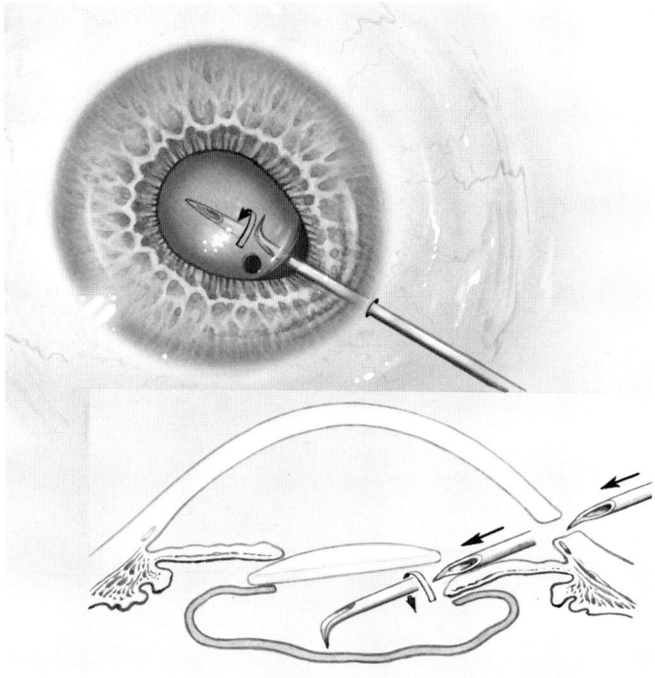

12.**7c** The tip of the needle is then turned horizontally to avoid scratching the intraocular lens, passed between the posterior surface of the lens and the posterior capsule, and across the pupil to engage the peripheral posterior capsule. *Inset:* The needle tip is then rotated posteriorly so that the capsule can be engaged.

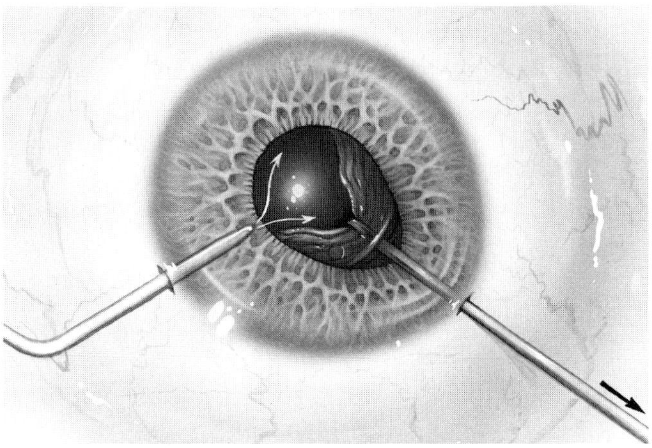

12.**7d** An infusion needle is inserted through the limbus to prevent the anterior chamber from collapsing. Once the posterior capsule is engaged by the bent needle, it is incised by drawing the needle back toward the limbal incision.

7e

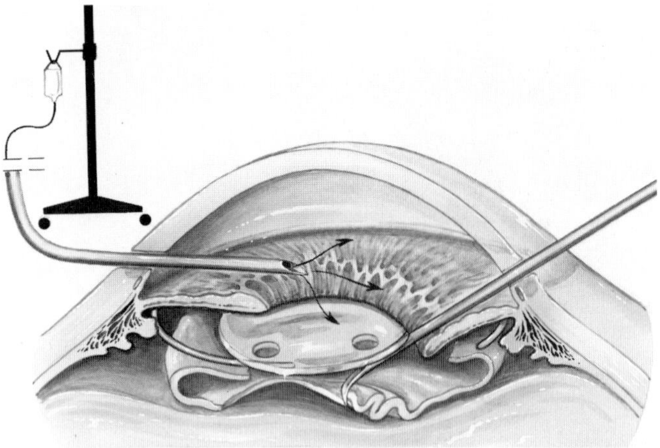

7g

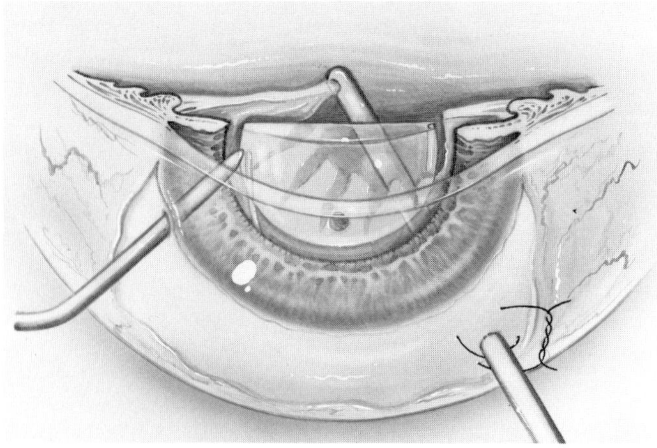

7f

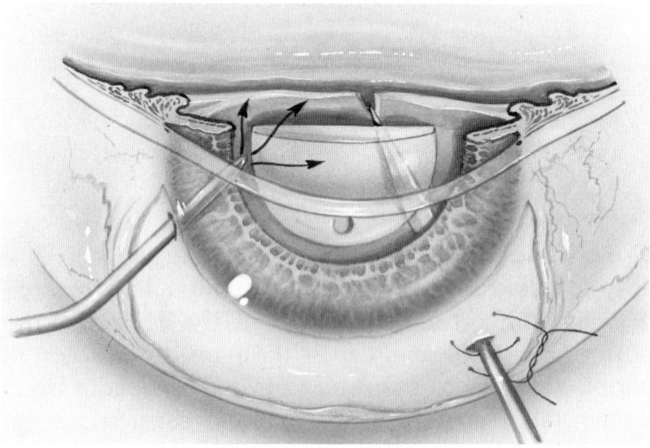

7h

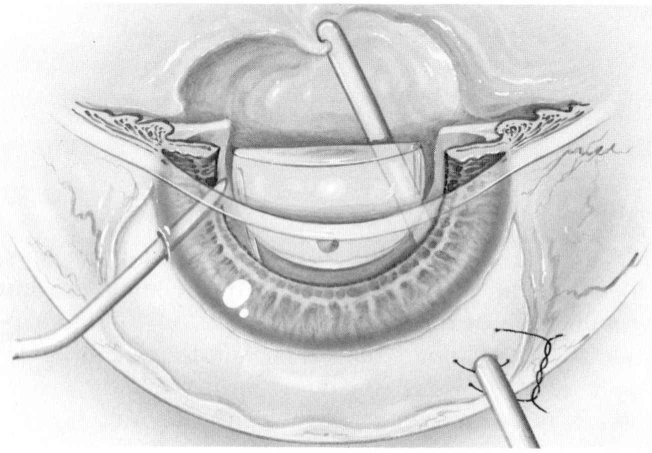

12.**7e** Additional passes are made with the bent needle to engage and clear capsule from the pupil.

12.**7f** Some tough posterior capsular membranes resist aspiration and cutting with the vitrectomy probe. An MVR knife is inserted through the pars plana and used to cut the membrane from behind, breaking it into smaller strips that can be aspirated into the cutting port of the vitrectomy probe. The infusion needle is retained in the anterior chamber to keep the eye firm while suction is being exerted by the vitrectomy probe.

12.**7g** The strips of membrane behind the lens are removed using the vitrectomy probe inserted through a sclerotomy in the pars plana.

12.**7h** After removing the posterior capsular membrane, an anterior vitrectomy is done to improve visualization of the peripheral and central fundus. If a total vitrectomy is needed, another sclerotomy is made for the endoilluminator. An infusion cannula is inserted into the lower temporal quadrant. The limbal incision is closed.

References

1. Clayman HM, Jaffe NS, Galin M. Intraocular lens implantation: techniques and complications. St. Louis: C V Mosby, 1983.
2. Michels RG. Vitreous surgery. St. Louis: C V Mosby, 1980.
3. Rice TA, Michels RG, Stark WJ, eds. Operative surgery: ophthalmic surgery. 4th ed. St. Louis: C V Mosby, 1984: 238–240. (Rob and Smith's operative surgery series.)
4. Wilkinson CP. Closed vitreous surgery for complications of intraocular lens implantation, I: indications. In: Blankenship GW, Stirpe M, Gonvers M, Binder S, eds. Basic and advanced vitreous surgery. Padua: Liviana, 1986: 135–140.
5. Wilkinson CP. Closed vitreous surgery for complications of intraocular lens implantation, II: techniques. In: Blankenship GW, Stirpe M, Gonvers M, Binder S, eds. Basic and advanced vitreous surgery. Padua: Liviana, 1986: 145–151.
6. Wilkinson CP. Closed vitreous surgery for complications of intraocular lens implantation, III: results and complications. In: Blankenship GW, Stirpe M, Gonvers M, Binder S, eds. Basic and advanced vitreous surgery. Padua: Liviana, 1986: 141–144.

13

Preexisting Cataract

Substantial lens opacities hamper preoperative assessment of the vitreous and fundus, as well as intraoperative visualization of the posterior segment.

Lensectomy or phacoemulsification is recommended in young patients whose cataract appears soft (7). Extracapsular cataract surgery with or without a posterior chamber intraocular lens is indicated in eyes with a hard nucleus that is not removed easily with the phacoemulsifiying probe. Implantation of an anterior chamber intraocular lens should be avoided in an eye that may need vitreoretinal surgery, because this type of lens tends to interfere with visualization during surgery.

Eyes with ischemic ocular disease, such as diabetic retinopathy, demand special consideration because they are prone to develop rubeosis iridis after cataract surgery (2). This complication is likely to occur when lensectomy and vitreoretinal surgery are combined in the same operation. In elective cases, eyes with ischemic ocular disease have prior removal of cataract, followed 3–6 weeks later by vitreoretinal surgery. Cataract and vitreoretinal surgery may be combined in the same session in emergency cases. In these eyes, supplemental panphotocoagulation of the fundus, including the periphery, should be carried out intraoperatively to prevent rubeosis iridis. Extracapsular cataract extraction, which leaves an intact posterior capsule, may minimize rubeosis iridis. If rubeosis iridis is present preoperatively, focal laser to the vessels in the filtration angle should be completed first. The temptation to place any type of intraocular lens must be resisted in these cases.

The hardness of the lens nucleus is judged traditionally by its color. A yellow appearance suggests a soft nucleus that may be removed successfully with a vitrectomy probe. A yellow-brown nucleus indicates moderate hardness that may be removed by phacoemulsification (4). A dark brown or black-brown lens indicates a very hard, large nucleus that is usually not amenable to phacoemulsification and is best removed through the cornea.

a

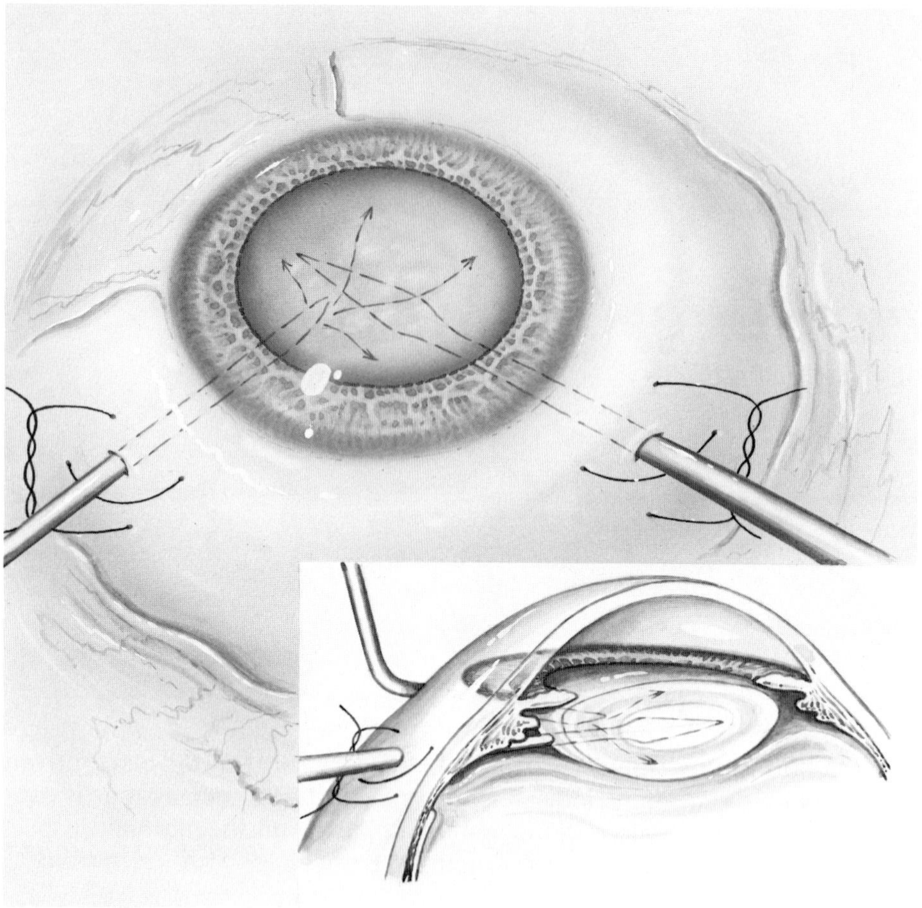

b

Removal of a Soft Lens

13.**1** A soft lens is removed through the pars plana (1,3,5,6,8: 111–114, 9).

a A bent 25-gauge infusion needle is inserted through the pars plana sclerotomy to penetrate the equator and nucleus of the lens. An MVR blade is introduced through the other sclerotomy, passing through the lens equator and nucleus. Little or no resistance as the blade penetrates the nucleus indicates a soft cataract that can be removed by lensectomy.

b The blade is rotated slowly to macerate the nucleus and cortex. The lens material is infused and hydrated with BSS Plus. The infusion pressure is decreased to avoid breakage of the posterior capsule.

a

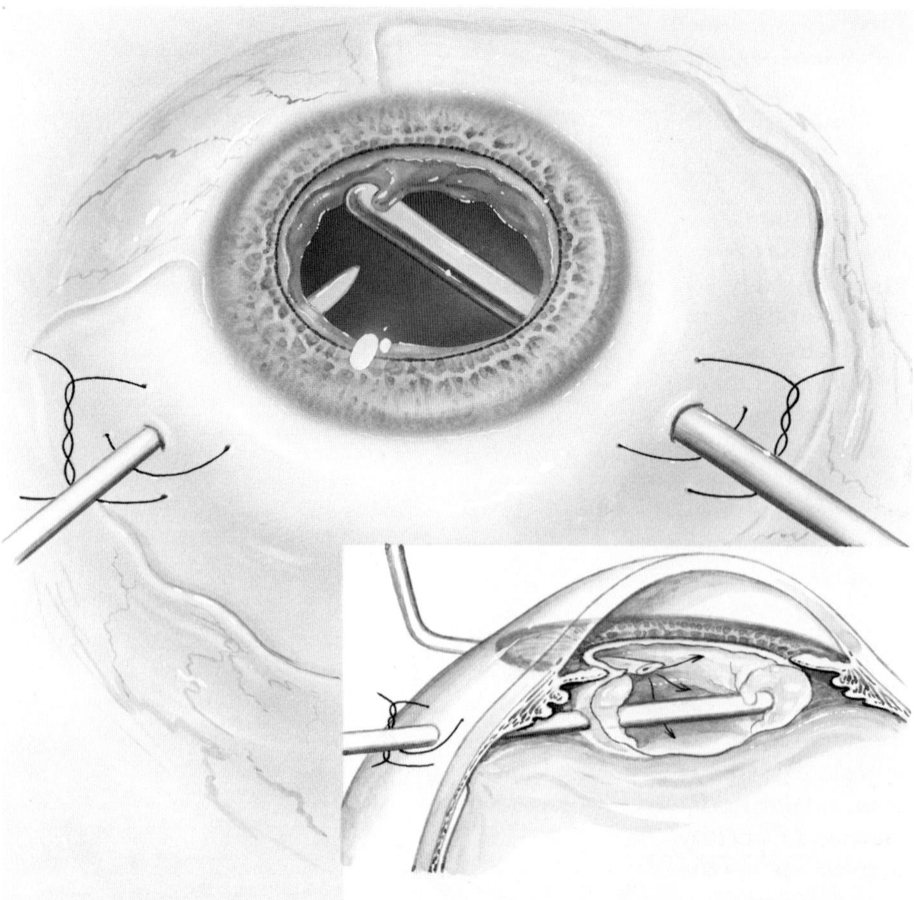

b

13.**2a** Withdrawal of the knife from the eye is followed by insertion of the vitrectomy probe through the incision. Lens material is aspirated using a high suction level without cutting. The nucleus of the lens is removed first. Fragmented nuclear materials may have to be pushed into the port with the infusion needle.

b When a central cavity has been created in the lens, peripheral cortical material is suctioned toward the central cavity, where it is removed.

Gentle depression of the sclera helps to ensure complete removal of the lens cortex from the periphery. All these maneuvers to remove the lens are carried out within the capsular bag. The posterior capsule is inspected, and residual opacities are aspirated gently. Using an

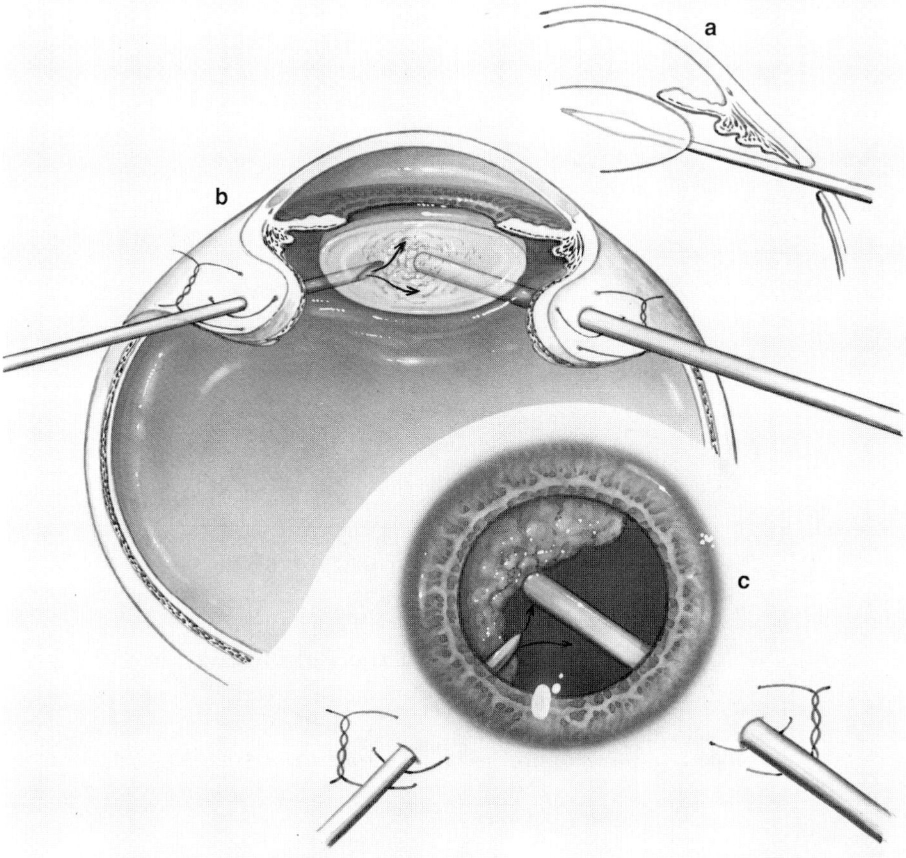

Removal of a Hard Lens

13.**3a** The blade enters the crystalline lens at the lens equator. The hardness of the nucleus and the feasibility of its removal with the vitrectomy probe can be determined at the time the MVR blade penetrates the lens.

b If there is a great deal of resistance to the knife during penetration of the nucleus of a hard lens, a phacoemulsifying probe is inserted instead of a vitrectomy probe.

c The nucleus is removed in a „coal-mining“ fashion inside the capsular bag. To avoid overheating the phacoprobe, it is operated at intervals to allow cooling. In addition, the capsular bag is infused with fluid at low pressure.

The lens is emulsified with a burst of ultrasonic energy, and the emulsified material is aspirated. These steps are repeated until all the lens material in the bag has been removed. If "lens milk" appears, the phacoemulsification probe should be removed immediately from the eye, or thermal damage to the sclera will result.

When all the nucleus has been removed, the cortex is suctioned to the center of the capsular bag and emulsified.

▷ MVR knife, the anterior capsule is incised into small, pie-shaped strips which are aspirated and cut from the center to the periphery using a vitrectomy probe. The infusion cannula is inserted into the inferior temporal quadrant in preparation for vitreoretinal surgery.

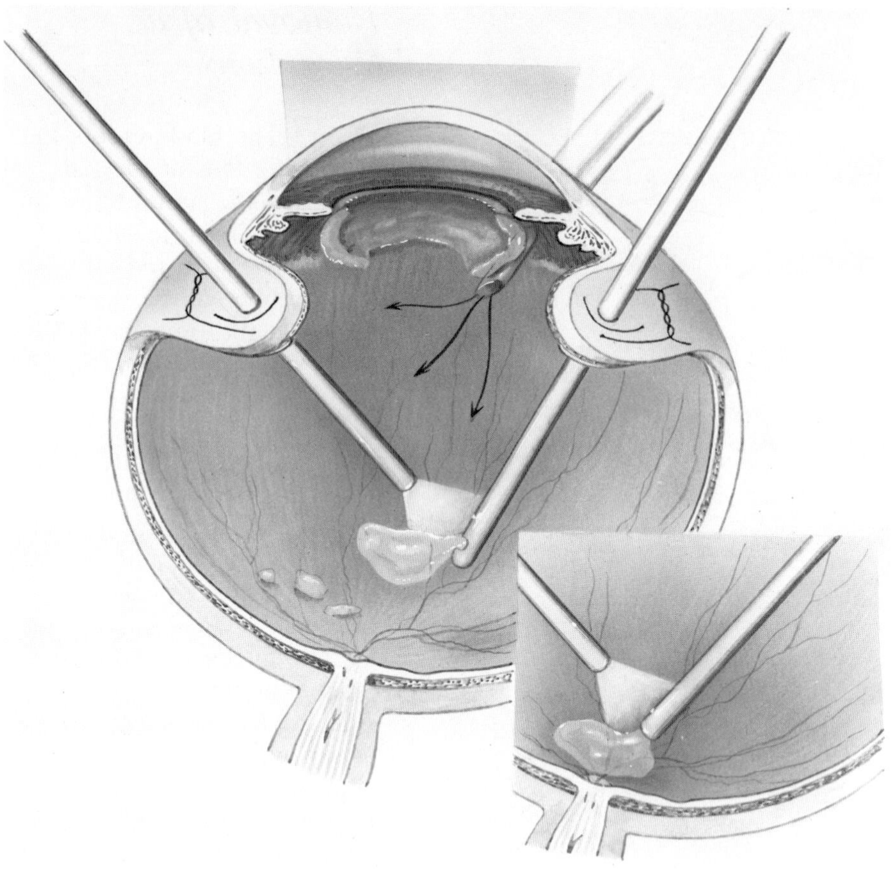

13.**4a** Fragmented cortical and nuclear lens material may inadvertently fall into the vitreous through a rupture in the posterior lens capsule. Any lens fragments trapped in vitreous gel are sucked carefully into the port of the vitrectomy probe. Large fragments are brought up to the anterior chamber, brought to rest on the iris, and aspirated out of the eye.

b Because the risk of retinal damage is great during lens aspiration with the vitrectomy probe, a flute needle is the instrument of choice for picking up large lens fragments resting on the retina. After the flute needle tip touches the material, the needle is vented to the atmosphere, creating a suction force that holds the lens material to it.

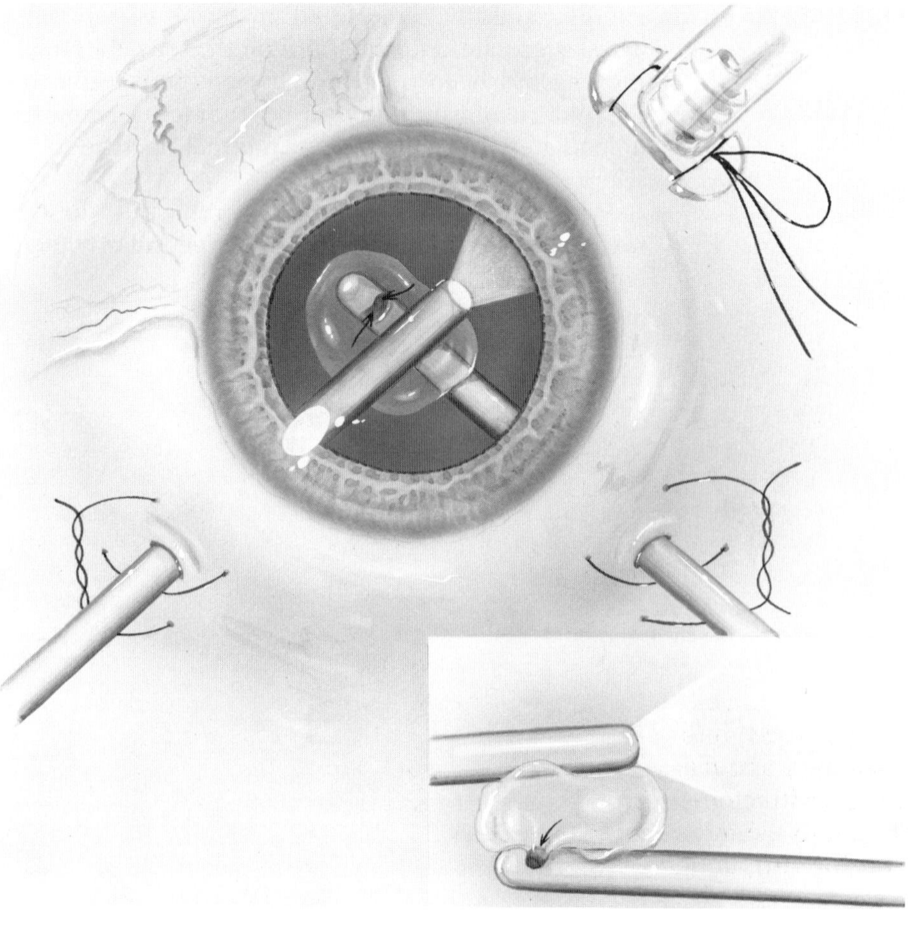

13.**5a, b** The lens is maneuvered into the anterior chamber, holding it and supporting it in place with the light pipe from behind. As soon as the lens fragment has been partially aspirated and secured in the cutting port of the probe, the light pipe is moved over the lens to assist in holding and crushing it into the cutting port. During this procedure, the probe should be in the continuous aspiration mode. **b** If fragments of a hard lens become dislocated posteriorly during phacoemulsification, they are removed after vitrectomy. The phacoemulsification probe is then reintroduced, and the fragments are brougth to the mid-vitreous for simultaneous sonification and aspiration.

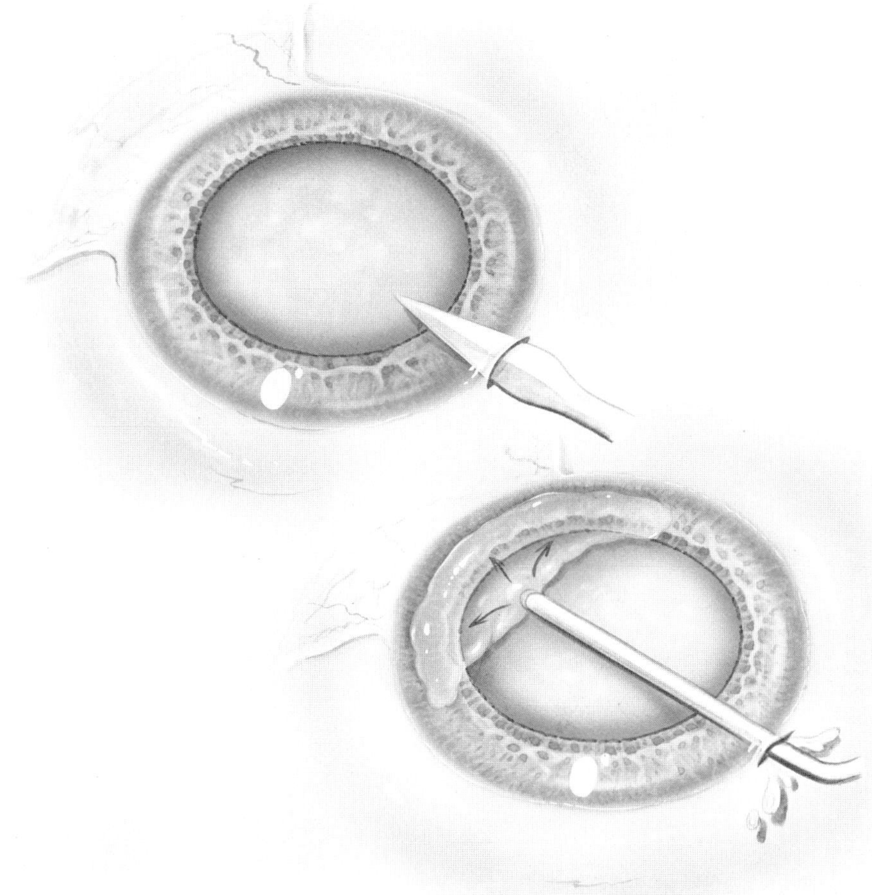

Removal of a Very Hard Lens

13.**6** A very hard cataract does not lend itself to phacoemulsification; therefore, extracapsular removal through a corneal incision is recommended (8: 116–118).

a The superior rectus tendon is imbricated with a 4–0 silk suture. A small limbal incision is made with an MVR blade or a Superblade knife to allow injection of 1% sodium hyaluronate into the anterior chamber with a 30-gauge bent needle.

b Sodium hyaluronate is first injected distal to the limbal incision to allow aqueous to exit from the eye. As injection is taking place, the needle is drawn slowly toward the incision until the anterior chamber is filled.

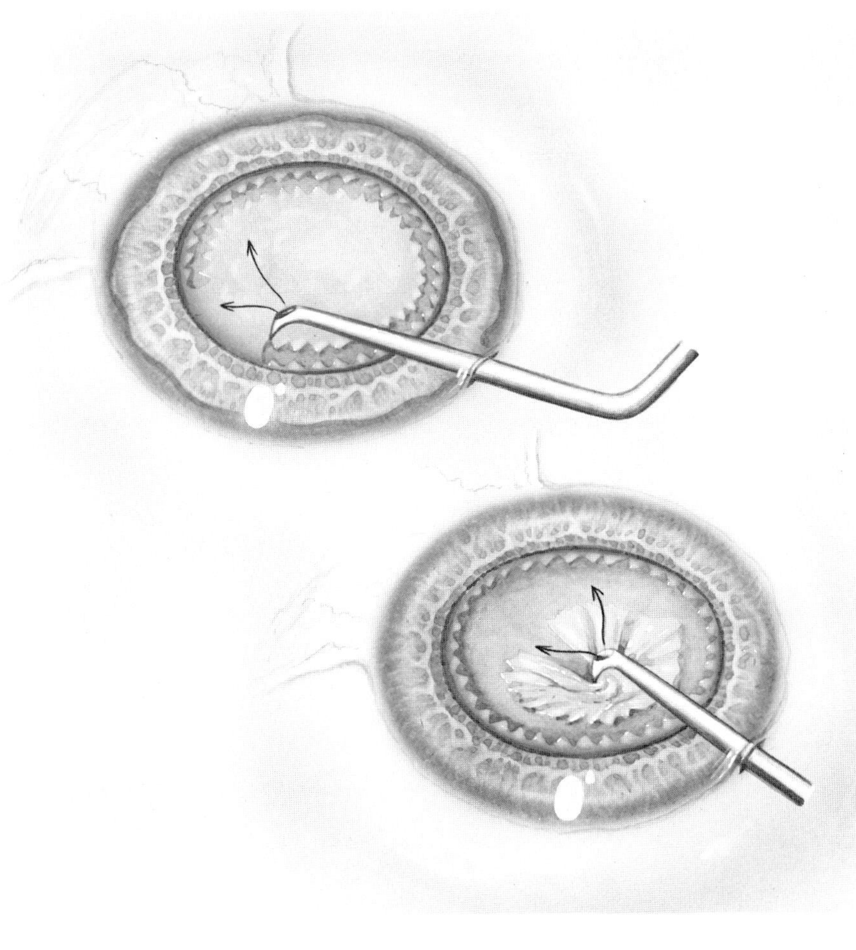

13.**7a** A 25-gauge needle made into a cystotome is inserted into the anterior chamber that has been filled with sodium hyaluronate. The cystotome is used to create a series of parallel perforations on the anterior capsule along the pupillary margin. To avoid a miotic pupillary reaction, the surgeon should be careful not to touch the iris.

b When the perforation has been completed, the cystotome is engaged at one end of the perforated capsule. The capsule is pulled toward the limbal incision, ripping the capsule through the perforation in one piece.

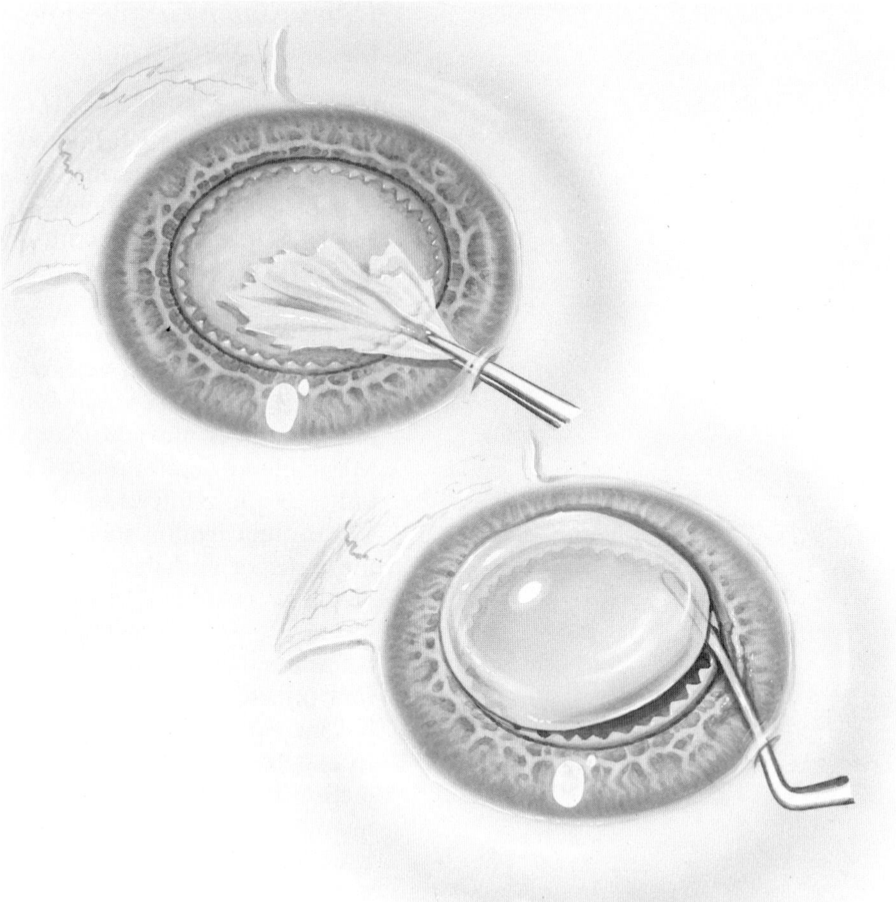

13.**8a** The torn capsule is grasped with a fine capsule forceps and removed from the eye through the small incision.

b The lens nucleus is separated from the cortex and dislocated anteriorly using a wire spatula inserted between the nucleus and the cortex.

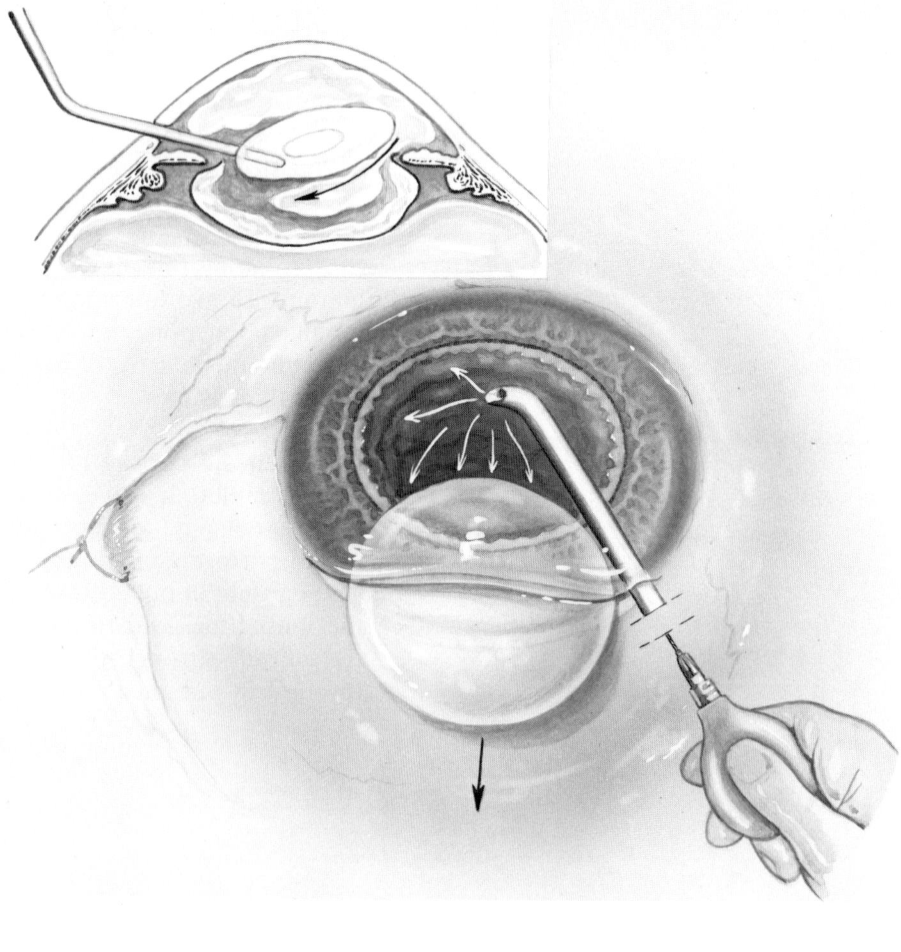

13.**9a** With a spatula the nucleus is dislocated into the anterior chamber by mechanically pushing along its side and rotating it. The sodium hyaluronate enters the space between the nucleus and the cortex and acts as a hydraulic wedge helping the dislocation.

b The limbal incision is enlarged to the approximate diameter of the nucleus. The nucleus is delivered from the anterior chamber by washing it out with the use of an irrigating tip attached to a bulb containing balanced salt solution.

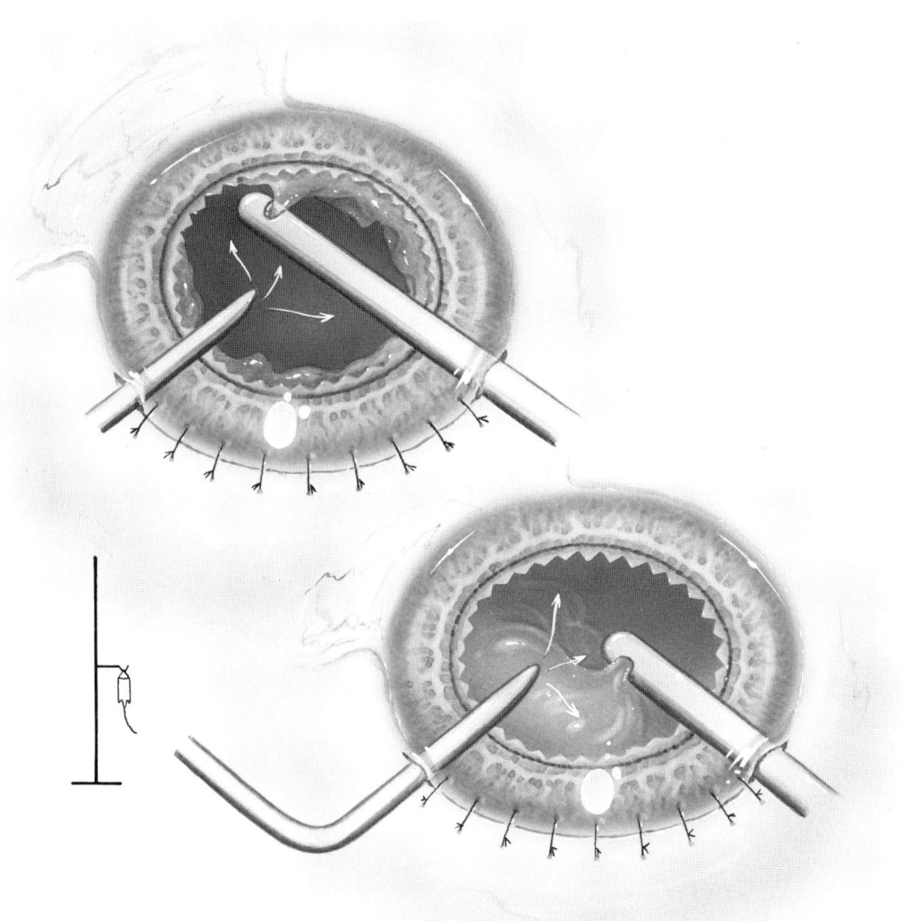

13.**10 a** The limbal incision is closed meticulously with multiple 10–0 polypropylene sutures. The 25-gauge infusion needle is inserted into the anterior chamber through one end of the closed limbal wound. The infusion pressure is set at a low level. The vitrectomy probe is inserted into the anterior chamber through the other end for the removal of cortical lens material. Suction is applied to peripheral cortical material to pull it to the center, where it is aspirated. This is repeated until all the cortical material has been removed.

b The posterior capsule is cleaned with gentle suction, the cutting port of the probe being positioned tangentially to the posterior capsule. The residual sodium hyaluronate is removed in a similar fashion.

References

1. Benson, WE, Blankenship GW, Machemer, R. Pars plana lens removal with vitrectomy. Am J Ophthalmol 1977; 84: 150–152.
2. Blankenship GW. The lens influence on diabetic vitrectomy results: report of a prospective randomized study. Arch Ophthalmol 1980; 98: 2196–2198.
3. Charles S. Vitreous microsurgery. 2nd ed. Baltimore: Williams and Wilkins, 1987: 44–47.
4. Girard LJ: Pars plana lensectomy by ultrasonic fragmentation: 1984 – part I: updated surgical technique. Ophthalmic Surg 1984; 15: 212–216.
5. Machemer R, Aaberg TM. Vitrectomy. 2nd ed. New York: Grune and Stratton, 1979: 146–151.
6. Michels RG. Vitreous surgery. St. Louis: C V Mosby, 1980: 150–161.
7. Peyman GA, Raichand M. Oesterle C, et al. Pars plicata lensectomy and vitrectomy in the management of congenital cataracts. Ophthalmology 1981; 88: 437–439.
8. Peyman GA, Schulman JA. Intravitreal surgery: principles and practice. New York: Appleton-Century-Crofts, 1986.
9. Scuderi G, Balestrazzi E, Picardo V, Moreno E, Crescenzi F. Pars plana lensectomy. In: Blankenship GW, Stirpe M, Gonvers M, Binder S, eds. Basic and advanced vitreous surgery. Padua: Liviana, 1986: 85–95.

14

Impaired Visualization of Posterior Segment: Intraocular Lens

Posterior chamber intraocular lenses may be covered by dense, fibrous membranes in eyes with diabetic rubeosis iridis, resolved endophthalmitis, or severe iridocyclitis. Because these membranes are usually thick and not amenable to photodisruption, removal of the membranes or of the intraocular lens may be necessary in rare instances before vitreoretinal surgery (1–3).

Persistent uveitis, malposition, or chronic endothelial cell loss may require the removal of an anterior chamber lens (2).

Posterior Chamber Intraocular Lens Removal

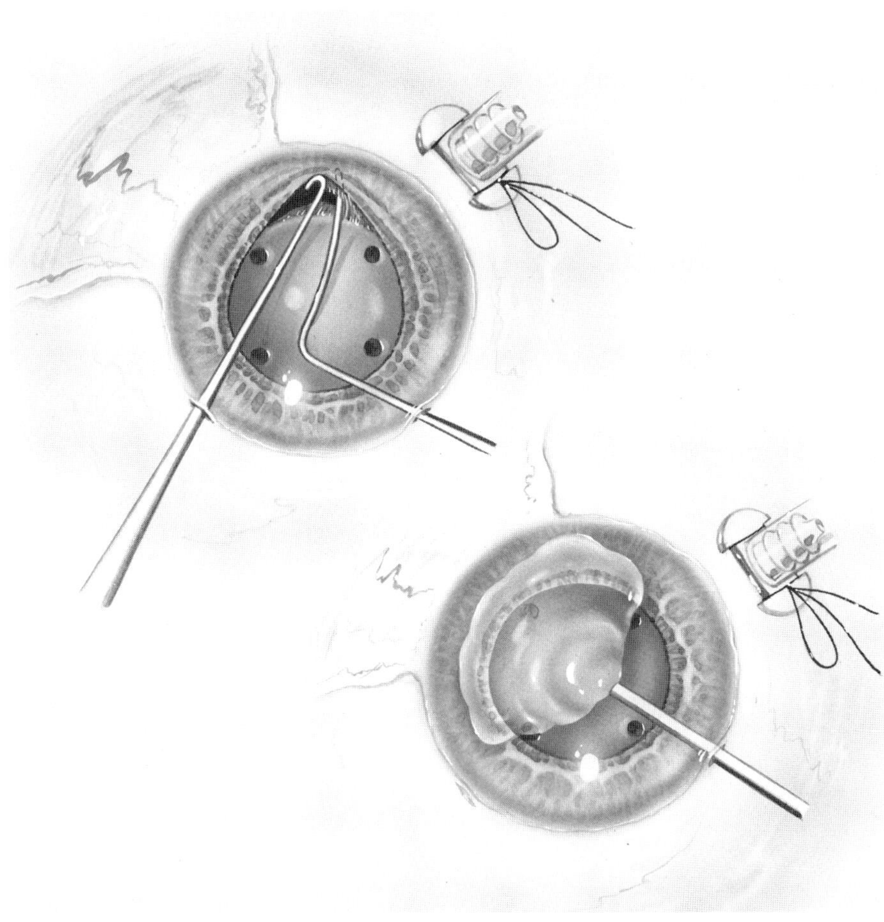

14.**1a** If vitrectomy is planned, an infusion cannula is inserted prior to intraocular lens removal. Two limbal incisions are made in the upper quadrants for insertion of a Kuglen iris lens manipulator and a Girard iris spatula. While the spatula is inserted between the iris and lens, the iris lens manipulator is used to push the iris margin away from the pupil to break iris adhesions to the lens.

b Sodium hyaluronate is then injected through one of the limbal incisions into the anterior chamber and underneath the iris to replace the aqueous in the anterior chamber.

c

d

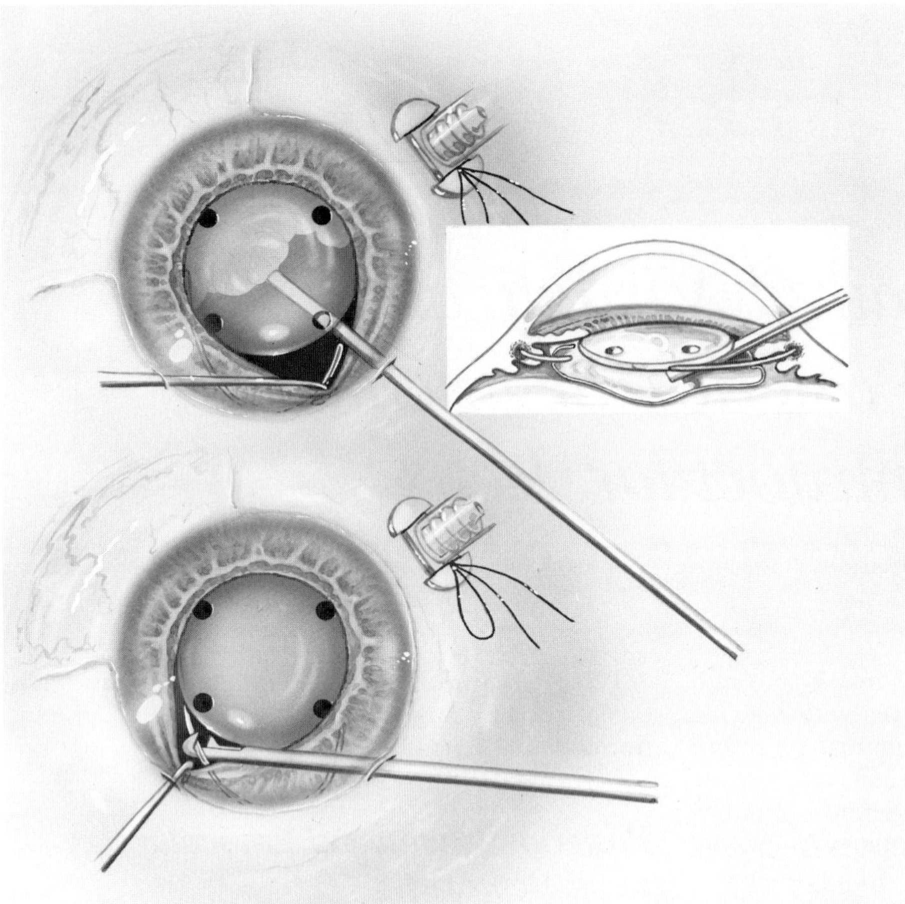

14.**1c** The needle is withdrawn slightly and placed behind the intraocular lens. Sodium hyaluronate is injected behind the intraocular lens to break adhesions between the lens and the capsular bag. *Inset:* Cross section shows posterior capsule separated from lens. The Kuglen iris lens manipulator is used to retract the superior iris margin and expose the upper edge of the lens implant.

d The irrigating needle is withdrawn from the anterior chamber and replaced with vertical-cutting scissors. With the upper iris margin retracted, the upper lens haptic is cut near the lens optic. The same procedure is done with the lower haptic, mobilizing the optical portion of the lens.

f

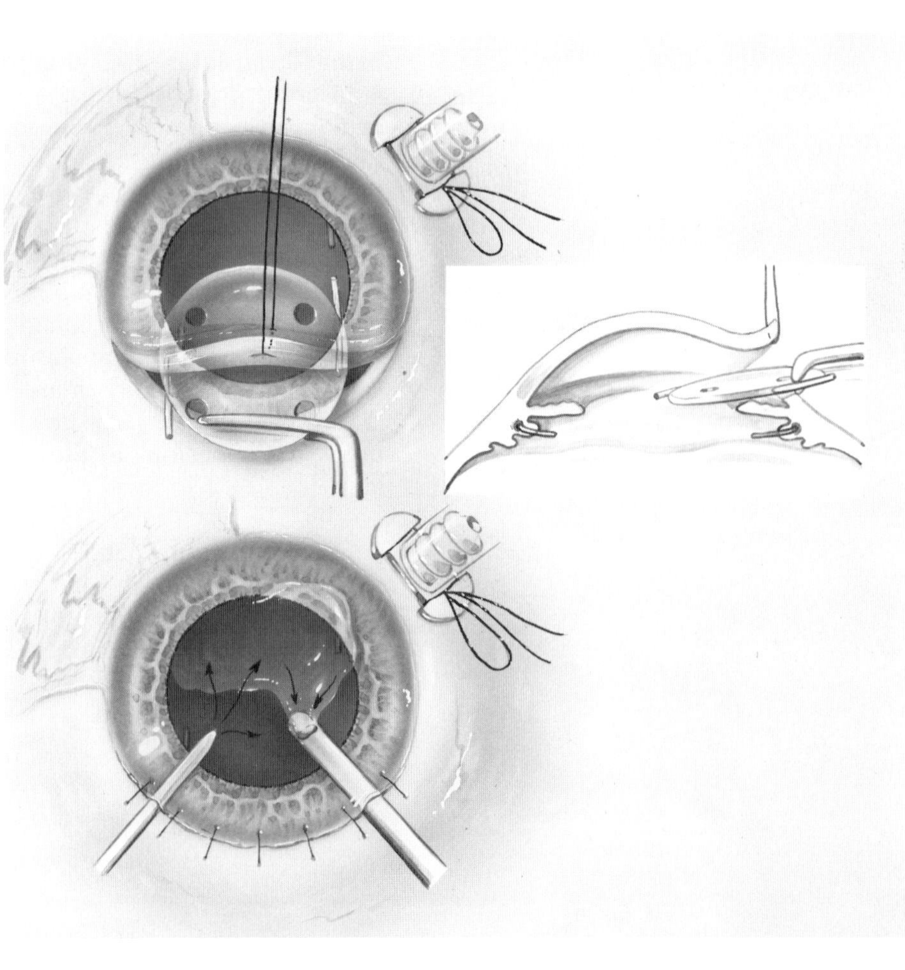

14.**1e** **Removal of lens optic.** The limbus is penetrated at 12 o'clock with a superblade. This incision is extended with scissors to the 2 and 10 o'clock meridians. The cornea is retracted with an 8–0 polyglactin suture placed in the 12 o'clock meridian. The superior edge of the optical part of the intraocular lens is exposed by retracting the superior iris behind it using the Kuglen iris retractor. *Inset:* With the superior edge of the optic exposed, it is grasped with a lens forceps and removed from the anterior chamber.

f The corneal incision is closed with multiple 9–0 polypropylene sutures. The anterior chamber is infused with BSS Plus solution while sodium hyaluronate is removed using the vitrectomy probe. With improved vitreous and fundus view, the surgeon can proceed with vitrectomy or scleral buckling.

Anterior Chamber Intraocular Lens Removal

An incorrectly fitted anterior chamber intraocular lens may cause recurrent anterior chamber and vitreous hemorrhage, as well as chronic iridocyclitis. These complications may necessitate removal of the lens.

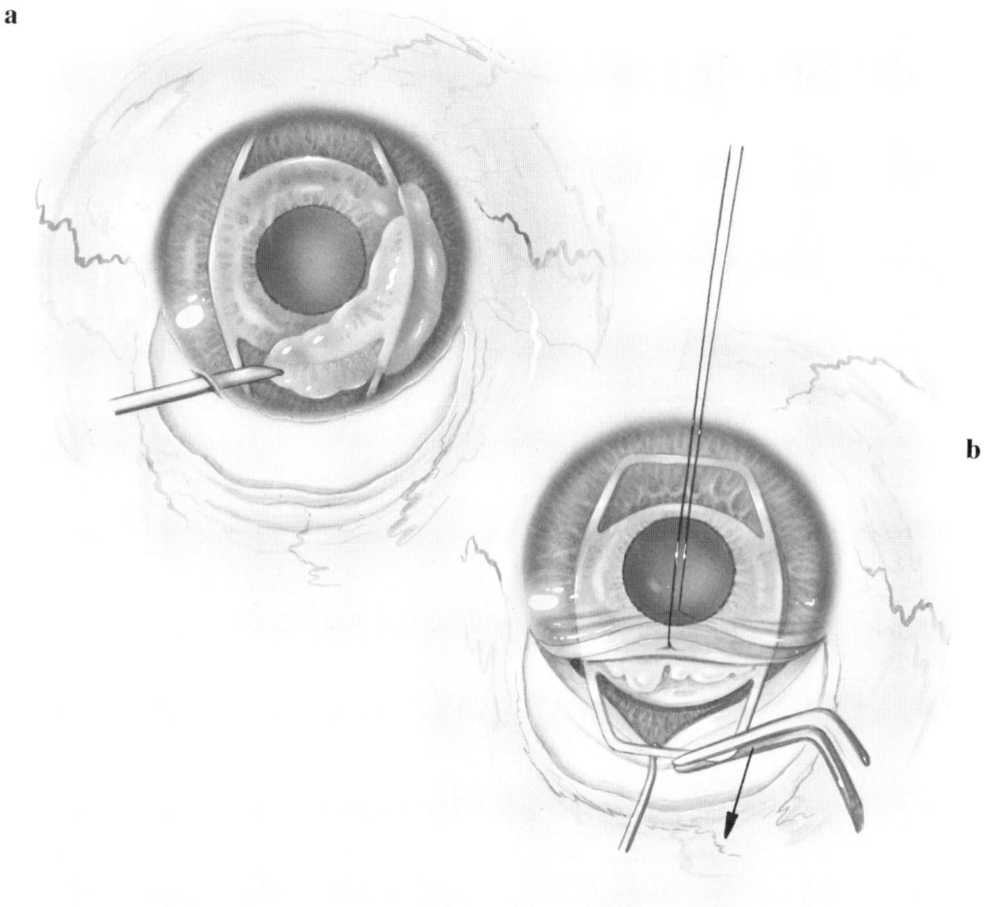

14.**2a** Sodium hyaluronate is injected into the anterior chamber through a limbal incision at 10 or 2 o'clock to facilitate lens removal and to protect the corneal endothelium.

b The incision is enlarged with corneal scissors to accomodate the diameter of the intraocular lens. An 8–0 polyglactin suture is placed at 12 o'clock for corneal traction. The limbal edge of the corneal wound is retracted with an iris hook, and the lens haptic at 12 o'clock is grasped with lens forceps. The lens is pushed inferiorly, tilted anteriorly, and lifted out of the anterior chamber. Finally, sodium hyaluronate is washed out of the anterior chamber with BSS Plus. The corneal incision is closed with multiple sutures. The illustrations do not show an infusion cannula, but if vitreous surgery is planned, an infusion cannula is placed at the outset, or after closure of the corneal incision with sutures.

3a

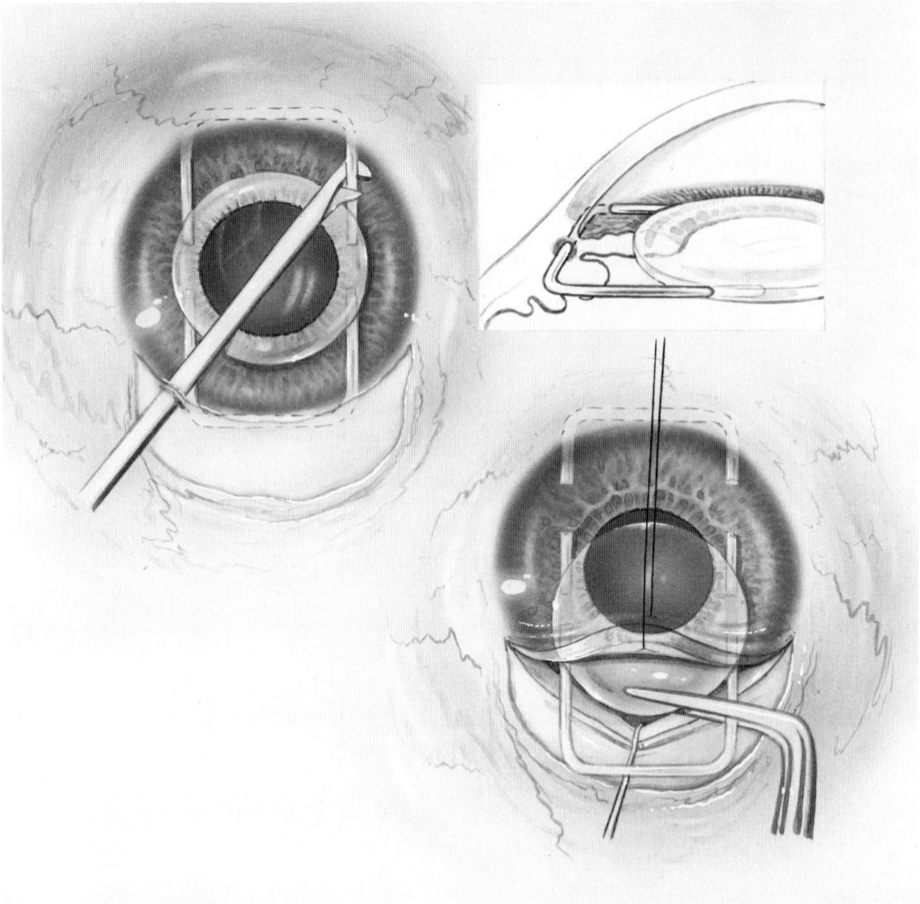

3b

4a

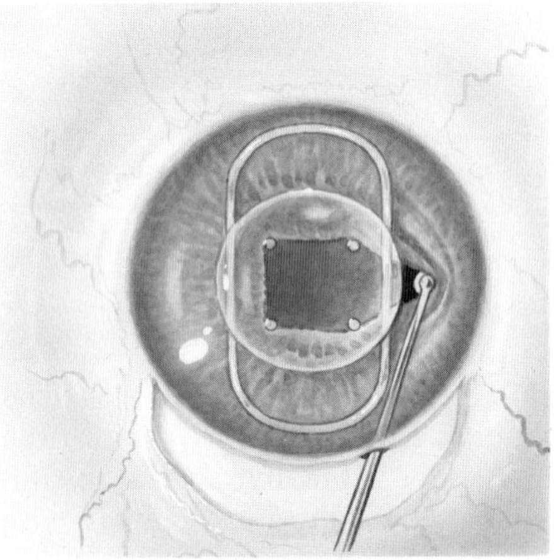

4b

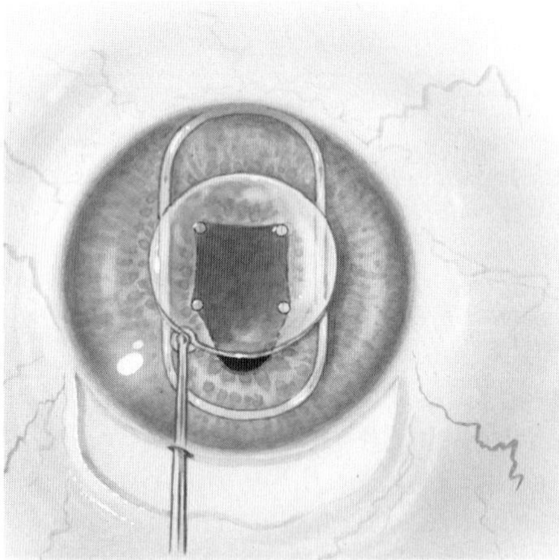

4c

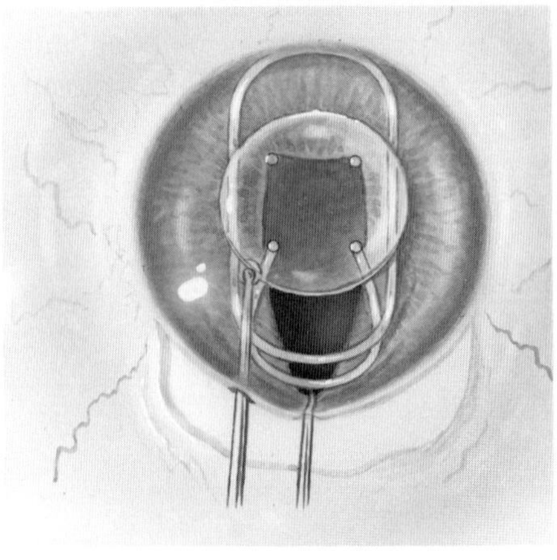

4d

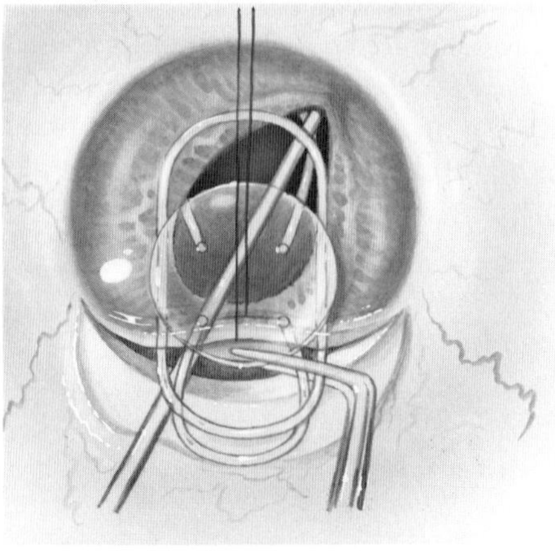

Fixed Haptics

Removal of an anterior chamber intraocular lens that has an encapsulated haptic requires a modification of the technique described in Figure 14.**2**. The inset at the upper right in Figure 14.**3** illustrates fibrous encapsulation around the haptic in the iridocorneal angle.

14.**3a** A limbal incision is made with a superblade in the 10 or 2 o'clock meridian through which sodium hyaluronate is injected into the anterior chamber. The lens haptic is cut close to the optical portion of the lens using vertical-cutting scissors. If gonioscopy has revealed fibrous encapsulation in both haptics, both are sectioned (inset).

b After the corneal incision is enlarged and the corneal traction suture is placed, the lens is grasped with lens forceps and removed from the anterior chamber. The cornea is sutured in the routine manner.

Removal of Iris Clip Intraocular Lens

14.**4a** Sodium hyaluronate is injected into the anterior chamber. The iris lens manipulator or hook is used to break any adhesions between the lens and the anterior vitreous face or iris.

b The iris manipulator is used to engage the lens optic by moving it form side to side. When the lens moves loosely, it is free of adhesions and can be removed.

c While the iris manipulator is held against the lens between the optic and the anterior and posterior haptics, an iris hook is introduced through the other limbal incision which has been enlarged slightly with corneal scissors. The iris is retracted superiorly, allowing the posterior loop of the haptic to become displaced anteriorly. The iris at 10 o'clock is retracted and then swept toward the opposite meridian to dislodge the posterior haptic into the anterior chamber.

d When both superior haptics have been relocated anteriorly, the iris hook and manipulator are withdrawn and the corneal incision is extended at both ends to permit removal of the lens. The anterior chamber is deepened with the injection of sodium hyaluronate. The iris manipulator is inserted under the intraocular lens, which is pushed downward to break any remaining iris adhesions to the haptics. The superior haptic is grasped with lens forceps and pulled out of the eye carefully in tandem with the iris manipulator. The corneal wound is closed after irrigating and aspirating the sodium hyaluronate from the anterior chamber.

References

1. Flynn HW. Vitrectomy in the management of dislocated crystalline lenses. In: Blankenship GW, Stirpe M, Gonvers M, Binder S eds. Basic and advances vitreous surgery. Padua: Liviana, 1986: 111–118.
2. Stark WJ, Terry AC, Stirpe M, Michels RG, Hamill MB, Gottsch JD, Rapoza PA. Surgical management of selected intraocular lens complications. In: Blankenship GW, Stirpe M, Gonvers M, Binder S, eds. Basic and advanced vitreous surgery. Padua: Liviana, 1986: 129–134.
3. Terry AC, Stark WJ. Removal of closed-loop anterior chamber lens implants. Ophthalmic Surg 1984; 15:575–577.

15

Vitreous Loss during Cataract Extraction

Loss of vitreous at the time of extracapsular extraction requires a modification of the surgical plan. If vitreous loss occurs during anterior capsulotomy or aspiration of equatorial cortical material, rupture of the zonules is suspected.

Vitreous loss during extraction of the lens nucleus indicates a break in the posterior lens capsule. Proper handling of this complication may allow implantation of either a posterior or an anterior chamber intraocular lens. In either case, removal of vitreous from the anterior chamber is mandatory (2–5).

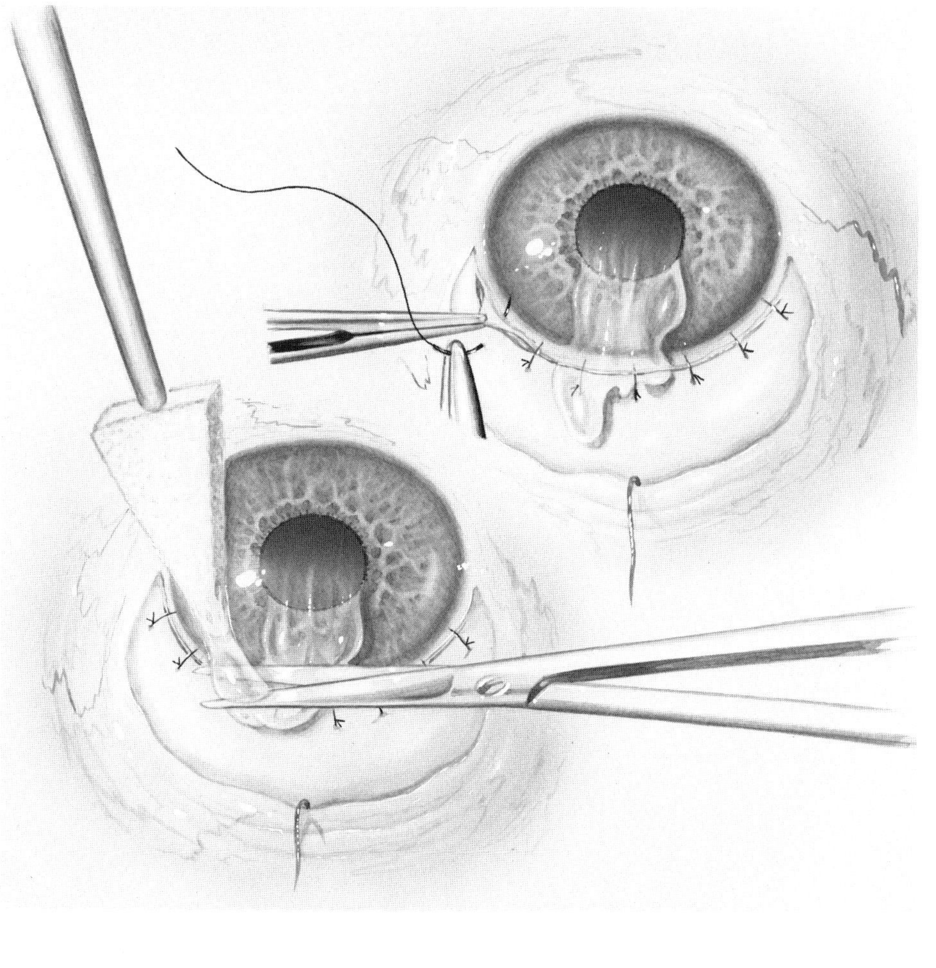

15.**1a** **Subluxated Cataract.** When the cataractous lens becomes inadvertently subluxated because of breakage of zonules during capsulotomy, vitreous may prolapse into the anterior chamber. The anterior chamber is infused with BSS Plus through an infusion needle inserted through the limbus. Prolapsed vitreous is removed with the vitrectomy probe, introduced through the limbal incision that was used for the capsulotomy. The lens is delivered intracapsularly through an enlarged corneal incision; then the corneal incision is closed with multiple sutures.

b After delivery of the lens, the anterior chamber usually contains vitreous gel which prolapses through the wound. Vitreous in the corneal wound is excised using a cellulose sponge and Vannas scissors.

c

d

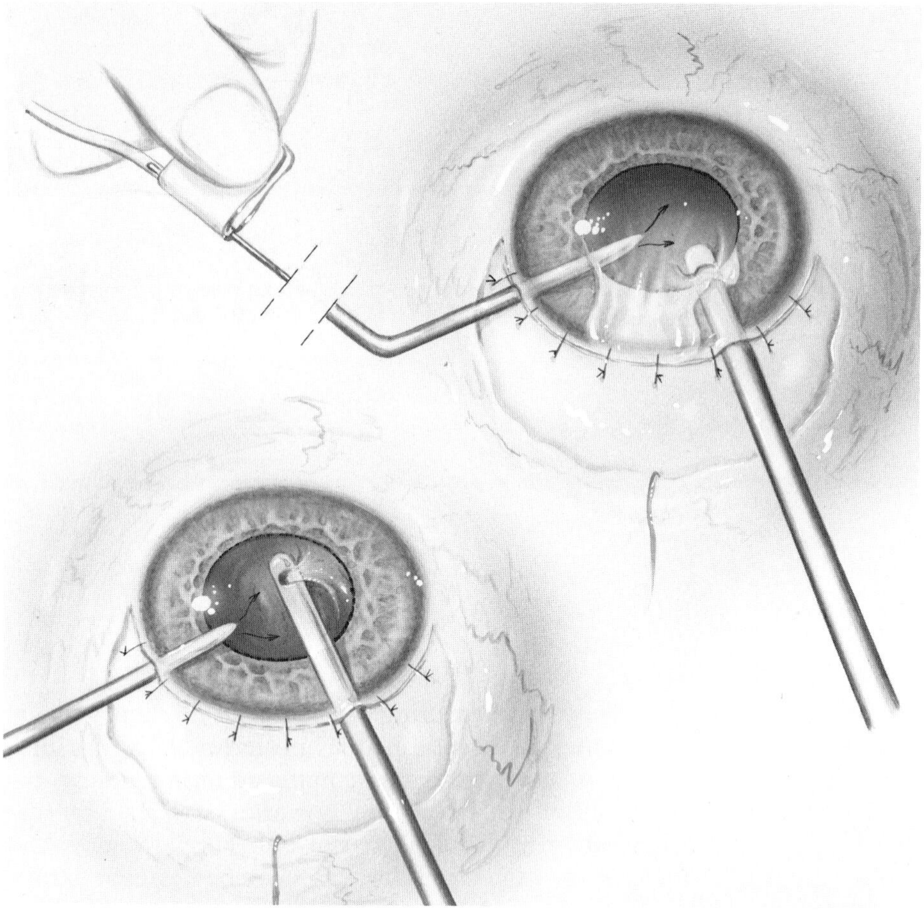

15.**1c** The anterior chamber is infused through a 20-gauge butterfly needle inserted between sutures near one end of the corneal incision. With the infusion pressure at a low level, the vitrectomy probe is inserted near the other end of the corneal incision. Vitreous between the superior margin of pupil and the corneal wound is removed first.

d Then the remaining vitreous in the pupil is resected.

e

f

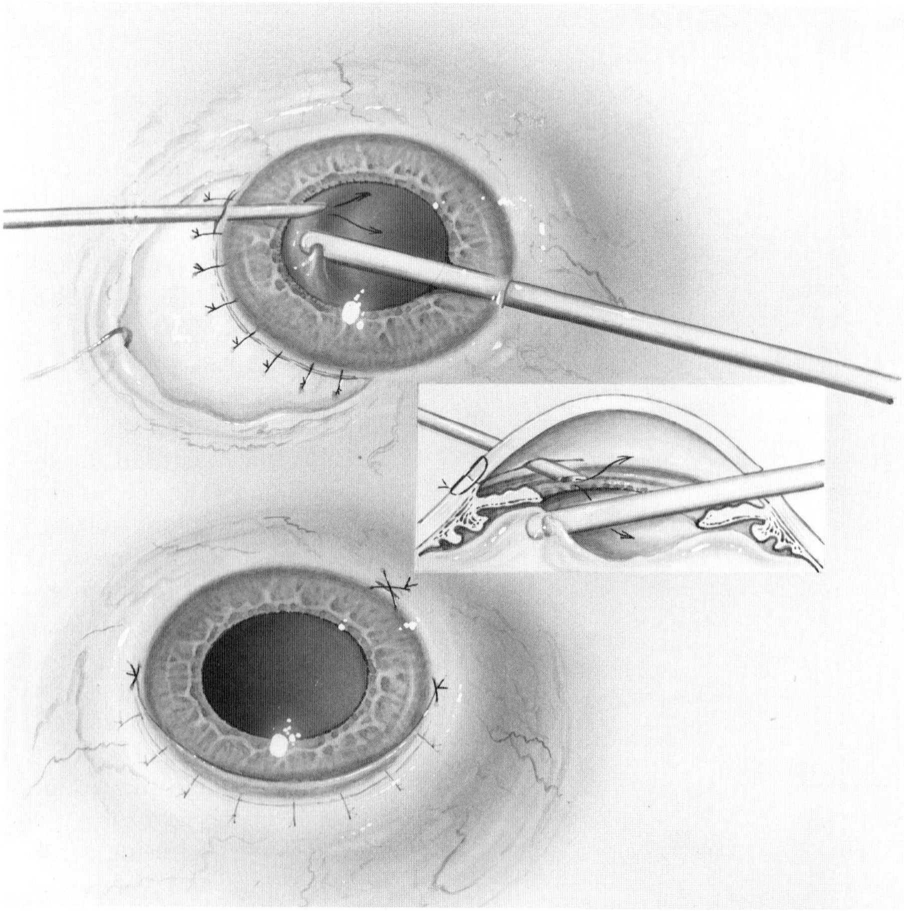

15.**1e** The vitreous beneath the iris in the upper quadrants is removed with the vitrectomy probe, inserted through a limbal incision in the inferior temporal quadrant. This location allows the probe to remove vitreous incarcerated in the corneal wound *(inset)*. Vitreous remaining incarcerated in the wound is swept toward the pupil with a Girard spatula, which is placed between the iris and incarcerated vitreous. Complete removal of these vitreous strands with the vitrector results in a round pupil.

f The corneal incisions and peritomy are closed in the routine manner.

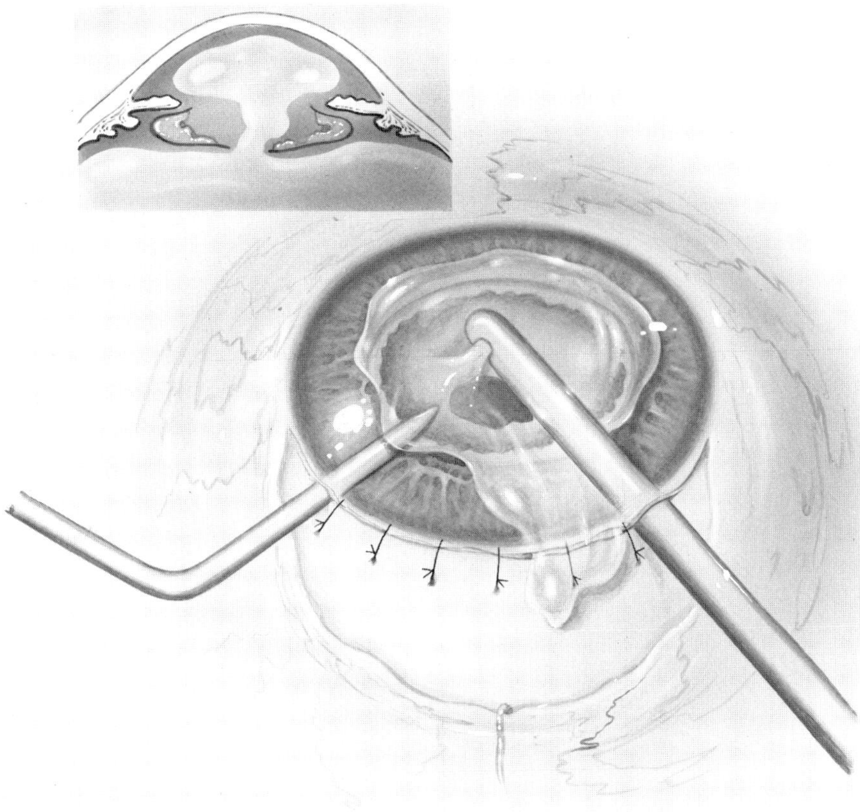

15.**2a** During extracapsular cataract extraction or phakoemulsification, a break may develop in the posterior capsule, resulting in vitreous prolapse into the anterior chamber and through the corneal incision *(below)*.

When this occurs, the corneal incision is enlarged to facilitate removal of the nucleus of the lens. Following extraction of the nucleus, the corneal incision is closed with multiple 9–0 polypropylene sutures. An infusion needle is introduced into the anterior chamber through one end of the corneal incision. The vitrectomy probe is inserted into the anterior chamber, and vitreous in front and behind the iris is excised.

b

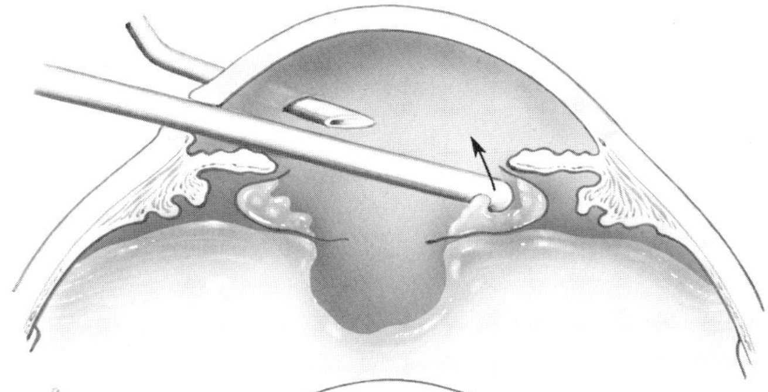

15.**2b** **Removal of lens cortex.** Residual equatorial lens cortex is removed by aspiration, using the vitrectomy probe. Continuous infusion in the anterior chamber hydrates the cortex, making it more easily visualized. Intermittent and gentle suction is used to aspirate cortex and avoid breaking the zonular ligaments. When the cortex becomes separated from the capsule, it is brought to the pupillary area and evacuated from the eye. Visualization of equatorial lens material can be improved using scleral depression.

c

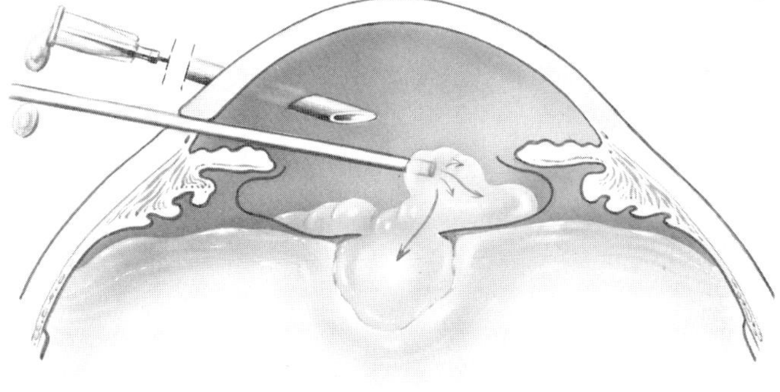

c Implantation of posterior chamber intraocular lens. If a posterior chamber lens is to be implanted, sodium hyaluronate is injected into the capsular bag, which becomes distended, facilitating intraocular lens insertion. Anterior chamber fluid is displaced into the infusion needle as the sodium hyaluronate is injected.

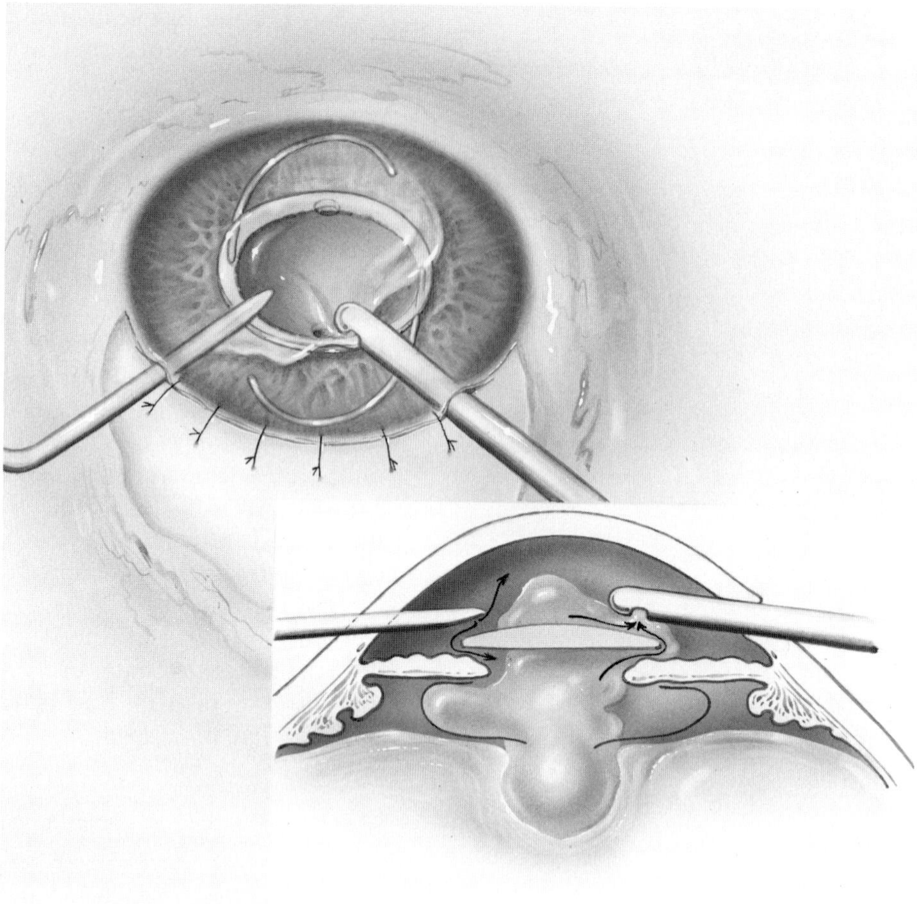

15.**2d, e** Implantation of either an anterior or a posterior chamber lens may be carried out, according to the surgeon's preference. In either case, the sodium hyaluronate and vitreous are removed from the anterior and posterior chambers with the vitrectomy probe and exchanged with BSS Plus at the end of the procedure (1).

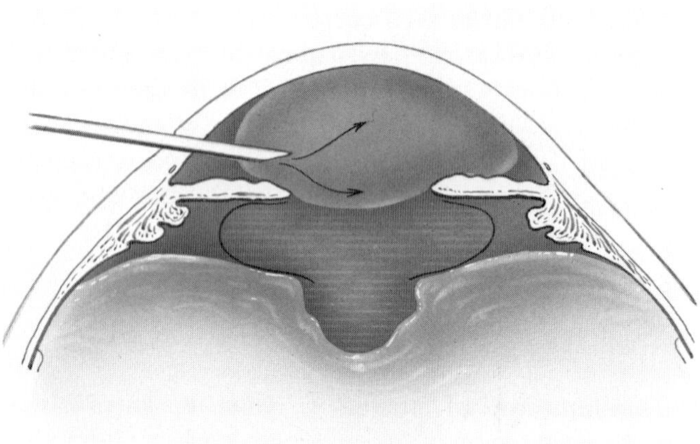

15.**3** The anterior chamber may be filled with sterile air or BSS Plus to normalize the intraocular pressure if an intraocular lens is not implanted.

References

1. Clayman HM, Jaffe NS, Galin M. Intraocular lens implantation: techniques and complications. St. Louis: C V Mosby, 1983: 281–282.
2. Machemer, R, Aaberg TM. Vitrectomy. 2nd ed. New York: Grune and Stratton, 1979: 163–166.
3. Michels RG. Vitreous surgery. St. Louis: C V Mosby, 1980: 200–206.
4. Peyman GA, Schulman JA. Intravitreal surgery: principles and practice. New York: Appleton-Century-Crofts, 1986: 133–135.
5. Rice TA, Michels RG, Stark WJ, eds. Operative surgery: ophthalmic surgery. 4th ed. St. Louis: C V Mosby, 1984: 165. (Rob and Smith's operative surgery series.)

16

Dislocated Lens and Intraocular Lens

Although dislocation of the lens into the vitreous may occur spontaneously in Marfan's syndrome, in most cases lens dislocation is a complication of ocular trauma, or results from rupture of the posterior capsule or lens zonules during cataract extraction (2, 4:653). In the presence of extensive liquefaction of the vitreous, the lens or portions of it may dislocate posteriorly. A lense – even an opaque lens – that is dislocated into the vitreous cavity and is freely moving need not be removed, unless it causes severe uveitis or glaucoma.

Indications: removal of the dislocated lens is indicated when it obstructs the visual axis, becomes adherent to the retina, or causes a violent inflammatory reaction in the eye. The lens may shrink and become cataractous without causing marked uveitis or severe glaucoma, but in many cases it causes severe uveitis and glaucoma that cannot be controlled medically. In such cases, lens removal is indicated, even though firm adhesions that develop between the lens and the retina make this a high-risk procedure (4:931–932).

The technique of removing a dislocated lens depends on its hardness. In young patients, the lens is usually soft and removed easily from the vitreous cavity or the anterior chamber by aspiration with the vitrectomy probe. Hard lenses are removed with a phakofragmentor (1,3). Small fragments of hard lens are aspirated, brought to the middle or anterior vitreous, and phakofragmented. Large fragments are brought to the anterior chamber to rest on the iris, then aspirated and phakofragmented. Very hard lenses are removed through a corneal section.

a

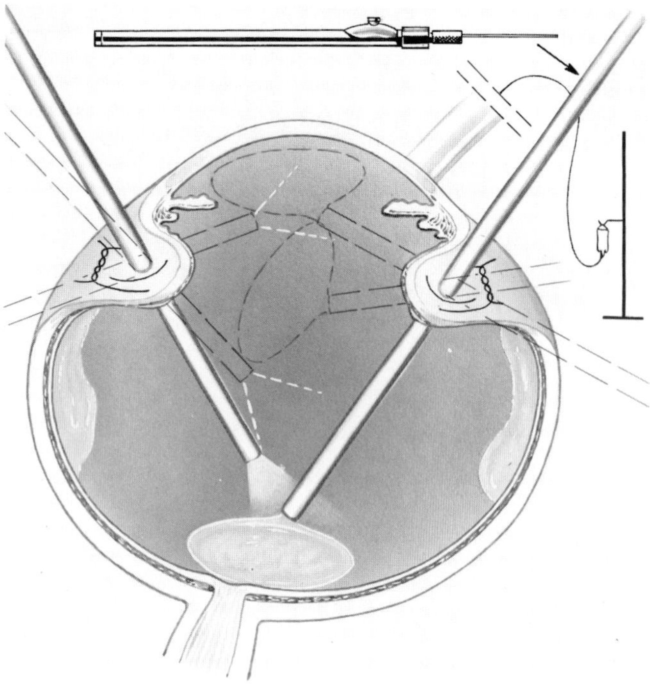

c

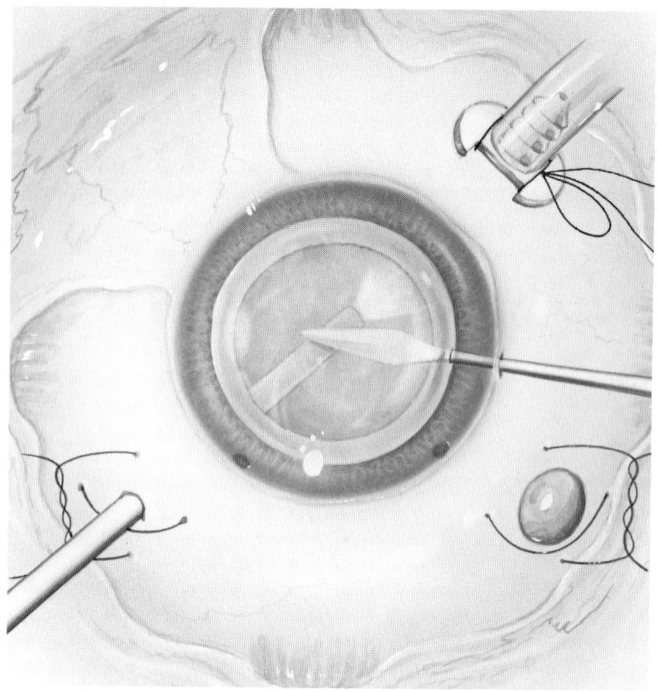

b

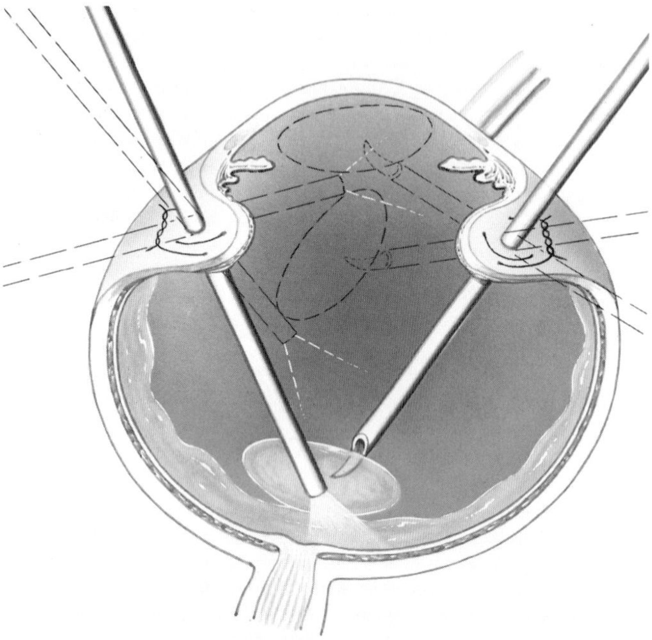

Dislocated Lens

16.**1a** In removing a dislocated hard lens, the routine preparatory steps for vitrectomy are completed. The pupil must be fully dilated with strong mydriatic drops. If the pupil does not dilate adequately, it is mechanically enlarged with sutures. An alternative method is to enlarge the pupil with an iridectomy at the 12 and 6 o'clock positions, made with the vitrectomy probe. The light pipe and vitrectomy probe are inserted into the vitreous cavity. The vitreous anterior to the dislocated lens is removed with the vitrectomy probe. The lens is sucked into the tip of the extrusion needle (instrument on the right) and brought into the anterior chamber. The holding capacity of the extrusion needle is increased by elevating the infusion bottle and thus the intraocular pressure. While the lens is held in place in the anterior chamber with both the light pipe and extrusion needle supporting it from behind, it is removed through a corneal section.

16.**1b** A dislocated lens with a very hard nucleus may not mold into the lumen of the extrusion needle, making it impossible to hold and bring it to the anterior chamber. Utilizing a 20-gauge needle bent 80° from its shaft, the lens is moved in front of the optic disc, or onto a layer of vitreous cortex overlying the nasal fundus. The light pipe is held against one side of the lens to stabilize it while it is impaled on the other side with the needle, and brought by the two instruments into the anterior chamber.

16.**1c** Providing the iris sphincter is intact, the pupil may be made to constrict by reducing intraocular pressure, by lowering the infusion bottle or by touching the iris sphincter with one of the instruments. If this fails, 1 ml of acetylcholine chloride is injected into the infusion line. Once the pupil is constricted, the light pipe is positioned behind the pupil to support the lens. The bent needle is withdrawn through the sclerotomy, which is closed with a plug. An MVR blade is introduced through the limbus to spear the lens cortex and nucleus, thereby firmly holding the lens in the anterior chamber.

d

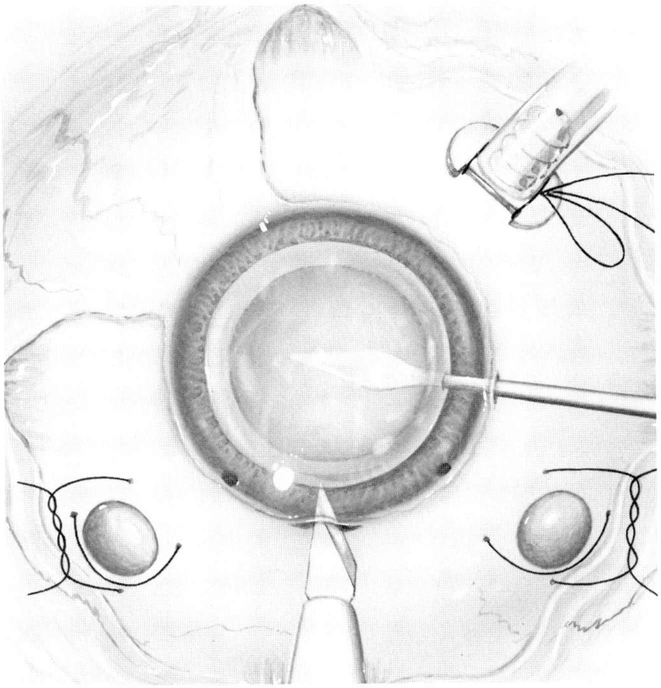

f

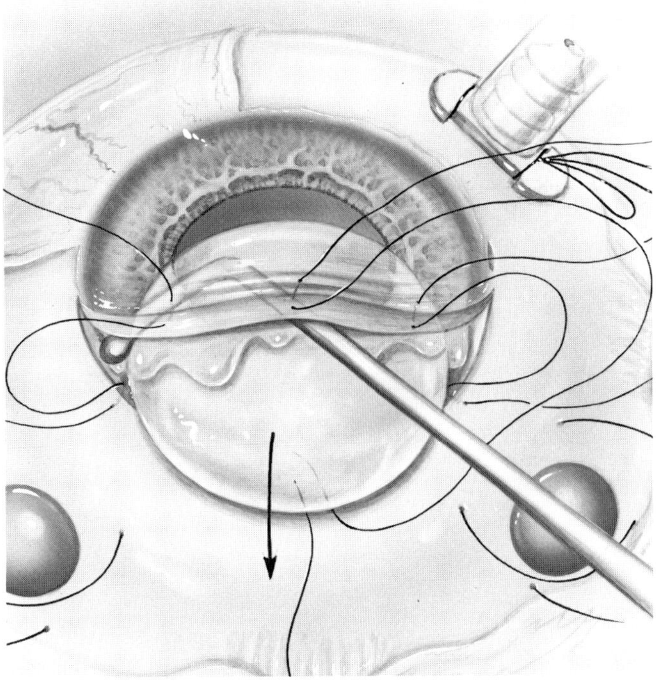

e

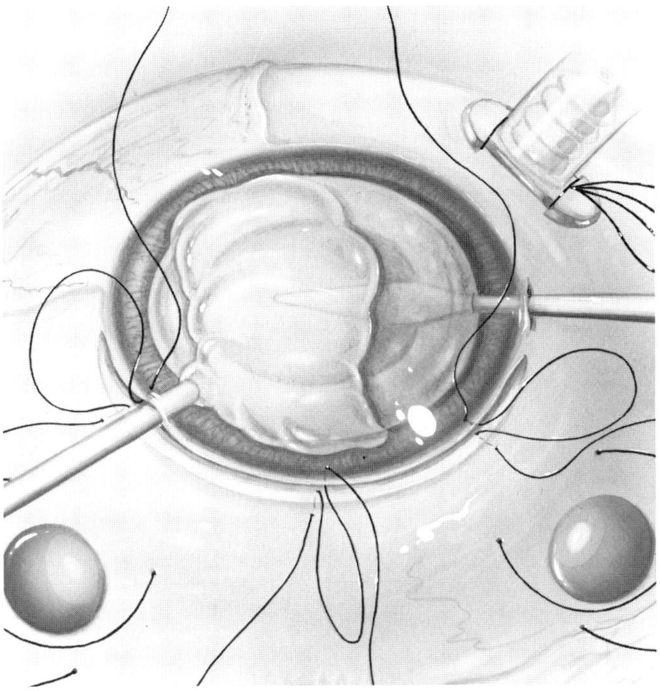

16.**1d** The light pipe is withdrawn, and the sclerotomy is closed with a plug. The assistant takes hold of the MVR knife to free the hand of the surgeon, who then makes a corneal incision with a superblade, and enlarges it with scissors.

16.**1e** Sodium hyaluronate is injected between the cornea and crystalline lens to protect the corneal endothelium. The infusion bottle is elevated to prevent hypotony. Corneal sutures may be placed before delivering the lens from the eye. The MVR knife is used as an aid to maneuver the lens toward the corneal section.

16.**1f** Following the removal of the lens using a muscle hook, the corneal section is closed with multiple 9–0 polypropylene sutures. The infusion bottle is lowered to reduce intraocular pressure during placement of the last two sutures. The surgeon reintroduces the light pipe and vitrectomy probe to remove any remaining vitreous gel. After sclerotomy closure and before conjunctival wound closure, the peripheral retina is inspected thoroughly.

2a

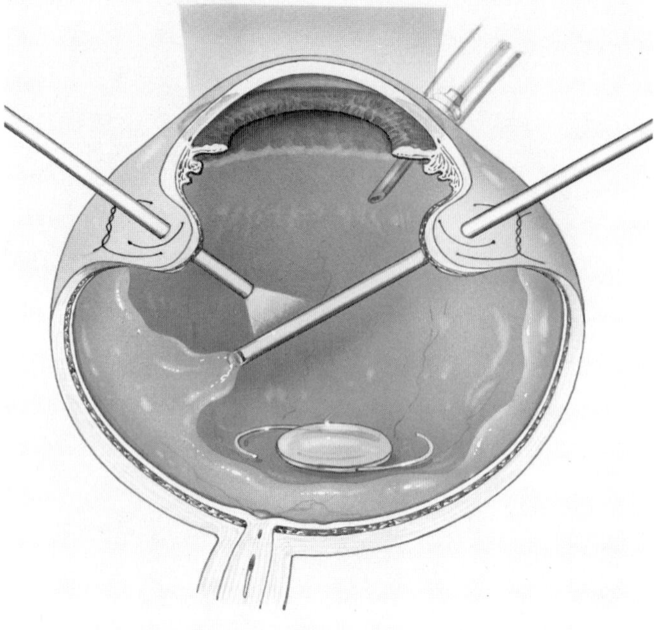

2c

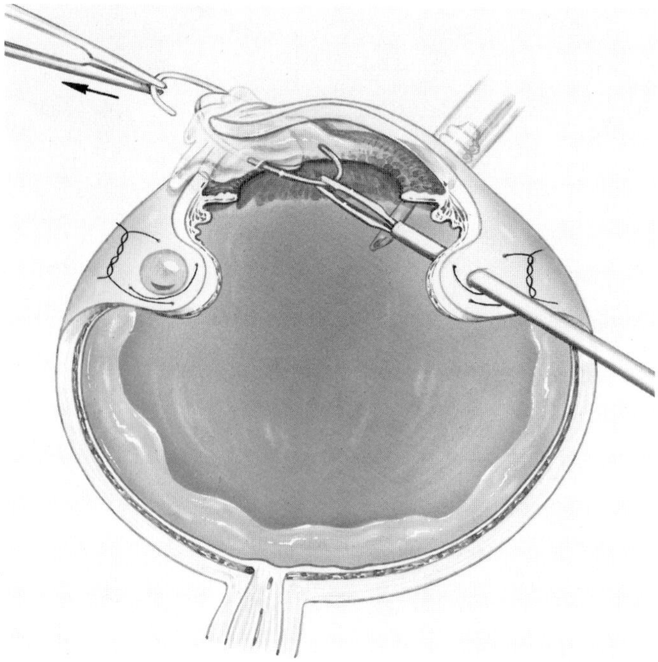

2b

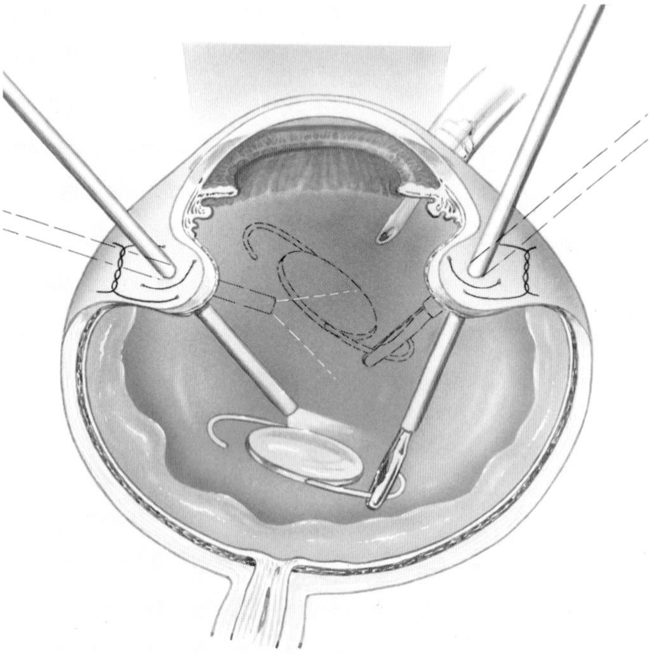

16.**2a** In most cases, a dislocated intraocular lens lies on the surface of the vitreous gel. If the lens is embedded in the vitreous and needs to be removed, a vitrectomy is performed first. The vitreous underlying the lens is left intact, to prevent the lens or its haptics from coming into contact with the retina (8).

16.**2b** One haptic is grasped with a vitreous forceps in such a manner that the other haptic is directed toward 12 o'clock and one surface of the optic faces the cornea. The lens is brought to the anterior chamber.

16.**2c** The limbal incision through which the cataract was removed and the intraocular lens was inserted is reopened. To protect the corneal endothelium during implant removal, the surface of the intraocular lens is coated with sodium hyaluronate injected into the anterior chamber. The haptic that is directed toward 12 o'clock is fed through the limbal incision and brought outside the eye, where it is grasped with forceps, and the lens is removed from the eye (5,6). The limbal incision is closed tightly with polypropylene sutures. Additional vitrectomy is performed to remove any blood in the vitreous and vitreous gel incarcerated in the limbal wound. The peripheral and central retina is checked for retinal breaks with indirect ophthalmoscopy and scleral depression.

Intraocular Lens

A dislocated intraocular lens is generally well tolerated (7). It can be left in the vitreous cavity unless it migrates to, or becomes fixed in, the vitreous along the visual axis. In cases in which it is not feasible to fixate the intraocular lens with a suture through the sclerotomy or the iris, the lens may have to be removed.

References

1. Charles S. Vitreous microsurgery. 2nd ed. Baltimore: Williams and Wilkins, 1987: 49–51.
2. Jensen D, Cross HE. Surgical treatment of dislocated lenses in the Marfan syndrome and homocystinuria. Trans Am Acad Ophthalmol Otolaryngol 1972; 76: 1491–1499.
3. Michels RG. Vitreous surgery. St. Louis: C V Mosby, 1980: 324–325.
4. Schepens CL. Retinal detachment and allied diseases. Philadelphia: W B Saunders, 1983.
5. Stark WJ, Michels RG, Bruner WE. Management of posteriorly dislocated intraocular lenses. Ophthalmic Surg 1980; 11: 495.
6. Stark WJ, Terry AC, Stirpe M, Michels RG, Hamill MB, Gottsch JD, Rapoza PA. Surgical management of selected intraocular lens complications. In: Blankenship GW, Stirpe M, Gonvers M, Binder S, eds. Basic and advanced vitreous surgery. Padua: Liviana, 1986: 129–135.
7. Wilkinson CP. Closed vitreous surgery for complications of intraocular lens implantation, I: indications. In: Blankenship GW, Stirpe M, Gonvers M, Binder S, eds. Basic and advanced vitreous surgery. Padua: Liviana, 1986: 135–140.
8. Wilkinson CP. Closed vitreous surgery for complications of intraocular lens implantation, II: techniques. In: Blankenship GW, Stirpe M, Gonvers M, Binder S. eds. Basic and advanced vitreous surgery. Padua: Liviana, 1986: 141–148.

17

Tractional Retinal Detachment

Diabetic Tractional Retinal Detachment

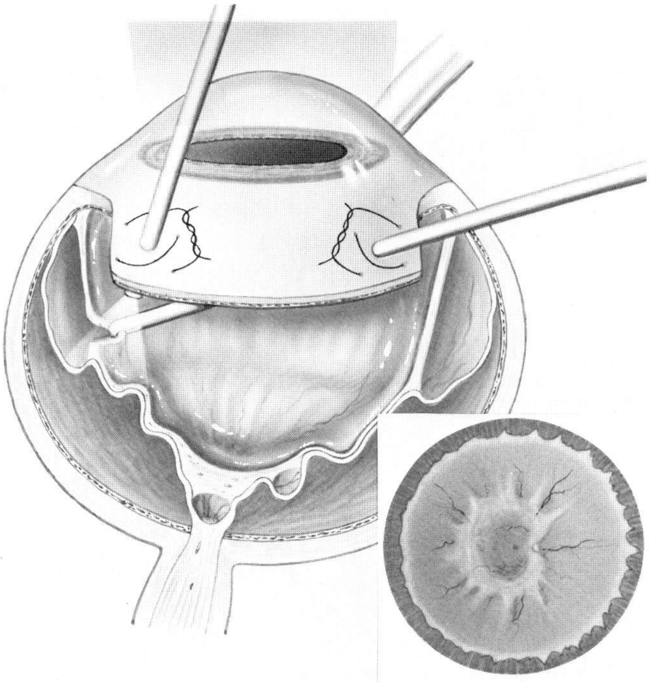

17.**1a** This fundus illustrates a classic complication of diabetic retinopathy characterized by fibrovascular proliferation along the vascular arcades, producing tractional retinal detachment in and around the posterior retina. Areas of proliferation are the site of firm adhesions of the vitreous cortex to the retina, which becomes detached when the vitreous cortex and the fibrovascular membrane undergo contraction (4,5,13). Surgical intervention is indicated when the macula becomes detached, when retinal detachment is associated with a retinal break, or when extensive vitreous hemorrhage occurs (1,9). Except for simple vitrectomy to release anteroposterior traction on the retina, surface membrane surgery is deferred in cases that have extremely active vascular proliferation. There are two surgical approaches to surface membrane surgery for diabetic tractional retinal detachment: circumcision and segmentation, and en bloc delamination.

The circumcision and segmentation surgical approach to diabetic tractional retinal detachment, in our experience, tends to reduce the risk of iatrogenic retinal breaks (8). The first step is removal of anterior-posterior traction membranes bridging the vitreous base and the detached posterior retina. The vitrectomy probe is used to circumcise the bridging membranes around the entire detached retina. This membrane contains cortical vitreous gel, which facilitates aspiration of the membrane into the cutting port of the vitrectomy probe.

b

d

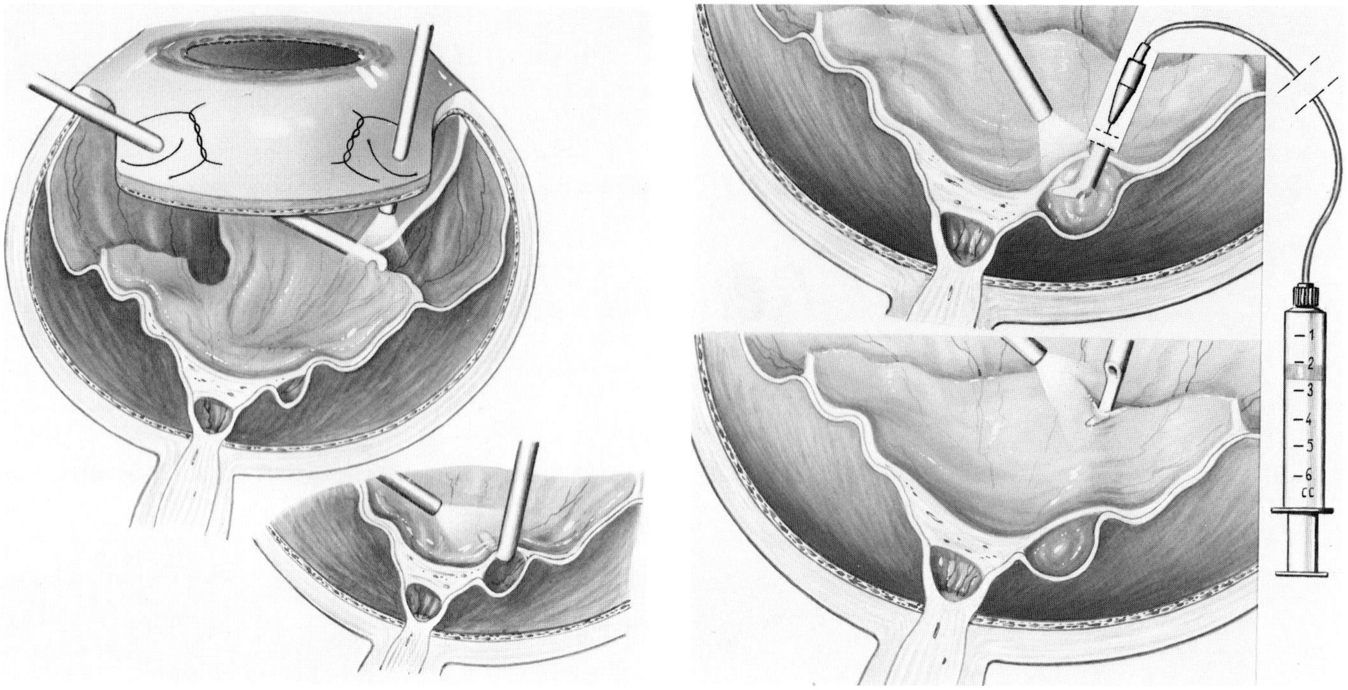

c

e

17.**1b** It is necessary to alternate the entry sites of the endoilluminator and vitrectomy probe to reach membranes otherwise poorly accessible from the initial entry sites.

c The circumcised, freely floating membranes near the equator and vitreous base are trimmed carefully with the probe. The surface membrane overlying the detached retina is examined around its edge for preexisting cleavage planes, which are probed with the dissecting vitreous cutter or vertical-cutting scissors.

17.**1d** The viscoelastic property of sodium hyaluronate makes it a good tool to delaminate large portions of the surface membranes. This substance serves as a hydraulic wedge that breaks tenuous vitreoretinal adhesions, separating membrane from retina, but leaving firm adhesions in place without causing iatrogenic retinal breaks.

The injection setup for sodium hyaluronate consists of a 6 ml syringe, short silicone tubing, 20-gauge irrigating needles with blunt tips, and a special spatula that has an irrigation aperture at the bottom of the spatula (see Chapter 3, p. 14).

e Additional membrane dissection is done with a vitreous spatula, isolating areas of residual vitreoretinal adhesions.

f

g

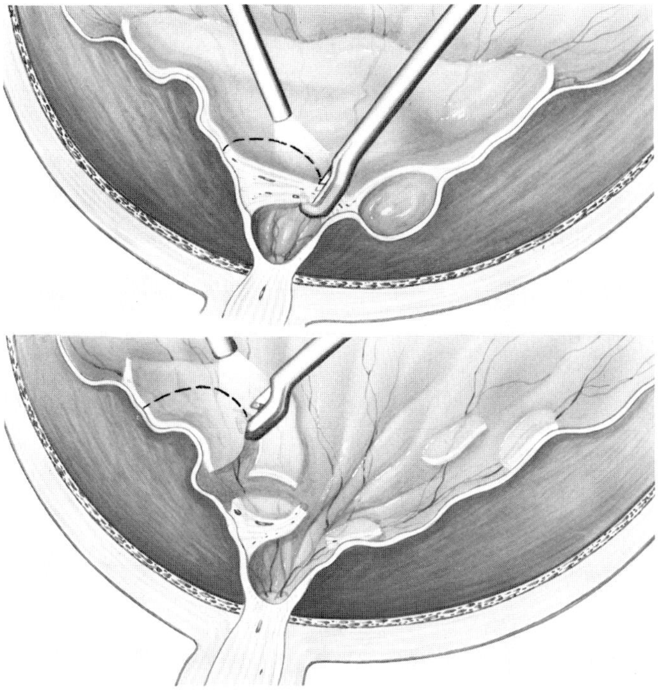

h

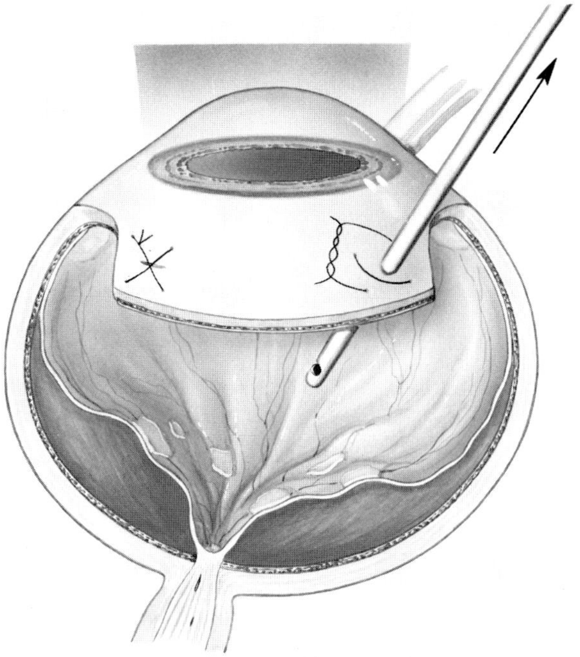

17.**1 f, g** After isolated vitreoretinal adhesions have been delineated, the elevated membranes around them are circumcised (broken line) with vertical-cutting scissors. The vitreous dissector-cutter is the preferred instrument, because its vertical configuration and remote-controlled cutting reduce the risk of exerting additional retinal traction and producing tearing during membrane cutting. In addition, the distal dissector portion of the scissors is specifically designed for atraumatic membrane separation from the retina in diabetic tractional retinal detachment.

17.**1 h** The vitrectomy probe is removed, and indirect ophthalmoscopy is done to check for retinal breaks. The next step depends on the extent and nature of retinal detachment. A limited detachment not involving the macula is left alone, because the retina usually reattaches spontaneously after several months. Extensive retinal detachment involving both posterior and peripheral retina benefits from external drainage of subretinal fluid, which is carried out in the quadrant of higher retinal elevation. Balanced salt solution is injected into the vitreous to restore intraocular pressure. Scleral resection may be necessary in areas of the fundus where thorough surface membrane surgery was not possible because of extreme atrophy of the underlying retina, or very firm adhesions to the retina.

Peripheral retinal breaks are treated with scleral buckling. Endolaser and gas tamponade are used in the treatment of posterior retinal breaks.

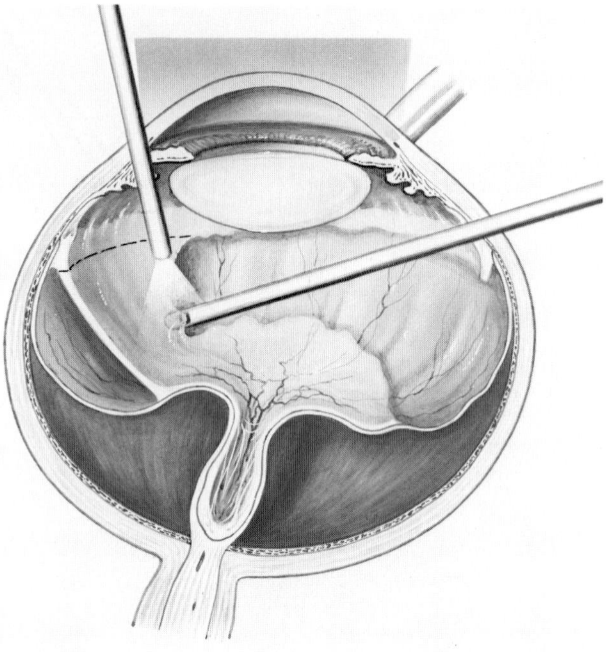

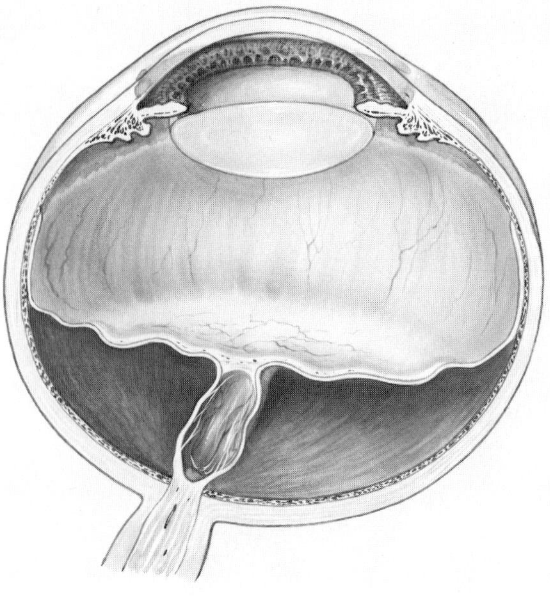

17.**2a** Table-top tractional retinal detachment is unique to diabetic retinopathy and is really an exaggerated type of posterior retinal detachment, produced by contracting extensive fibrovascular tissue on the posterior retina. Surgery is indicated when the neovascularization process has become inactive or is declining. It requires advanced instrumentation and sometimes a two-stage procedure.

The initial step is vitrectomy of posterior-anterior membranes, circumcising them around the edge of the "table-top" retinal elevation.

17.**2b** In some cases a tunnel of a narrow funnel-shaped retinal detachment extends between the table-top membrane and the optic disc and the posterior pole.

c

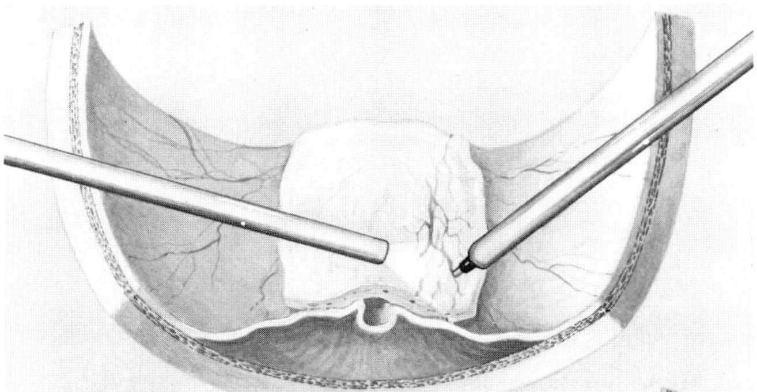

d

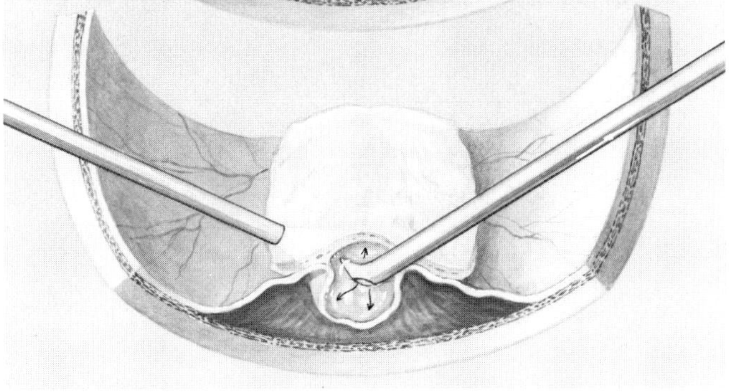

e

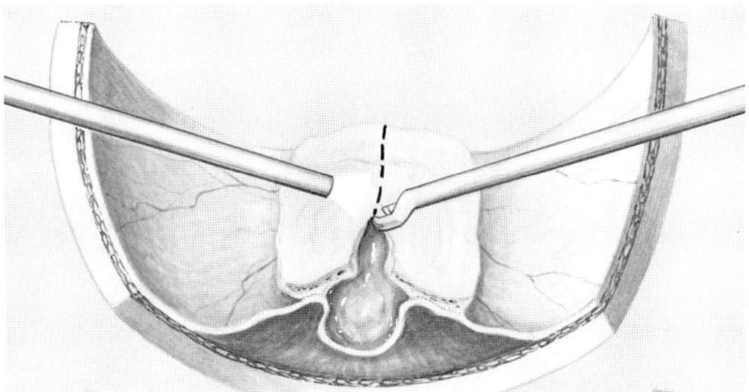

f

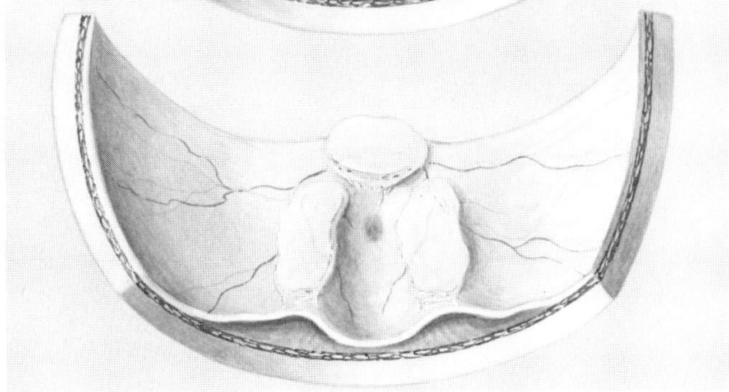

17.**2c** Trampoline-like membranes affect the posterior retina in varying degrees of severity, depending on the extent of vitreoretinal adhesions. New-formed blood vessels are closed with the endodiathermy probe. The fine tip of the probe allows pinpoint coagulation, which is done systematically from small to large blood vessels.

d Trampoline-like surface membranes are separated gently from the retina by injecting sodium hyaluronate under the membrane.

17.**2e** Through hydraulic dissection, the tunnel underneath the membrane is enlarged, permitting the membrane to be segmented with less risk of retinal damage. The vitreous dissector-cutter is used for this precarious dissection and cutting procedure, because the rounded, probe-like tip and cutting block for the blade does not move when the blade is closed against it by remote control.

f To relieve macular distortion and dragging, the membrane attachment to the optic disc is carefully circumcised.

a

b

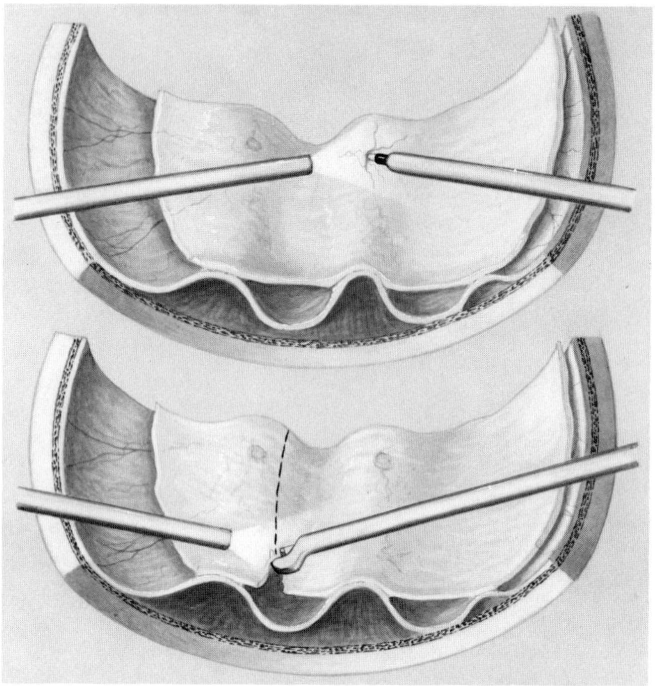

17.**3a** Very adherent membranes require membrane delamination and segmentation. The basic steps of hemostasis (**a**) and membrane sectioning (**b**) are done first.

b The membrane bridging the retinal elevations which extend along the temporal arcades is cut with the vitreous dissector-cutter to relieve traction extending across the posterior pole.

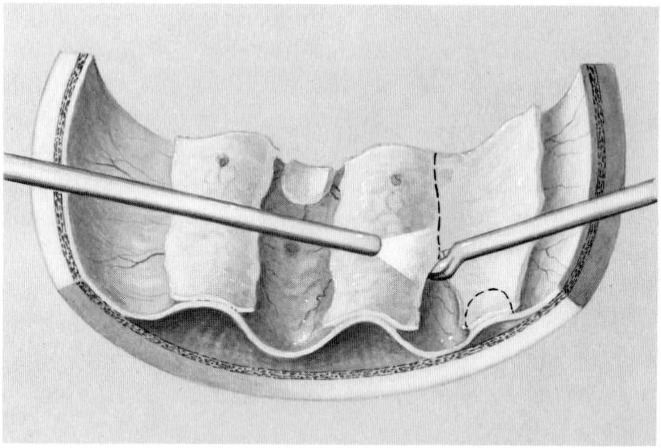

17.**3c** After circumcision of membrane around the optic disc and sectioning of other bridging membranes (vertical broken line), isolated vitreoretinal adhesions are circumcised (curved broken line, lower right).

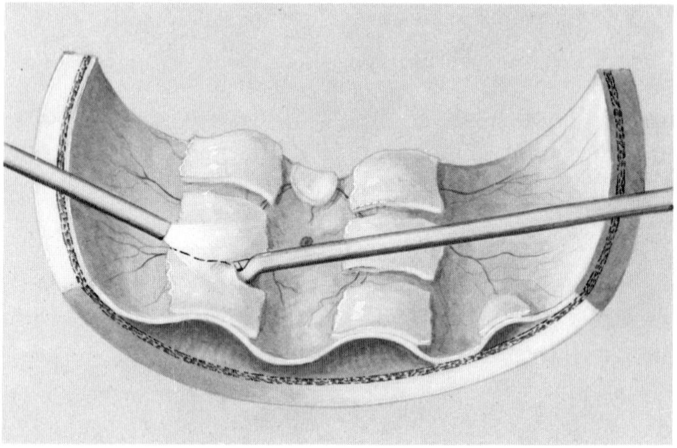

17.**3d** Large sheets of membranes are cut into small segments. The site of the membrane to be segmented is explored with a blunt spatula, which is used to undermine the space between the membrane and the retina. Then the membrane is sectioned with the membrane cutter.

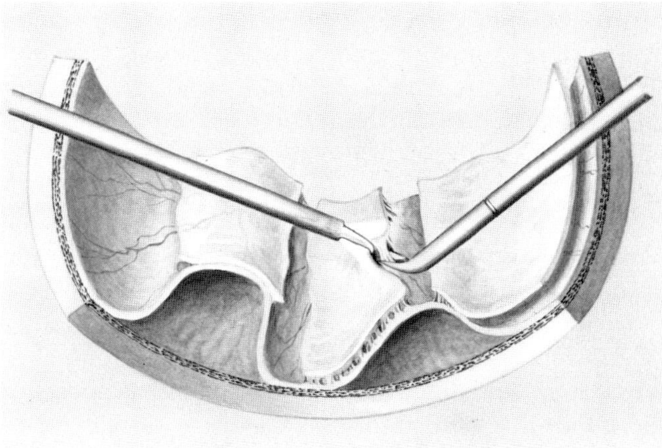

17.**4a** A tissue micromanipulator, which has a pick as well as aspiration and illumination capabilities, may be used with the Sutherland scissors for delaminating vascularized membranes. It sucks membrane edge, holds and fixates it, and coagulates potential bleeding vessels.

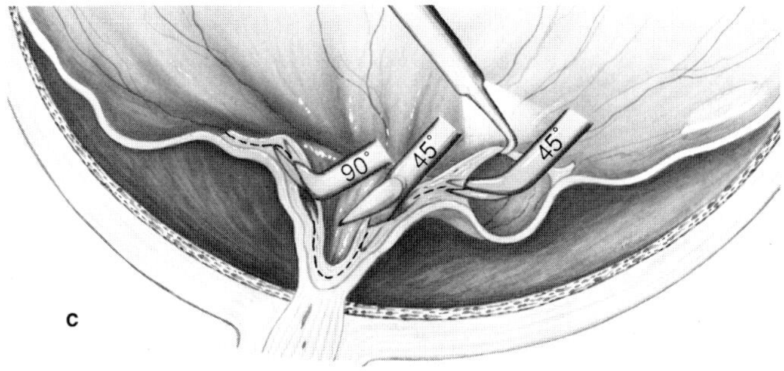

c

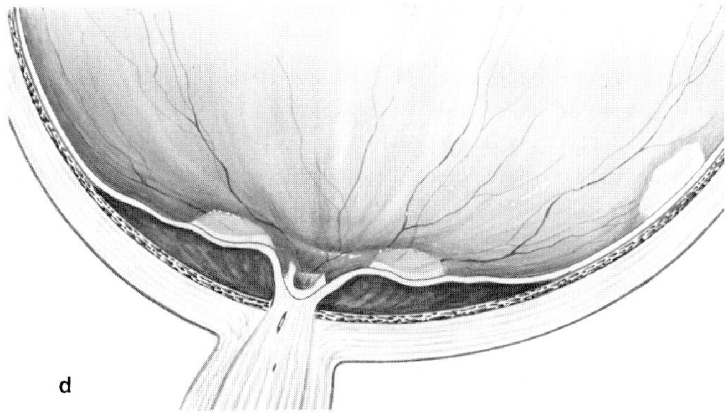

d

b

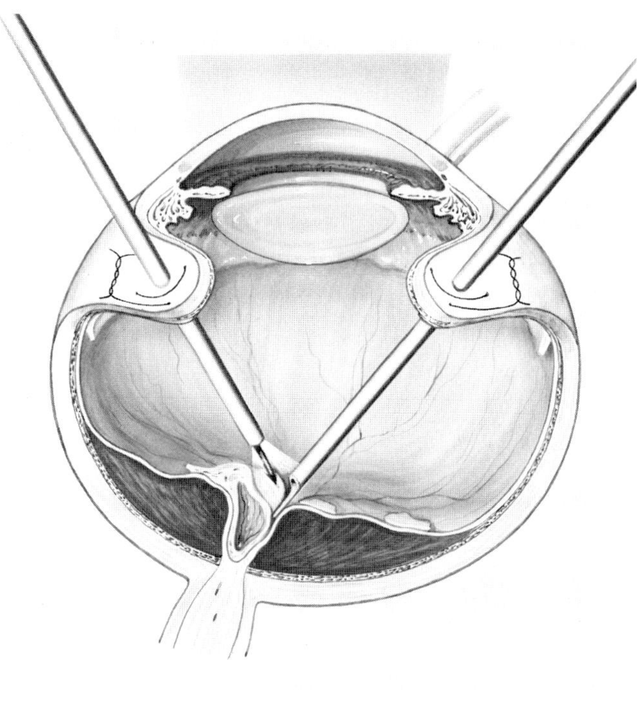

e

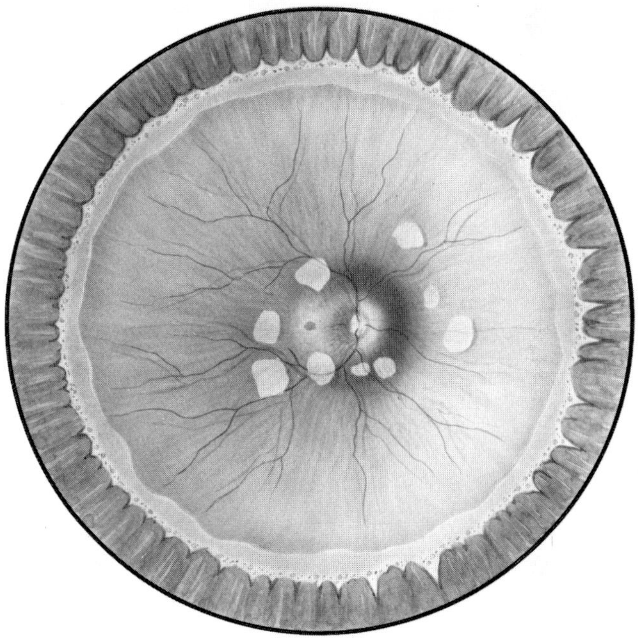

17.**4b** Delamination of membranous stalk lining a funnel-shaped detachment around the optic disc is difficult to accomplish with curved Sutherland scissors. A needle knife, MVR blade, or 20-gauge needle (see Chapter 3) is used in combination with the micromanipulator to retract the stalk from the retina; connecting strands are sliced with the needle knife. Bleeding vessels are coagulated with the diathermy mode of the micromanipulator.

17.**4c** Sutherland scissors of different blade angulations should be readily available for complicated tractional retinal detachments involving the retina around the optic disc.

d Membranes that are difficult to delaminate should be left alone, as were the three segments of membrane shown here.

17.**4e** This fundus illustrates a case of table-top diabetic tractional retinal detachment 6 months after successful vitreoretinal membrane surgery. Multiple techniques (surface membrane sectioning, segmentation, and delamination; external subretinal drainage; and air injection) produced retinal reattachment. Small pieces of membrane left on areas of vitreoretinal adhesion after circumcision usually shrink further with time.

Another surgical approach to diabetic tractional detachment is en bloc dissection of the vitreous (2). The first step is a core vitrectomy, which preserves the detached membranous cortical vitreous. The next step is to open an area between the posterior detached retina and the equator in the elevated cortical membrane. The light pipe with pick is inserted through this opening, and is used to retract the cut edge of the membrane from the retina. The blade of the Sutherland scissors is closed to dissect, then opened to split and cut the tissues connecting membranes and retina. This procedure is repeated until all adhesions have been released. The entire vitreous is finally removed with the vitrectomy probe.

Surface membranes on the retina located between the posterior pole and equator are sometimes unresectable, so that the retina remains foreshortened and detached after subretinal fluid drainage. If relaxing retinotomy is deemed inadvisable, scleral resection may be performed (3,12).

5a

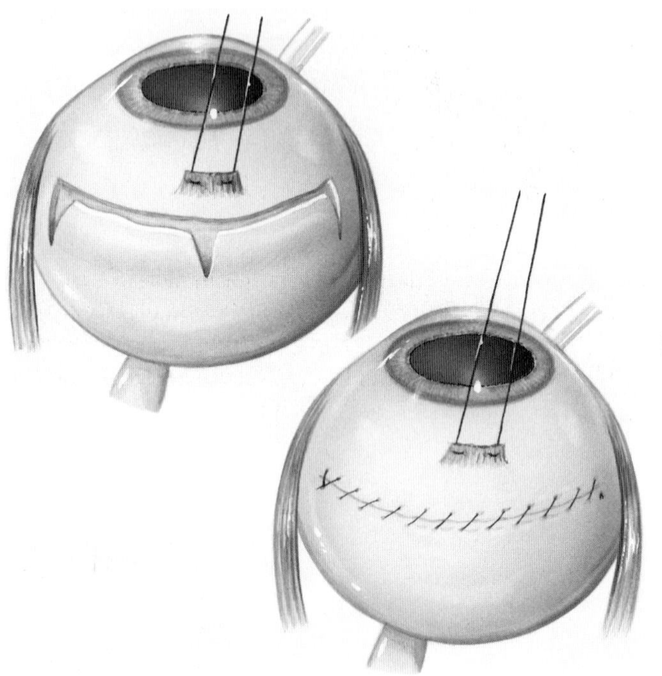

b

17.**5a** Scleral resection requires adequate scleral exposure: a complete conjunctival peritomy, traction sutures on the recti muscles, and, if necessary, temporary disinsertion of the rectus muscle in the center of the proposed resection. The area to be resected is outlined with a marking pencil. The area, which measures 3–5 mm in width, should straddle the equator of the globe and extend to cover the quadrants with unresected membranes.

Using a hockey-stick shaped scarifier, a perpendicular scleral groove is cut on the sclera along the anteriorly located linear mark and extended to cover the quadrants with unresected surface retinal membranes. A radial incision is made to connect to the posterior mark at each end of the groove. The scleral flap is dissected, leaving a thin layer of sclera on the choroid, and extended to the posterior mark. The scleral flap is cut along the posterior mark, leaving a posterior scleral edge which is later approximated to the anterior scleral edge.

b If extensive subretinal fluid is present in the region of the scleral bed, sclerochoroidotomy is made there to drain the fluid externally. Otherwise, drainage is made outside the resection in the area of maximum retinal elevation and the sclerotomy is closed with a 5–0 nylon suture. The running 5–0 nylon suture is pulled up and tied permanently. Then the intraocular volume is restored with an injection of balanced salt solution. The disinserted rectus muscle is reattached, and the conjunctiva is closed.

Tractional Retinal Detachment after Vitreous Loss

Tractional retinal detachment can occur after incarceration and loss of vitreous through a corneal or scleral wound (10,11: 138–142). The advent of extracapsular cataract surgery, and the ability of anterior segment surgeons to perform anterior vitrectomy for vitreous loss during cataract surgery or penetrating ocular injury, have reduced the prevalence of tractional detachment in these eyes.

Tractional retinal detachments progress very slowly; therefore, elective vitrectomy is indicated only when there is documented progression of the retinal detachment posterior to the equator to threaten the macula. When traction produces retinal breaks, early vitrectomy is indicated.

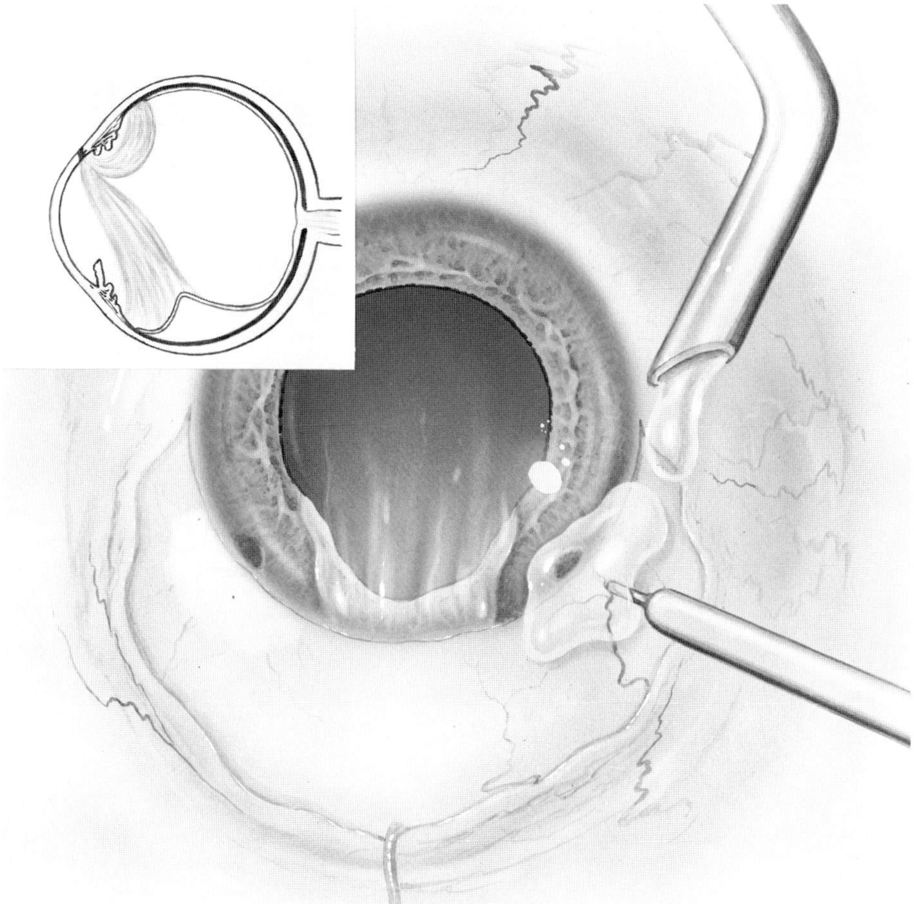

17.**6a** *Inset:* cross section of an eye with a tractional retinal detachment. Vitreous is incarcerated in the corneal wound, pulling and detaching the inferior retina. The incarcerated vitreous consists of two components: an inferior leaf that is connected with the inferior retina, and a superior leaf that is continuous with the gel behind the upper iris.

After a 270° limbal peritomy, hemostasis is accomplished with minimal tissue damage using light diathermy applied under a stream of BSS Plus solution.

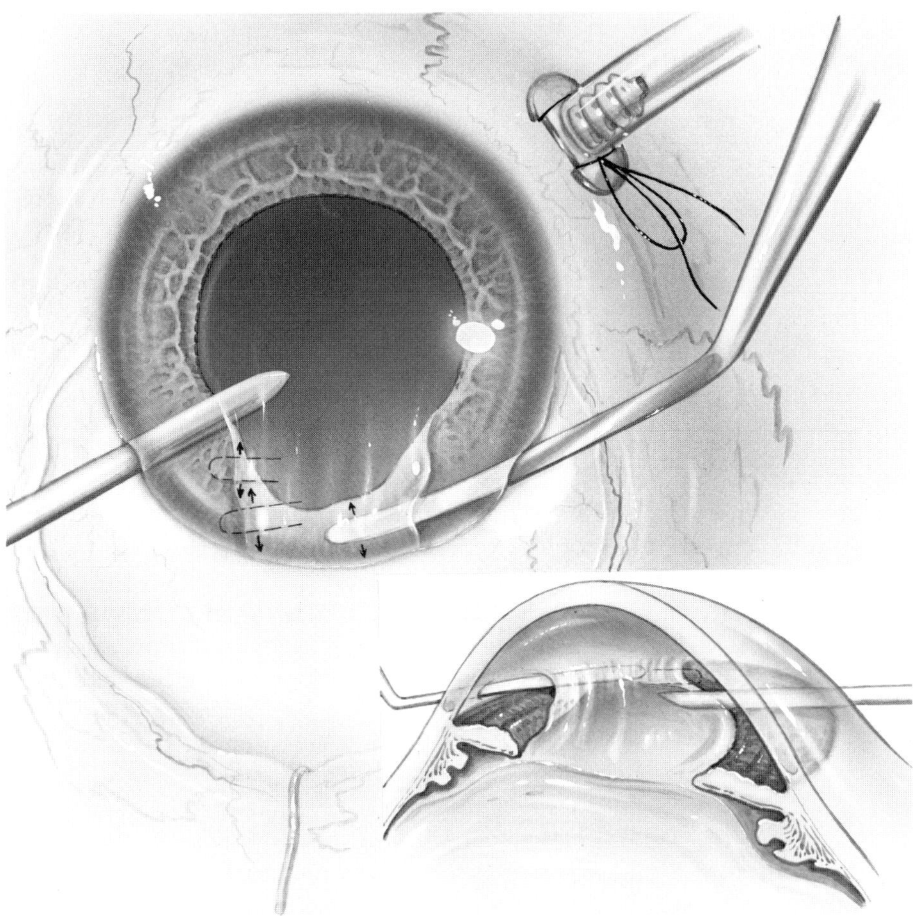

17.**6b** The anterior chamber is infused with BSS Plus solution through a bent 25-gauge needle inserted at 10 o'clock through the limbus. The condensed vitreous is separated from the anterior surface of the iris using blunt dissection with a fine cyclodialysis spatula inserted into the anterior chamber through a limbal incision in the 2 o'clock meridian (right eye).

Inset: the tip of the spatula is directed peripherally under the vitreous near the chamber angle, and swept both centrally and peripherally to isolate the vitreous from the iris.

6c

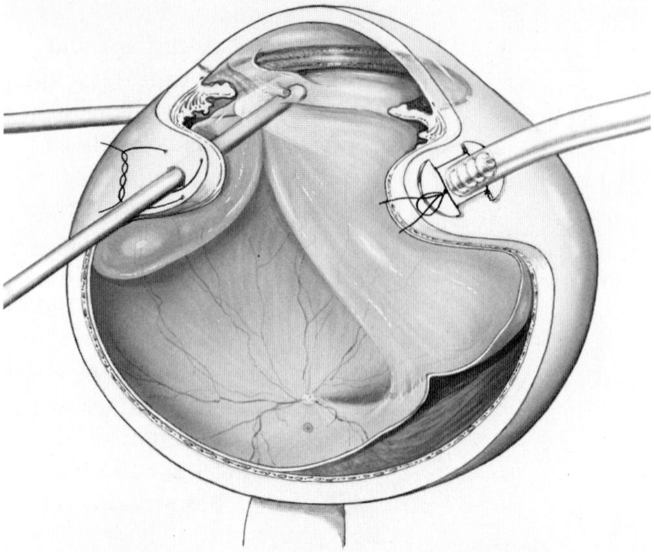

6e

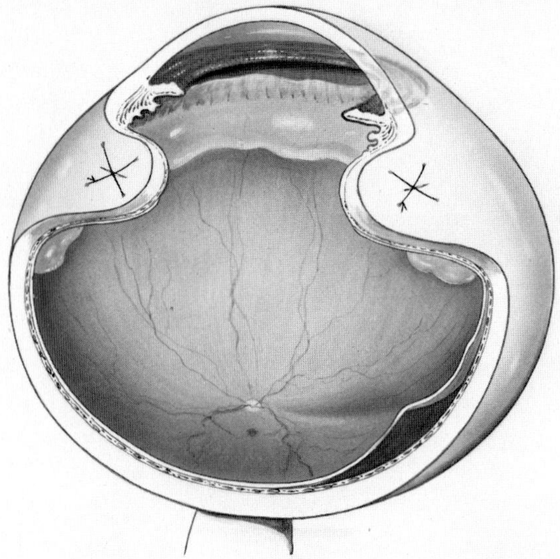

6d

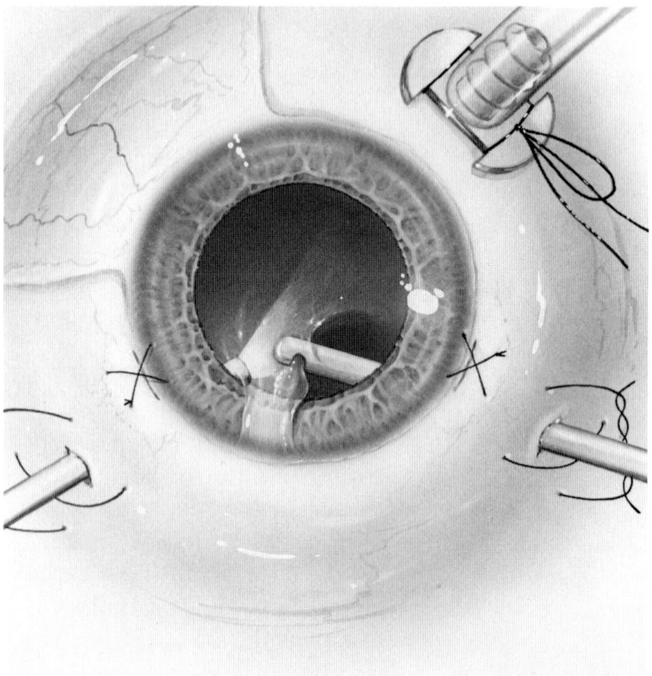

17.**6c** The two instruments are withdrawn from the anterior chamber, and the limbal incisions are closed with 8–0 nylon sutures. An infusion line to the vitreous is established through a cannula through the pars plana inferotemporally. The cutting frequency of the vitrectomy probe is increased to reduce traction on the vitreous and retina. The vitrectomy and endoilluminator probes are inserted through the sclerotomies in the pars plana into the anterior portion of the vitreous cavity.

17.**6d** The portion of the inferior leaf within the pupil is removed first (see Fig. 17.**6a**). With the port of the vitrectomy probe parallel to the plane of the iris, the superficial portion is removed next. Finally, the remaining vitreous gel, including anterior portions of the superior leaf, is removed.

17.**6e** After the incarcerated anterior vitreous gel has been removed, the vitrectomy proceeds posteriorly until all of the vitreous gel has been removed.

The entire retina is inspected under the operating microscope, and then with indirect ophthalmoscopy and scleral depression, to search for iatrogenic retinal breaks. If breaks are found, they are treated with endolaser or external cryoapplications.

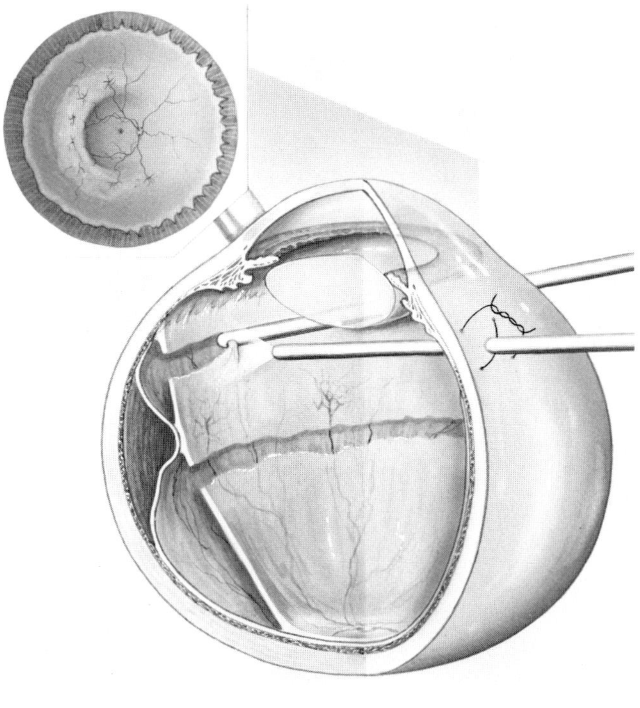

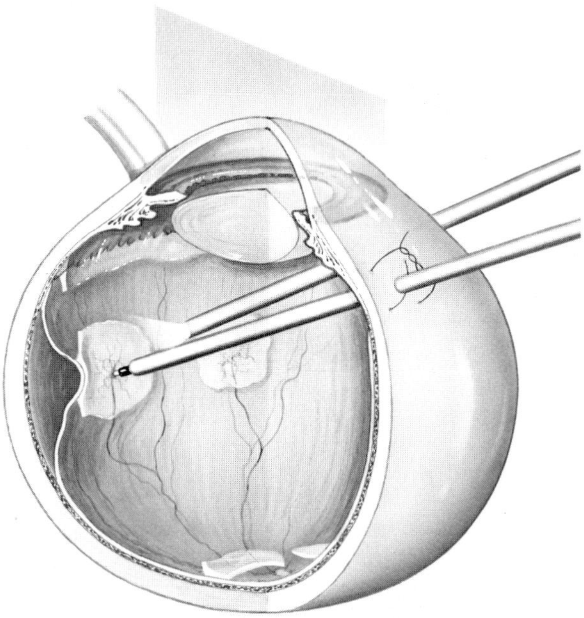

Sickle Cell Disease

17.**7a** Vitrectomy and membrane resection are indicated when one or more of the following conditions exist: (1) vitreous hemorrhage that has not cleared within six months; (2) recurrent vitreous hemorrhage; and (3) progressive tractional retinal detachment threatening or involving the macula.

In eyes with sickle cell disease, fibrovascular proliferation, which usually occurs in the mid-periphery of the fundus, may produce tractional retinal detachment (*inset*) (11: 327–335). The potential for complications during vitrectomy in these patients is higher because the retina is thin and atrophic at the base of the sea fans.

The vitreous changes in tractional retinal detachment in eyes with sickle cell disease are different from those in diabetic tractional detachment. The major difference is in the vitreous cortex, which becomes membranous and detached anterior and posterior to its attachment to the elevated retina. In addition, the cortical membrane may be firmly adherent to the optic disc, which may be elevated.

The surgical procedure includes removal of the central vitreous to permit visualization of the retina and to provide a clear visual axis. The cortical membrane originating from the detached retina and the vitreous base is completely resected in a 360° arc with the vitrectomy probe. The cortical membrane bridging the vitreous base and the area of detached retina is circumcised with either the vitrectomy probe or the vertical-cutting scissors.

Removal of the cortical vitreous in the area of the sea fans is desirable to eliminate a scaffold for future neovascular growth (6).

17.**7b** Active neovascular proliferation at the membrane epicenters is meticulously coagulated with endodiathermy after membrane segmentation. The vitreous is often very tightly adherent to these epicenters or sea fans, so that excessive traction on them easily results in retinal tears or vitreous hemorrhage (14). The segmented membrane around the epicenter is trimmed only if this can be done safely with the vitrectomy probe.

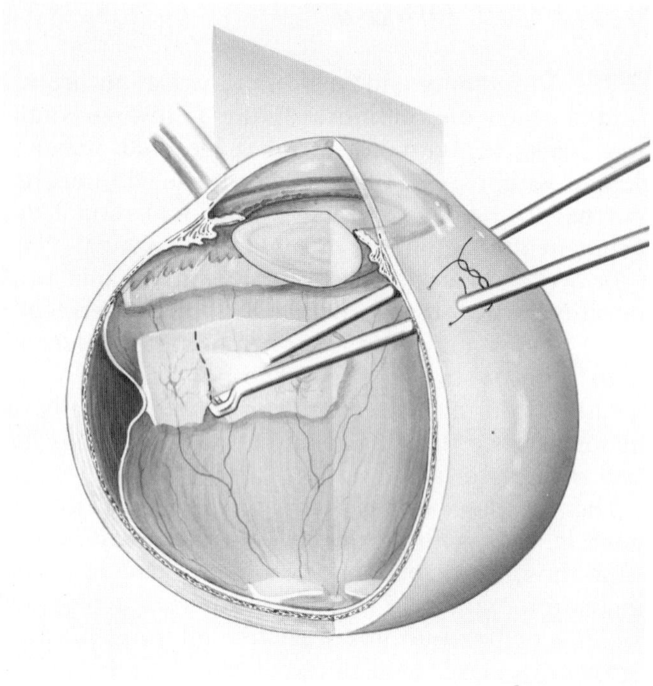

17.**7c** The site of fibrovascular proliferation is usually the epicenter of a membranous adhesion to the elevated retina. The fibrovascular sheet between the epicenters is undermined with a vitreous spatula and sectioned with vertical-cutting scissors. This segmentation of the surface membrane reduces tangential traction on blood vessels, and minimizes recurrent vitreous hemorrhage.

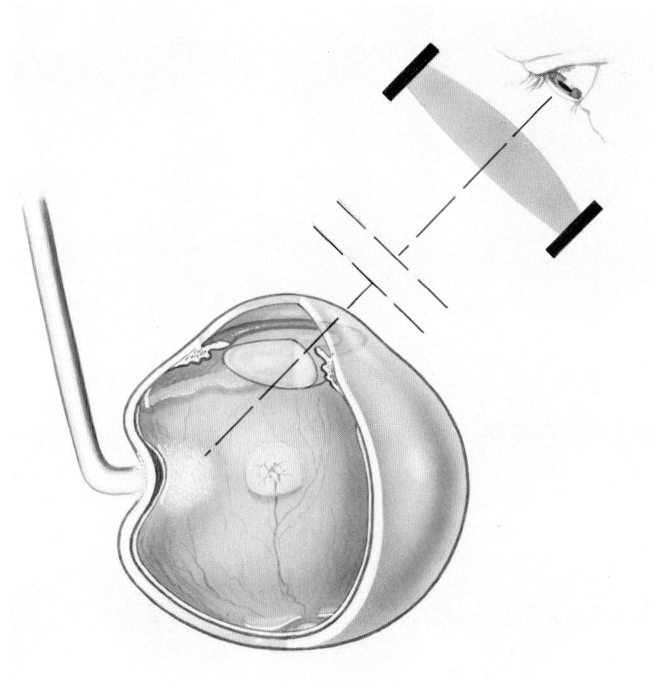

17.**7d** When actively growing neovascular proliferation is so close to the retina that it may not be safely closed with endodiathermy, the neovascular membrane is treated with cryoapplications using the freeze-thaw technique, applied three times (7).

References

1. Aaberg TM. Clinical results in vitrectomy for diabetic traction retinal detachment. Am J Ophthalmol 1979; 88: 246–253.
2. Abrams GW, Williams GA. "En bloc" excision of diabetic membranes. Am J Ophthalmol 1987; 103: 302–308.
3. Charles S. Vitreous microsurgery. 2nd ed. Baltimore: Williams and Wilkins, 1987: 111–114.
4. Charles S, Flinn CE. The natural history of diabetic extramacular traction retinal detachment. Arch Ophthalmol 1981; 99: 66–68.
5. Cohen HB, McMeel JW, Franks EP. Diabetic traction detachment. Arch Ophthalmol 1979; 97: 1268–1272.
6. Goldbaum MH, Peyman GA, Nagpal KC, et al. Vitrectomy in sickling retinopathy: report of five cases. Ophthalmic Surg 1976; 7(4): 92–102.
7. Lee CB, Woolf MB, Galions SO, Goldbaum MH, Stevens TS, Goldberg MF. Cryotherapy of proliferative sickle retinopathy, part I: single freeze-thaw cycle. Ann Ophthalmol 1975; 7: 1299–1308.
8. Machemer R, Aaberg TM. Vitrectomy. 2nd ed. New York: Grune and Stratton, 1979: 71–76.
9. Michels RG. Vitrectomy for complications of diabetic retinopathy. Arch Ophthalmol 1978; 96: 237–246.
10. Michels RG. Vitreous surgery. St. Louis: C V Mosby, 1980: 309–318.
11. Peyman GA, Schulman JA. Intravitreal surgery: principles and practice. New York: Appleton-Century-Crofts, 1986.
12. Schepens CL. Retinal detachment and allied diseases. Philadelphia: W B Saunders, 1983: 696–701.
13. Tolentino FI, Schepens CL, Freeman HM, Vitreoretinal disorders: diagnosis and management. Philadelphia: W B Saunders, 1976: 432–441
14. Welch RB, Goldberg MF. Sickle-cell hemoglobin and its relation to fundus abnormality. Arch Ophthalmol 1966; 75: 353–362.

18

Retinal Breaks without Retinal Detachment

Retinal breaks without retinal detachment occur in approximately 7.8% of the population, or approximately 16 million persons in the United States (12). The incidence of retinal detachment is about 1:9000 persons per year; therefore it is obvious that all retinal breaks do not require treatment. In deciding whether prophylactic treatment is advisable, the following factors should be considered (1, 4, 5, 7, 8, 10, 17):

- *Type of retinal break:* retinal tear, retinal dialysis, retinal hole
- *Size, location, and number of retinal breaks*
- *Other significant ocular findings:* high myopia, vitreous hemorrhage, retinopathy of prematurity, cataractous changes, lattice degeneration
- *Systemic syndromes predisposing to retinal detachment:* Marfan's syndrome, Ehlers-Danlos syndrome, Wagner's syndrome, atopic dermatitis

Type of retinal break: peripheral retinal breaks may be classified into three types: retinal tears, retinal dialyses, and retinal holes. Each type has a different predisposition to cause a retinal detachment.

Retinal tear: in most cases, a retinal tear forms at the site of an abnormal, isolated vitreoretinal adhesion or along an irregularity in the posterior vitreous base. As the vitreous gel undergoes liquefaction and collapse, a posterior vitreous detachment develops that extends anteriorly to exert traction on this adhesion, resulting in the formation of a retinal tear (6, 18, 19: 394–397). Following vitreous detachment, fluid vitreous comes in to contact with the retinal tear to promote the development of a retinal detachment. For these reasons, retinal tears show the greatest predisposition to retinal detachment; we therefore treat all retinal tears prophylactically.

Retinal dialysis: a retinal dialysis is a slit-like retinal break that occurs at the ora serrata. The most common type of dialysis occurs in the inferotemporal quadrant in young males. A traumatic form of dialysis develops superonasally after bluntocular trauma, or inferotemporally after direct trauma to that quadrant. Retinal detachment caused by a dialysis tends to progress slowly and pose less of an immediate threat to the macula; nonetheless, dialyses ultimately cause retinal detachments and prophylactic treatment is therefore indicated.

Retinal hole: small, asymptomatic retinal holes located near the ora serrata and not associated with vitreoretinal degeneration rarely require treatment unless there is a history of retinal detachment in the fellow eye or in the family. Treatment is also indicated if an eye with a retinal hole is phakic or pseudophakic.

Size, location, and number of retinal breaks: the larger and greater the number of retinal breaks, the stronger and more urgent are the indications for treatment. Retinal detachment resulting from retinal breaks located superiorly, temporally, and especially posterotemporally, pose a greater threat to the macula than those located nasally, anteriorly, and inferiorly.

Other significant ocular findings: retinal breaks in eyes with high myopia, vitreous hemorrhage, or retinopathy of prematurity have a greater predisposition for retinal detachment. Treatment is indicated when retinal breaks occur in eyes with a developing cataract, because the ability to visualize an early detachment decreases as the lens becomes more cataractous.

Lattice degeneration: lattice degeneration occurs in approximately 6.4% of eyes in the general population (15). This degeneration has a propensity for bilaterality. Both sexes are affected equally. Lattice degeneration occurs as oval or spindle-shaped areas of retinal thinning, 0.5–1.5 DD wide, varying in length from 2 DD to an entire quadrant. Lattice lesions extend parallel to the ora serrata and are located between the ora serrata and the equator. White interlacing lines of sheathed or occluded vessels are seen frequently within the lattice.

Most forms of lattice are benign and nonprogressive; only 1% of eyes develop retinal detachment (16). The benign form of lattice is located near the ora serrata, and is usually located in the inferotemporal quadrant. It is not associated with vitreoretinal traction, and therefore requires no treatment. Retinal holes may develop in approximately 23% of eyes with lattice degeneration. The holes are usually small, round or oval-shaped, and located within or adjacent to the lattice lesions (2). Retinal holes are much less likely to cause retinal detachment than retinal tears; however, if there is a history of retinal detachment in the family or the fellow eye, we tend to treat eyes with multiple holes in lattice degeneration. Retinal tears develop along the posterior margin or at the ends of the lattice as a result of traction from vitreous membranes. Treatment of the retinal tears associated with lattice degeneration should be undertaken without delay, because retinal detachments tend to develop rapidly in these eyes (19: 40–350).

Systemic syndromes predisposing to retinal detachment: retinal breaks found in patients with Marfan's syndrome, Wagner's syndrome, Ehlers-Danlos syndrome, and atopic dermatitis should be treated, because of the poor prognosis associated with retinal detachments that develop in patients with these connective tissue diseases.

Choice of treatment modality: according to the location of the retinal breaks: treatment of retinal breaks without detachment utilizes cryopexy, photocoagulation, or scleral buckling.

Cryopexy is preferable for treating retinal breaks located anterior to the equator (3,9,11,13). Transconjunctival cryoapplications are used in the prophylactic treatment of retinal dialyses, anterior retinal holes surrounded by localized retinal detachment, retinal holes in multiple areas of lattice degeneration, and small anterior retinal tears. Visualization and treatment of retinal breaks near the ora serrata is easier using indirect ophthalmoscopy and scleral depression with the cryoprobe than using photocoagulation through the mirror of a Goldmann three-mirror lens. We prefer photocoagulation to cryopexy for lesions located in the region of, or posterior to, the equator.

Photocoagulation is preferable for the treatment of posterior retinal breaks, because it can be done without the conjunctival incision that would be required for cryopexy. Treatment of retinal breaks is done using an argon laser and Goldmann three-mirror contact lens. The pupil is dilated as widely as possibly. Only topical anesthesia is used.

The retinal break is surrounded on all sides with three to four rows of applications 500 μ in diameter applied for 0.2 seconds.

After photocoagulation or cryotherapy, an antibiotic ointment is instilled, and the eye is patched for 6 hours (if the patient is not monocular). The patient is instructed to report any visual field loss immediately and to return for reexamination in two weeks, at which time the laser or cryopexy lesions should be pigmented.

If adequate pigmentation is noted, the patient is reexamined two, three, and six months later.

Scleral buckling is used in treating large retinal tears, retinal tears associated with a substantial amount of vitreous hemorrhage, and multiple retinal tears associated with severe lattice degeneration.

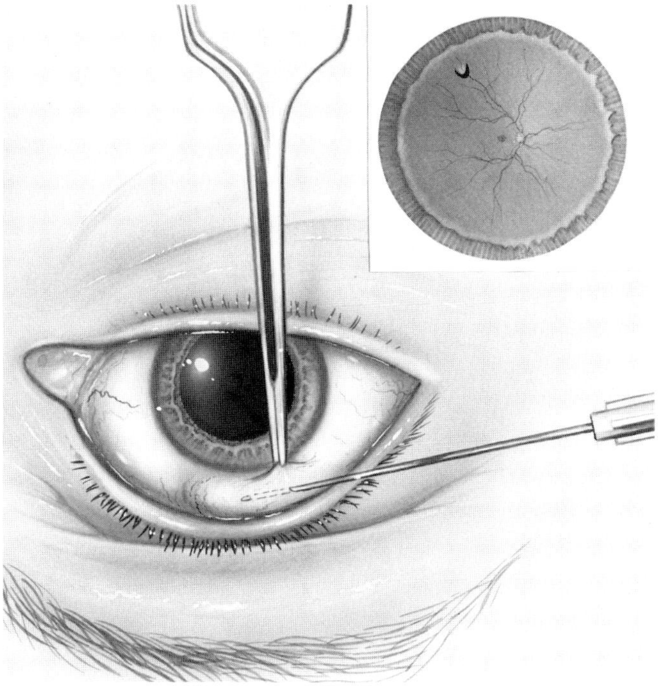

18.**1a** **Retinal tear without detachment.** *Inset:* Small superotemporal retinal tear located near the ora serrata.

The perilimbal superotemporal conjunctiva is grasped using smooth Bishop-Harmon forceps. Then 0.1–0.2 ml of 1% xylocaine is injected under the conjunctiva using a short 30-gauge needle on a tuberculin syringe.

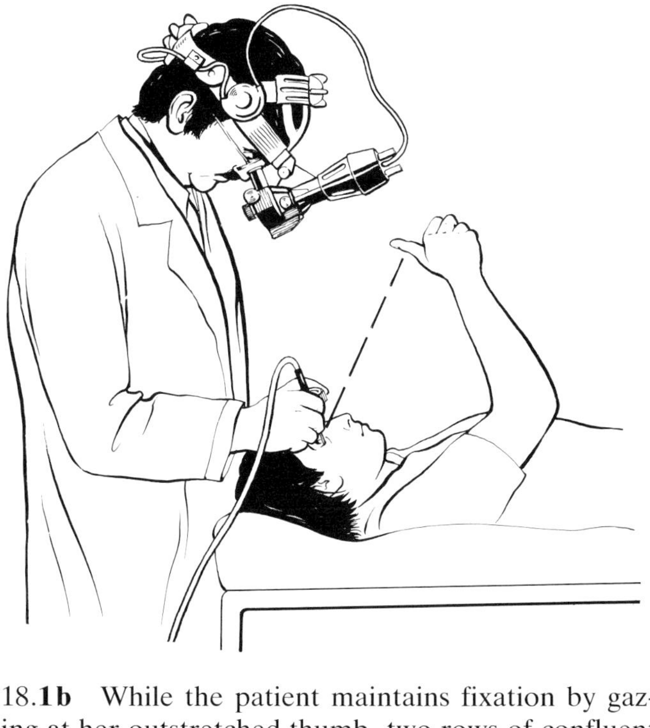

18.**1b** While the patient maintains fixation by gazing at her outstretched thumb, two rows of confluent cryoapplications are placed surrounding the retinal tear.

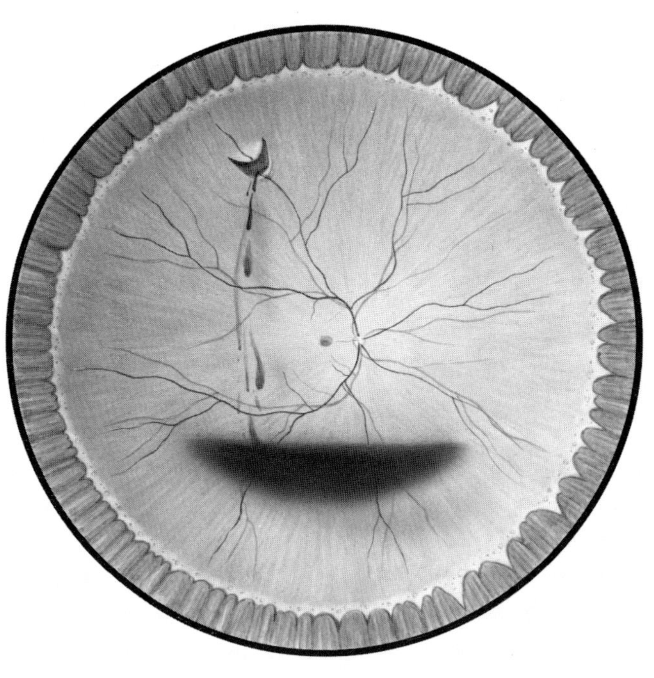

18.**2a** **Retinal tear associated with vitreous hemorrhage**. superotemporal equatorial retinal tear bridged by a retinal vessel that has ruptured to cause vitreous hemorrhage which has settled inferiorly (14).

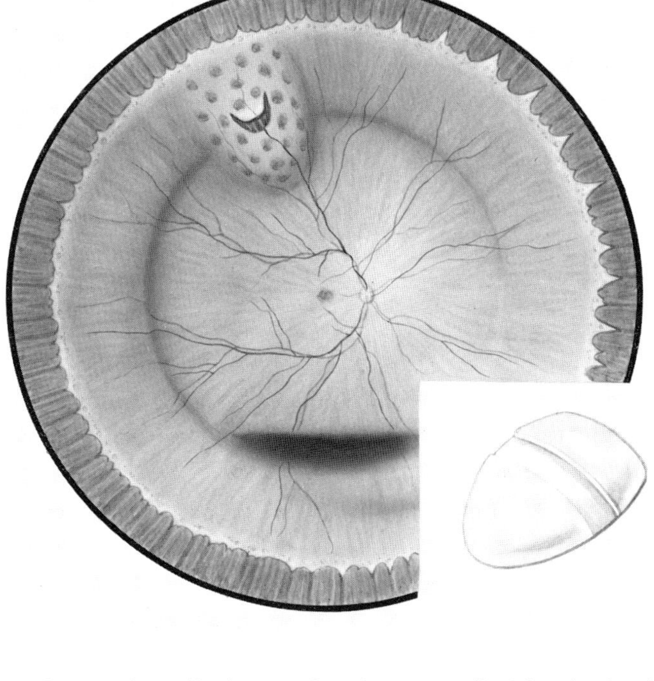

18.**2b** After diathermy has been applied in the bed of the scleral pocket, as described in Chapter 21, traction to the blood vessel and retinal tear are relieved with a scleral buckle produced with a wedge-shaped implant (*inset*). The indentation extending around the fundus in the region of the equator was produced by an encircling element, which ensures a more permanent buckling effect.

References

1. Bensen WE. Prophylactic therapy of retinal breaks. Surv Ophthalmol 1977; 22: 41–47.
2. Byer NE. A clinical definition of lattice degeneration of the retina and its variations. Mod Probl Ophthalmol 1975; 15: 58–67.
3. Chignell AH. Retinal detachment surgery. New York: Springer, 1980: 133–136.
4. Chignell AH, Shilling JS. Prophylaxis of retinal detachment. Br J Ophthalmol 1973; 57: 291–298.
5. Cockerham WD, Freeman HM. Molehills, mountains and prophylaxis of retinal detachment. Arch Ophthalmol 1968; 79: 655–656.
6. Davis MD. Natural history of retinal breaks without detachment. Arch Ophthalmol 1974; 92: 183–194.
7. Freeman HM. Surgery of the retina and vitreous. In: Jaffe NS, ed. Atlas of ophthalmic surgery. New York: Gower (in press).
8. Kanski JJ. Retinal detachment: a color manual of diagnosis and treatment. London: Butterworths, 1986: 45–50.
9. Lincoff HA. The prophylactic treatment of retinal detachment. Arch Ophthalmol 1961; 66: 48–60.
10. Morse PH. Vitreoretinal disease: a manual for diagnosis and treatment. Chicago: Year Book Medical Publishers, 1979: 121–135.
11. Morse PH, Scheie HG. Prophylactic cryoretinopexy of retinal breaks. Arch Ophthalmol 1974; 92: 204–207.
12. Nussbaum JJ, Freeman HM. Peripheral retinal breaks and degeneration. In: Fraunfelder FT, Roy FH, eds. Current ocular therapy, 2. Philadelphia: W B Saunders, 1985: 471–473.
13. Ramsay RC, Eifrig DE. Outpatient freezing of retinal breaks. Am J Ophthalmol 1973; 76: 782–785.
14. Robertson DM, Curtin VT, Norton EWD. Avulsed retinal vessels with retinal breaks: a cause of recurrent vitreous hemorrhage. Arch Ophthalmol 1971; 85: 669–672.
15. Rutnin U, Schepens CL. Fundus appearance in normal eyes, III: peripheral degenerations. Am J Ophthalmol 1967; 64: 1042–1062.
16. Schepens CL. Retinal detachment and allied diseases. Philadelphia: W B Saunders, 1983: 1097–1101.
17. Sigelman J. Retinal diseases, pathogenesis, laser therapy and surgery. Boston: Little, Brown, 1984: 203–229.
18. Tasman WS. Posterior vitreous detachment and peripheral retinal breaks. Trans Am Acad Ophthalmol Otolaryngol 1968; 72: 217–224.
19. Tolentino FI, Schepens CL, Freeman HM. Vitreoretinal disorders: diagnosis and management. Philadelphia: W B Saunders, 1976; 394–397.

19

Rhegmatogenous Retinal Detachment: Pneumatic Retinopexy

Pneumatic Retinopexy without Conjunctival Incision

Hilton and Grizzard have defined the indications for pneumatic retinopexy as retinal detachments with one retinal break, or a group of breaks, no larger than one clock hour and located in the superior eight hours of the fundus. Contraindications include grade C or D proliferative vitreoretinopathy, mental incompetence, or severe glaucoma (1,2,4). We follow these indications and contraindications, and use pneumatic retinopexy primarily in patients in whom severe systemic illness precludes general anesthesia.

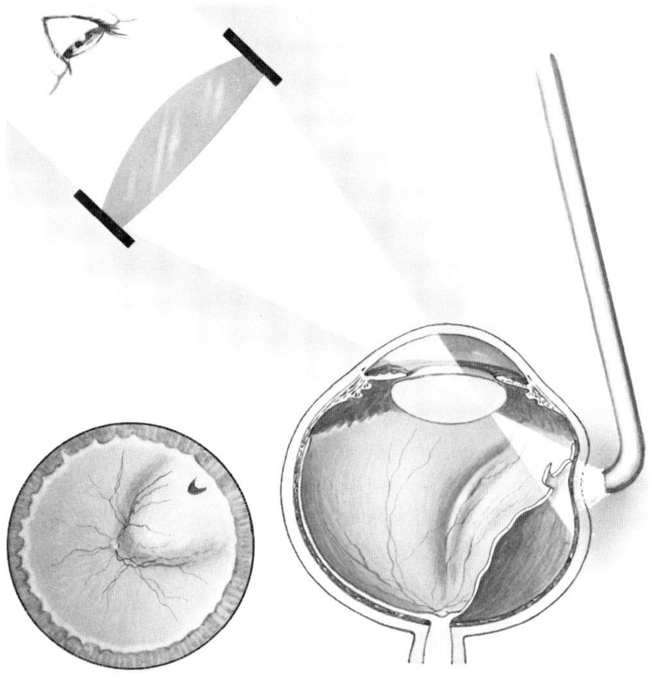

19.**1** Lower left shows a temporal retinal detachment with a superior temporal retinal tear extending less than one clock hour. Gentamicin is given topically hourly for 5 hours preoperatively. The pupil is maximally dilated using 5% phenylephrine hydrochloride three times at 5-minute intervals. Retrobulbar anesthesia is given using 1% xylocaine. The retinal break is treated with two rows of contiguous cryoapplications applied under indirect ophthalmoscopic control (right).

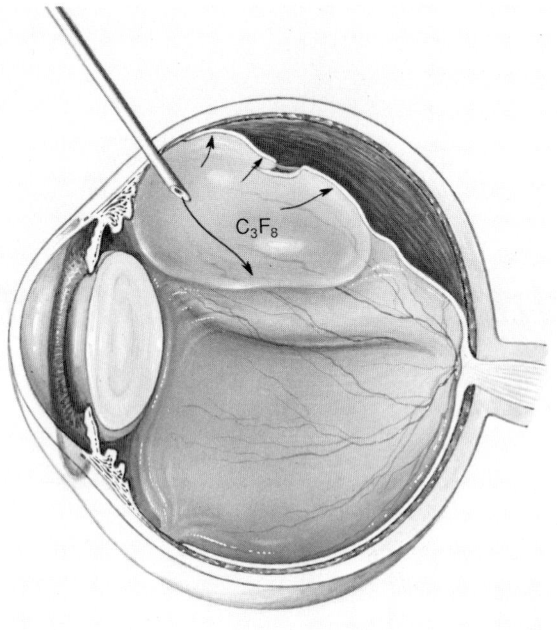

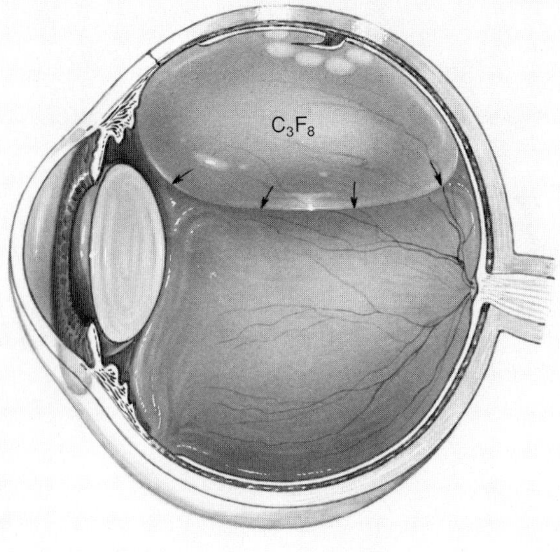

19.**2** **Injection of gas into the vitreous cavity.** Intraocular pressure is lowered to near zero with intermittent indentations of the sclera using the cryoprobe. A wire lid speculum is inserted, and the conjunctiva and cornea are treated with three drops of a solution containing equal parts of povidone-iodine solution and balanced salt solution. After 3 minutes, the pars plana injection site is dried with a sterile cotton stick applicator. Then 0.3 ml of perfluoropropane gas is drawn through a Millipor filter into a tuberculin syringe with a 1/2-inch 30-gauge needle. The patient's head is positioned so that the injection site is uppermost, and the injection is made 0.4 mm posterior to the limbus. A large bubble of gas forms and floats superiorly to tamponade (small arrows) the retinal break and detached retina. As the needle is withdrawn from the eye, the needle track is covered immediately with a sterile cottontipped stick applicator to prevent loss of gas.

The patient's head is rotated to move the gas bubble away from the injection site, and the cotton applicator is removed. The central artery is examined with indirect ophthalmoscopy, and the intraocular pressure is measured 5 and 10 minutes after the injection. If the central artery is closed and does not begin to pulsate within 4 minutes, a paracentesis of the anterior chamber or aspiration of gas or fluid from the vitreous cavity is performed.

If ophthalmoscopy reveals multiple gas bubbles that might pass subretinally, a thump is applied to the uppermost part of the globe using a cotton-tipped applicator to promote the coalescence of the bubbles into a single bubble. This thump is performed by flexing a cotton-tipped applicator and then releasing its tip to firmly strike the pars plana.

Topical antibiotic is instilled, and the eye is patched.

19.**3** Following this, the patient's head is positioned so that the gas bubble moves superotemporally to close the retinal break and maximize the tamponade effect of the bubble.

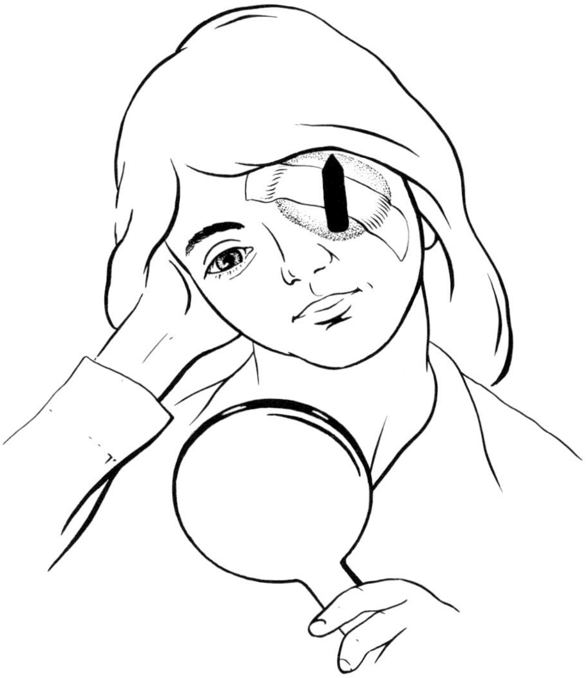

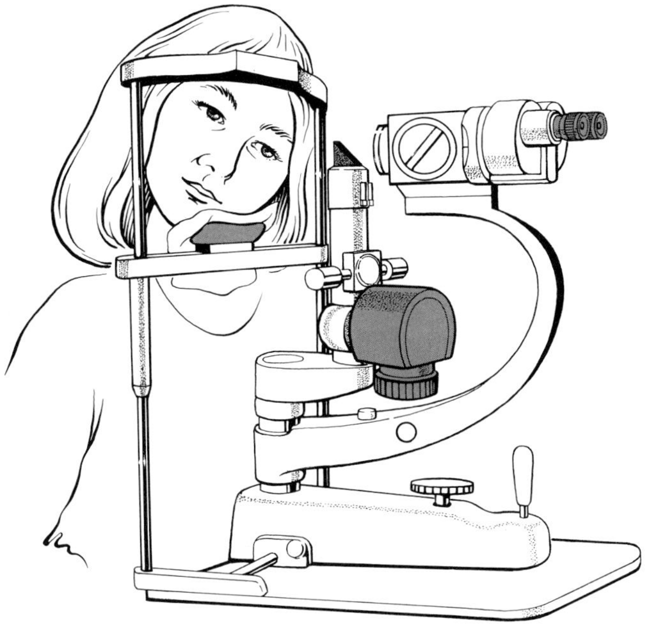

19.4 **Postoperative management.** The patient is instructed to position the head so that the retinal break is uppermost for 16 hours a day for 5 days. The meridian of the retinal break is marked with a arrow made from colored tape and stuck to the eye patch. The patient can easily position the head at the appropriate angle by pointing the arrow toward the ceiling, with periodic use of a hand-held mirror. With proper positioning so that the retinal break is tamponaded by the gas bubble, the retina is usually reattached by the first postoperative day. The intraocular tension is measured at 1/2, 1, 6 and 24 hours postoperatively. Topical steroid drops are prescribed three times a day. Follow-up examinations are at 1, 2, 4, 8, and 16 days. The patient is allowed to return to work 2 weeks after surgery.

19.5 **Cryoapplication or laser photocoagulation for a retinal break.** If the retinal break is too posterior to be reached by the cryoprobe in the conjunctival cul-de-sac, one may either make a conjunctival incision to pass the probe posteriorly to reach the retinal break, or treat the break with laser photocoagulation 2 days after the gas injection, when the retina is usually reattached. The patient's head is tilted 45° to move the bubble away from the retinal break so that it can be visualized adequately.

Subretinal Gas

If multiple gas bubbles are present in the vitreous cavity following pneumatic retinopexy, some bubbles may pass subretinally (3). A moderate or large amount of subretinal gas will produce a bullous detachment, with the retina dragged toward the position of the gas bubbles. With the patient in the supine position, the retina will be moved toward the lens. The detached retina overlying the gas bubbles has a pearly, opalescent appearance, the result of light reflected from the subretinal gas bubbles. A small bubble of subretinal gas may be difficult to identify, especially when viewed through a large bubble, and thus may escape detection as the cause of a persistent retinal detachment.

Management of subretinal gas should start with positioning the patient's head to allow the gas to pass into the vitreous cavity. If multiple bubbles are present, and positioning fails to deliver the bubbles through the retinal break, an attempt is made to form one subretinal bubble using the thump technique. If the subretinal bubble exits through the retinal break, another thump is done to coalesce this bubble with one in the vitreous cavity. If the subretinal gas cannot be removed by positioning and the retinal break remains open, surgery is indicated. If the subretinal bubble is small, or can be positioned away from the retinal break, a scleral buckle is made to close the retinal break. If the bubble is large, it may be evacuated during the drainage of subretinal fluid. Vitrectomy for the purpose of subretinal gas removal and gas-fluid exchange can be hazardous because the retina may be pulled toward the lens. Insertion of the infusion cannula, vitrectomy probe, extrusion needle, or endoilluminator through a displaced retina may produce a large retinal break. This can be avoided by positioning the eye to allow the intravitreous gas to rise to the area where the instrument is to be inserted, thus displacing and moving the subretinal bubbles away from the penetration site. A complete fluid-air exchange is performed, during which an attempt is made to remove the subretinal gas using the extrusion needle.

References

1. Dominguez DA. Cirurgia precoz y ambulatoria del desprendimento de retina. Arch Soc Esp Oftalmol 1985; 48: 47–54.
2. Hilton GF, Grizzard WS. Pneumatic retinopexy: a two-step outpatient operation without conjunctival incision. Ophthalmology 1986; 93: 626–641.
3. McDonald HR, Abrams GW, Irvine AE, et al. The management of subretinal gas following attempted pneumatic retinal reattachment. Ophthalmology 1987; 94: 319–326.
4. Poliner LS, Grand GM, Schoch LH, et al. New retinal detachment after pneumatic retinopexy. Ophthalmology 1987; 94: 315–318.

20

Rhegmatogenous Retinal Detachment: Episcleral Buckling

The choice of episcleral or intrascleral buckling technique is usually influenced by the surgeon's training; both techniques are effective. This chapter deals with episcleral buckling.

Soft, sponge-like materials have been used effectively for scleral buckling to provide external tamponade for retinal breaks (2, 5, 6, 8, 9, 10, 14). These materials are nonabsorbable, provide a permanent implant, and are commercially available as silastic sponge or hydrophilic acrylate implant. (See chapter on implants.)

Silastic sponges are used mainly for episcleral buckling. Hydrophilic acrylate implants are used for either episcleral or intrascleral buckling, and have the advantage of being devoid of dead air spaces, which can trap bacteria and serum fluids and therefore promote bacterial growth (12, 13, 15). Solid silicone rubber has no air spaces, and is also used in episcleral buckling.

a

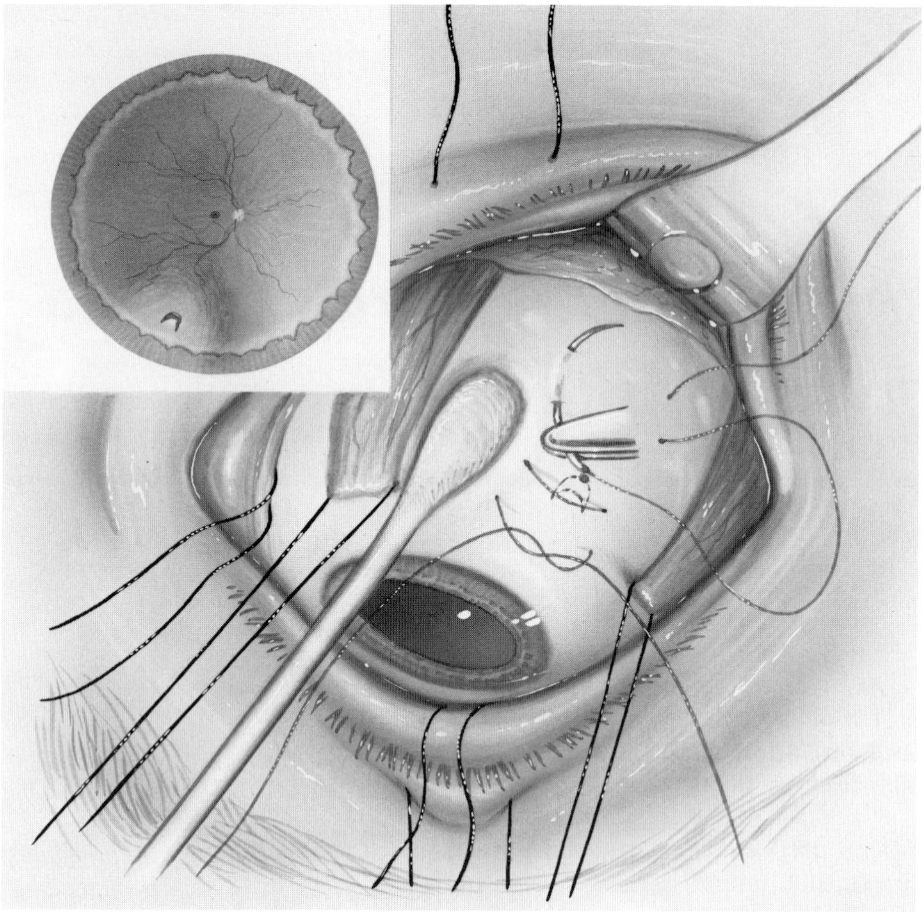

Radial Buckle and Placement of Scleral Mattress Suture

20.**1a** *Inset:* rhegmatogenous retinal detachment in the lowr temporal quadrant caused by a retinal tear at 7 o'clock. Two 5–0 monofilament mattress sutures (Dermalon #1693) are placed anterior and posterior to the localizing mark on the sclera. The separation of the scleral bites of the suture depends on the width of the implant selected. A good rule is to place the sutures one and a half times as far apart as the width of the implant, so that for a 7 mm implant, for example the sutures are placed 10.5 mm apart (1). To obtain a deep and secure scleral mattress suture, the globe is stabilized with a cotton swab pressed against the globe. The scleral bites may be directed radially or equatorially, depending on the thickness of the sclera and exposure of the globe. In this illustration, the needle bite is directed at right angles to the mattress suture because of weak thin sclera near the inferior rectus muscle.

b

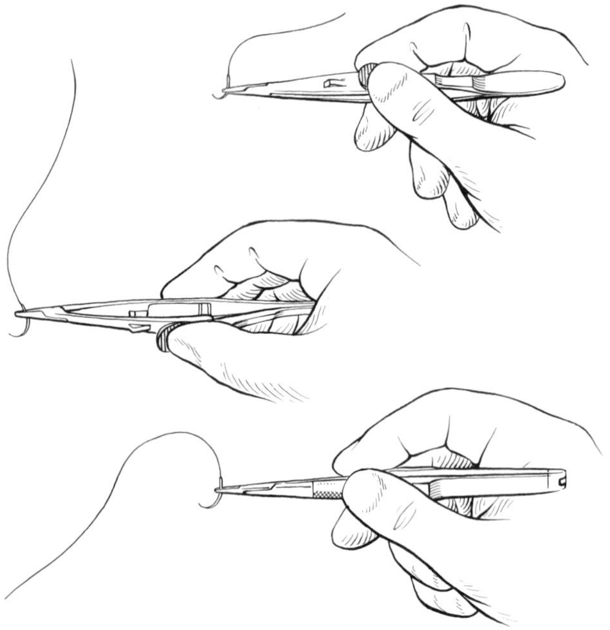

20.**1b** Proper placement of mattress sutures is a crucial factor in producing an effective and lasting episcleral buckle. In the restricted space at the posterior aspect of the globe, proper handling of the needle holder helps in placing deep and secure mattress sutures. The usual method of handling the needle holder is "over the hand" in a manner similar to that in which a pen is held. The other method is "under the hand", in which the needle holder is held like a knife.

A locking needle holder is held over the hand (top) and under the hand (center). A nonlocking needle holder is held over the hand (bottom). The surgeon should master both methods.

c

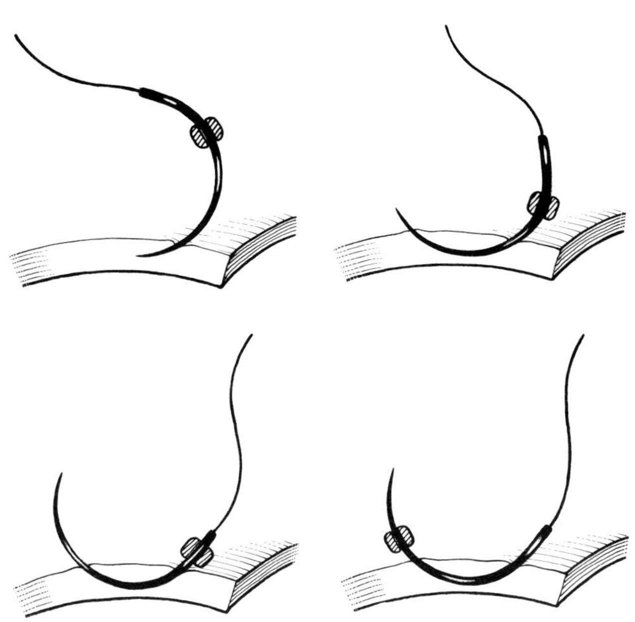

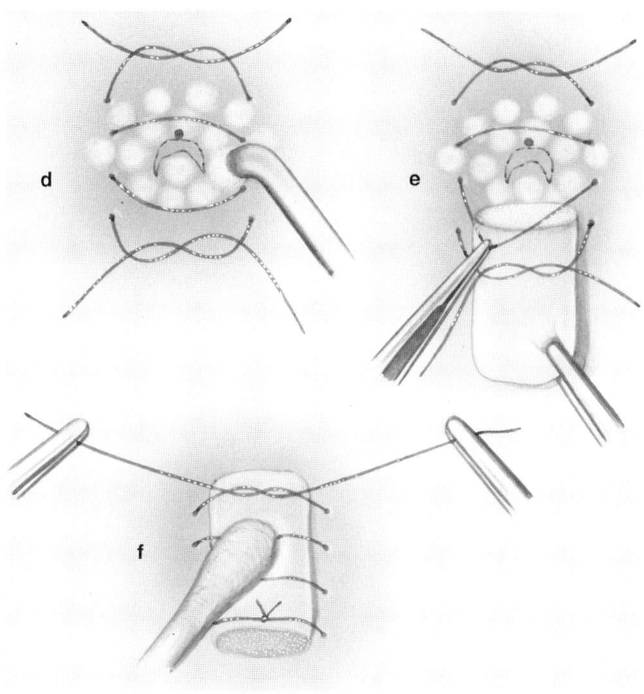

20.**1c** **Insertion of suture needle on sclera** (11). The posterior third of the needle is grasped with the tips of the needle holder. This location provides some mechanical advantage during scleral penetration. To obtain adequate depth of penetration, the needle point penetrates the sclera at a 45° angle (top left). The needle is pushed down until the jaws of the needle holder are on the sclera (top right). The jaws grasp the tail of the needle, which is pushed farther down (bottom left) to increase the length of the needle point outside the sclera. This exposed end of the needle is grasped with the holder and pulled through the sclera (bottom right).

20.**1d** **Cryoapplications** (3, 4). While visualizing with indirect ophthalmoscopy, the retinal tear is surrounded with contiguous cryoapplications. The probe must be held in such a manner that only the tip and not the shaft indents the sclera. After each application the surgeon keeps the probe in place until the iceball has thawed; then, watching retinal landmarks, the surgeon gently slides the probe to place the next contiguous application. Application over the break should be avoided, to minimize dispersion of retinal pigment epithelial cells into the vitreous.

Indentation of the sclera with the cryoprobe can be helpful in deciding whether it is necessary to drain subretinal fluid. If the retinal break closes, it indicates that the break can be closed with an episcleral implant, and therefore drainage of subretinal fluid is not attempted at this stage in the operation (7).

e **Placement of implant.** A piece of hydrophilic acrylate implant, 7 mm in diameter, is cut to fit under the mattress sutures, which are temporarily tied.

f **Securing the episcleral implant.** The sutures are pulled up with forceps while the assistant pushes the implant against the sclera with a cotton swab. The anterior mattress suture and then the posterior mattress suture are tied temporarily. Before the sutures are tied permanently, the fundus is examined to check that the indendation underlies the retinal tear.

If the retinal break cannot be closed by indentation with the cryoprobe or the scleral buckle, or if a retinal fold extends posteriorly from the break, subretinal fluid drainage is performed under the posterior part of the radial implant. The mattress sutures are untied to expose the sclera. A sclerochoroidotomy is made posterior to the retinal break. The choroid is diathermized lightly and penetrated with a needle electrode. When drainage has ceased, the mattress sutures are pulled up snugly and tied.

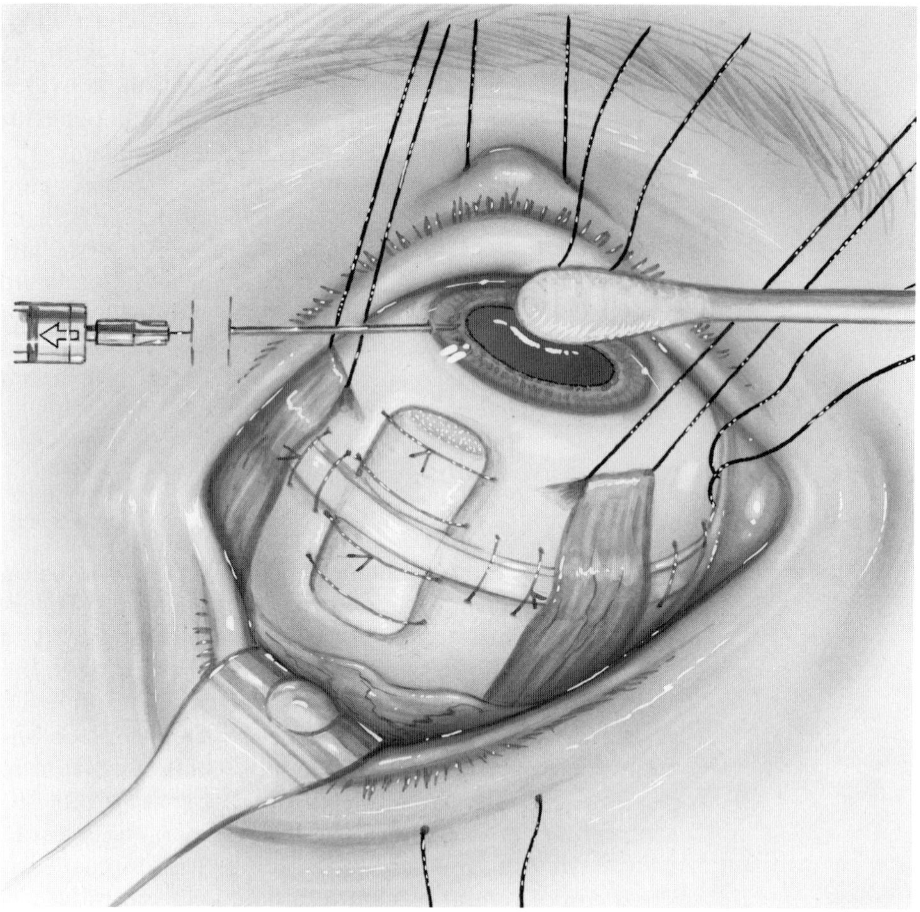

20.1g Radial episcleral implant and encircling band. In the presence of marked vitreous base contraction, as evidenced by a circumferential retinal fold at the posterior vitreous base, a silicone rubber encircling element is added to produce a more permanent buckling effect and to relieve some of the traction. The band is placed over the center of the implant and around the equator of the globe. Anchoring mattress sutures are placed on each side of the implant and in each of the other quadrants. The two ends of the encircling band are joined with a clove hitch. If the intraocular pressure is excessively high, the band is loosened. Intraocular pressure can be reduced further by aspirating aqueous from the anterior chamber with a 30-gauge needle attached to a tuberculin syringe. A cotton swab is pushed against the central cornea to squeeze aqueous out of the posterior chamber and into the anterior chamber.

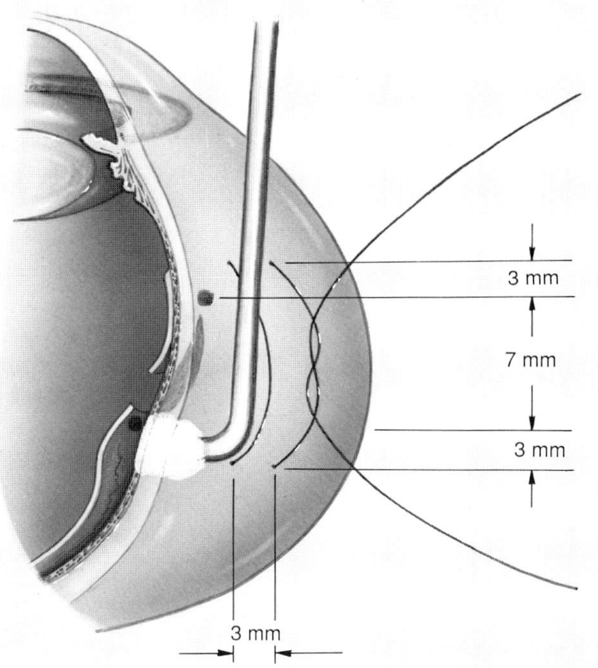

Equatorial Episcleral Buckling

20.**2a** When multiple retinal breaks are present in more than one quadrant, an equatorially oriented episcleral implant is used. If the vitreous base is severely contracted in four quadrants, the implant is made to extend around 360°.

Prevention of gutter phenomenon in equatorial episcleral buckling. The posterior portion of a retinal tear may be supported and closed with a round equatorial buckle but remain open anteriorly, allowing vitreous fluid to leak into the subretinal space anterior to the buckle. The unsupported retina anterior to the buckle may serve as a gutter along which subretinal fluid leaks posteriorly around the buckle. To prevent this gutter phenomenon, the anterior and posterior borders of the retinal breaks are localized and marked with diathermy. The anterior-posterior width of the break (7 mm) is measured to determine the size of the implant, which should be twice the width of the break. The scleral bite of the mattress suture is placed so that it will be 3 mm from the anterior and posterior edges of the implant. The distance between the arms of the mattress suture is at least 3 mm. Light to moderate cryoapplications are applied around the retinal break. Since cryotreatment weakens the sclera, it should not be applied over the mattress suture tracks.

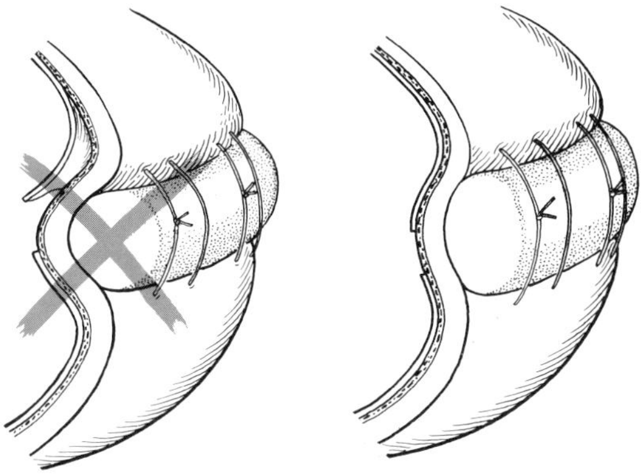

b c

20.**2b** **Selection of implant shape.** A round, equatorially oriented implant may close only the posterior part of a retinal tear, allowing vitreous fluid to leak anterior to the scleral buckle. The elevated retina anterior to the tear may serve as a gutter along which subretinal fluid can leak posteriorly around the buckle.

c An oval-shaped implant offers support both anteriorly and posteriorly, and is preferable for large retinal tears.

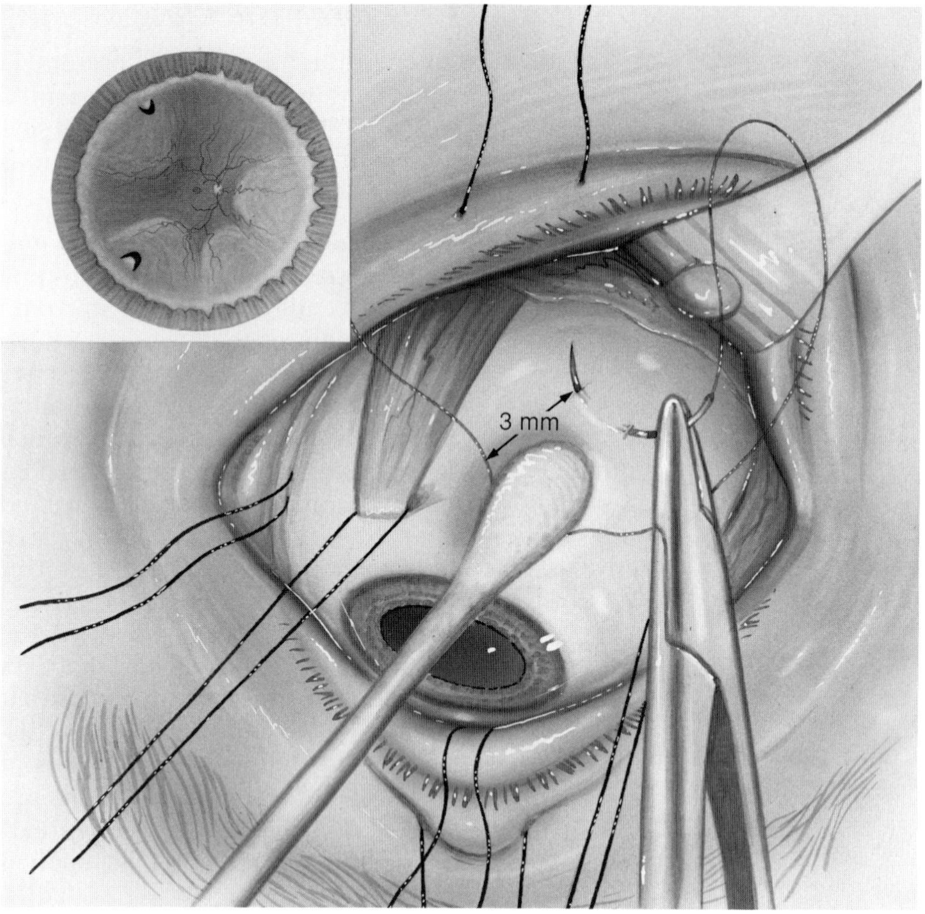

20.**2d** *Inset:* fundus sketch shows total retinal detachment. Severe vitreous base contraction is present, requiring a 360° scleral buckle.

The globe is stabilized with a cotton swab while a mattress suture is placed parallel to the equator. The arms of the suture are 3 mm apart. Two mattress sutures are placed in each quadrant.

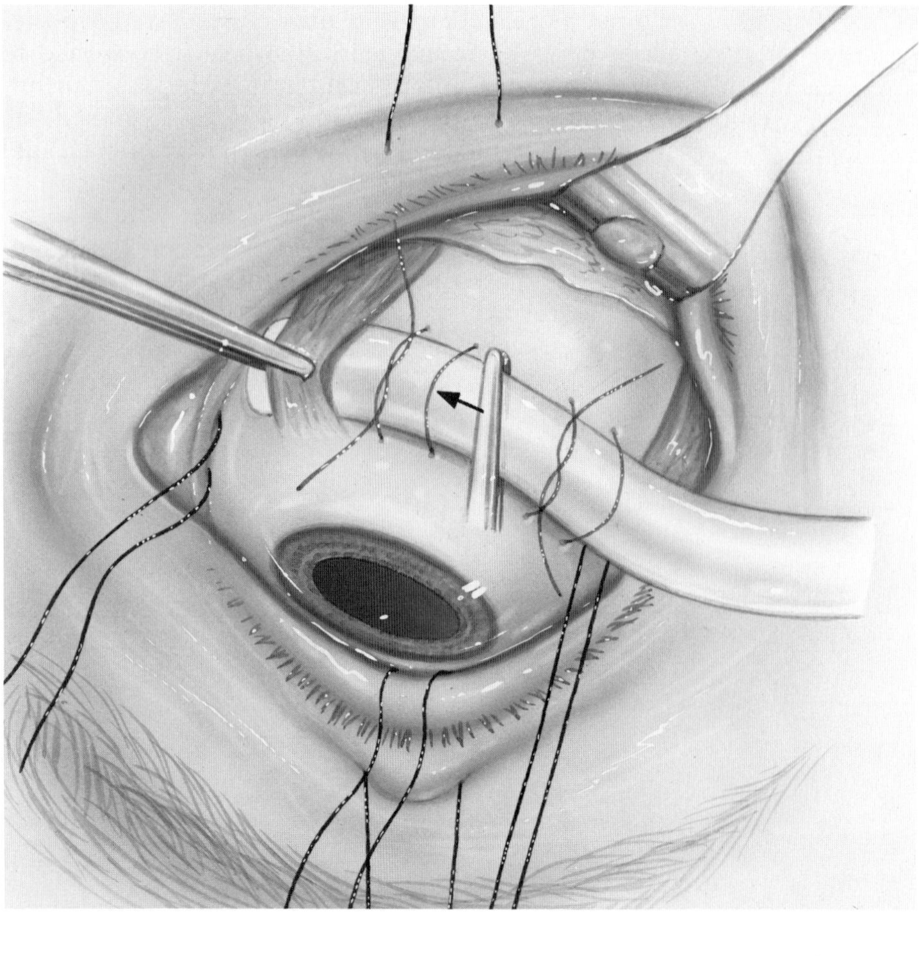

20.**2e** **Placement of equatorial implant.** The mattress sutures are tied temporarily. The hydrophilic acrylate implant is held with a toothless, heavy-duty utility forceps, and inserted under the mattress sutures and the recti muscles.

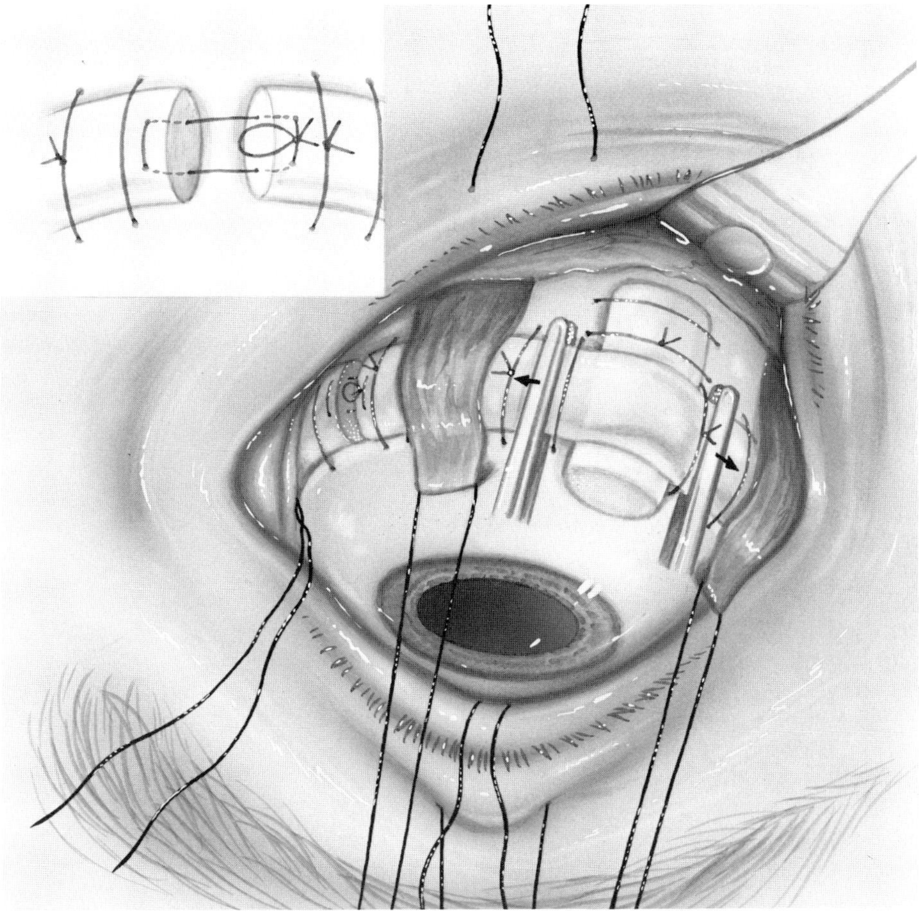

20.2f Meridional implants under the buckle. *Inset:* the ends of the implant are cut parallel with straight scissors, and joined with a mattress suture.

A meridional implant may be necessary to close a retinal break that remains gaping open following drainage of subretinal fluid. A radial implant is placed in the meridian of the retinal breaks, underneath the equatorial buckle, and anchored posteriorly with a mattress suture. The equatorial implant is stretched in opposite directions on each side of the radial implant to increase the indentation in the sclera over the retinal break.

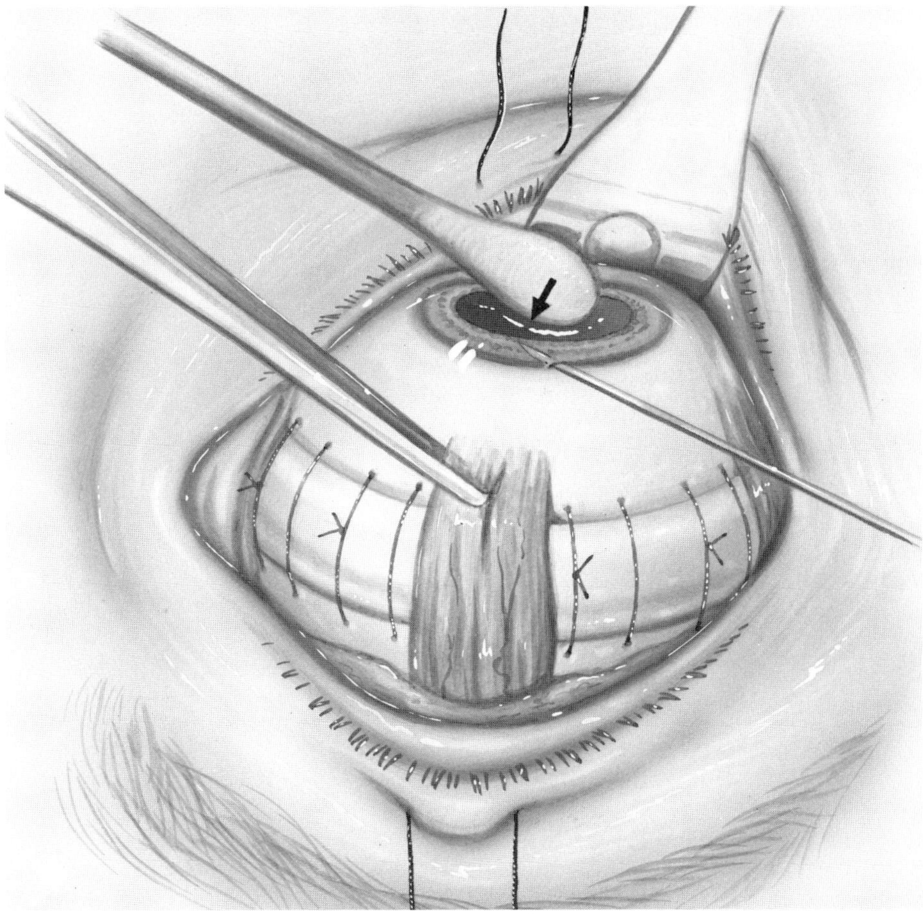

20.**2g** Mattress sutures that anchor the ends of the equatorial buckle are tied permanently. To lower the intraocular pressure, aqueous is removed from the anterior chamber using a 30-gauge needle on a tuberculin syringe. The central cornea is depressed with a cotton swab to displace the aqueous peripherally.

References

1. Benson WE. Retinal detachment: diagnosis and management. Hagerstown, MD: Harper and Row, 1979: 111–116.
2. Chignell AH. Retinal detachment surgery. New York: Springer, 1980: 111–136.
3. Curtin VT. Management of retinal detachment. In: Duane TD, Jaeger EA, eds. Clinical ophthalmology. Philadelphia: Harper and Row, 1983: 1–23.
4. Freeman HM. Surgery of the retina and vitreous. In: Jaffe NS, ed. Atlas of ophthalmic surgery. New York: Gower (in press).
5. Kanski JJ. Retinal detachment: a colour manual of diagnosis and treatment. London: Butterworths, 1986: 93–127.
6. Lincoff H. Full-thickness scleral buckling with silicone sponge implant. In: McPherson A, ed. New and controversial aspects of retinal detachment. New York: Harper and Row, 1968: 293–296.
7. Lincoff H, Kreissig I. The treatment of retinal detachment without drainage of subretinal fluid (modifications of the Custodis procedure, part VI). Trans Am Acad Ophthalmol Otolaryngol 1972; 76: 1221–1233.
8. Lincoff H, Kreissig I, Goldbaum M. Selection of patients for non-drainage operations. In: Pruett RC, Regan CDJ, eds. Retina congress. New York: Appleton-Century-Crofts, 1976: 397–411.
9. McPherson A, Moura R. Full-thickness scleral buckling with cryoapplication and silicone sponge in retinal detachment surgery: a review of 447 cases. In: Pruett RC, Regan CDJ, eds. Retina congress. New York: Appleton-Century-Crofts, 1972: 325–353.
10. Morse PH. Scleral buckling with soft silicone sponge and lamellar scleral dissection. Ann Ophthalmol 1975; 7: 731.
11. Morse PH. Vitreoretinal disease, a manual for diagnosis and treatment. Chicago, Year Book Medical Publishers, 1979: 159–164.
12. Refojo MF, Leong F-L. A poly(methyl acrylate-co-hydroxyethyl acrylate) hydrogel implant material of strength and softness. J Biomed Mater Res 1981; 15: 497–508.
13. Refojo, MF, Natchiar G, Liu HS, et al. New hydrophilic implant for scleral buckling. Ann Ophthalmol 1980; 12: 88–92.
14. Rice TA, Michels RG, Stark WJ, eds. Operative surgery: ophthalmic surgery. 4th ed. St. Louis: C V Mosby, 1984: 274–275. (Rob and Smith's operative surgery series.)
15. Tolentino FI, Refojo MF, Schepens CL. A hydrophilic acrylate implant for scleral buckling: technique and clinical experience. Retina 1981; 1: 182–286.

21

Rhegmatogenous Retinal Detachment: Intrascleral Buckling

Intrascleral buckling involves a scleral undermining for the placement of an implant beneath scleral flaps (1, 7, 10). We prefer scleral undermining for retinal detachments with marked vitreous base condensation manifested by multiple or large retinal tears in two or more quadrants. Scleral undermining permits the use of diathermy, which is less likely than cryoapplications to produce dispersion of pigment epithelial cells through the multiple tears, which would increase the risk of proliferative vitreoretinopathy (2). Burying an anteriorly placed implant under scleral flaps reduces the likelihood of implant erosion in comparison with an episcleral sponge.

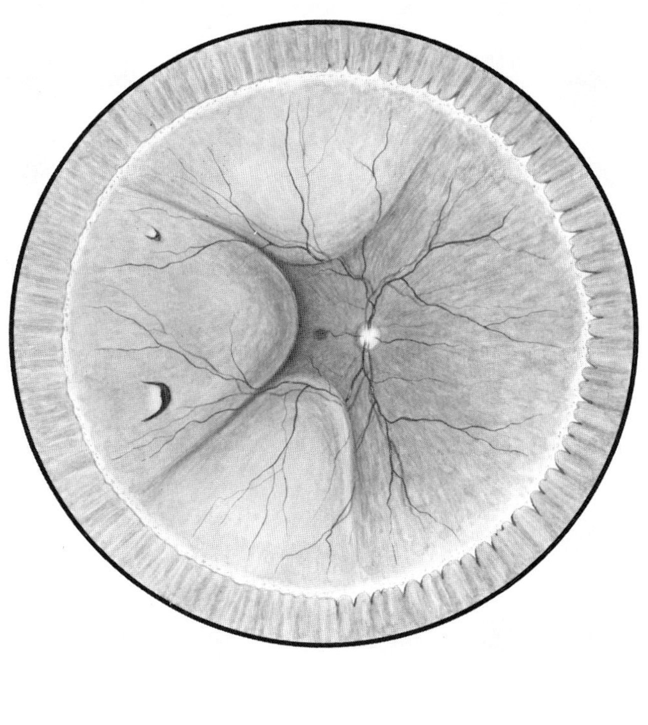

21.**1** **Primary rhegmatogenous retinal detachment.** Bullous temporal retinal detachment with retinal breaks in the 8 and 10 o'clock meridians of the right eye. A detailed fundus drawing is made using the binocular indirect opthalmoscope and scleral depression. A painstaking effort should be made preoperatively to find all retinal breaks. Suspicious lesions should be examined with higher magnification obtained using a + 14 condensing lens or biomicroscopy with the Goldmann three-mirror contact lens.

2

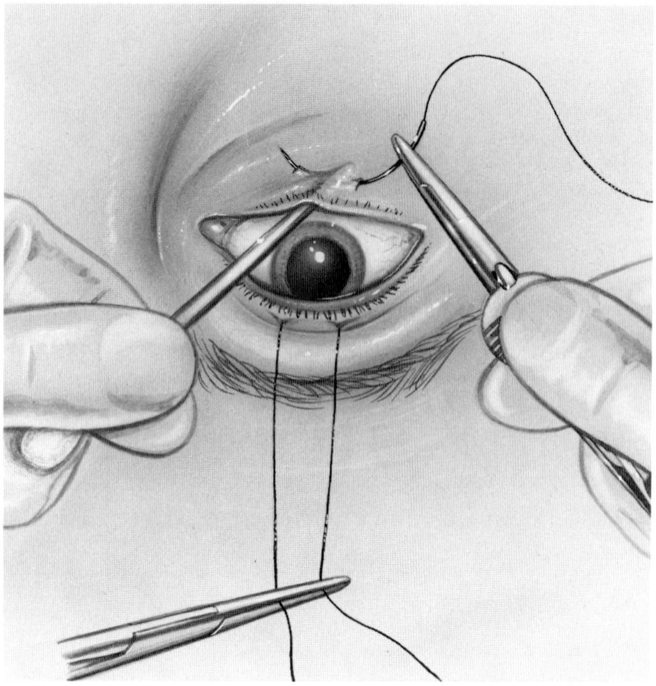

3

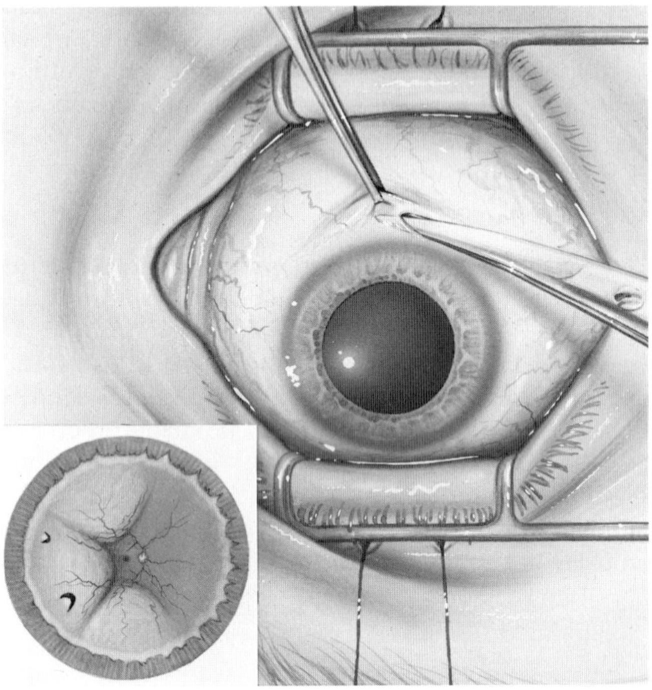

4

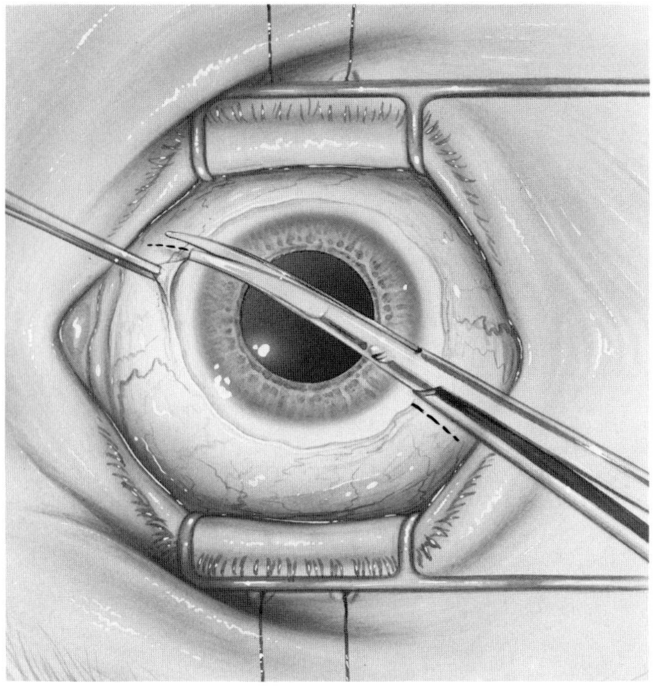

5

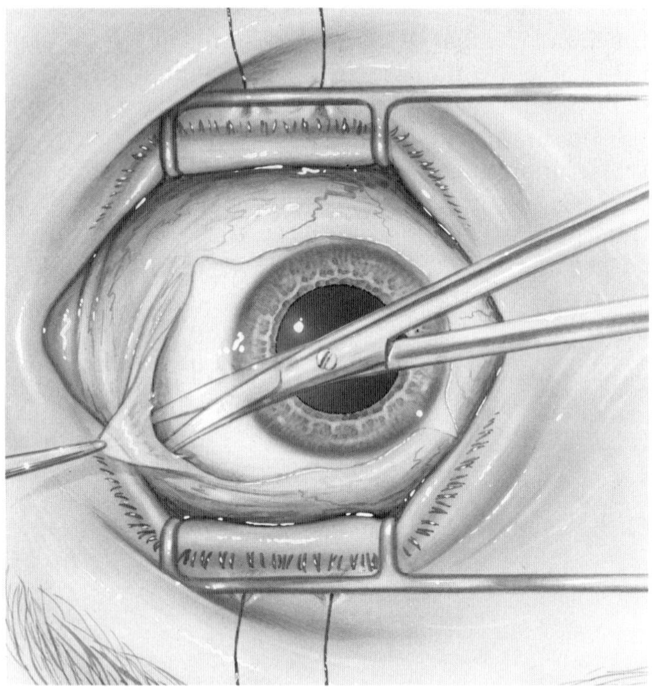

21.**2** **Lid sutures.** While the lid is tented away from the globe with a cotton-tipped applicator, a 4–0 silk traction suture mounted on a tapered needle is passed through the tarsal plate about 2 mm from the lash line.

21.**3** **Limbal peritomy.** The lids are retracted with a wire lid retractor. A limbal peritomy is begun by grasping both Tenon's capsule and the conjunctiva as close to the limbus as possible using toothed Bishops forceps. The tips of curved iris scissors should reach the plane of the sclera before the peritomy is extended around the limbus (6).

21.**4** **Relaxing incisions.** A radial relaxing incision approximately 8 mm long is made through the conjunctiva and Tenon's capsule in oblique meridians (2 and 8 o'clock or 10 and 4 o'clock). These incisions prevent tearing of the conjunctiva during exposure of the globe. To prevent symblepharon formation, the incisions are made away from the horizontal meridian.

21.**5** **Exposure of the anterior sclera.** By spreading the tips of the scissors, Tenon's capsule is separated from the sclera around 360°. Care must be taken to avoid damaging the vortex veins.

6

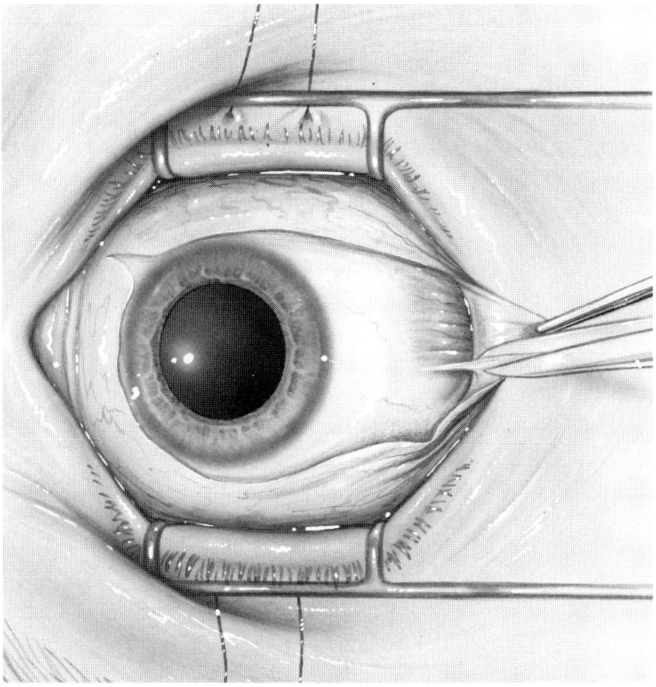

8

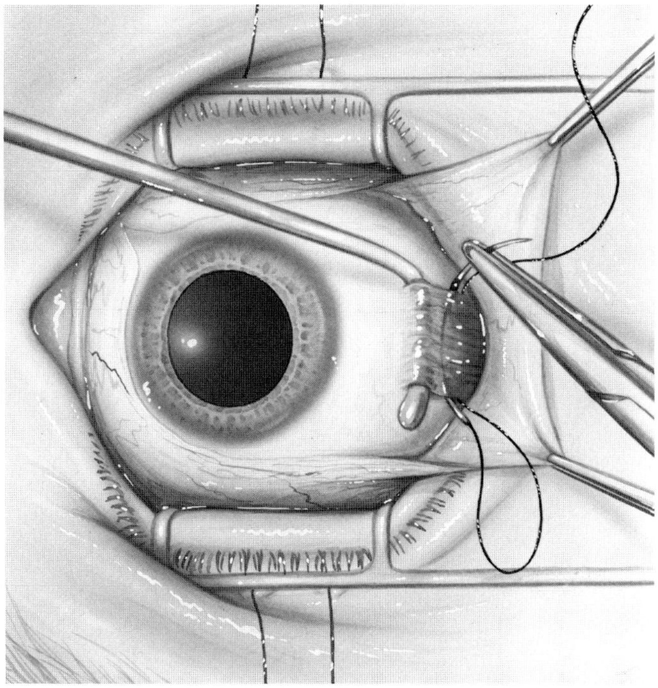

7

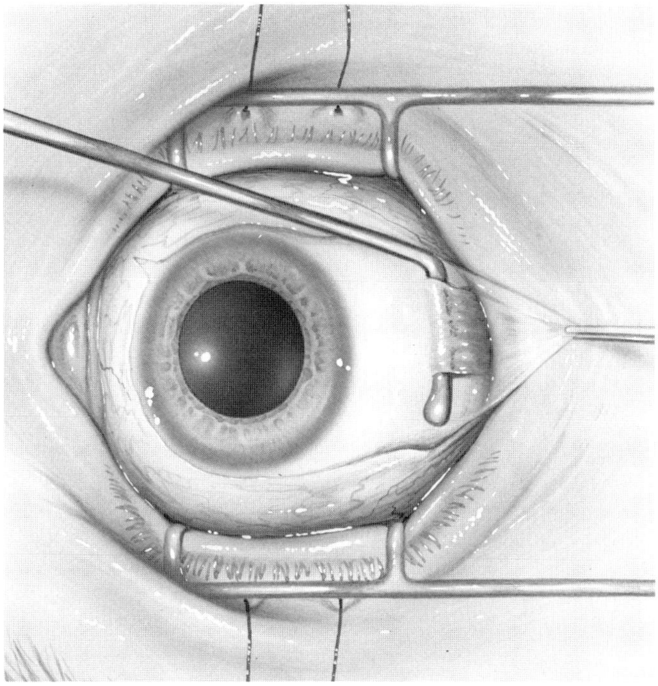

9

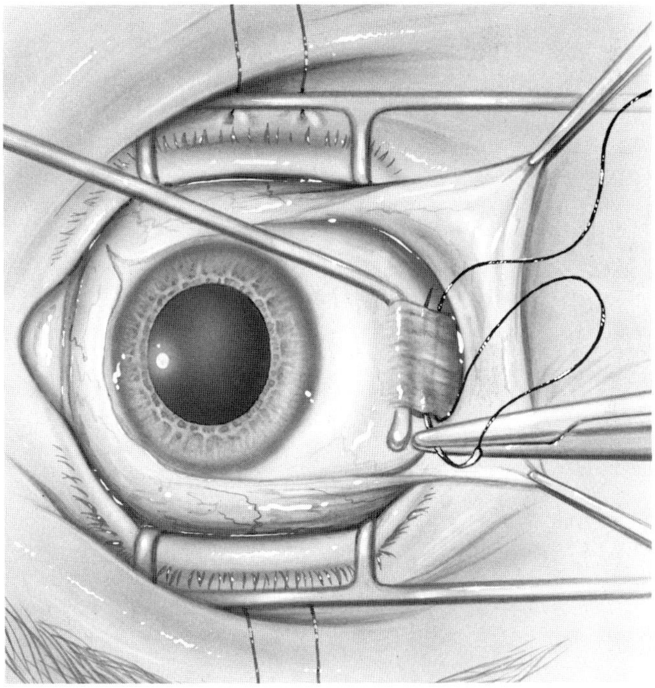

21.**6** **Isolation of muscle margins.** Adhesions of Tenon's capsule to the sheath of the extraocular muscles are cut. This dissection is done near Tenon's capsule to avoid cutting the muscle belly, which would result in hemorrhage and scaring. The inferior and superior margins of the muscle are isolated from their connective tissue adhesions by twirling a cotton-tipped applicator along each margin.

21.**7** **Isolation of muscle tendons.** Tenon's capsule and conjunctiva are retracted, and the insertion of the rectus muscles is isolated using a muscle hook.

21.**8** **Muscle bridle sutures.** The needle of a 4–0 black silk suture is grasped near its tip using a Kalt needle holder. While the muscle hook retracts the tendon from the sclera, the needle is passed under the muscle.

21.**9** After the needle has passed over the superior border of the muscle, it is grasped again, and the suture is withdrawn to produce a bridle suture around the muscle. The arms of the bridle suture are cut approximately 4 inches long.

When isolating the superior rectus tendon, care is taken to avoid trapping the tendon in the superior oblique muscle; the muscle hook is passed along the underside of the superior rectus muscle.

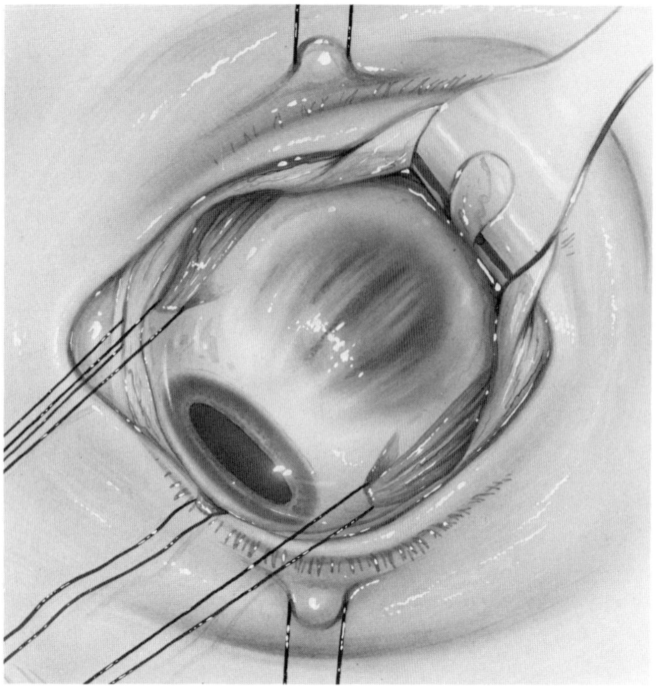

21.**10** **Inspection of the sclera.** Inspection of the sclera is important to identify thinned sclera in anterior dehiscences or anterior staphyloma (3). Failure to recognize thin sclera may result in perforation or rupture of the globe during localization of the retinal breaks.

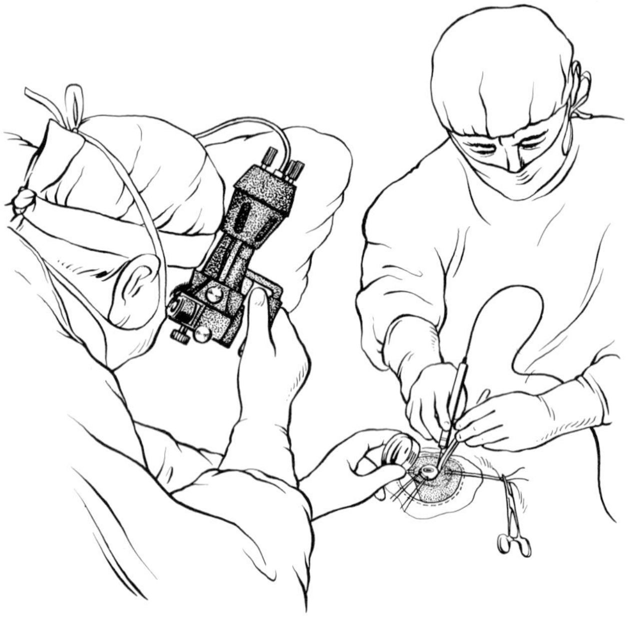

21.**11** **Localization of the retinal breaks.** Localization of the retinal breaks is performed with the aid of an assistant. The surgeon localizes the retinal break using an indirect ophthalmoscope mounted on flexible arms that are attached to a mobile stand. A 20 diopter aspheric lens is used for ophthalmoscopy. The surgeon positions himself in the meridian opposite the retinal break, e.g. standing on the left side of the patient in the 2 o'clock meridian when localizing the retinal break in the 8 o'clock meridian of the right eye.

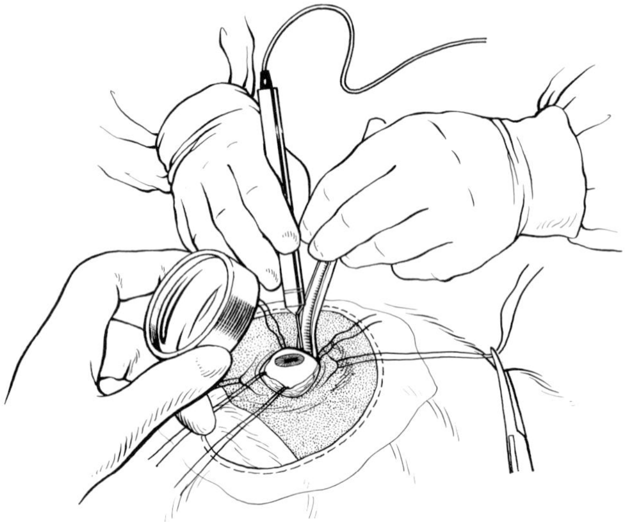

21.**12** The assistant positions the Arruga retractor in the meridian of the retinal break. Care must be taken to refrain from inserting the retractor too deep, to avoid damaging the vortex veins or producing excessive pressure on the globe, causing elevation of intraocular pressure and edema of the corneal epithelium.

13

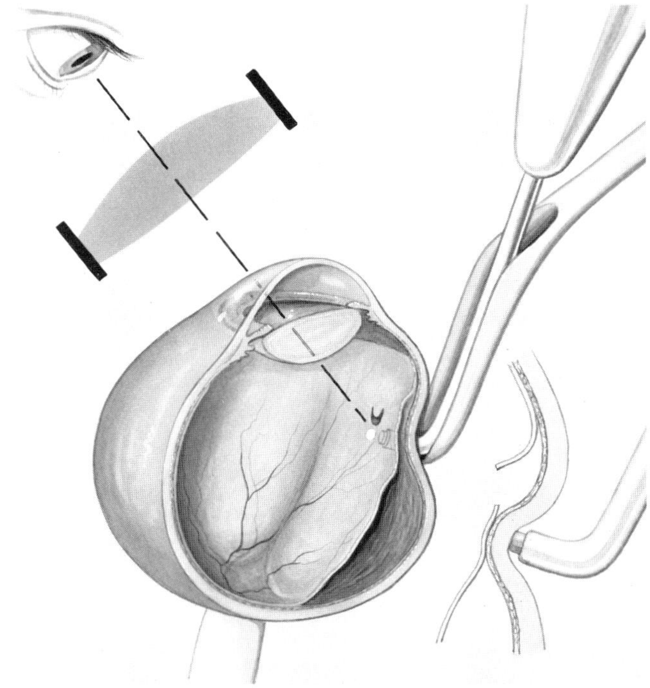

14

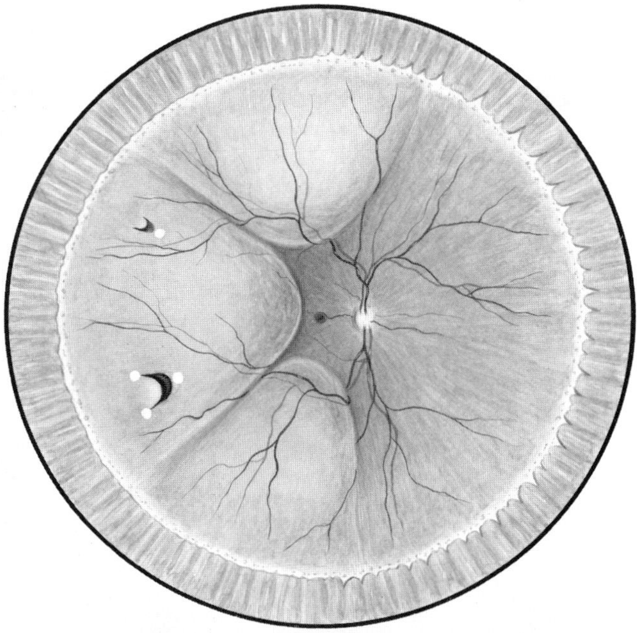

21.**13** The sclera exposed by the retractor is dried with a sponge. Using the blunt diathermy electrode, the assistant carefully indents the sclera in the meridian of the retinal break. The surgeon directs the assistant to move the electrode so that its indentation corresponds with the posterior edge of the retinal break. *Inset:* the surgeon then instructs the assistant to make a diathermy mark by pressing on the diathermy microswitch. If the retina is not too highly elevated and the sclera is dry, a white mark will appear on the retina within a few seconds.

21.**14** When a horseshoe tear is 3 disc diameters or more in size, as in the retinal tear in the 8 o'clock meridian, it is desirable to localize the anterior horns of the tear.

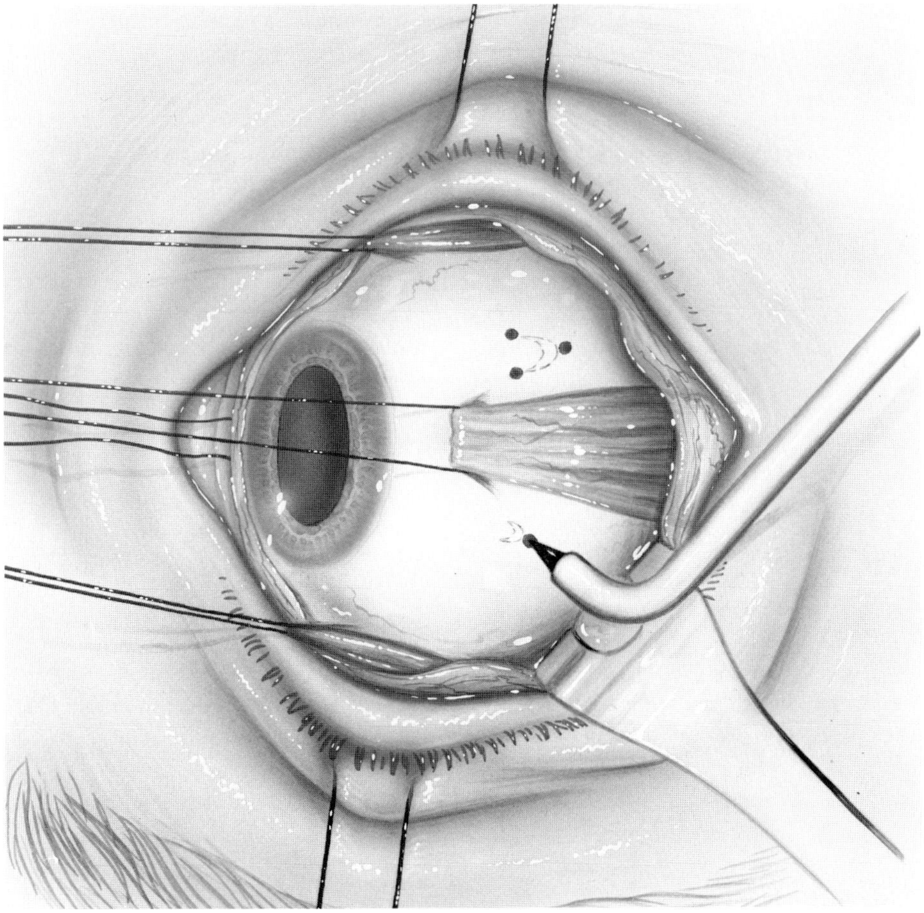

21.**15** To prevent the localizing diathermy marks on the sclera from fading or becoming unrecognizable, they are strengthened using a blunt, conical diathermy electrode.

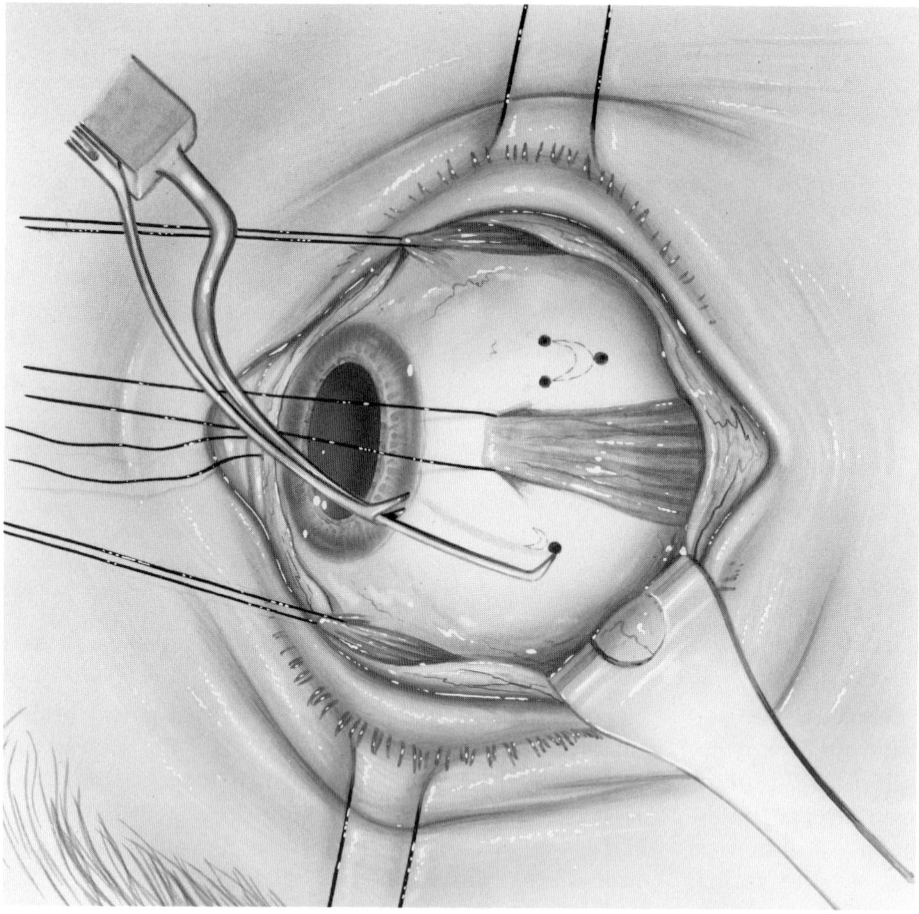

21.**16** The distance of the localizing marks from the limbus is measured using the Amsler marker. This information is helpful in deciding the location of the circumferential incision for the lamellar scleral dissection.

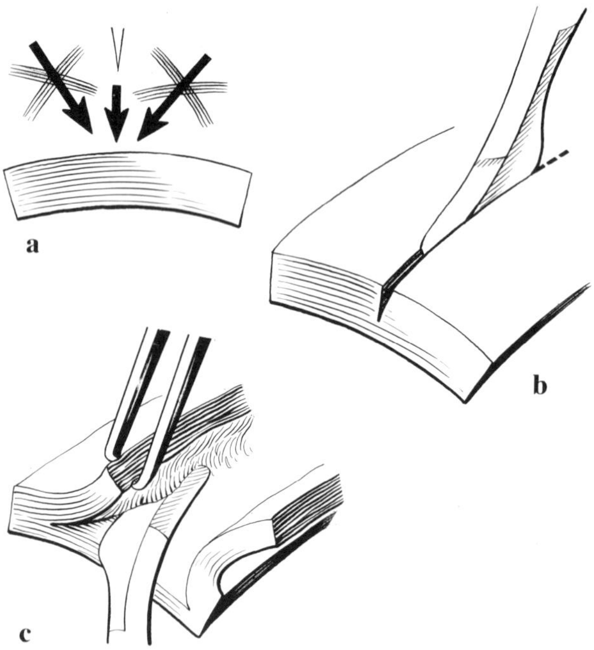

21.**17** **Scleral undermining. a** It is important that the scleral incision be made at right angles to the surface of the sclera, so that a uniform depth of the undermining can be maintained.

b The incision should extend approximately two-thirds of the thickness of the sclera.

c The lips of the incision are undermined using the Grieshaber scarifier. The edge of the incision is retracted with toothed forceps, and the sclera is peeled away, keeping the blade of the scarifier tangential to the scleral bed.

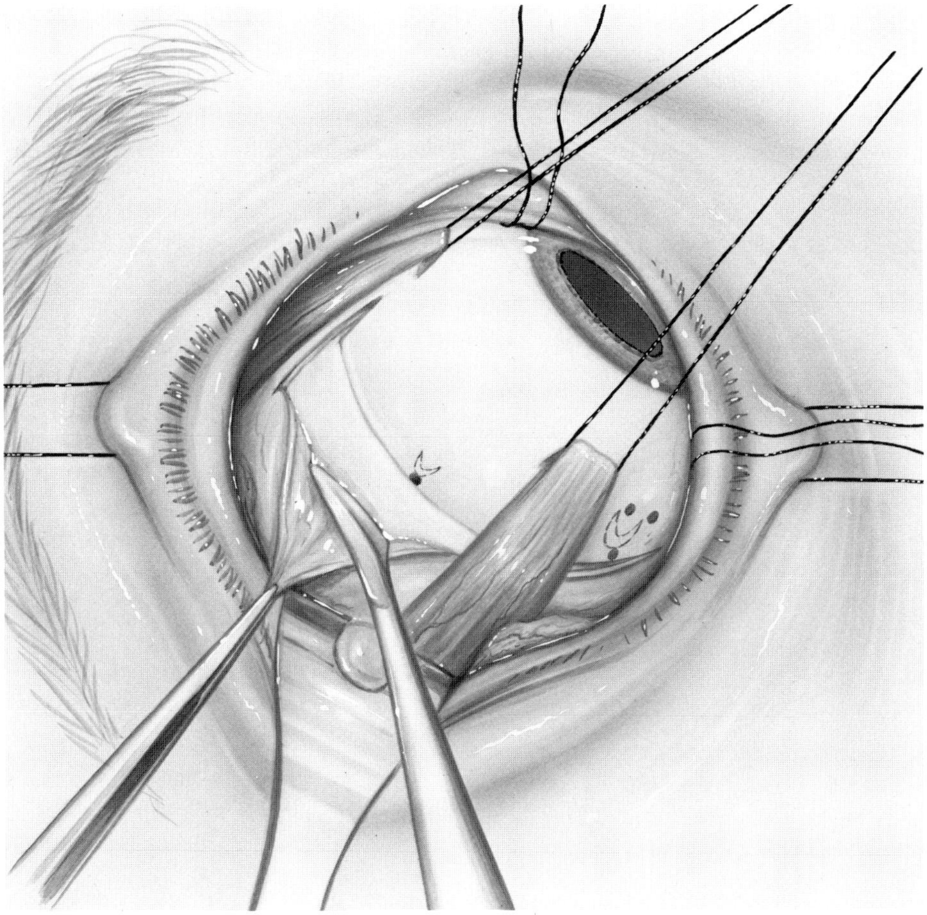

21.**18** A circumferential incision is made joining the diathermy marks at the posterior edge of the retinal breaks. A 12 mm radial incision is made approximately 6 mm lateral to the retinal break. The posterior flap is then dissected to a width of 6 mm.

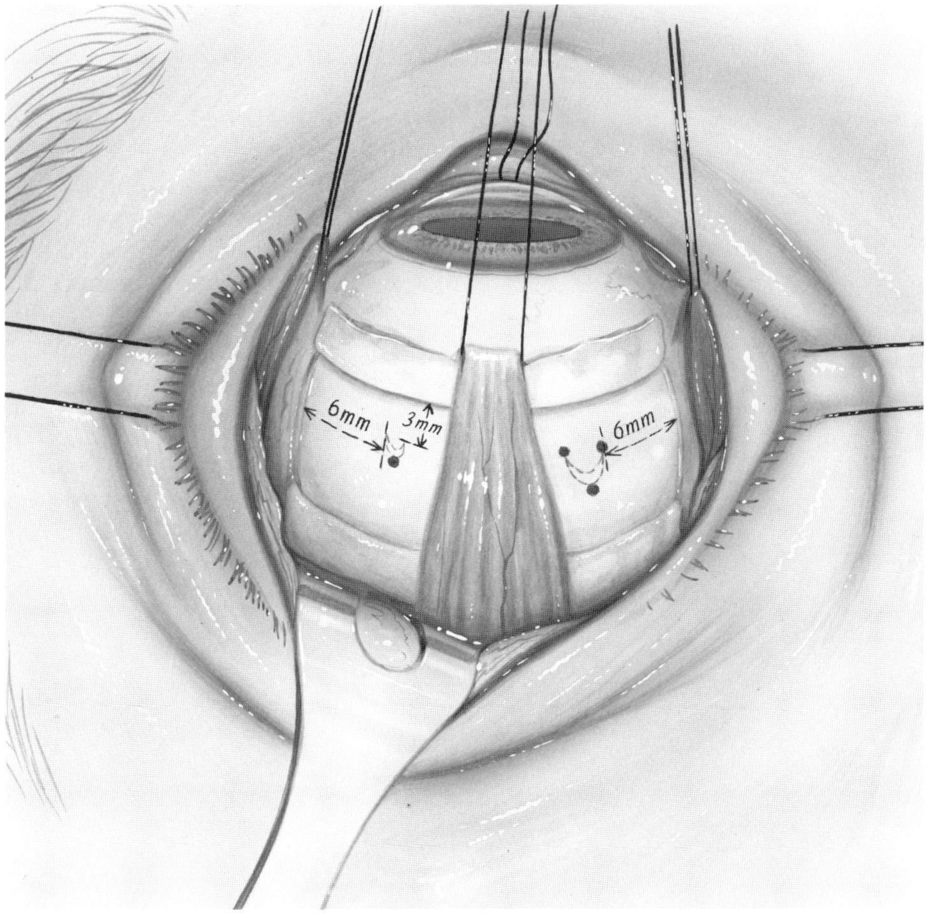

21.**19** The undermining should extend 3 mm anterior to the anterior edge of the retinal break, 6 mm equatorially beyond the edge of the retinal break, and 6 mm posterior to the posterior edge of the break.

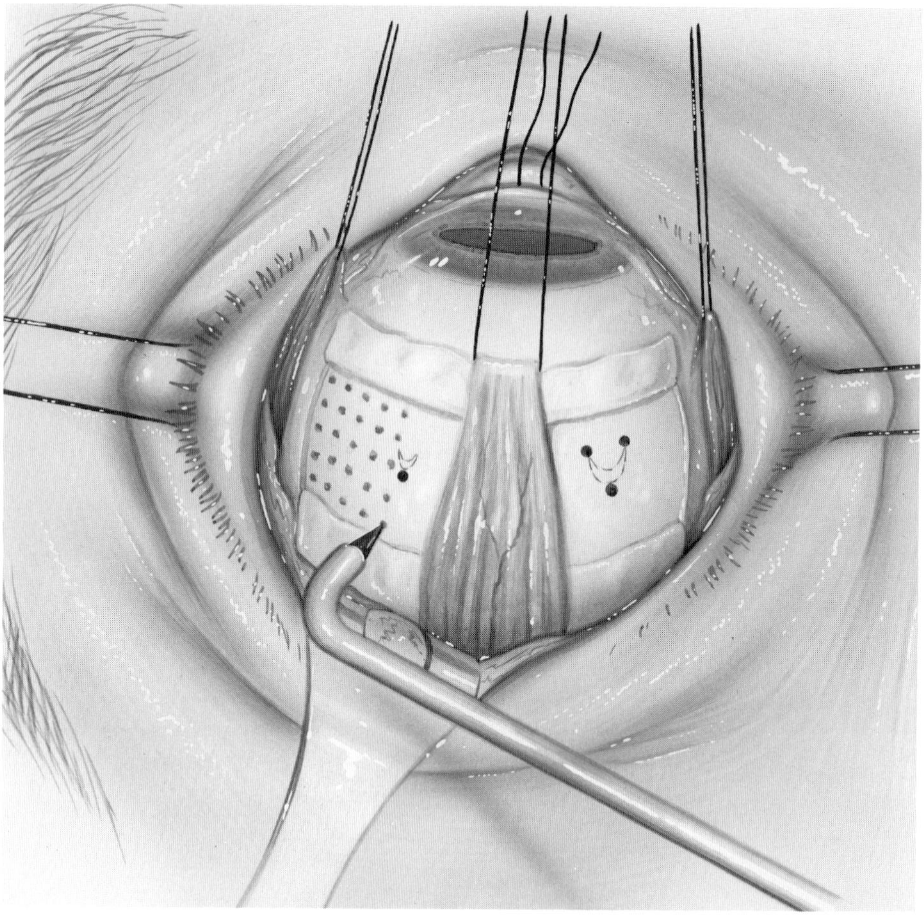

21.**20** **Application of diathermy.** Either diathermy or cryoapplications can be used, depending on the surgeon's preference. Diathermy is applied in the lamellar scleral dissection using a blunt conical electrode. Applications are made with slight pressure on sclera that has been dried with a cotton sponge applicator. Test diathermy applications are made and monitored ophthalmoscopically to determine the proper application time and intensity setting. If the retina is attached or only slightly elevated, a diathermy mark will be visible on the retina. A slight gray-yellow reaction is desirable; an excessively strong diathermy may produce a hole in the retina through which the charred choroid is visible.

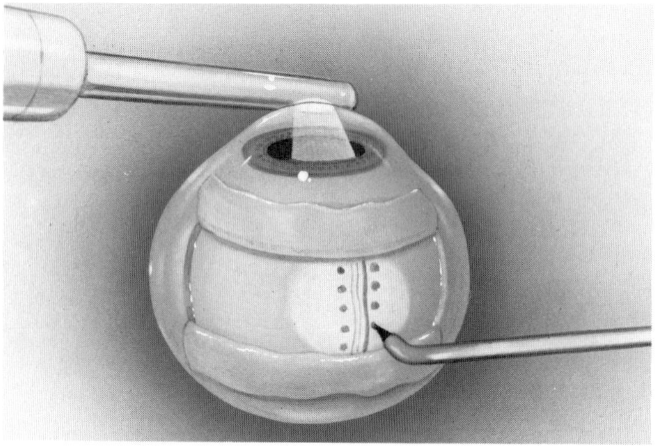

21.**21** **Transillumination of the long posterior ciliary vessels and nerve.** To avoid diathermizing the long posterior ciliary artery and long ciliary nerve, they are transilluminated with a hand-held transilluminator. The operating room is darkened, and the light aperture of the transilluminator is applied to the cornea near the limbus in the meridian opposite the vessel to be transilluminated. The artery appears as a thin red line; the nerve is lined by two parallel pigmented lines, which are the pigmented epineurium. A row of diathermy applications is made 1 mm on either side of the artery and nerve.

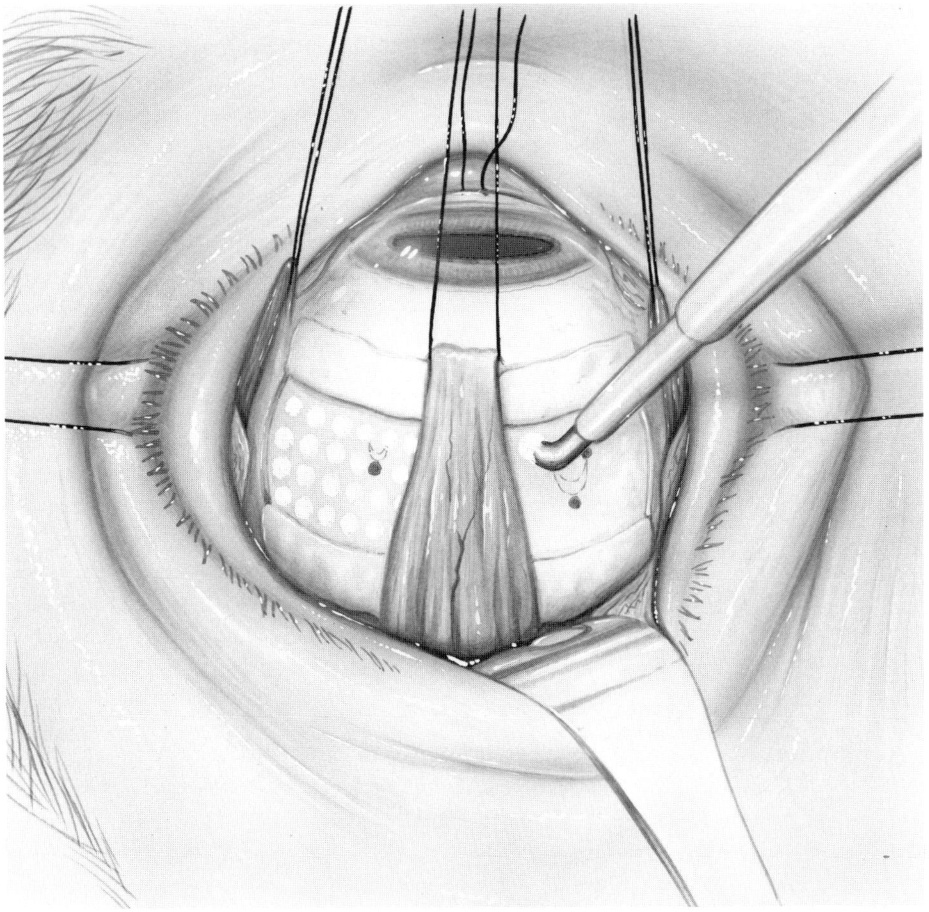

21.**22** **Cryoapplications.** When cryoapplications are used rather than diathermy, the optimum application time should be determined ophthalmoscopically by applying the cryoprobe with gentle indentation to provide test spots on attached or shallowly detached retina. A desirable color of the test spot is a slight yellowing of the retina or an orange glow. Once the optimum timing of cryoapplications is determined, parallel rows are applied under direct observation.

Care must be taken to hold the probe steady until the tip has become thawed, and to keep the area to be treated free of pooling of irrigating solution, which freezes and can result in tearing of adjacent vortex veins. Excessively long applications are undesirable because they may cause dispersion of pigment epithelial cells, which may collect at the posterior pole. In eyes with thin sclera, extra care must be taken to allow the ice ball that fixes the probe to the thin sclera to melt; otherwise, scleral rupture can occur as a result of inadvertent movements of the probe.

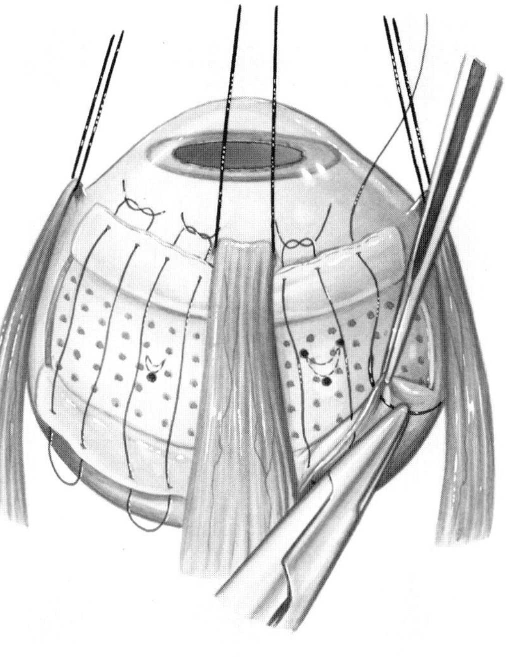

21.**23** **Suturing the flaps of the scleral undermining.** Blue polyester 4–0 sutures with a cutting needle are used to close the scleral flaps. The double arms of the suture are placed 2 mm apart in a radial fashion and 1.5 mm from the edge of the scleral flap. Two mattress sutures are placed in each quadrant, but preferably not under the muscles. A suture is placed in the meridian of the larger reginal tear so that if an additional radial implant is needed following drainage of subretinal fluid, the suture will identify that meridian.

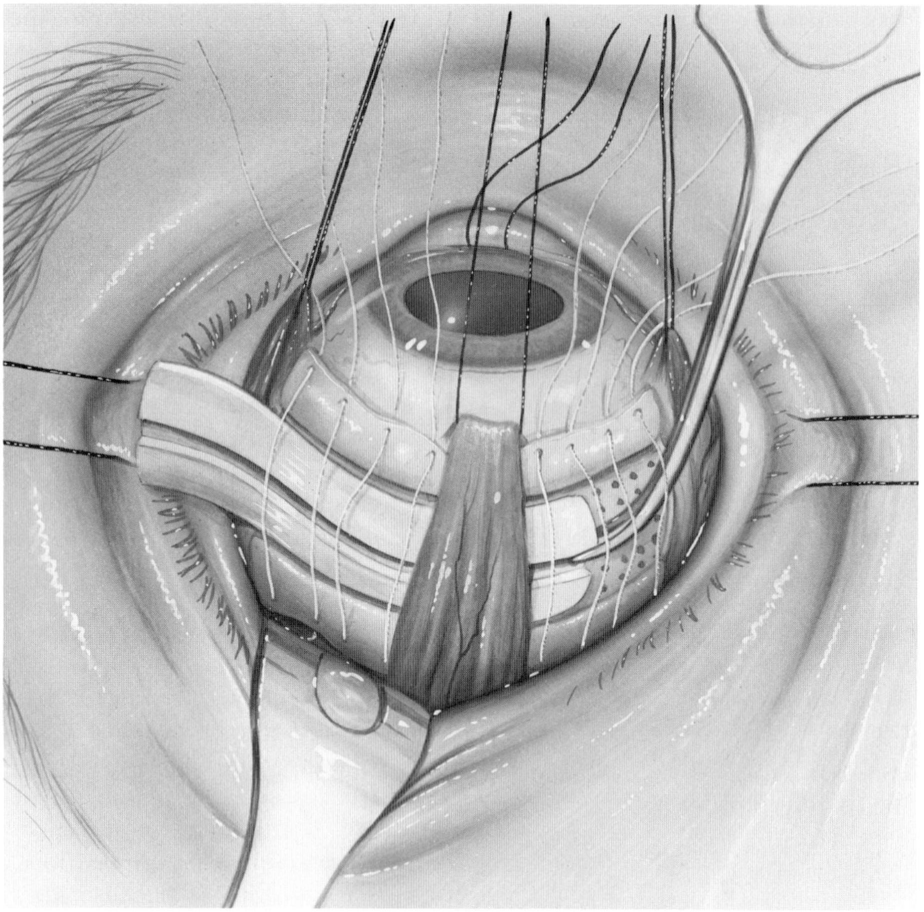

21.**24** **Placement of the implant.** The implant is 3 mm narrower and 3 mm shorter than the undermining, so it will produce an adequate indentation of the sclera. The sharp edges are trimmed to prevent scleral erosion. The implant is rinsed in a saline solution containing 5000 units of polymyxin B sulfate. Using a curved, smooth Bishop's forceps, the implant is inserted beneath the mattress sutures and recti muscles. Insertion of the band is begun where one intends to join both ends, usually in a quadrant opposite the scleral buckle. The preferable location for the joint is superonasal.

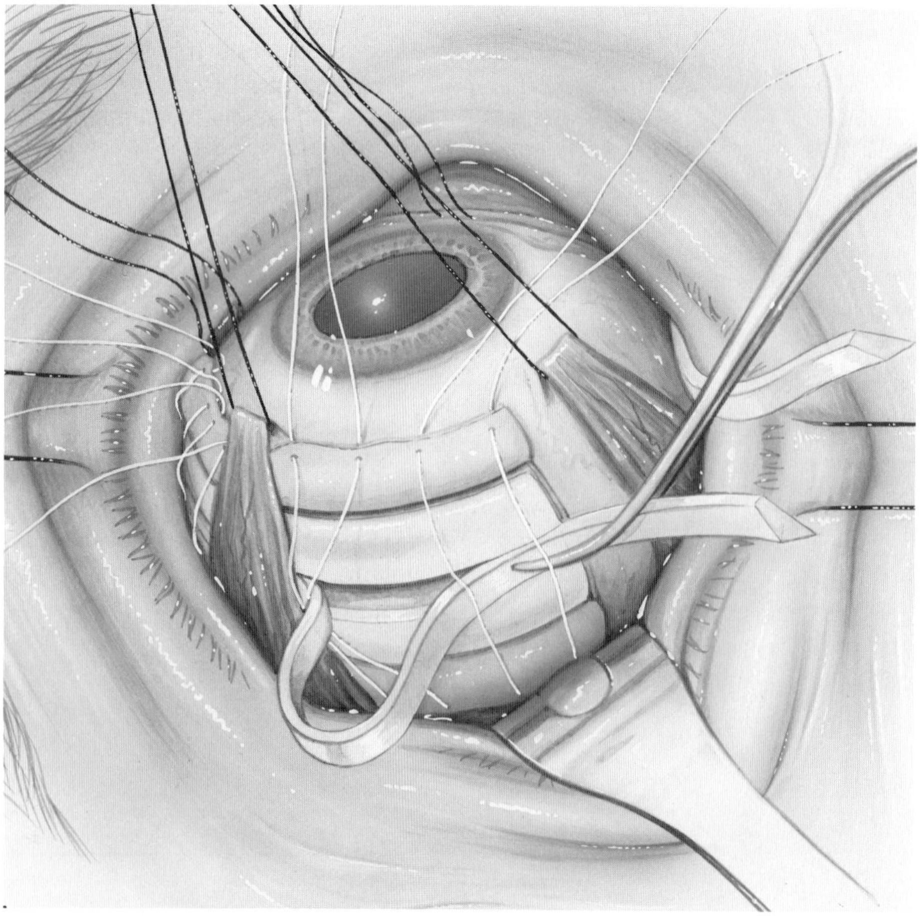

21.**25** **Placement of encircling element.** The ends of the encircling element are beveled so that it can be passed under the sutures more easily; then it is placed in the groove of the implant, under the mattress sutures and beneath all recti muscles.

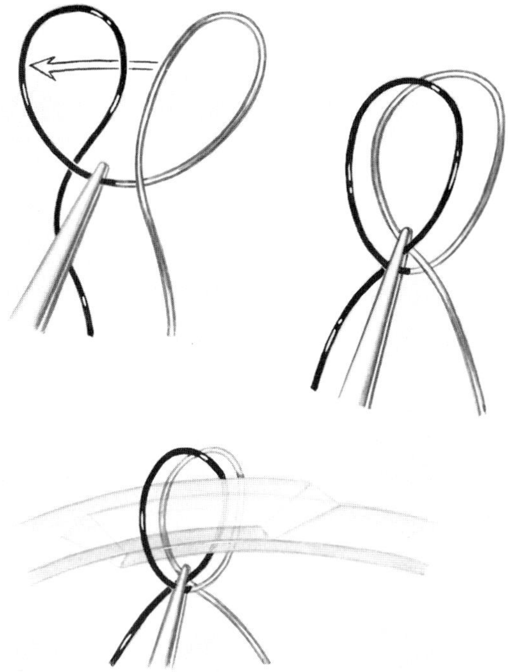

21.**26** **Joining the ends of the encircling element.** The ends of the encircling element are joined using a clove hitch knot made from a 4–0 polyester suture. In making the clove hitch, the second loop (gray) is placed behind the first loop (black), and held in a straight hemostat. The clove hitch is then placed around one end of the encircling element, and the other end is threaded through the loop.

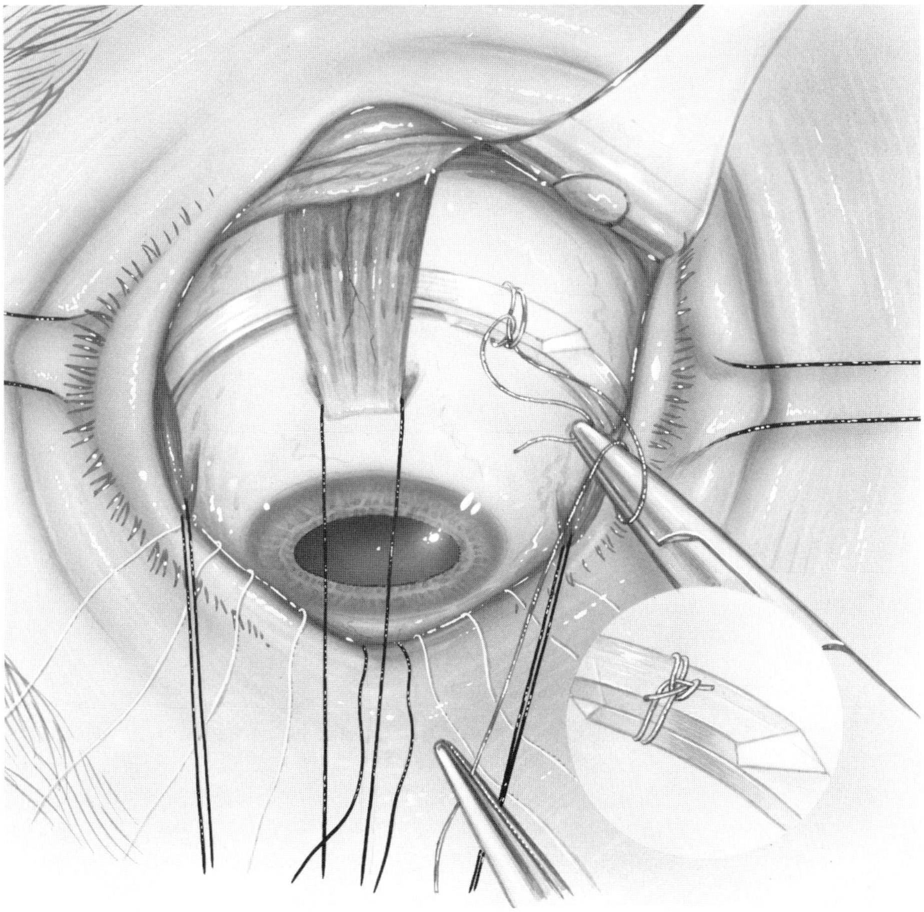

21.**27** The clove hitch is moderately tightened, and then secured with a surgeon's knot.

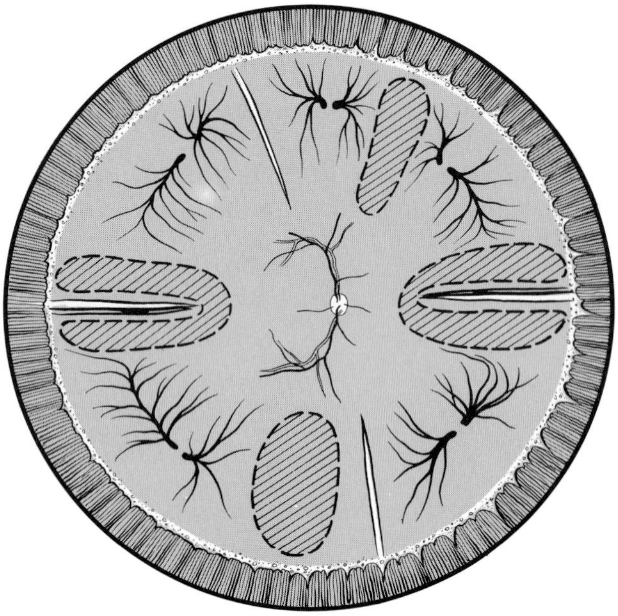

21.**28** **Drainage of subretinal fluid.** Not all retinal detachments require drainage of subretinal fluid. If the retinal break is located anteriorly and there is no evidence of preretinal organization, drainage of subretinal fluid may be unnecessary.

The shaded areas show desirable locations for drainage of subretinal fluid where there are fewer choroidal blood vessels. Tributaries of the vortex vein system are more sparse anterior to the equator and near the 3 and 9 o'clock meridians. Drainage in the horizontal meridians must be avoided due to the location of the long posterior ciliary arteries.

The usual number of choroidal systems is one in each quadrant, but variations are not uncommon. The illustration shows three choroidal systems inferiorly.

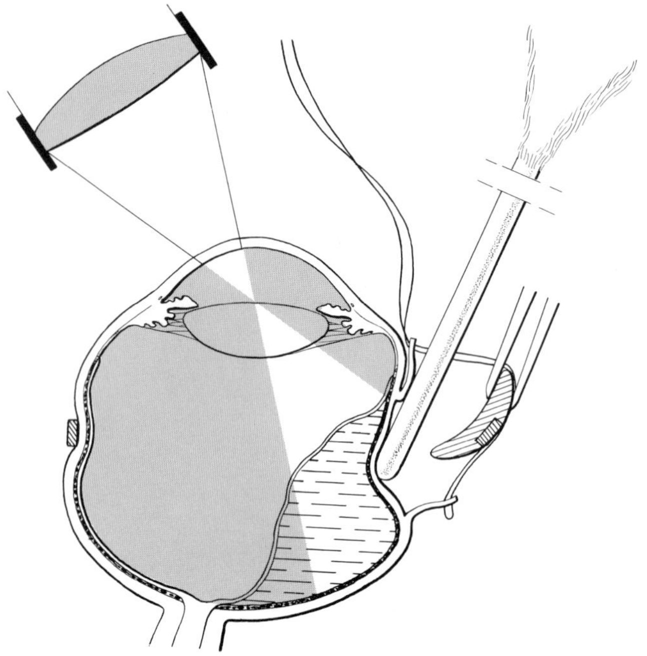

21.**29** The prime consideration in selecting the site for drainage of subretinal fluid is the abundance of subretinal fluid. This must be checked by indirect ophthalmoscopy just prior to making the sclerotomy for drainage. In most cases, draining subretinal fluid in the scleral undermining carries less risk of complications. The implant is moved aside, permitting indentation with a cotton-tipped applicator to confirm that adequate subretinal fluid is present.

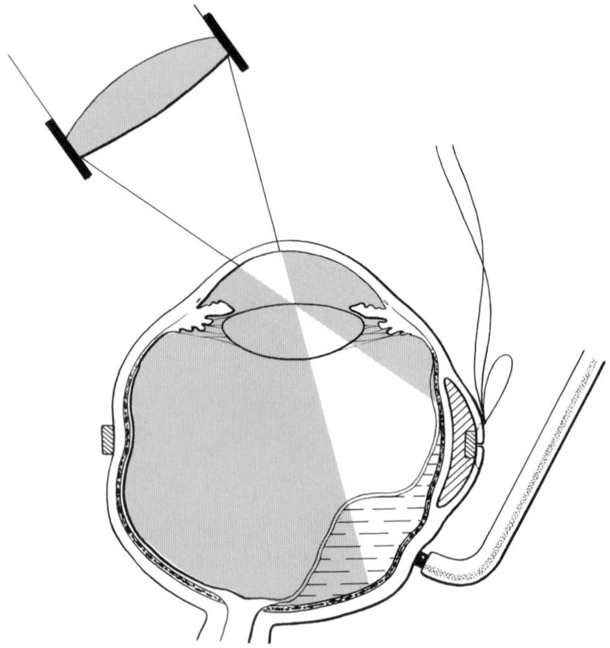

21.**30** When minimal fluid is present over the scleral buckle, it is preferable to drain subretinal fluid posterior to the buckle. Under indirect ophthalmoscopic control, a localizing mark for the sclerotomy for draining fluid is made posterior to the undermining.

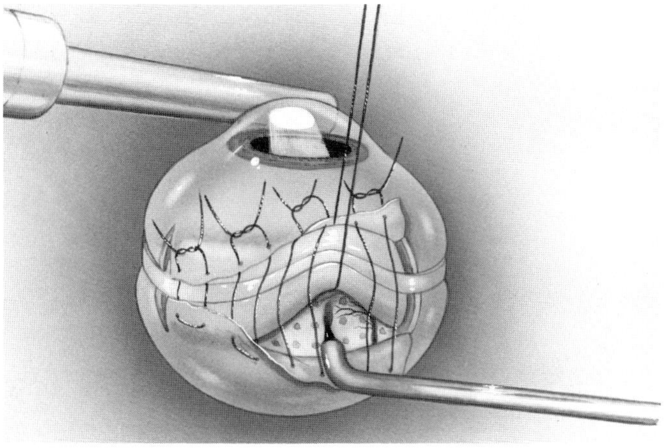

21.**31** Using a 4–0 black suture, the assistant retracts the implant to expose the intended sclerotomy site. To avoid hemorrhage during perforation of the choroid for drainage of subretinal fluid, transillumination is used to identify choroidal blood vessels (4). The operating room is darkened, and the meridian selected for perforation is examined with the aid of a hand-held transilluminator. A diathermy mark is made in an area that appears devoid of choroidal blood vessels.

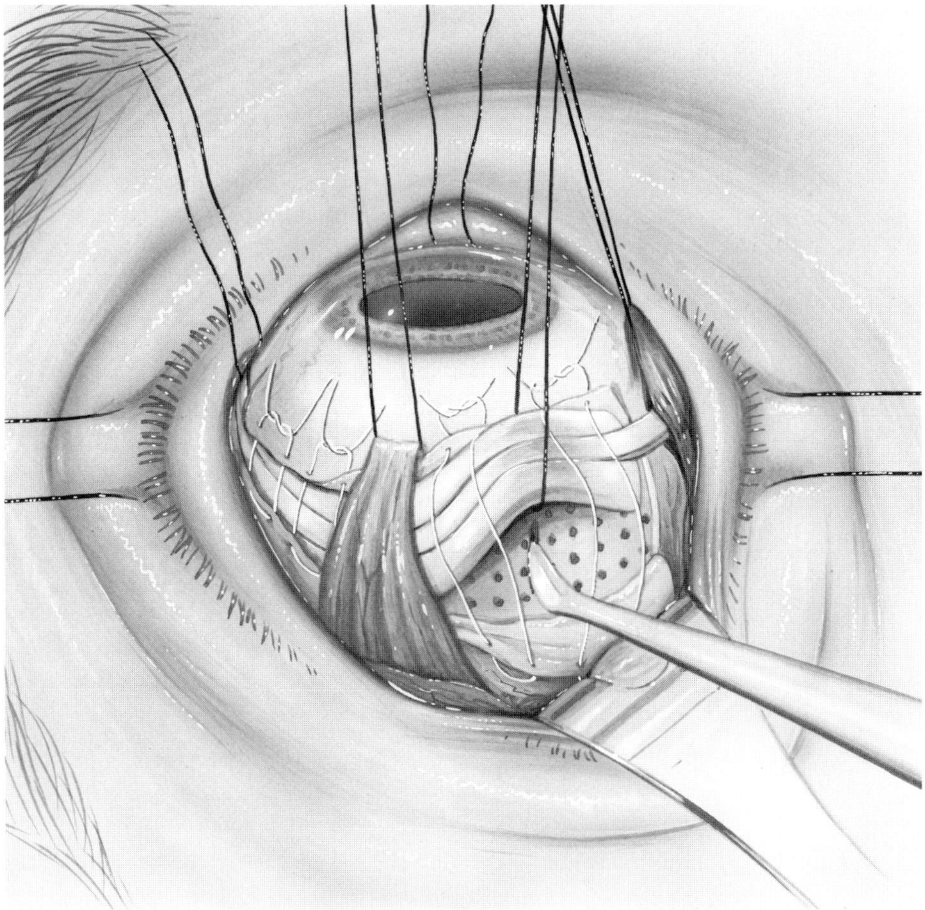

21.**32** A radial sclerotomy 4 mm long is made through the diathermy mark using the Grieshaber scarifier. The incision must be made as perpendicular as possible, because shelved incisions tend to close and hinder the egress of subretinal fluid.

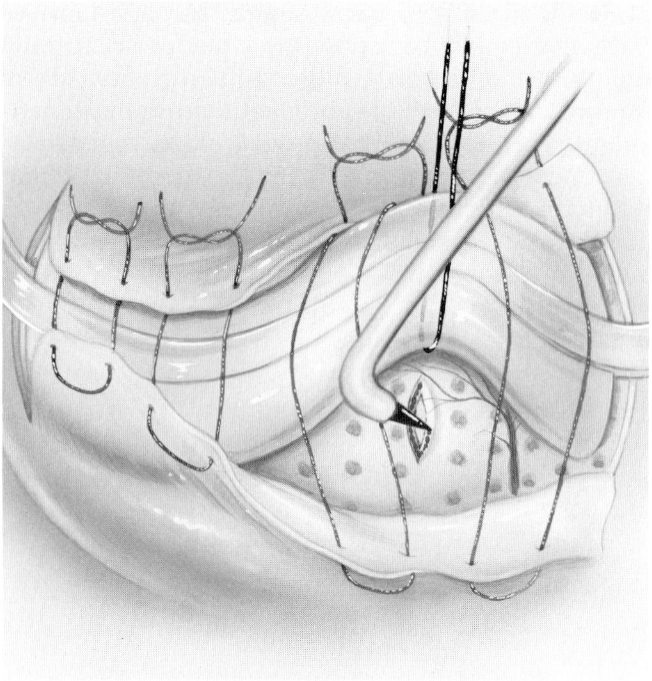

21.**33** By applying diathermy to its edges, the sclerotomy is made to gape to expose a knuckle of choroid that can be examined by transillumination.

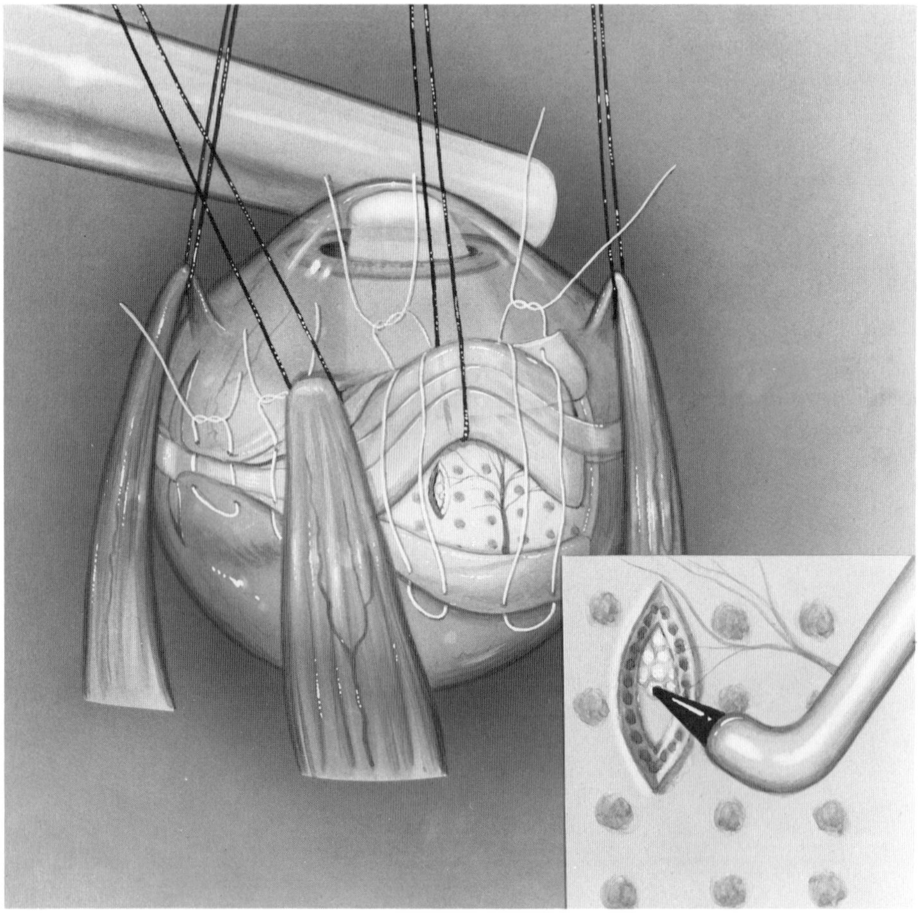

21.**34** *Inset:* to avoid bleeding from small tributaries of the choroidal blood vessels, multiple confluent diathermy applications are placed on the exposed choroid, using a blunt conical electrode with a current setting lower than that used on the sclera.

The choroid is then examined by transillumination, and if patent blood vessels are visible, additional diathermy is applied until the vessels appear obliterated.

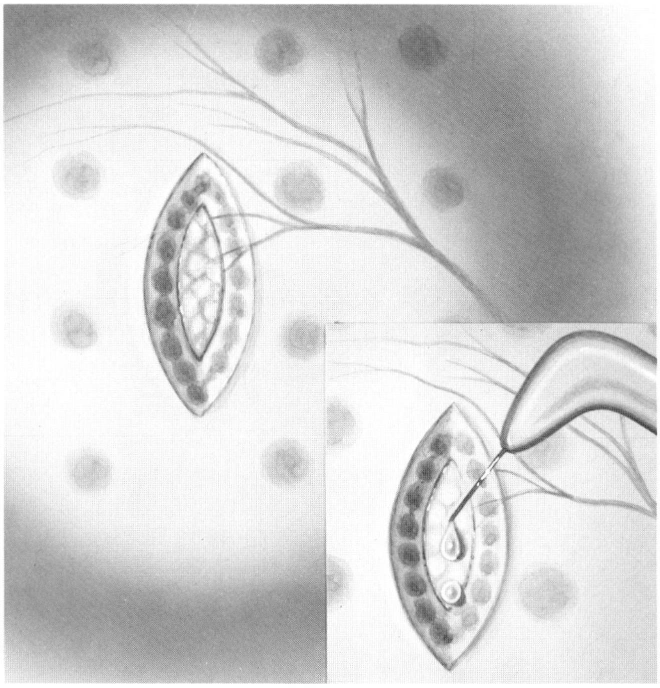

21.**35** If transillumination reveals the choroid to be free of patent blood vessels (**a**) perforation is made using a sharp diathermy electrode (**b**). The needle is entered tangentially to avoid perforating the retina. Slow spontaneous drainage of subretinal fluid, avoiding pressure on the globe, is desirable. If the globe become hypotonous, some of the mattress sutures of the lamellar scleral bed are tightened. When most of the subretinal fluid has been drained, flecks of pigment may appear in the escaping subretinal fluid. As soon as the fluid stops, the sclerotomy is covered with the implant.

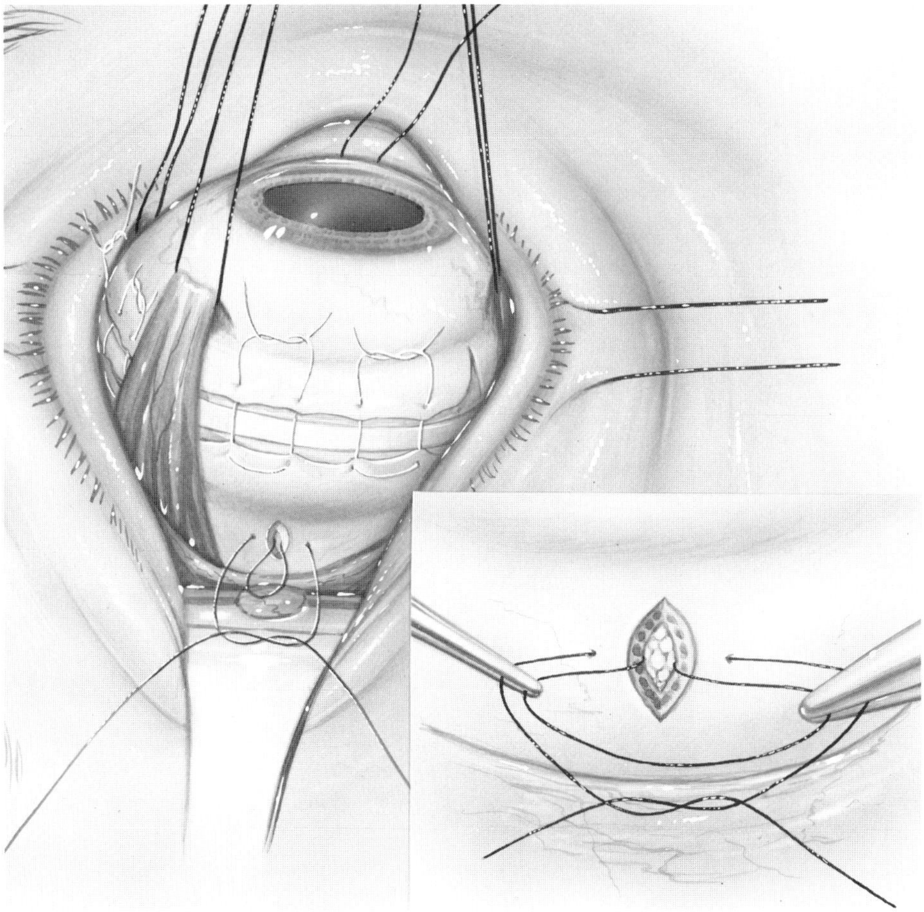

21.**36** When it is necessary to perform drainage of subretinal fluid posterior to the scleral undermining, a 5 mm radial sclerotomy is made. Diathermy is applied to the edges of the sclerotomy, and a 4–0 polyester sutures is placed in its lips. With the aid of the assistant, the sutures are retracted to cause further gaping of the sclerotomy, so that the exposed choroid can be examined by transillumination and confluent applications of diathermy can be applied to it.

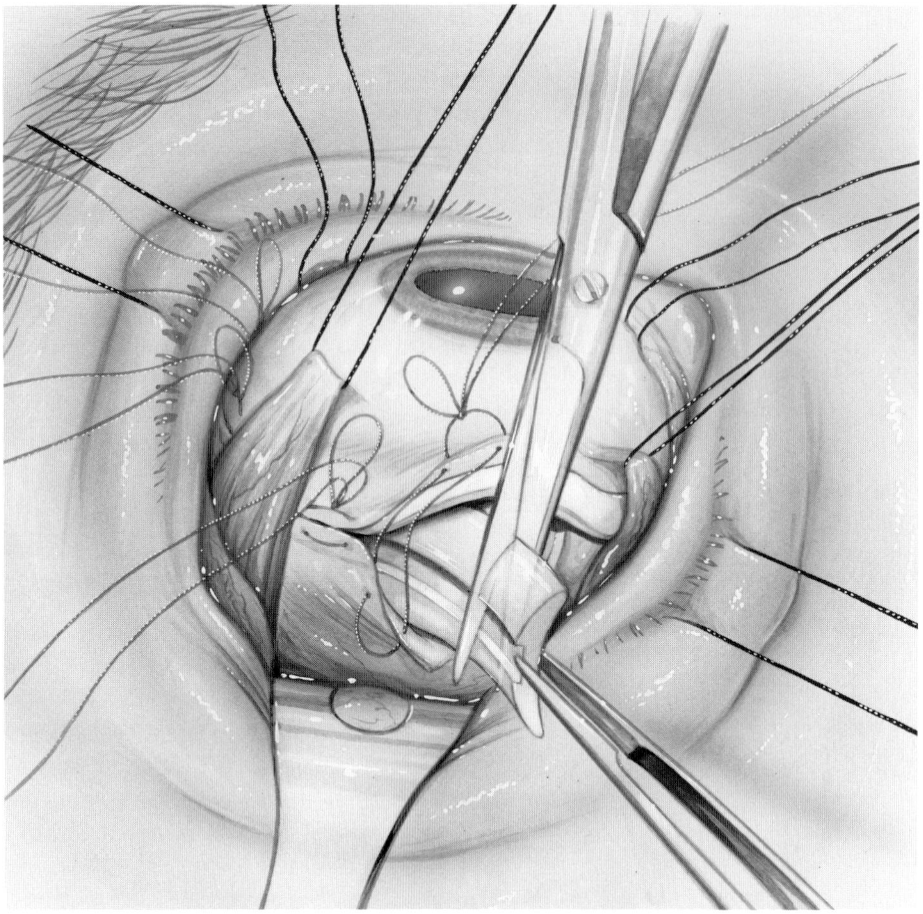

21.**37** **Closure of the lamellar scleral undermining.** If indirect ophthalmoscopy reveals that the retinal breaks are closed, or are well situated on the scleral buckle, the mattress sutures of the scleral flaps are temporarily closed with a slipknot. Any implant that extends beyond the undermining is cut off with straight scissors. The mattress sutures are then loosened, so that the implant can be cut 3 mm shorter than the circumferential length of the undermining.

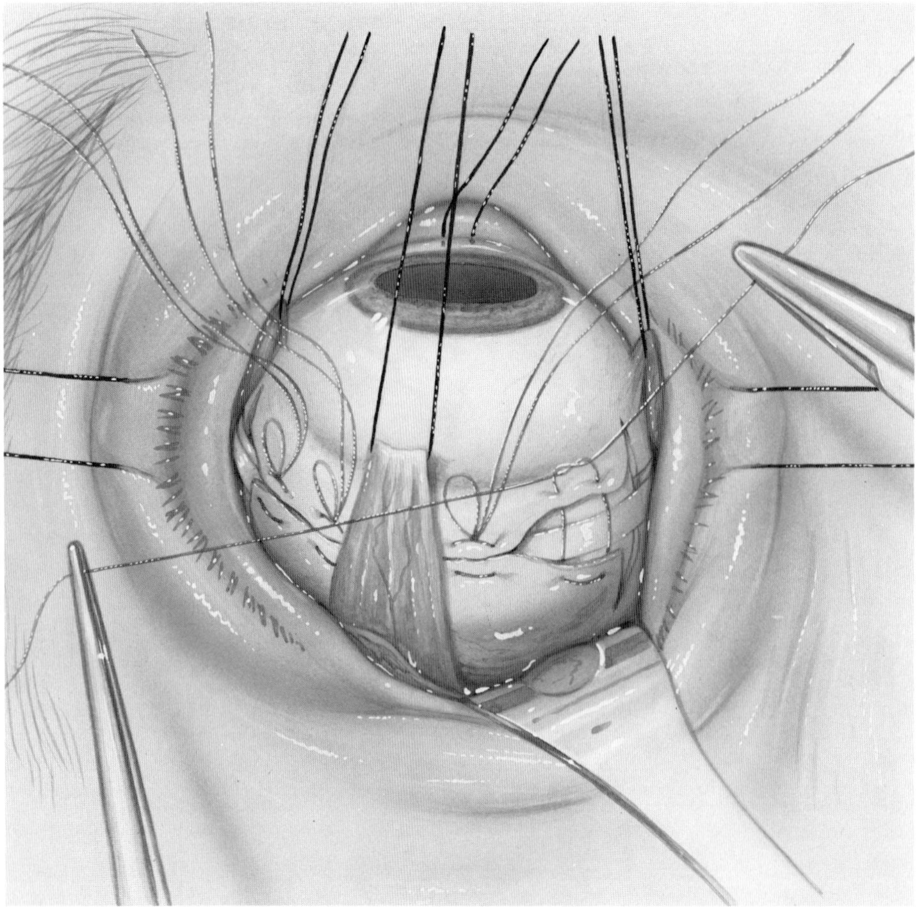

21.**38** After the ends of the implant are trimmed, all of the mattress sutures are closed with a slip knot.

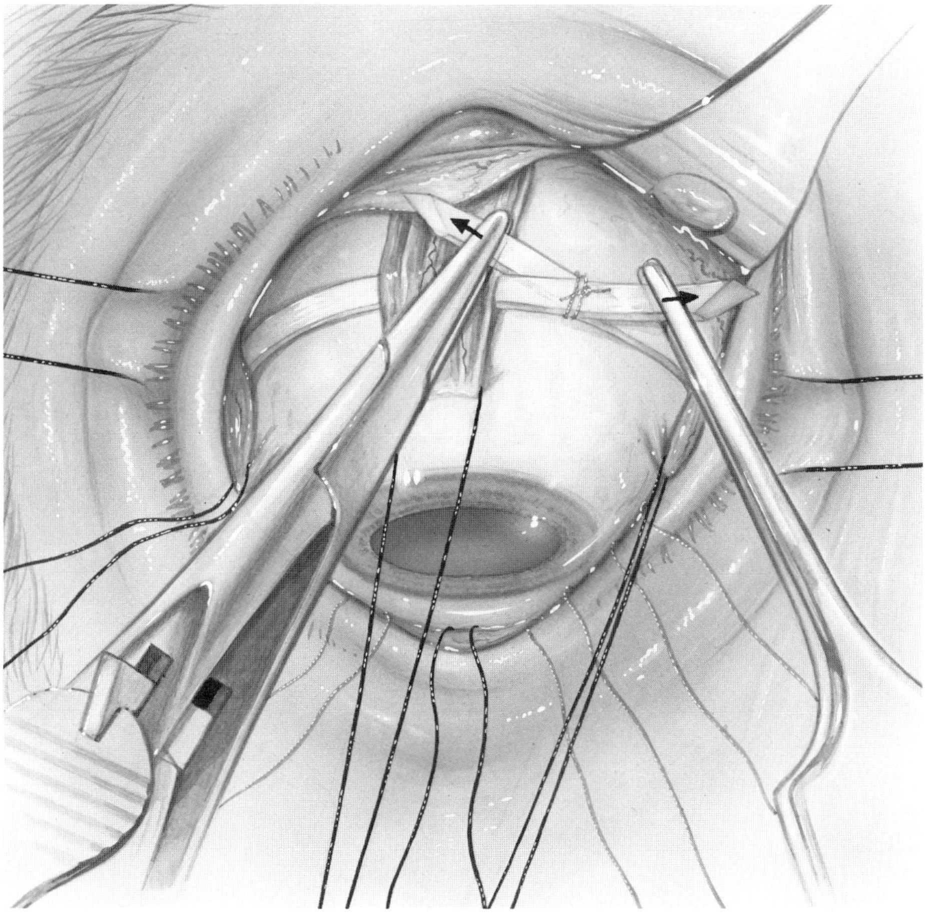

21.**39** The encircling band is tightened by grasping the ends with smooth forceps and a Kalt needle holder and pulling in opposite directions. The encircling band is tightened enough to relieve hypotony.

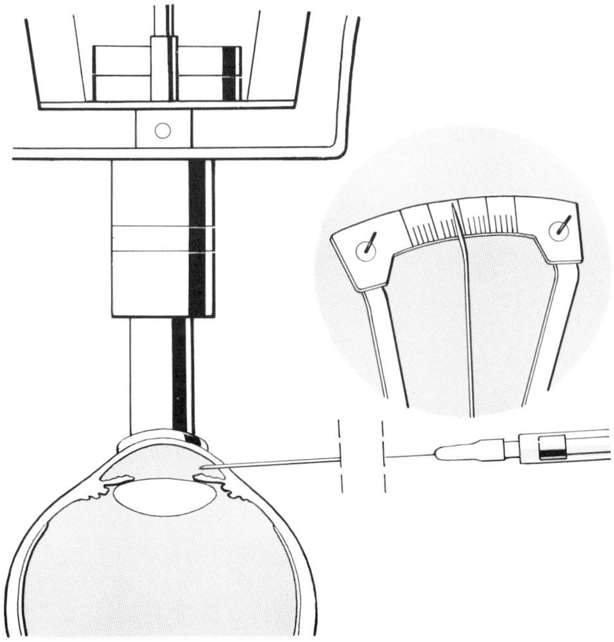

21.**40** **Measurement of intraocular pressure.** Intraocular pressure is measured using a sterile Schiøtz tonometer. A desirable level is 15 mmHg. If the eye is hypotonous, intraocular pressure may be raised by thightening the mattress sutures and the encircling band, or by injecting saline using a short 30-gauge needle inserted through the limbus or the pars plana.

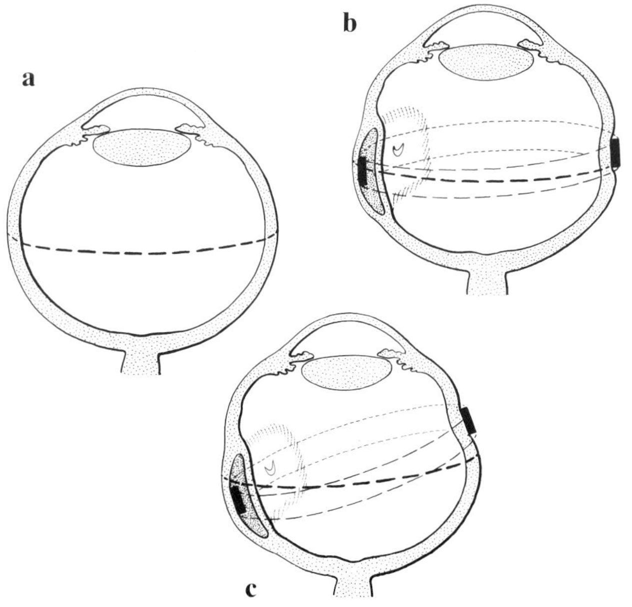

21.**41** **Anchoring the encircling element.** To prevent the encircling element from slipping anterior or posterior to the equator (**a,** broken line), it must be anchored along the greatest circumference of the globe. In **b,** the greatest circumference is at the equator. In **c,** the greatest circumference is achieved by anchoring the implant anterior to the equator opposite the intrascleral implant.

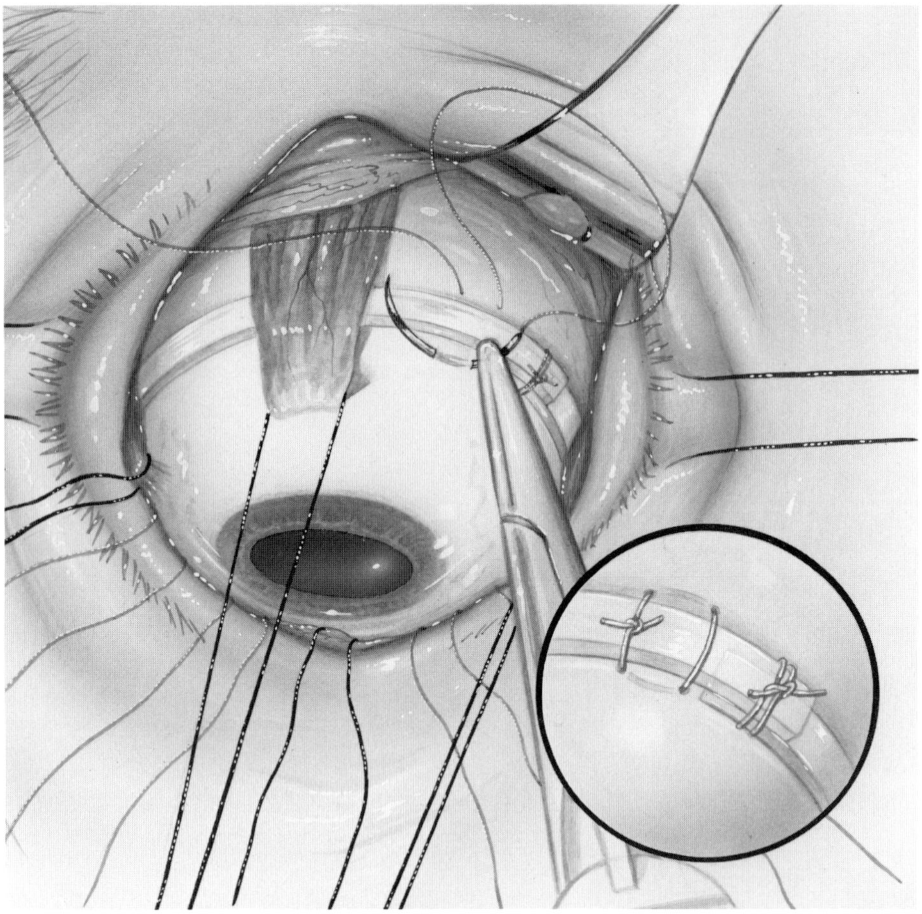

21.**42** After the ends of the encircling element have been trimmed, it is anchored in each quadrant along the greatest circumference of the globe using a 4–0 polyester suture with a spatula cutting needle.

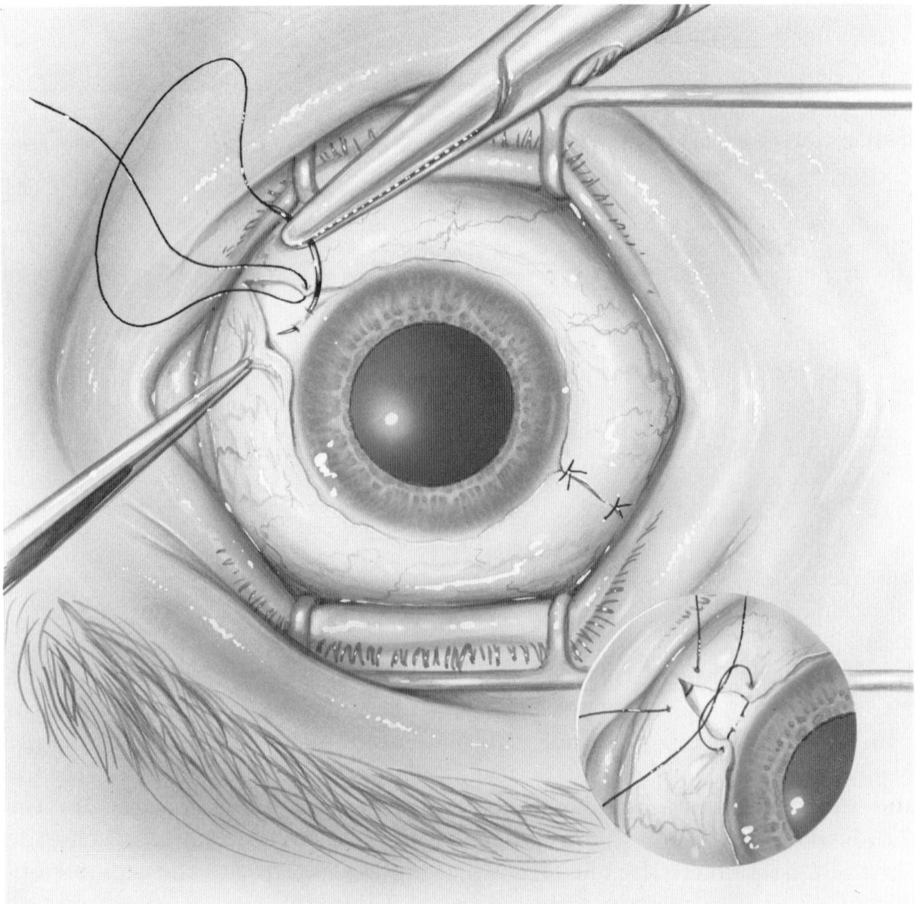

21.**43** **Closure.** The globe is irrigated with an antibiotic solution. Then the relaxing conjunctival incisions are closed with a radial 5–0 plain gut suture. *Inset:* Tenon's capsule and conjunctiva are anchored near the limbus using an episcleral bite.

Problem Cases

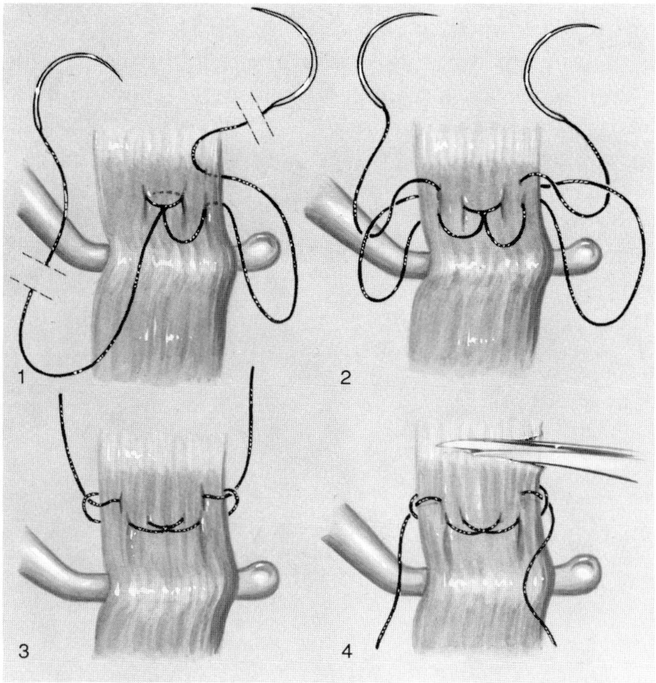

21.**44a** Detachment of a rectus muscle during surgery for retinal detachment. In rare situations in which adequate exposure is unobtainable far posteriorly, e.g. when the globe is large in a normal-sized or small, bony orbit, it may be necessary to detach one muscle.

1. A 6–0 polyglactin suture is passed through the middle third of the muscle with a double-armed suture tied with a single knot.
2, 3. Each needle is passed through the outer quarter of the muscle and locked.
4. The tendon is cut 1–2 mm from its insertion.

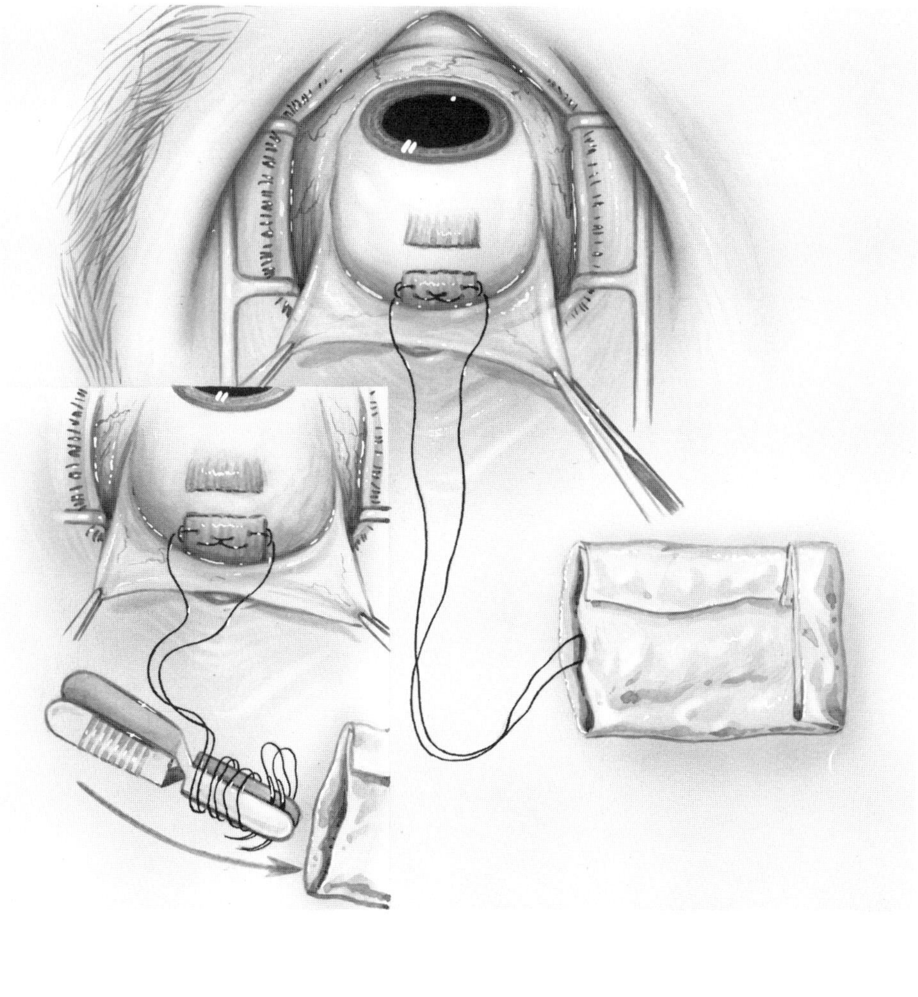

21.**44b** The needles of the double-armed suture are placed between small clamps, and the sutures are rolled around the clamp (lower left) and placed in the suture package, which is tucked under an edge of the drape (lower right).

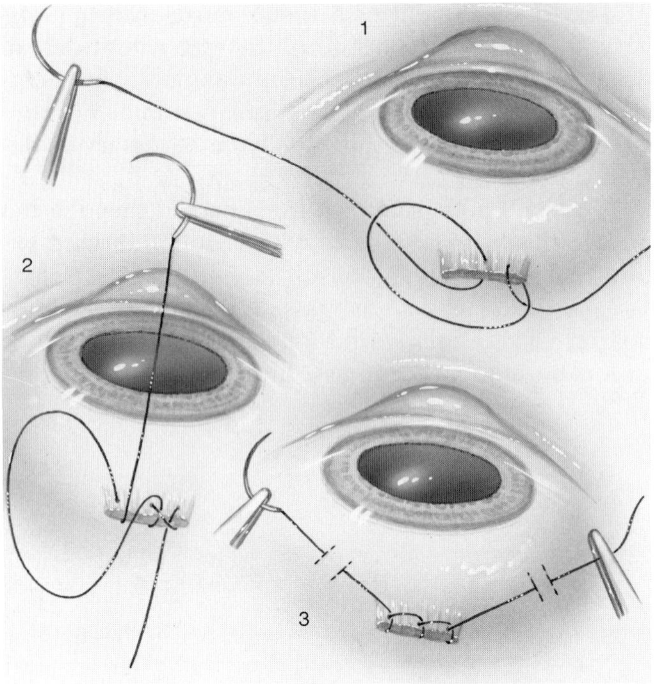

21.**44c** 1, 2. Using a 4–0 black silk suture on a spatula needle, three locking scleral bites are placed through the muscle tendon.

3. The suture is locked on the tendon by drawing the suture ends laterally. The arms are cut 4 inches long and tied in a knot.

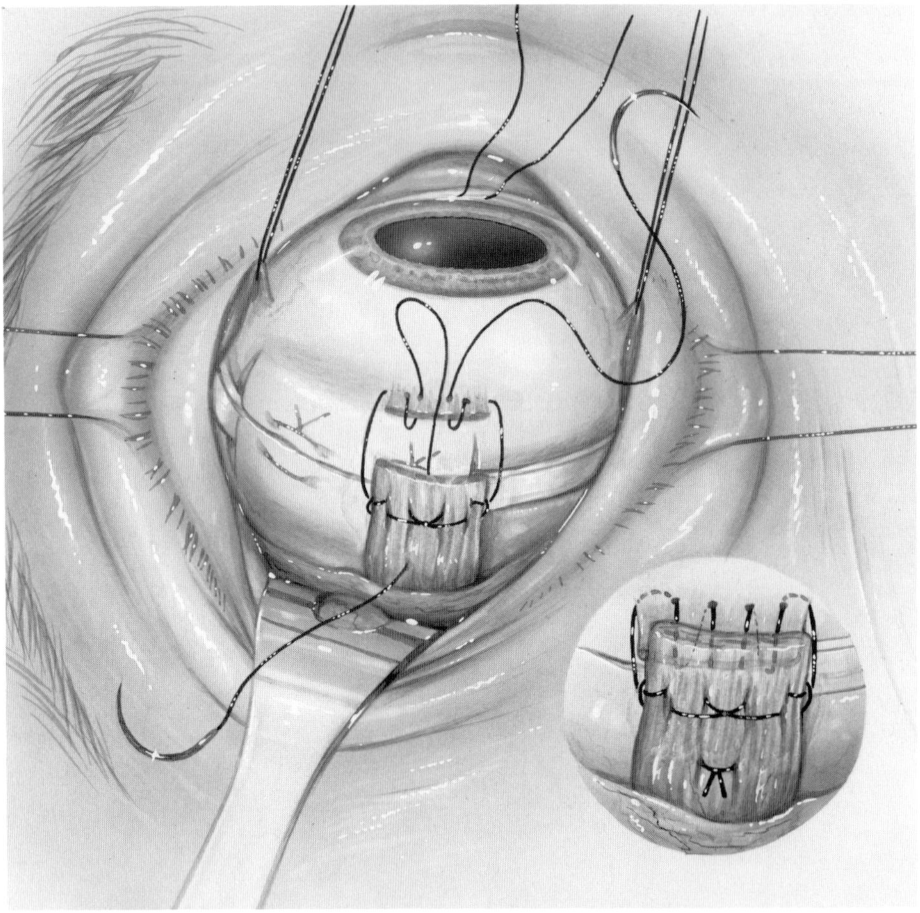

21.**45** **Reattachment of muscle.** Each needle of the double-armed suture is passed through the superficial layers of the sclera at each end of the muscle stump. A second bite is made in the sclera to prevent the suture from slipping.

Inset: Each suture is passed through the muscle belly and tied with a knot.

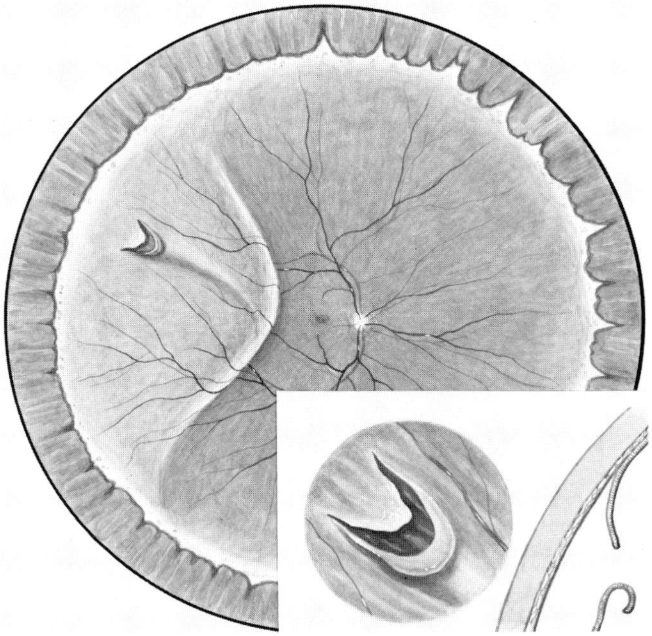

21.46 **Intrascleral buckling with wedge implant for horseshoe tear with a tendency to fishmouth.** Fishmouth refers to the tendency of certain retinal breaks to open more widely following the drainage of subretinal fluid (9). The fishmouth phenomenon occurs more frequently when it is necessary to use a circumferentially-oriented scleral buckle to encompass multiple retinal tears. Breaks that have a tendency to fishmouth are large equatorial horseshoe tears with a rolled posterior edge (inset) and a radial fold extending posteriorly from the tear.

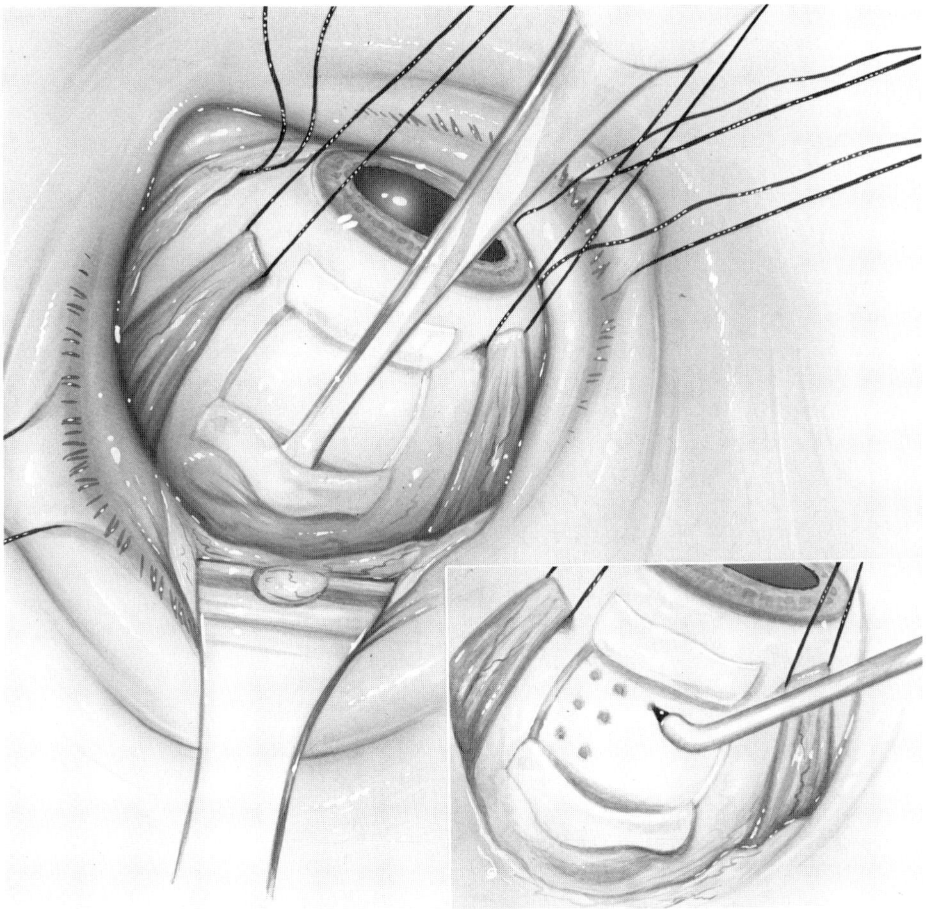

21.**47** Both anterior horns and the posterior edge of the retinal tear are localized with indirect ophthalmoscopy. A circumferential incision for the scleral undermining is made, passing through the posterior diathermy mark and extending 4 mm beyond both horns to the ora serrata. The posterior portion of the bed is made like a pouch to house the edge-shaped implant (8). The pouch is extended 6 mm posterior, with posterior and lateral margins conforming to the shape of the implant.

Inset: diathermy applications are placed under the anterior flap using a blunt conical electrode.

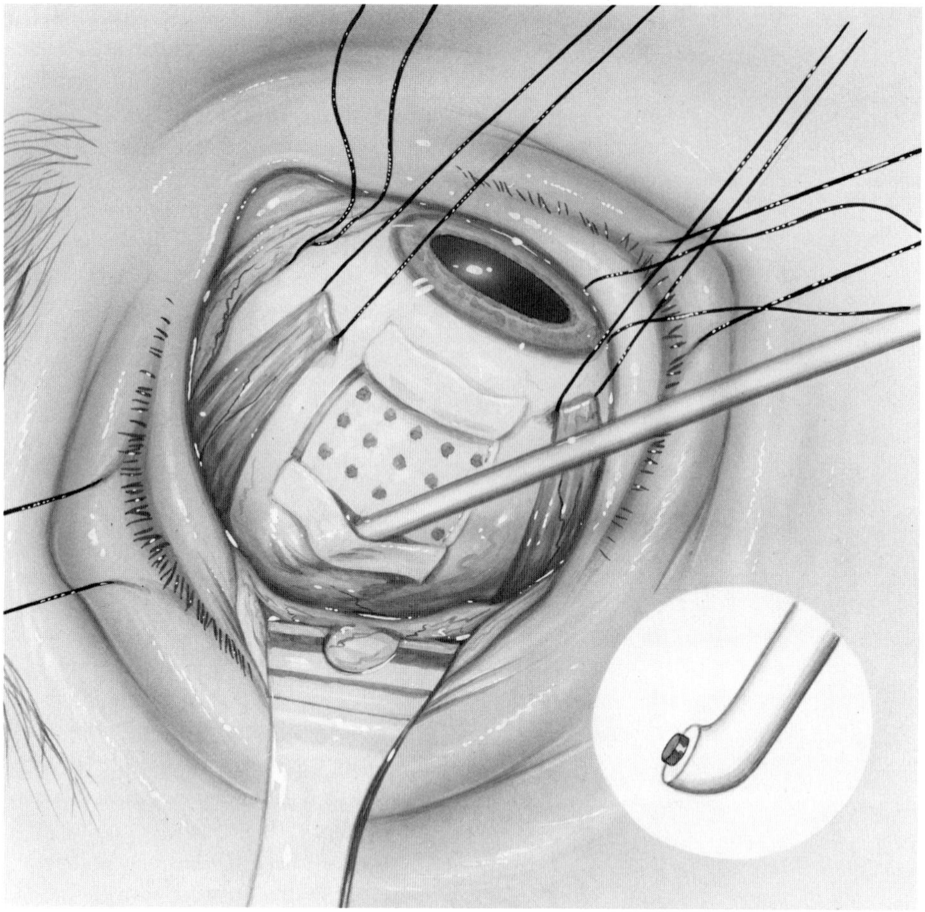

21.**48** Applications within the pouch are made using the short flat diathermy electrode (inset).

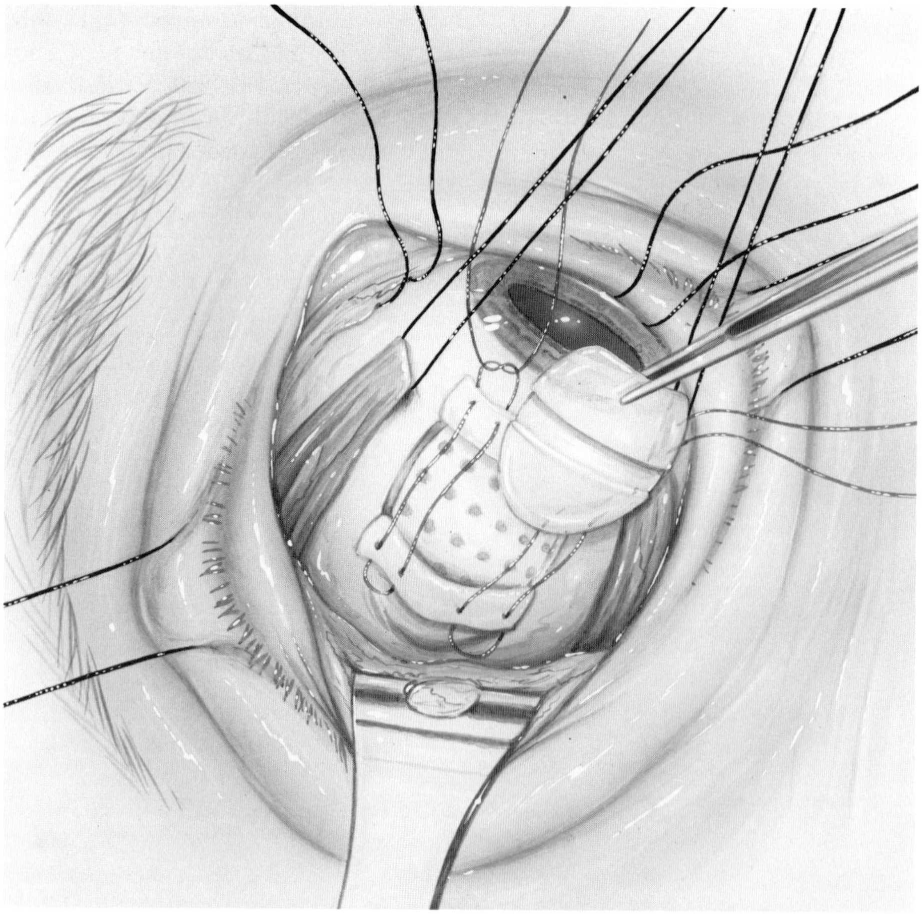

21.**49** The anterior edge of the wedge implant is trimmed so that the implant will be 4 mm shorter than the undermining. The implant is placed in the pouch, and if the fit is tight laterally, the undermining is extended so that the pouch is at least 3 mm wider than the implant. This will allow for a greater indentation of the implant following drainage of subretinal fluid. The encircling band is placed around the globe and in the groove of the wedge implant. Subretinal fluid is drained in the scleral undermining if the detachment is limited to one quadrant, or outside the undermining if the detachment involves more than one quadrant.

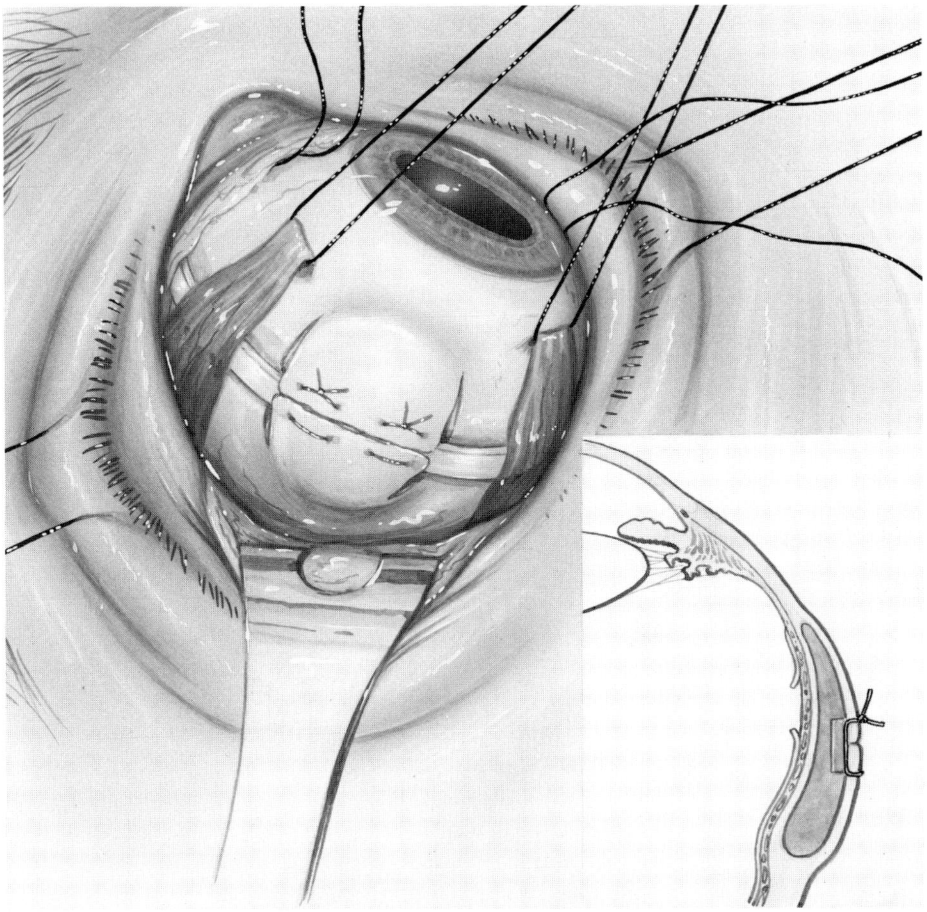

21.**50** Following drainage of subretinal fluid, the sutures are closed, and the encircling band is anchored on the greatest circumference of the globe. The cross section illustrates how the wedge-shaped configuration of the implant, with its convex, blunt, rounded tip, tends to produce an indentation that counteracts fishmouthing of the retinal break and radial folding of the retina.

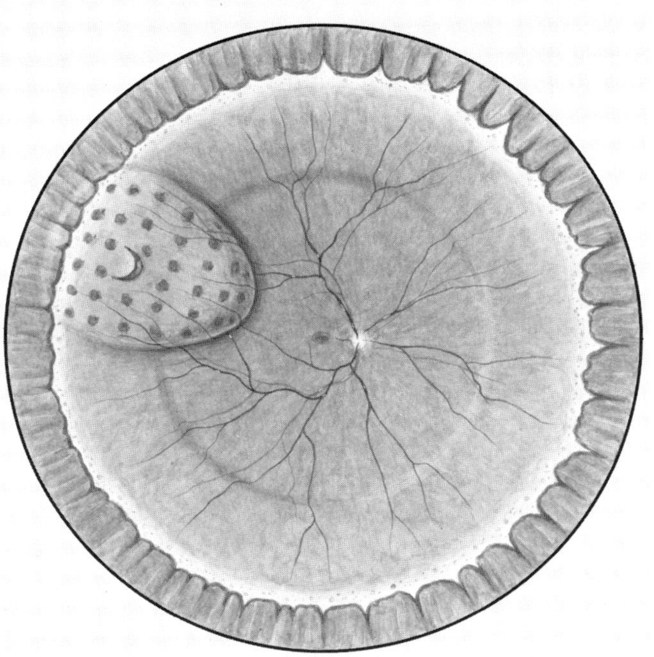

21.**51** A wedge-shaped indentation is produced, with the horseshoe tear smoothly situated on it. A lesser equatorial indentation extending clockwise from the 11 to 9 o'clock meridian is the result of the encirling band, which assures a more permanent buckling effect from the wedge-shaped silicone rubber implant.

52

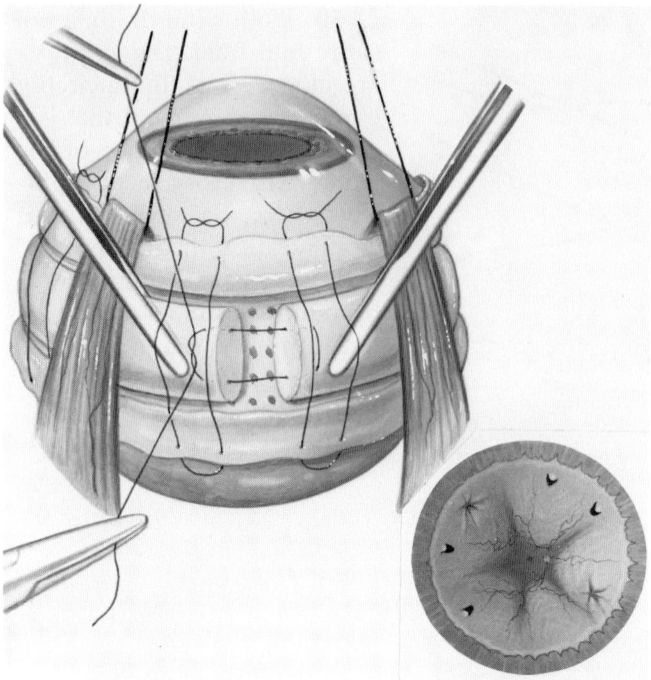

54

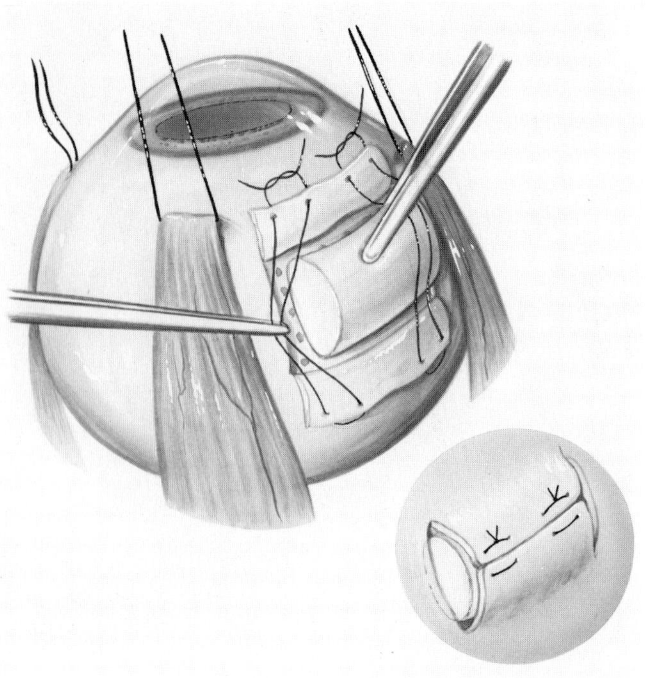

53

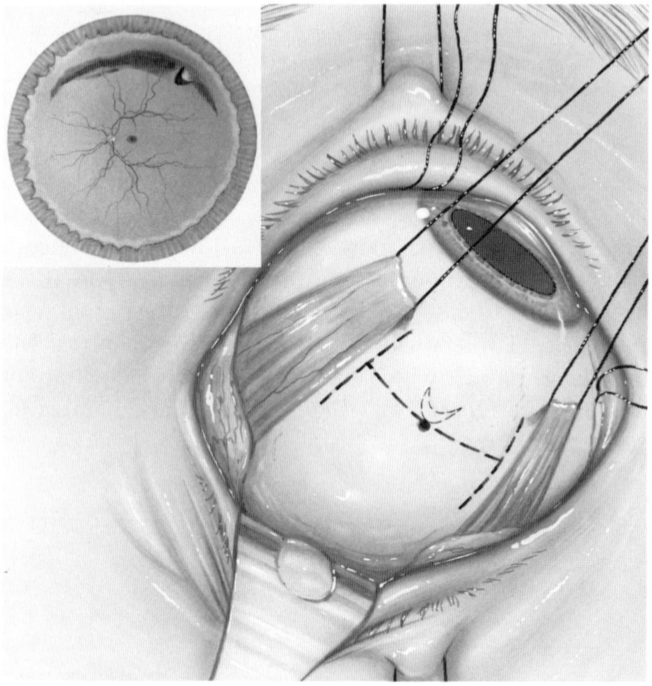

21.**52** *Inset:* total retinal detachment with multiple horseshoe tears, which have a tendency to fishmouth.

With multiple large retinal tears, there may be an increased tendency for proliferative vitreoretinopathy if extensive cryoapplications are used. In this type of case, we prefer to use diathermy, which results in less dispersion of pigment epithelial cells. A lamellar scleral undermining is made to extend clockwise from the 7 to the 4 o'clock meridian.

An elliptical hydrophilic acrylate implant reduces the chance of fishmouthing. The ends of the implant are joined with a mattress suture.

21.**53** **Intrascleral buckle with hydrogel implant for an anterior retinal tear.** If a retinal tear is located far anteriorly, there is less risk of protrusion or extrusion if a hydrophilic acrylate implant is buried under scleral flaps. Because the implant has no dead spaces that can harbor infection, it can be buried under a scleral flap like a solid silicone implant.

Inset: a localized retinal detachment caused by a retinal tear with strong localized vitreous traction.

A scleral groove is made along the localizing mark, and extended at least 1½ clock hours on each side of the retinal tear. Radial incisions are made at the end of the groove to create posterior and anterior scleral flaps.

21.**54** Diathermy or cryo is applied to the bed of the lamellar scleral undermining. Two mattress sutures are placed on the scleral flaps. *Inset:* sutures are tied to close the flaps over the implant. If subretinal fluid is not drained, 500 mg of acetazolamide is given intravenously to reduce the intraocular pressure.

The intrascleral hydrophilic acrylate buckle may be combined with an encircling silicone rubber band. In this case, a grooved hydrophilic acrylate implant is used with a # 240 silicone band to relieve marked vitreous traction. The scleral bed is made 10 mm wide to accommodate a 7 mm implant, which is cut 3 mm shorter than the equatorial length of the undermining.

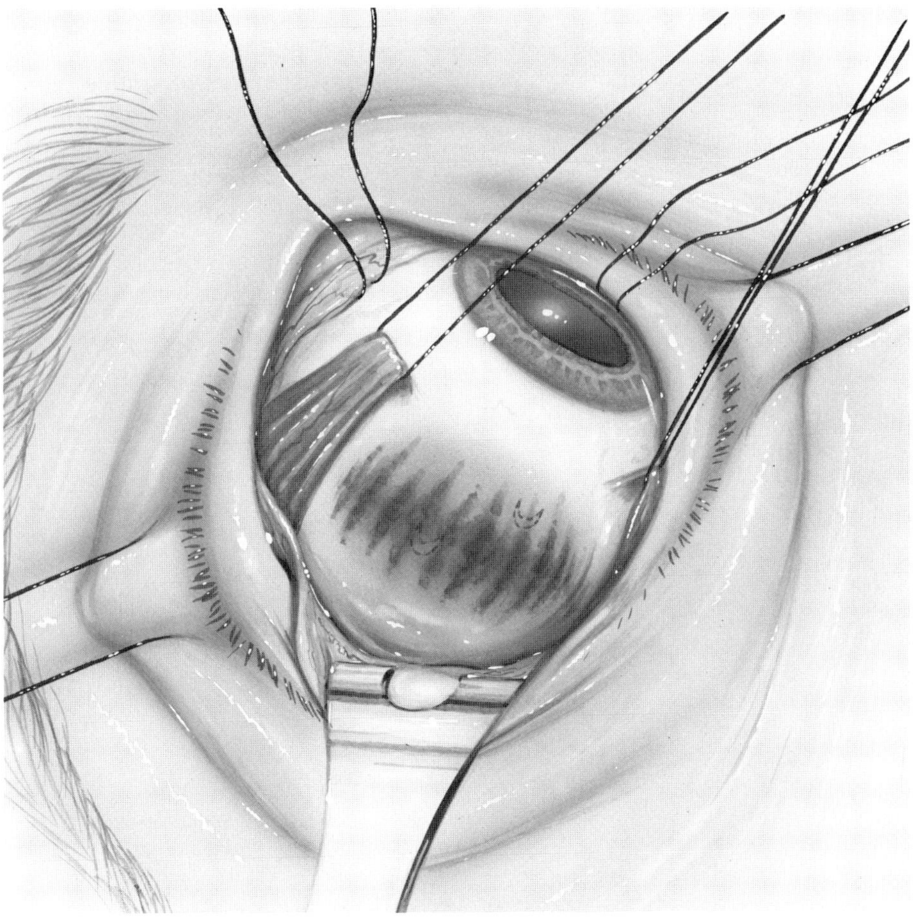

21.**55** **Intrascleral buckling with miniflaps for scleral dehiscences and anterior staphyloma.** Scleral dehiscences and anterior staphyloma have been found in 13% of eyes with primary rhegmatogenous retinal detachment. Scleral dehiscences are elliptically shaped, meridionally oriented, thinned areas of sclera through which choroid is partially visible. They are usually associated with an anterior staphyloma, i.e. a large round or oval-shaped area of thinned sclera that bulges. Dehiscences and anterior staphyloma are usually located in the equatorial region of the superotemporal quadrant. The broken lines outline the location of horseshoe-shaped retinal tears.

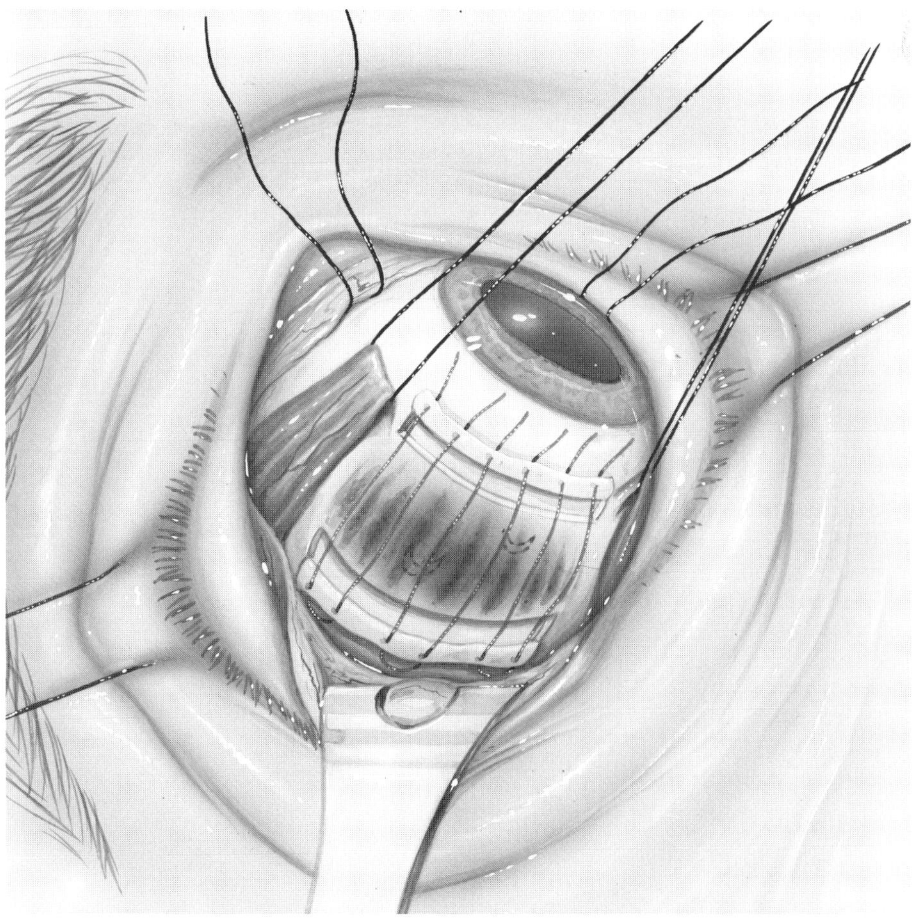

21.**56** To avoid perforating thin sclera, the retinal breaks in areas of thinned sclera are localized with gentle pressure, using a cotton-tipped applicator rather than a localizing electrode. Short scleral flaps (miniflaps) are dissected anterior and posterior to the thinned sclera (5). These flaps have the advantage of making suture placement easier and safer, because the sclera in these eyes tends to vary considerably in thickness. Cryoapplications are placed between the scleral underminings, and 4–0 polyester mattress sutures are placed every 30° along the miniflaps. Subretinal fluid is drained as described in Figures 21.**28**–21.**36**.

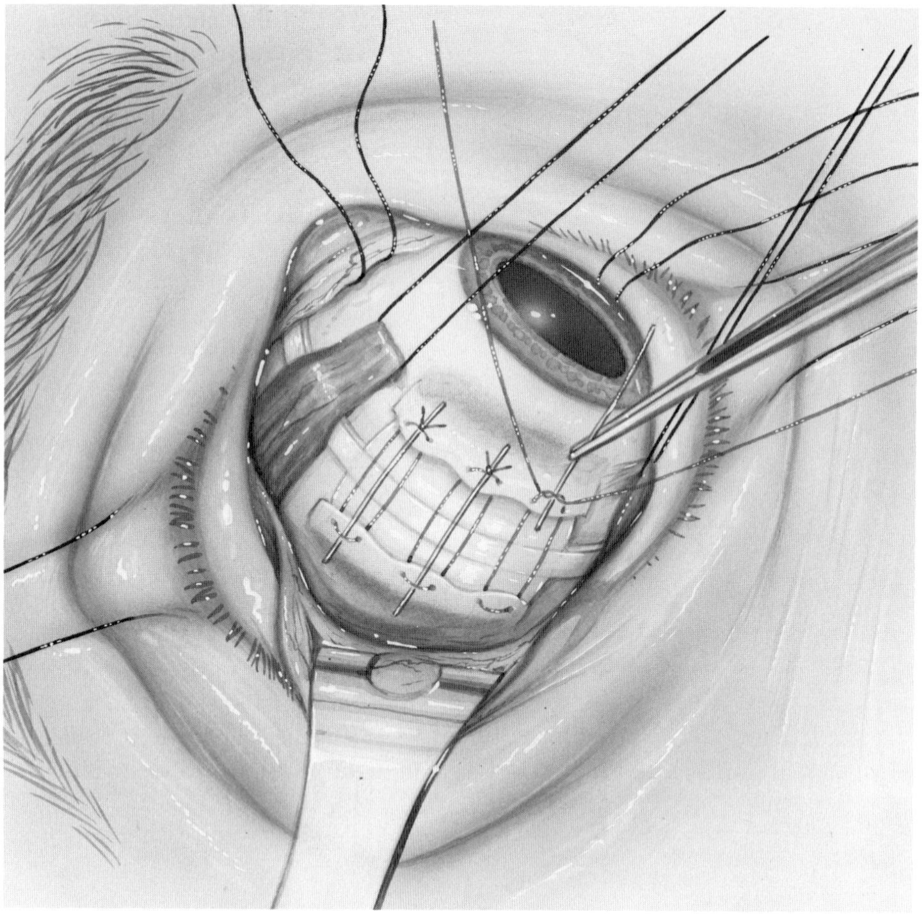

21.**57** To prevent sutures from pulling through the miniflaps, reinforcement sutures of 000 plain gut are inserted beneath the posterior loop and the knot of the mattress suture.

References

1. Benson WB. Retinal detachment: diagnosis and management. Philadelphia: Lippincott, 1988: 113–152.
2. Campochiaro PA, Kaden IA, Vidaurri-Leal J, et al. Cryotherapy enhances intravitreal dispersion of viable retinal pigment epithelial cells. Arch Ophthalmol 1985; 103: 434–436.
3. Faris B, Freeman HM, Schepens CL. Scleral dehiscences, anterior staphyloma, and retinal detachment, part 1: incidence and pathogenesis. Trans Am Acad Ophthalmol Otolaryngol 1975; 79: 851–853.
4. Freeman HM, Schepens CL. Innovations in the technique for drainage of subretinal fluid: transillumination and choroidal diathermy. Mod Probl Ophthalmol 1975; 15: 119–126.
5. Freeman HM, Schepens CL, Faris B. Scleral dehiscences, anterior staphyloma, and retinal detachment, part 2: surgical management. Trans Am Acad Ophthalmol Otolaryngol 1975; 79: 854–857.
6. King LM Jr, Schepens CL. Limbal peritomy in retinal detachment surgery. Arch Ophthalmol 1974; 91: 295–298.
7. Morse PH. Vitreoretinal disease: a manual for diagnosis and treatment. Chicago: Year Book Medical Publishers, 1979: 137–203.
8. Pruett RC. The fishmouth phenomenon, I: clinical characteristics and surgical options. Arch Ophthalmol 1977; 95: 1782–1787.
9. Pruett RC. The fishmouth phenomenon, II: wedge scleral buckling. Arch Ophthalmol 1977; 95: 1782–1787.
10. Schepens CL. Retinal detachment and allied disease. Philadelphia: W B Saunders, 1983: 374–435.

22

Complications of Scleral Buckling

Intraoperative Complications

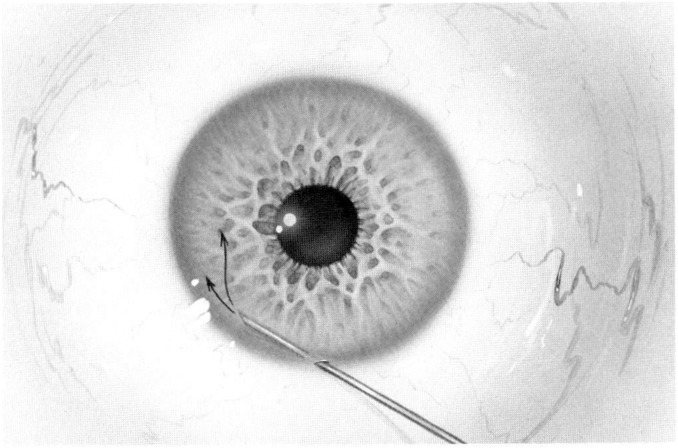

22.**1** **Miosis during surgery.** If the pupil becomes miotic during surgery, it may be dilated by an injection into the anterior chamber of 0.1 ml of the following solution:

Phenylephrine hydrochloride	50 mg
Homatropine hdydrobromide	25 mg
Procaine hydrochloride	25 mg
Distilled water	1 ml

The solution is drawn through a short 30-gauge needle attached to a tuberculin syringe. Care must be taken that no air bubbles are present in the syringe or needle. To prevent damage to the corneal endothelium by the mydriatic solution, the bevel of the needle is directed toward the plane of the iris.

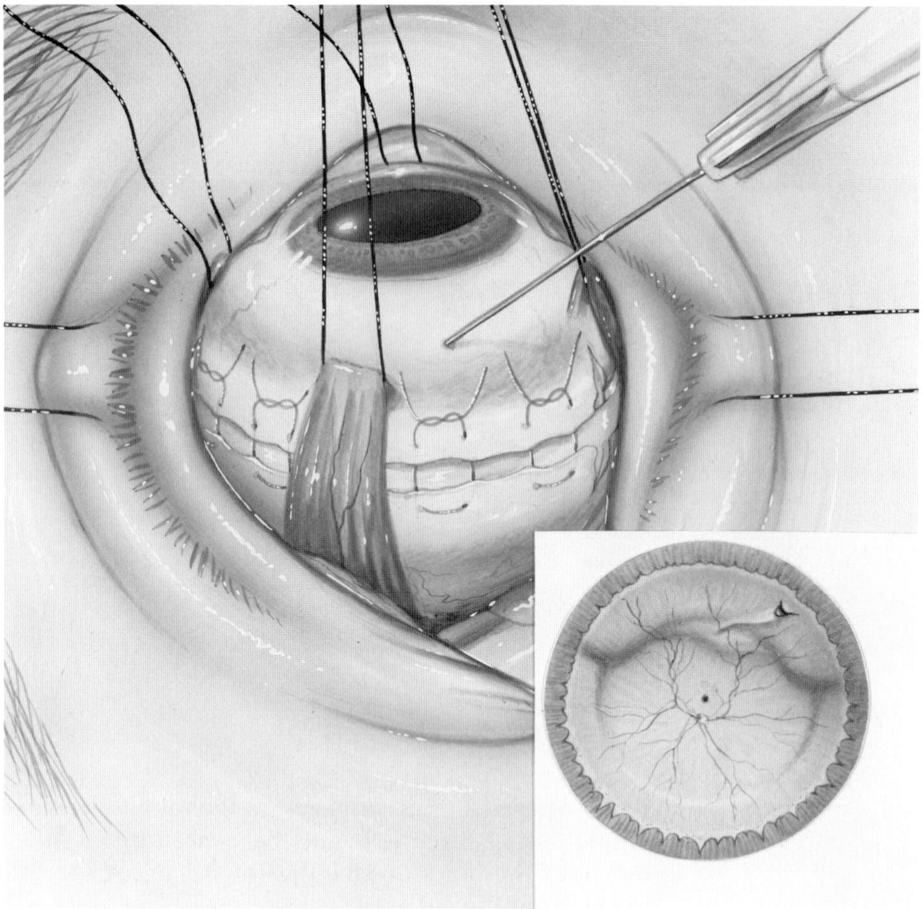

22.**2** **Meridional fold following subretinal fluid drainage.** *Inset:* meridional fold extending from the retinal break posteriorly over the scleral buckle, following the drainage of subretinal fluid. In some cases, this fold is a result of an excessively high buckle which can be lowered by loosening the mattress sutures of the scleral undermining and injecting saline or air into the vitreous cavity. Injection is made with a 30-gauge needle through the pars plana in phakic eyes, or through the limbus in aphakic eyes (13: 452–453).

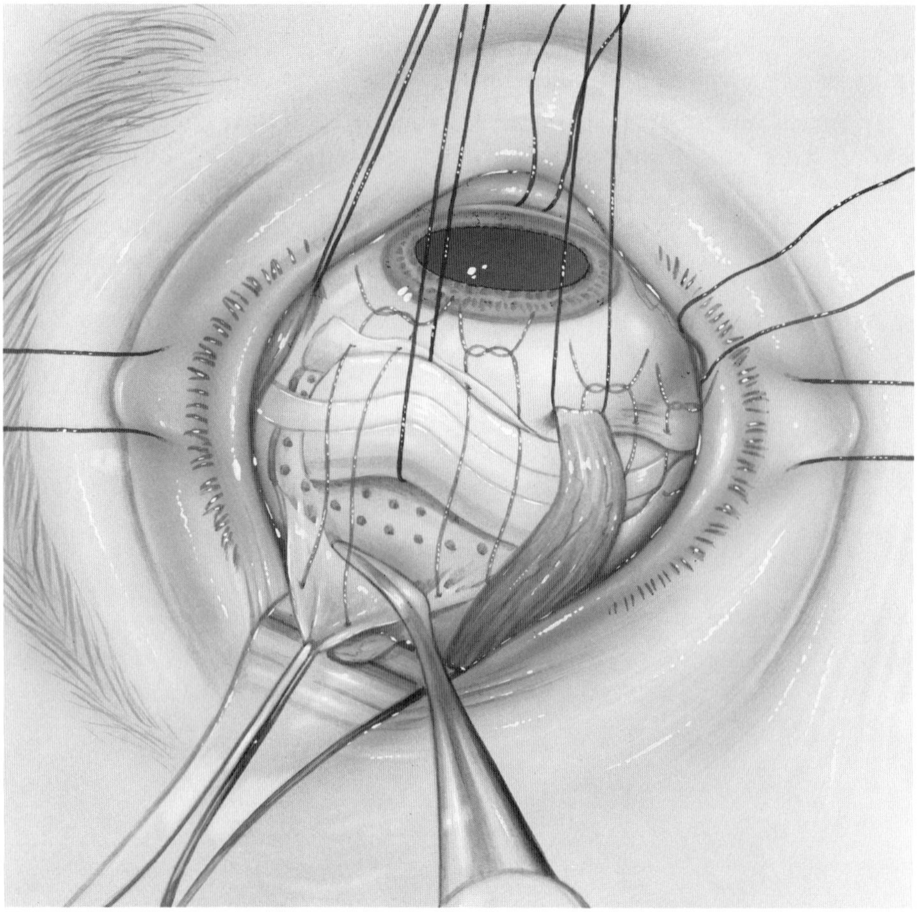

22.**3a** If the meridional fold extending posteriorly from an open retinal break cannot be flattened with air or saline injection, the scleral undermining is extended 4 mm posteriorly in the meridian of the fold and 8 mm circumferentially. Exposure is obtained by retracting the implant anteriorly with a 4–0 black silk suture. Diathermy is applied in the extended scleral undermining.

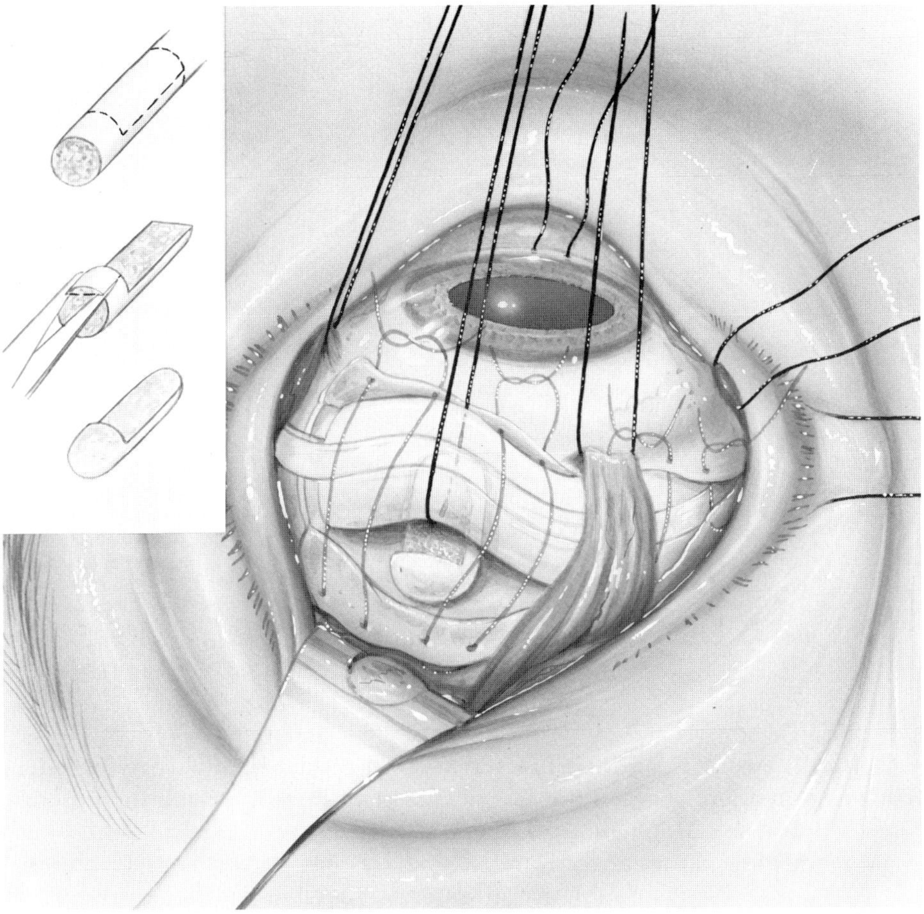

22.**3b** A meridional implant is fashioned from a cylindrical hydrophilic acrylate sponge 5 mm in diameter. A semi-cylindrical section 4 mm long is cut from a 7 mm section of the rod. The remaining 3 mm is trimmed to a diameter of 4 mm. The flat portion fits under the flat solid silicone rubber implant, and the 3 mm portion produces a radial indentation posterior to the buckle. The silicone rubber implant is retracted, and the meridional implant is inserted beneath it. Proper positioning of the implant under the retinal fold is determined by indirect ophthalmoscopy.

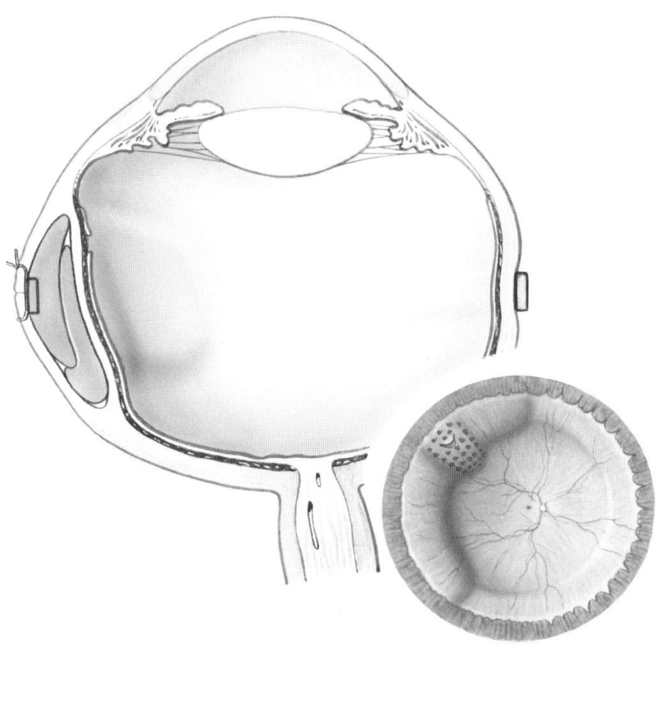

22.**3c** A solid silicone rubber meridional implant may be used to flatten a meridional fold. *Inset:* this meridional implant produces a broader, less convex indentation of the sclera than a meridional implant fashioned from a sponge. See Fig. 3.**35a, b** for illustrations of the variety of solid silicone rubber meridional implants.

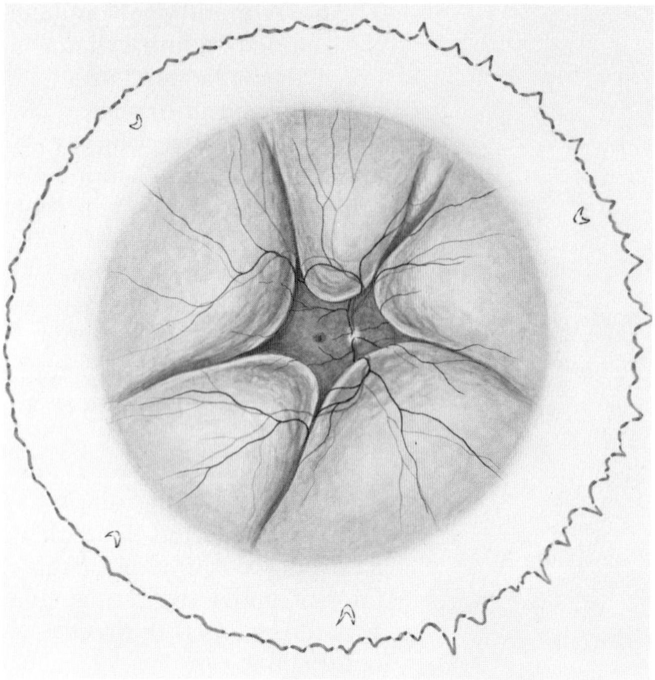

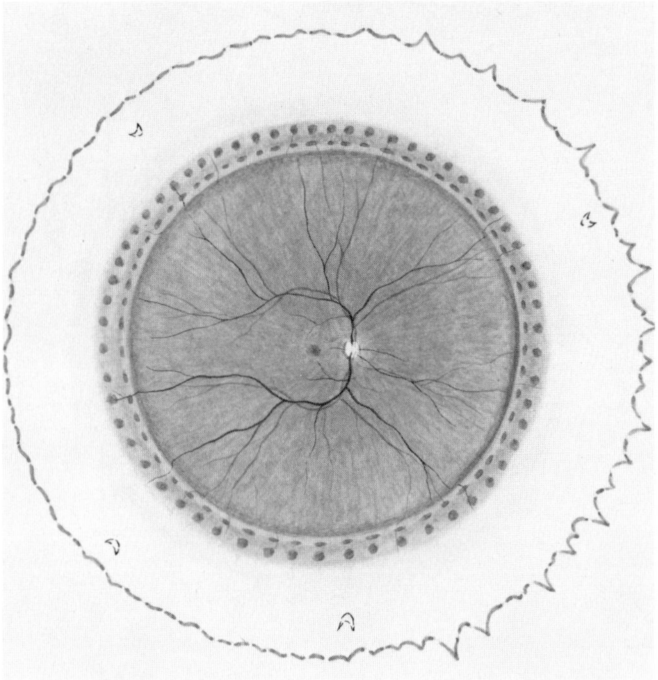

22.**4a** **Failure to visualize retinal breaks.** In some eyes, the retinal breaks cannot be visualized because of capsular remnants or a pupil that will not dilate due to synechiae to an intraocular lens. Marked scleral depression under anesthesia may be rewarding in the search for retinal breaks.

22.**4b** In this case, the peripheral retina (white) and the ora serrata and retinal breaks (broken lines) could not be visualized with indirect ophthalmoscopy and scleral depression. If no retinal breaks can be visualized, and a total retinal detachment is present, an equatorial scleral buckling is made to extend around 360° of the globe and far enough posteriorly so that the posterior third of the buckle will be visible (2). Care must be taken to avoid treatment over the long posterior ciliary arteries, which are visualized by transillumination through the pupil.

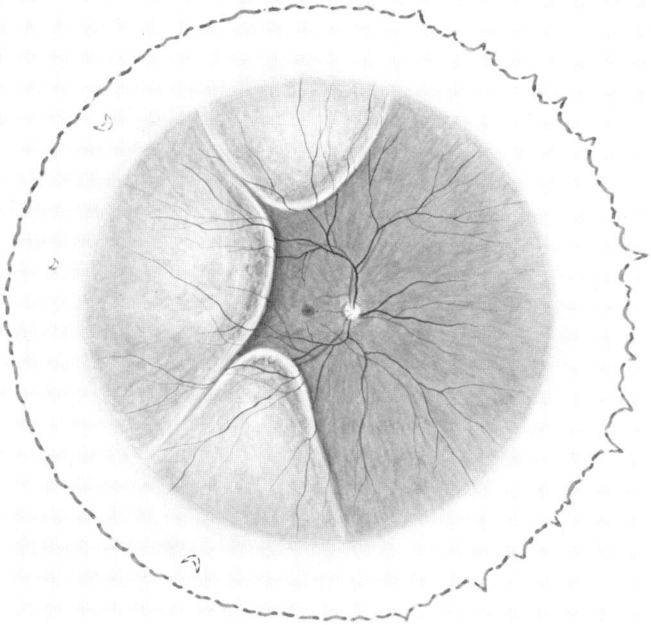

22.5a **Partial retinal detachment in which retinal breaks are not visible.** Fundus view of a retinal detachment in which the retina is detached from the 6 to the 12 o'clock meridian. The ora serrata (broken line) and retinal breaks in the 7, 9, and 10 o'clock meridians are not visible by indirect ophthalmoscopy.

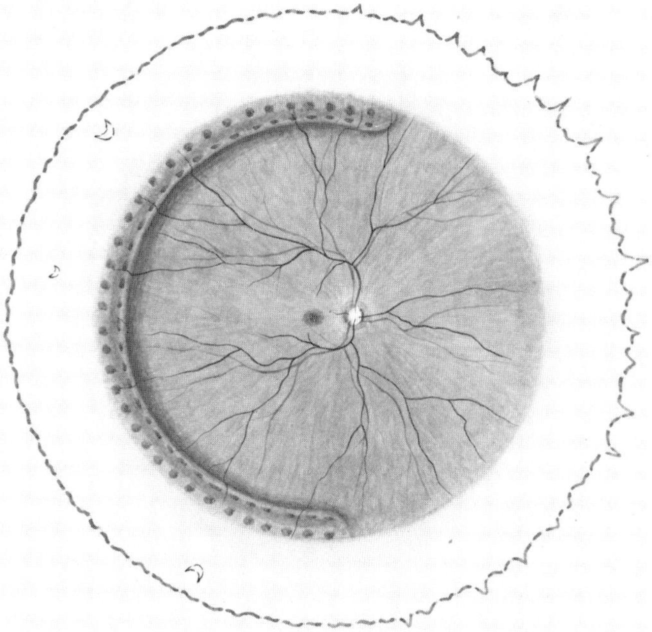

22.5b An equatorial scleral buckling is made extending over the circumference of the retinal detachment from the 6 to 12 o'clock meridians. The buckle is made to extend far enough posteriorly so that the posterior third of the buckle is visible.

6a

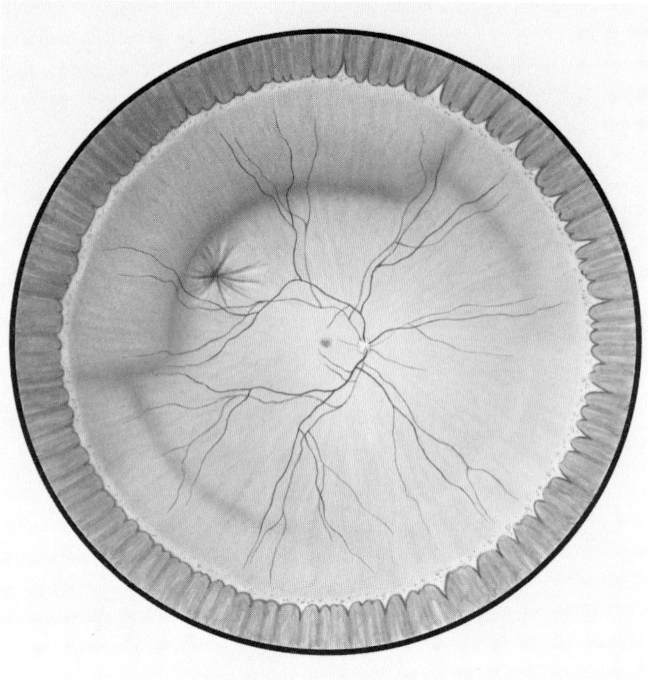

6c

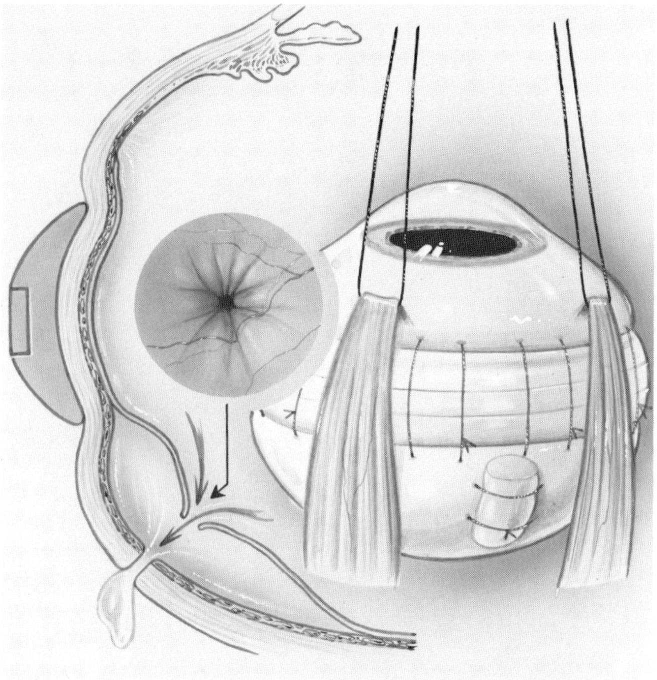

6b

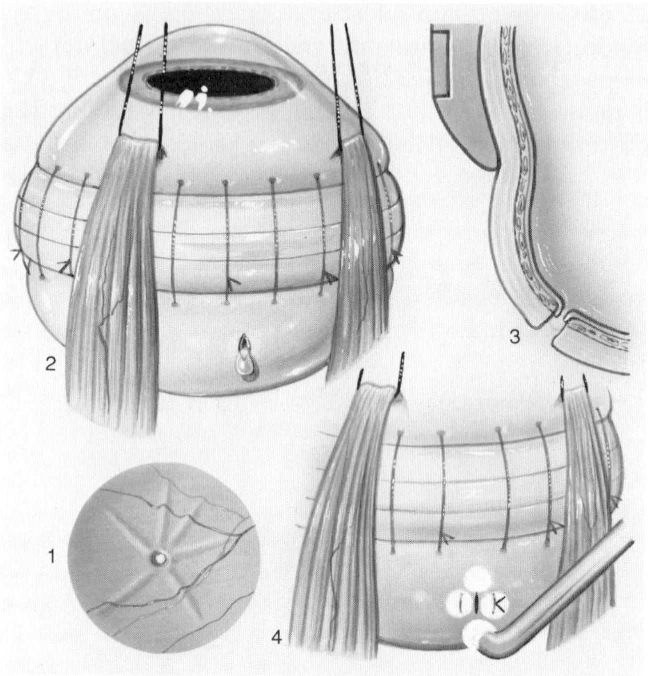

22.**6a Drainage complications: retinal incarceration.** A sudden cessation of drainage of subretinal fluid may be the result of incarceration of retina in the perforation site (13: 981–982). This complication tends to occur in cases with shifting subretinal fluid. No pressure should be exerted on the globe to promote further drainage until after indirect ophthalmoscopy has been performed. Folds radiating from the region of the perforation site indicate that the retina is incarcerated in the choroidal perforation. As long as these folds do not communicate with a retinal breaks to prevent it from being closed, no treatment is indicated. If subretinal fluid was drained through a sclerotomy posterior to the buckle, the sclerotomy suture is closed and tied permanently.

22.**6b Drainage complications: retinal hole.** If (1) indirect ophthalmoscopy reveals a retinal hole in the center of star-shaped retinal folds at the perforation site, and (2) fluid continues to ooze from the sclerotomy, treatment is indicated.

3 Cross section illustrates a retinal incarceration in the sclerotomy and a retinal hole.

4 The sclerotomy is closed with a mattress suture and surrounded by cryoapplications. If the sclerotomy is located in the scleral undermining, cryoapplications or a suture are not used.

22.**6c Drainage complications: vitreous loss.** *Left:* vitreous gel prolapsing through an iatrogenic hole at the perforation site.
Center: the retinal hole is elevated and surrounded by radial retinal folds and detached retina. Cryoapplications are applied around the sclerotomy.
Right: a sponge is sutured to the sclera to produce a buckle to close the retinal break and flatten the retinal folds.

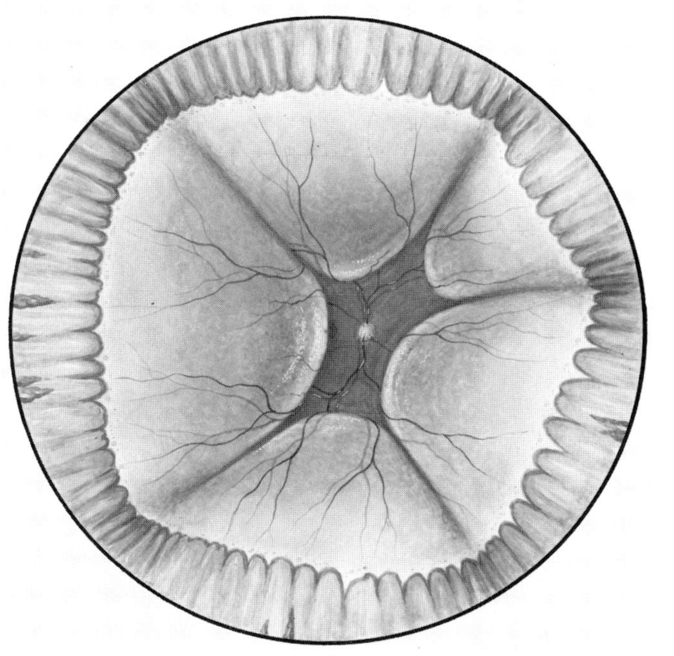

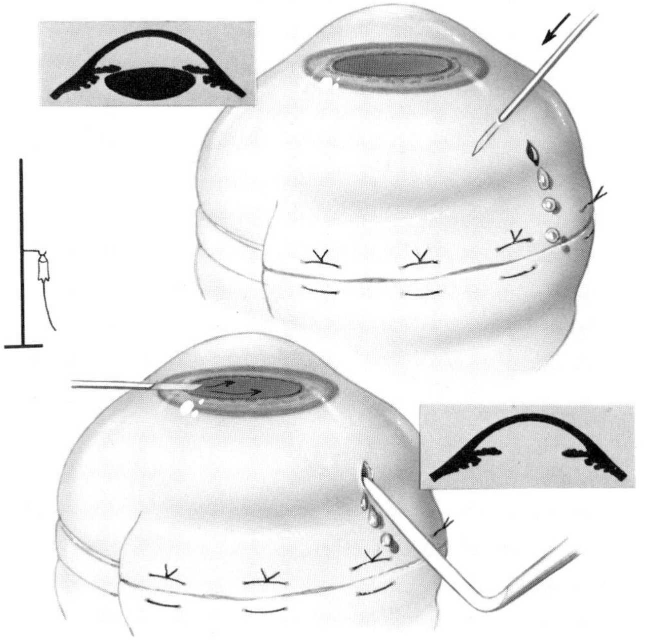

Postoperative Complications

22.7a **Postoperative choroidal detachment.** Choroidal detachment occurs in varying degrees of severity in approximately 24% of eyes following scleral buckling surgery for retinal detachment (4). The majority of postoperative choroidal detachments are transudative; very few are hemorrhagic. Small choroidal detachments often pass unnoticed, because they affect only the region of the pars plana ciliaris and the retinal periphery, and subside spontaneously (13: 1001–1009). Postoperative choroidal detachment appears as a solid, immobile, orange-brown elevation of the fundus. The detachment extends beyond the ora serrata, making the extreme fundus periphery visible without scleral depression. The choroidal elevation may be single or multilobular. It may progress in an annular direction around the entire fundus periphery, or extend posteriorly to obscure the macula or optic disc.

Management of postoperative choroidal detachment. Most postoperative choroidal detachments subside spontaneously and require no treatment. When the choroidal elevation extends posterior to the equator and around the entire fundus periphery to result in a shallowing of the anterior chamber, 100 mg of prednisone is given daily orally for 5 to 7 days. Drainage of subchoroidal fluid is indicated when the choroidal detachment involves the macula, or when temporal and nasal detachments extend posteriorly until they come in contact. These are termed "kissing" choroidal detachments (1).

22.7b *Top:* **drainage of subchoroidal fluid in a phakic Eye.** The inset (left) indicates that the eye is phakic. A radial sclerotomy is made 8 to 10 mm posterior to the limbus in the meridian of the most marked choroidal elevation. It is important to avoid profound hypotony during the drainage of subchoroidal fluid, because this may incite choroidal hemorrhage or recurrence of the choroidal detachment. After approximately 0.5 ml of fluid has been drained, BSS Plus solution is injected through the pars plana ciliaris 4 mm posterior to the limbus, using a 30-gauge needle. Additional subchoroidal fluid is drained, and BSS Plus solution is injected into the vitreous cavity until indirect ophthalmoscopy reveals that the choroidal elevation has disappeared.

Below: **drainage of subchoroidal fluid in an aphakic eye.** *Inset (right):* in the aphakic or pseudoaphakic eye, infusion during drainage of subchoroidal fluid is accomplished through a bent 25-gauge needle attached to an intravenous infusion bottle. Care must be exercised to keep the infusion bottle at a level that does not produce ocular hypertension, which can cause an incarceration or hole in the uvea overlying the sclerotomy. Additional subchoroidal fluid may be released using an iris spatula inserted tangentially into the sclerotomy.

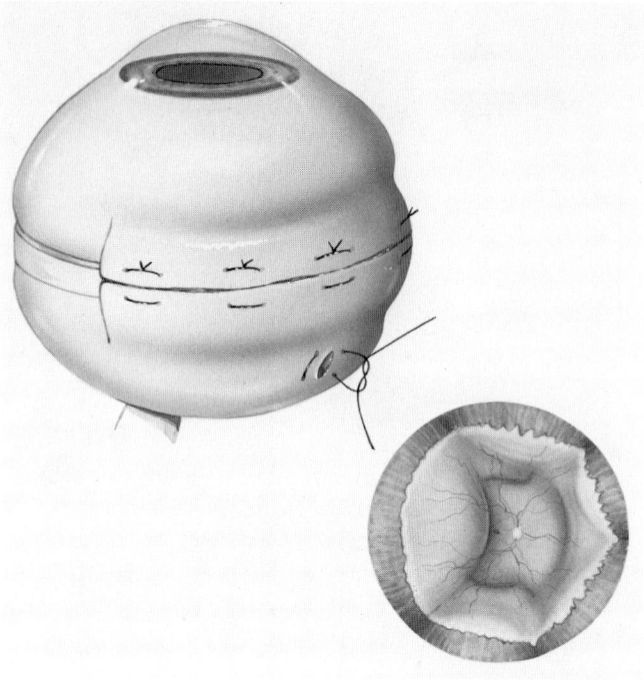

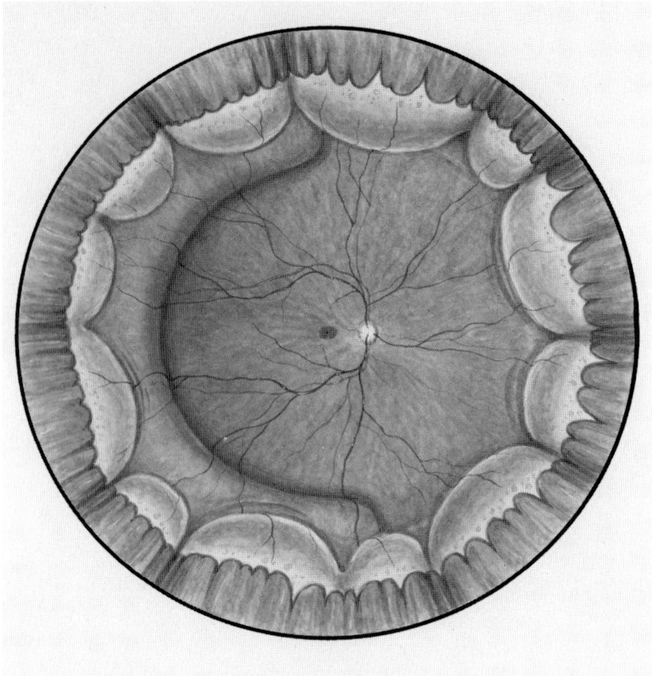

22.**7c** **Posterior drainage of subchoroidal fluid.** In cases in which insufficient subchoroidal fluid is drained through an anterior sclerotomy, it may be necessary to make a sclerotomy posterior to the scleral buckle. A mattress suture is placed across the sclerotomy prior to the release of subchoroidal fluid. The infusion bottle must be kept very low to prevent retinal incarceration or a retinal hole at the site of the postertior sclerotomy.

22.**7d** **Angle-closure glaucoma.** Routine postoperative biomicroscopy of the anterior segment and measurement of the intraocular pressure are important in detecting an early shallowing of the anterior chamber that may flatten within a few days. Subsequent elevated intraocular pressure may produce corneal edema and a masking of closure of the filtration angle. Ophthalmoscopy may reveal a rather shallow annular choroidal elevation.

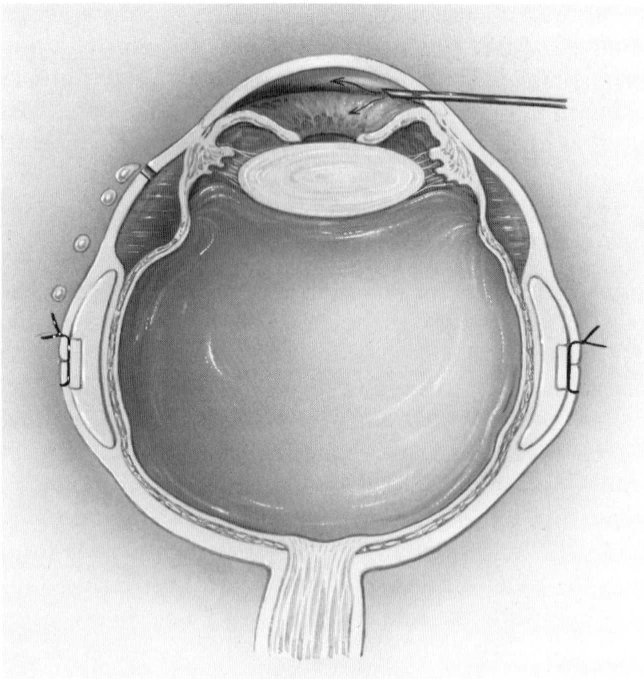

22.**8** An annular peripheral choroidal detachment may elevate the ciliary body around the scleral spur, bringing the iris root against the filtration angle to shallow and then close the filtration angle (13: 1007–1011). Introcular pressure should be measured by applanation rather than by Schiøtz tonometry because of the reduction in scleral rigidity (10). The anterior chamber can be of almost normal depth centrally, despite closure of the angle. A 4-day trial of medical therapy with acetazolamide and systemic steroids should be made, after which surgical intervention is indicated to prevent synechiae formation (15: 165).

Using a fine-bladed # 5 paracentesis knife, a bevelled incision is made through the limbus into the anterior chamber. The incision tract is marked with fluorescein so that it can be identified later for the injection of saline to deepen the anterior chamber. Radial sclerotomies are made 3 to 4 mm posterior to the limbus and 180° apart. The inner aspect of the sclerotomy incision should be 2 mm in length to achieve optimal drainage of subchoroidal fluid. The fluid may be loculated; a cyclodialysis spatula is therefore inserted into the sclerotomy and swept clockwise and anticlockwise to release additional fluid. Saline is injected into the anterior chamber through the preplaced incision. If the anterior chamber fails to deepen, additonal sclerotomies are made in the remaining two quadrants (C. D. Belcher, personal communication). Ophthalmoscopy and gonioscopy may be attempted, to determine if the choroidal detachment has disappeared and the angle has been openend. However, in most cases, corneal edema precludes a clear view.

Implant exposure. Implants and sutures used in scleral buckling may erode through Tenon's capsule and conjunctiva to become exposed and secondarily infected. Implant exposure may occur when the implant is located too far anteriorly, is too bulky, inadequately sutured to the sclera, or poorly covered by Tenon's capsule. The signs and symptoms of an infected implant include conjunctival ecchymosis, purulent discharge, a fistulous tract, granuloma, pain, tenderness, and, rarely, a sterile endopthalmitis. As a general rule, topical or systemic antibiotics will not eradicate this type of infection. If the exposed implant or sutures become infected, they should be removed (3, 5–9, 11, 12, 13: 1025–1036, 14, 15: 166, 16).

Implant erosion. A solid rubber implant with a sharp edge that has not been trimmed may erode through the sclera. Implant erosion may also occur when the underlying sclera has been repeatedly or excessively treated with diathermy or croyapplications. In rare instances, erosion may result from an excessively tight encircling element.

The main goal of implant removal in eyes with scleral erosion is to relieve the pressure exerted by the implant against the sclera. Cutting the encircling band alone may be sufficient to stop the progression of scleral erosion. The band is cut at both ends of the scleral buckle, an ideal location because the band is resting on the implant, easy to identify, and safe to cut. If an intrascleral implant has caused sclerochoroidal erosion, it may be removed without opening the sclera completely. The band and mattress at both ends of the buckle are cut. The entire implant is removed with forceps by sliding it out of the intrascleral space. It the band must be removed, anchor sutures and the joint of the band are located. The sutures are removed, and the band is pulled out gently at the joint.

Anesthesia for implant removal. Although some cases of implant removal can be operated under local anesthesia, general anesthesia is preferred, because retrobulbar and regional anesthetic agents do not readily infiltrate scarred or infected periorbital tissues, and therefore fail to provide adequate anesthesia. Before starting the procedure, the previous operative reports should be reviewed to account for all implant materials and sutures that were used during previous scleral buckling procedures.

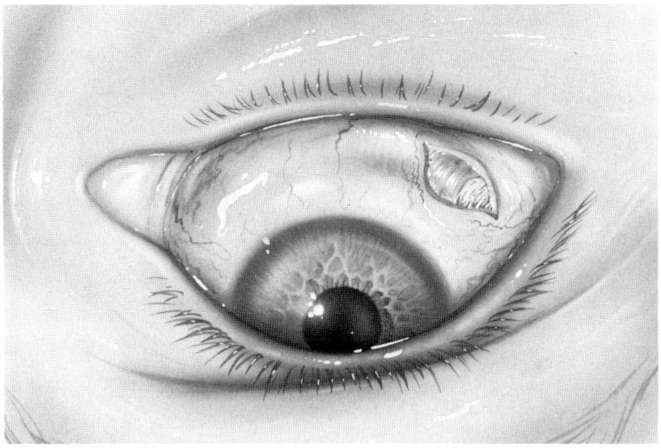

22.9 a **Removal of exposed silastic sponge.** A silastic episcleral implant in the inferior quadrant is infected and associated with a fistulous tract through the conjunctiva. The end of the implant is exposed by the erosion of the conjunctiva. The surgical plan is to expose the entire implant to allow removal of all sutures.

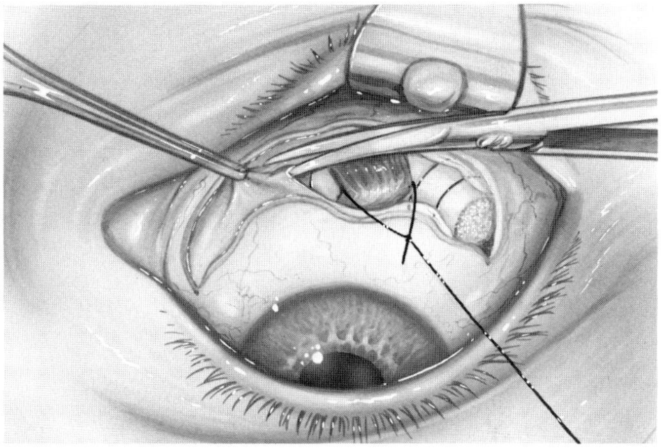

22.9 b Conjunctiva and Tenon's fascia over the sponge and inferior rectus muscle are grasped with toothed forceps and cut with curved iris scissors. To improve exposure of the operative field, a bridle suture is inserted under the tendon of the inferior rectus muscle. The mattress sutures anchoring the episcleral implant are cut with scissors or a knife and then removed with forceps. The sponge is then gently extracted. The lower quadrants of the orbit are irrigated with an antibiotic solution. Tenon's fascia and conjunctiva are closed in separate layers.

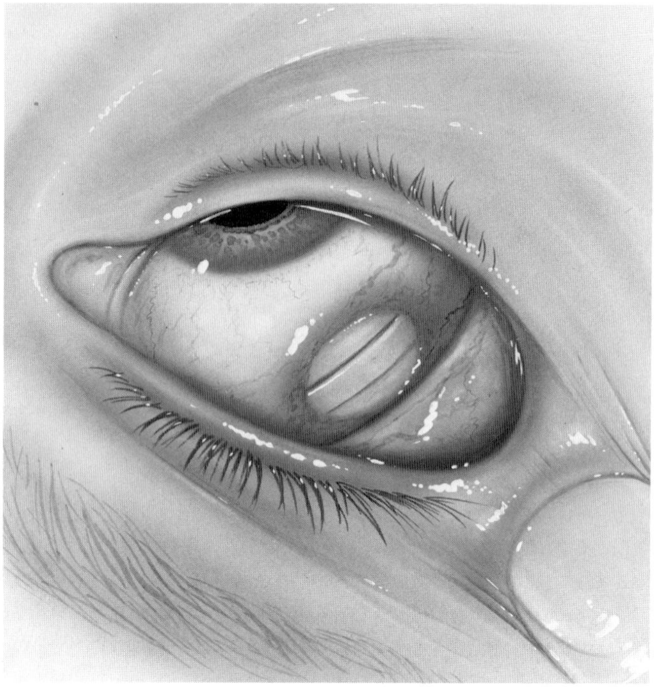

22.**10a** **Removal of infected, exposed silicone rubber implant.** A solid silicone rubber implant is exposed following erosion and infection of the scleral flaps and conjunctiva. Removal of the infected intrascleral implant requires complete exposure of the globe to recover all nonabsorbable materials, including sutures. All sutures must be removed, because any remaining suture may serve as a focus for reinfection.

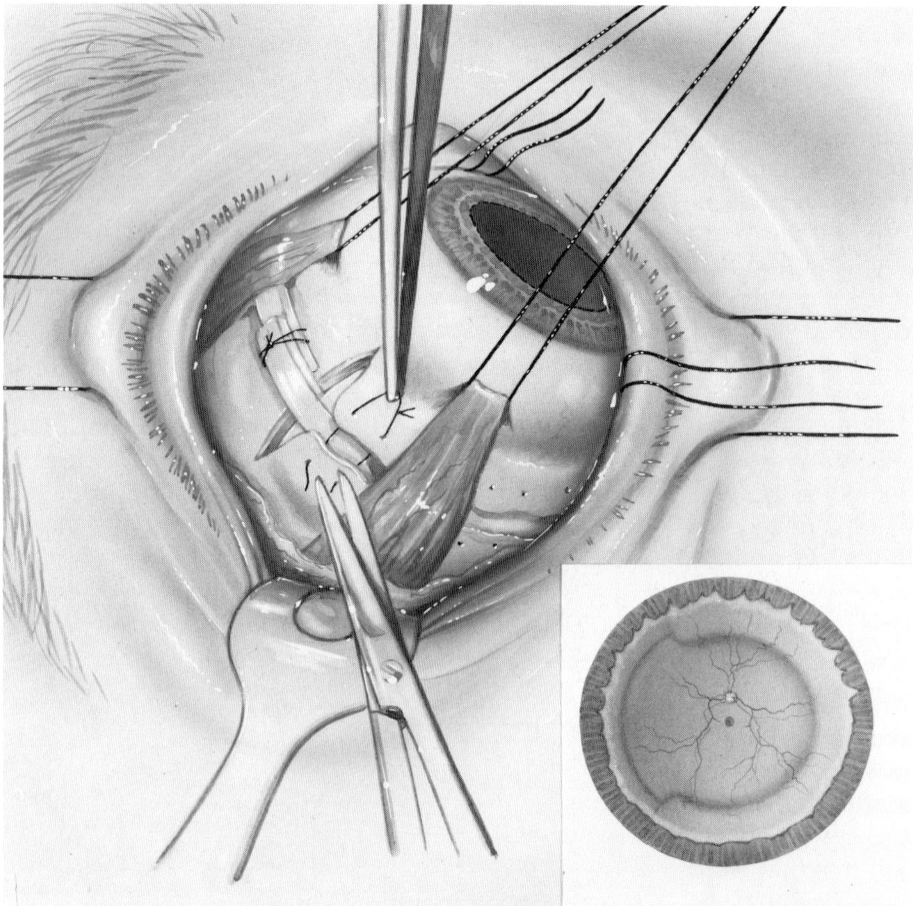

22.**10b** *Inset:* the implant extends from 2 to 10 o'clock.

The line of the previous peritomy is reopened with scissors. Traction sutures of 4–0 black silk are placed around or through the tendons of the recti muscles. Sharp dissection is used to expose and remove all of the sutures in the scleral flaps and those anchoring the encircling element. An effort should be made to account for all the sutures mentioned in the sketch or report form the previous operation.

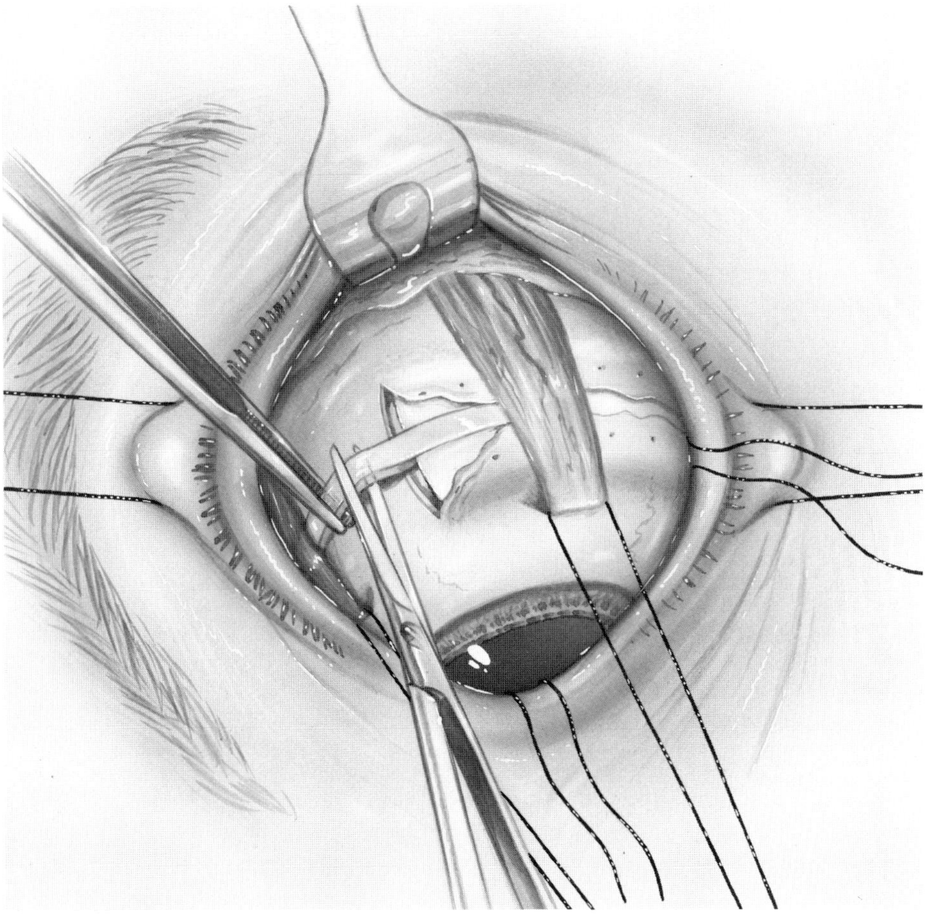

22.**10c** The other end of the buckle is exposed to allow cutting of the encircling band.

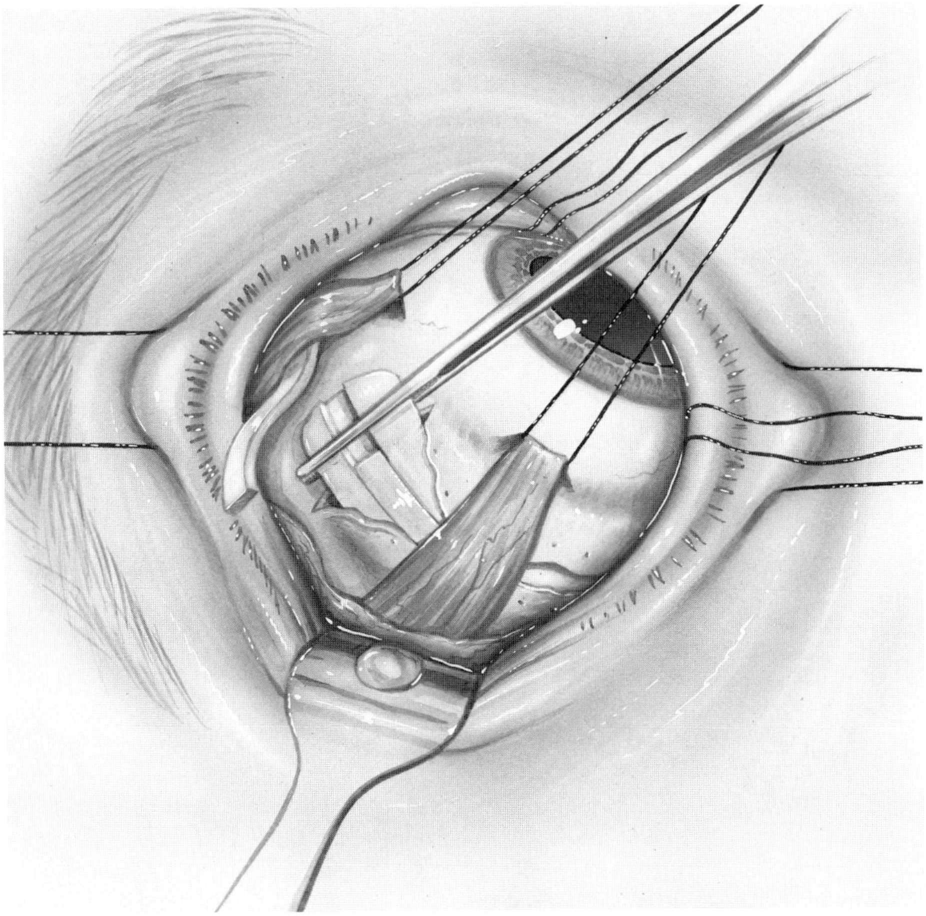

22.**10d** The encircling band at the other end of the buckle is cut with scissors. The anterior and posterior flaps are partially opened, permitting the implant to be grasped and removed. Antibiotic solution is irrigated in the space vacated by the implant. After the encircling element is removed, Tenon's fascia and conjunctiva are closed in separate layers with absorbable polyglactin sutures.

References

1. Bell FC, Stenstrom WJ. Atlas of the fundus periphery. Philadelphia: W B Sauders, 1983: 50–51.
2. Freeman HM, Dobbie JG, Friedman MW, Johnston GP, Jungschaffer OH, McPherson AR, Nicholson DH, Spalter HF, Wilkinson CP, Tasman WS. Pseudophakic retinal detachment. Mod Probl Ophthalmol 1979; 20: 345–353.
3. Hahn YS, Lincoff A, Lincoff H, Kreissig I. Infection after sponge implantation for scleral buckling. Am J Ophthalmol 1979; 87: 180–185.
4. Hawkins WR, Schepens CL. Choroidal detachment and retinal surgery: a clinical and experimental study. Am J Ophthalmol 1966; 62: 812–819.
5. Hilton GF, Wallyn RH. The removal of scleral buckles. Arch Ophthalmol 1978; 96: 2061–2063.
6. Kanski JJ. Retinal detachment: a color manual of diagnosis and treatment. London: Butterworths, 1986: 147–148.
7. Langston R, Lincoff HA, McLean JM. Scleral abscess, II: the experimental production in animals. Arch Ophthalmol 1965; 74: 665–668.
8. McMeel JW. Infections and retina surgery, II: incidence and significance of positive wound site cultures. Arch Ophthalmol 1965; 74: 45–47.
9. McMeel JW, Naegele DF, Pollalis S, Badrinath SS, Murphy PL. Acute and subacute infections following scleral buckling operations. (Symposium: postoperative endophthalmitis.) Ophthalmology 1978; 85: 341–349.
10. Pemberton JW. Schiøtz applanation disparity following retinal detachment surgery. Arch Ophthalmol 1969; 81: 534–537.
11. Rice TA, Michels RG, Stark WJ, eds. Operative surgery: ophthalmic surgery. 4th ed. St. Louis: C V Mosby, 1984: 308–309. (Rob and Smith's operative surgery series.)
12. Russo CE, Ruiz RS. Silicone sponge rejection: early and late complications in retinal detachment surgery. Arch Ophthalmol 1971; 85: 647–650.
13. Schepens CL. Retinal detachment and allied diseases. Philadelphia: W B Saunders, 1983.
14. Schwartz PL, Pruett RC. Factors influencing retinal redetachment after removal of buckling elements. Arch Ophthalmol 1977; 95: 804–807.
15. Sigelman J. Retinal diseases: pathogenesis, laser therapy and surgery. Boston: Little, Brown, 1984.
16. Ulrich RA, Burton TC. Infections following scleral buckling procedures. Arch Ophthalmol 1974; 92: 213–215.

23

Giant Retinal Breaks

Giant retinal breaks have been defined as retinal breaks that extend 90° or more around the circumference of the fundus (14). The surgical techniques are based on those that have resulted in an improvement in results over the 30% success rate reported 25 years ago (1–5, 15–29). This chapter deals with giant retinal breaks of the following varying degrees of severity:

A. **Giant retinal break with an inverted retinal flap,** treated with lensectomy, vitrectomy, fluid-air exchange, endolaser, and air-gas exchange.

B. **Giant retinal breaks with an inverted retinal flap and mild proliferative vitreoretinopathy** (PVR), treated with lensectomy, vitrectomy, fluid-air exchange, retinal suturing, scleral buckling, and air-gas exchange.

C. **Giant retinal break with severe PVR,** treated with lensectomy, vitrectomy, membrane peeling, retinal screws, and fluorosilicone oil.

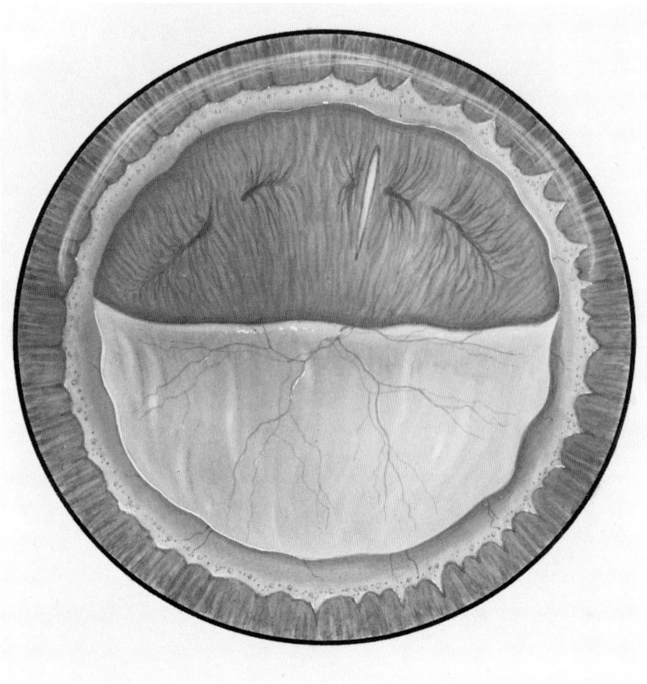

Giant Retinal Break with Inverted Retinal Flap

23.**1** Superior giant retinal break with a mobile posterior retinal flap that is inverted over the optic disc. The giant retinal break is located at the posterior border of the vitreous base. The anterior edge of the giant break, ora serrata, and pars plana ciliaris are detached from 9:30 to 3 o'clock. There is no evidence of PVR.

2a

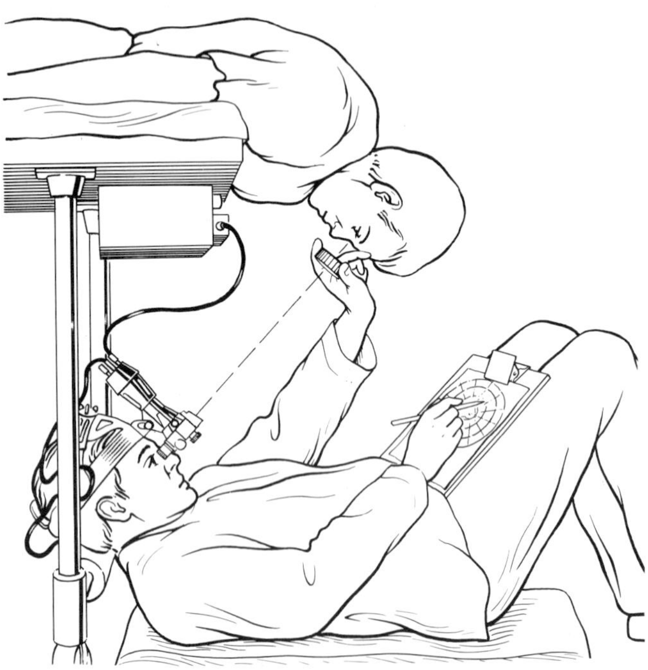

2b

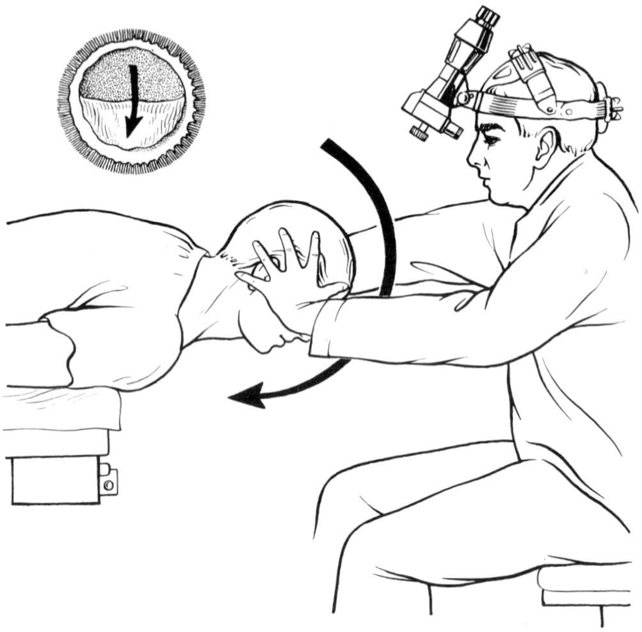

23.**2a** **Preoperative ophthalmoscopic examination.** With the patient in supine position, a detailed large fundus drawing is made of both eyes. Examination of the involved eye with the patient in prone position is important to determine the extent to which an inverted flap is capable of unfolding. In addition, examination with the patient prone is helpful in identifying where the posterior retinal flap may not unfold completely because of fixed radial folds, or a rolled posterior edge due to contraction of preretinal tissue (13).

23.**2b** **Preoperative head movements to unfold the retinal flap.** When a retinal flap does not unfold with prone positioning, it may be made to unfold as a result of certain rapid movements of the head (8). The patient is placed in prone position with his or her head and shoulders extending over the edge of the examining table. Head movements consists of a fast component, a pause, and a slow return component. The fast component is made in the same direction in which the flap is folded.

Inset: when the giant break is superior, the inverted retinal flap is folded downward; the fast component is therefore made in the downward direction by rapidly flexing the neck. The examiner's hands guide the patient's head into the flexed position.

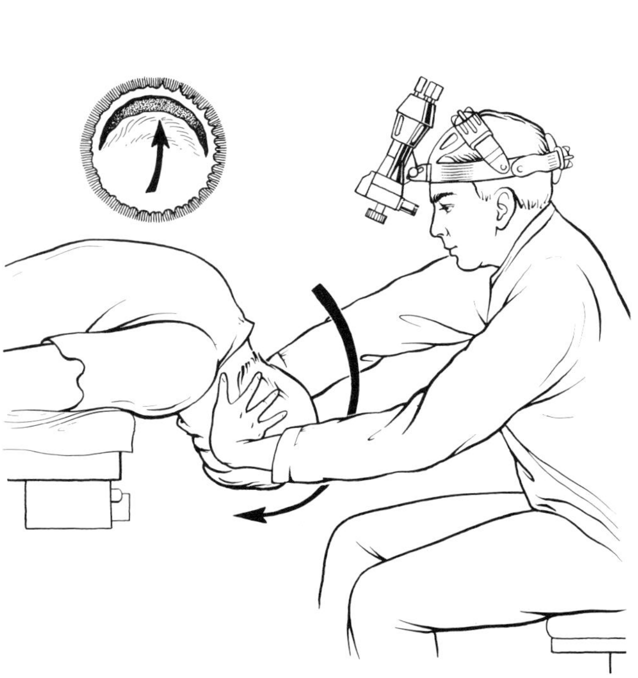

23.**2c** During the rapid neck flexing and the pause at the end of the head movement, the flap tends to unfold (see inset).

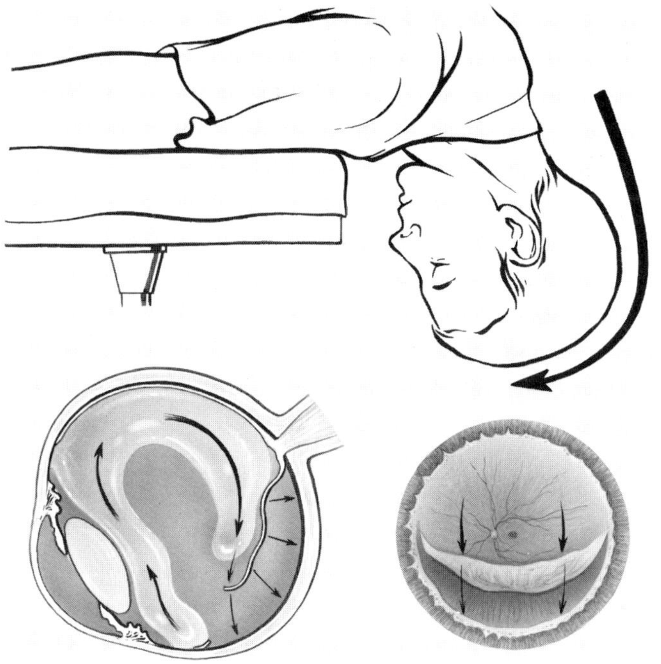

23.**2d** The pause at the end of the fast component lasts for a count of three, allowing time for inertial movements of the fluid portion of the vitreous to unfold the flap. During this time, when the head is held motionless, vitreous continues to move in a circular direction within the globe and impinges upon the retinal flap to unfold it (large arrows, lower insets). Then the head is returned very slowly to the hyperextended position of the neck (see Fig. 23.**2b**). Ophthalmoscopy is done before and after three to four exercises to determine the flap's status and whether the tear has extended circumferentially or nasally.

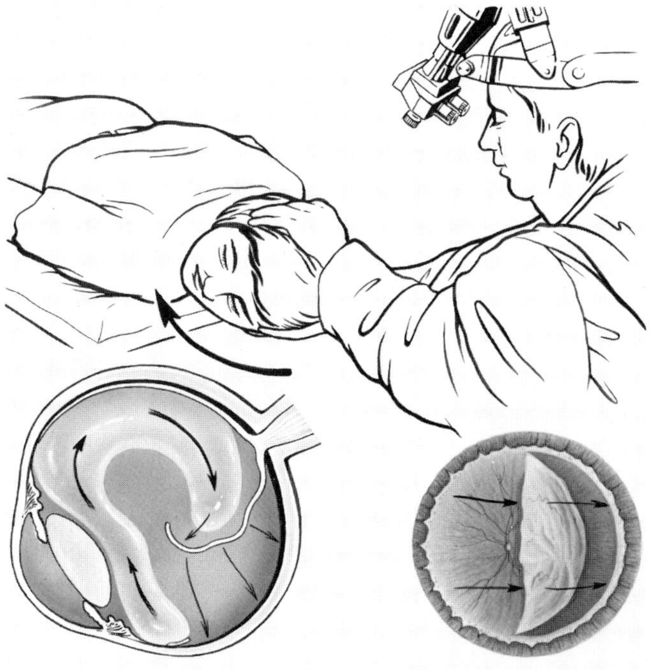

23.**2e** The patient in prone position has a temporal giant retinal break in the left eye. The posterior flap of a temporal giant break tends to be folded nasally, and the fast component is therefore performed by rotating the head toward the shoulder on the side opposite the affected eye. The arrow indicates the direction of the fast component. The insets show the inertial movements of the vitreous during the pause at the end of the rotational movement toward the right shoulder. The vitreous impinges on the posterior retinal flap to unfold it. A slow rotational return movement is made so that the face is in the direction of the left shoulder.

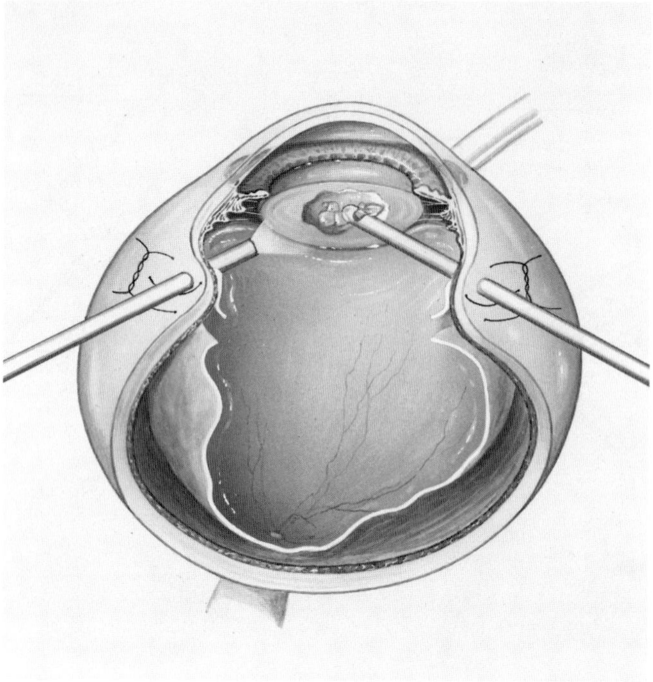

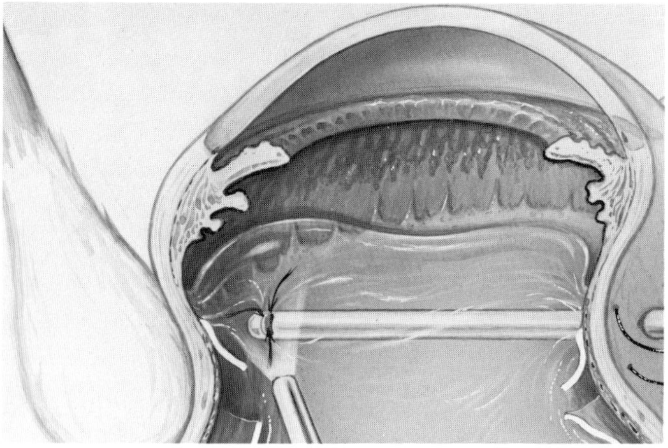

23.**3a** **Operative technique.** Patients with an inverted posterior retinal flap are operated on a power-driven, multi-positional operating table. This giant-tear operating table makes it possible to unfold the retinal flap utilizing the effects of gravity by rotating the patient to any inclination in the supine or prone position. We prefer to unfold a mobile retinal flap using gravity and an expanding intravitreous bubble of air, rather than manipulating the flap with an instrument, which may produce hemorrhage, wrinkling, or a tear in the flap.

The patient is held in position by heavy web canvas straps attached to the sides of the table and extending across the patient's legs, thighs, abdomen, and chest. The head is held firmly against the table by two Kerlix bandages 4½ inches wide. One bandage is passed over the patient's chin, the other over the forehead. Foam rubber padding 2 inches thick is placed beneath the straps to prevent undue pressure on the body. Surgery is performed under general anesthesia. After endotracheal intubation, the nose and pharynx are packed with gauze to absorb and prevent nasal and pharyngeal secretions from contaminating the operative field. Prior to rotation, extra-long tubing is used to connect the patient to the anesthesia machine.

A limbal peritomy is performed, and bridle sutures are passed under the tendons of the recti muscles. A lensectomy is performed to make room for injection of as large a bubble of gas as possible and to permit a thorough vitrectomy of the vitreous base and anterior hyaloid (12).

23.**3b** To lessen the incidence of iatrogenic retinal breaks during vitrectomy involving the vitreous base, low suction and short intermittent cutting are used while keeping the peripheral retina visualized with scleral depression. Following vitrectomy, the entire fundus periphery is examined with indirect ophthalmoscopy and scleral depression, to determine if the giant retinal break has extended circumferentially and to detect any retinal tears that may have been produced during vitrectomy (11).

A thorough vitrectomy of the vitreous base is performed, because the major problem in most giant retinal breaks is vitreous base traction. If not relieved, contraction of the vitreous base may cause an extension of the giant break or an elevation of its ends, resulting in redetachment of the retina or formation of retinal tears elsewhere in the fundus periphery.

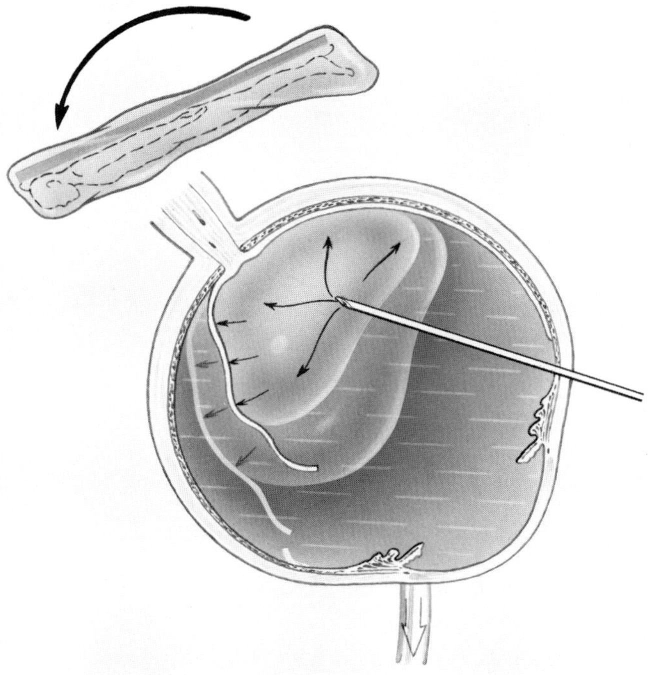

23.**3c** The patient with a superior giant retinal break is rotated counterclockwise to prone position, with the head 30–40° below the horizontal (inset). (Patients with a nasal or temporal giant retinal break are rotated to the horizontal position; patients with an inferior giant retinal break are rotated so that the head is 30–40° above the horizontal meridian.) Prior to rotation to the prone position to unfold a superior retinal flap, the infusion line is clamped near the eye and disconnected from the three-way stopcock so that the intraocular pressure will not fall as the patient's head is rotated upward.

Air from a 20 ml plastic syringe is injected by the scrub nurse through a Micropore filter connected to 6 inches of plastic tubing. To accomplish this, tubing is attached to a long, 30-gauge needle held by the surgeon. The needle tip is passed through the pars plana and directed under indirect ophthalmoscopic control over the optic dis. To prevent air from passing behind the retinal flap, air is injected in front of the optic disc. As the air bubble expands toward the fundus periphery, it tends to unfold the flap smoothly. To drain fluid from the eye during air injection, the tubing of the infusion cannula is clamped and disconnected from the stopcock. A 25-gauge needle is connected to the tubing using a female adapter. The needle's small bore prevents rapid egress of fluid from the eye after the clamp has been removed.

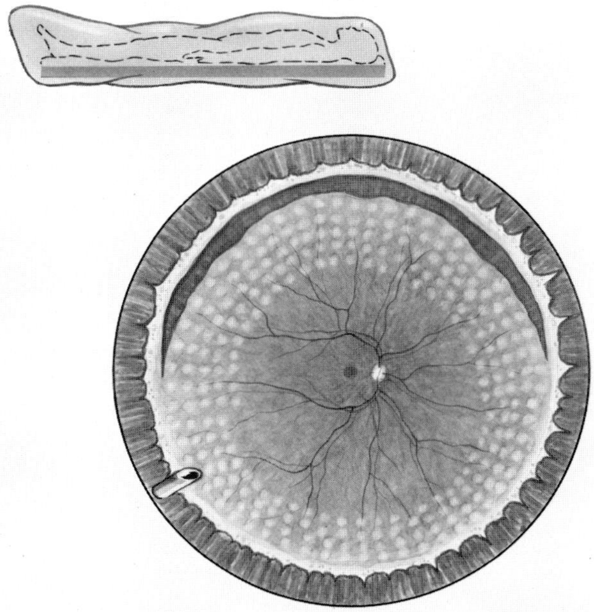

23.**3d** Following a complete fluid-air exchange, the infusion tubing is clamped, the 25-gauge needle is removed, and the infusion tubing is re-connected to the air pump set at a pressure of 30 mmHg. The patient is rotated to supine position, and indirect ophthalmoscopy is performed to determine if the retinal flap is unfolded. If the entire retina is reattached, endolaser is applied in 6 to 8 rows around the entire fundus periphery. Prior to closure of the conjunctiva, air is exchanged for a 20% mixture of C_3F_8 and air, lavaging 50 ml through the vitreous cavity over a period of 2 minutes. Supplemental fluid-gas exchanges are done postoperatively to maintain a large gas bubble for approximately three weeks, during which time laser applications may be added to ensure a strong chorioretinal adhesion posterior to the giant retinal break.

4a

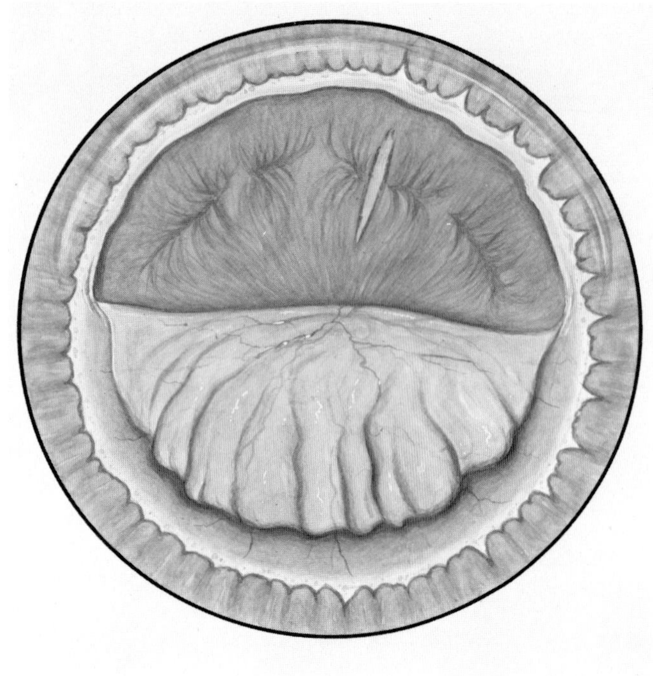

4c

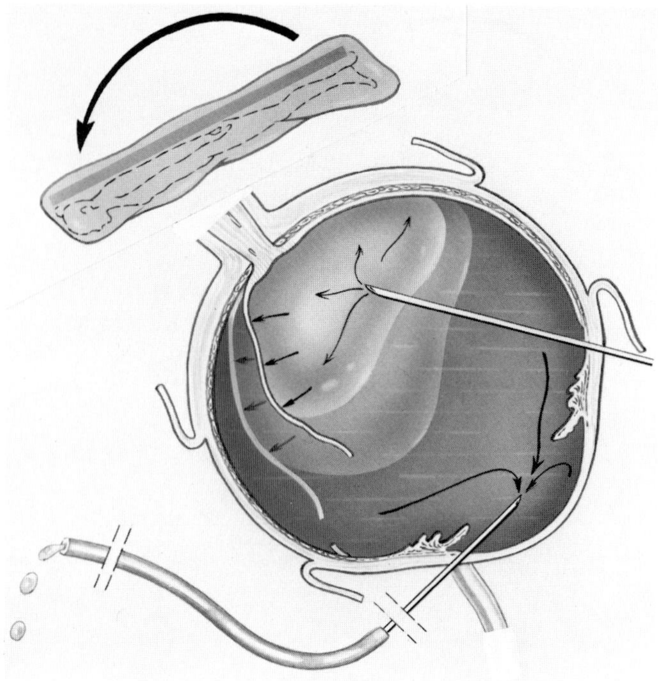

4b

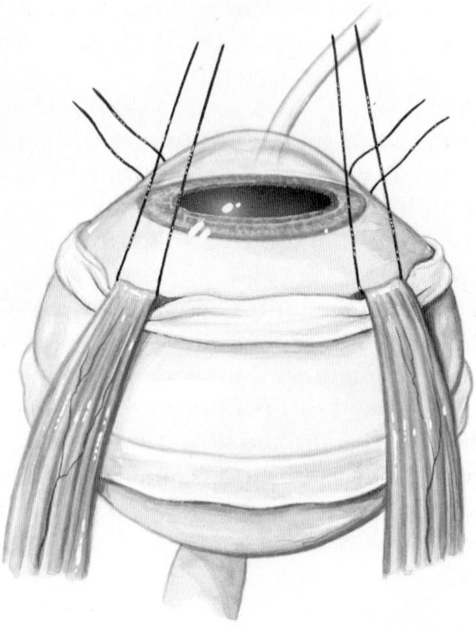

23.**4b** Lensectomy and vitrectomy are performed as previously described. A lamellar scleral undermining is made so that the thin, relatively long needle used for retinal suturing can be passed through the thin bed of sclera. Lamellar scleral undermining is made approximately 11 mm wide, straddling the equator and extending approximately two-thirds of the scleral depth.

23.**4c** The infusion line is clamped so that the intraocular pressure remains constant while the patient is rotated to prone position (inset). A fluid-air exchange is performed to unfold the posterior retinal flap. The transscleral retinal sutures are passed through rather than under the retinal flap. To accomplish this, the retina must be firmly tamponaded against the pigment epithelium. To tamponade the posterior edge of the giant retinal break, the fluid-air exchange must be nearly total. By rotating the head of the operating table upward, the air bubble floats superiorly, enabling additional fluid to be drained from the inferior portion of the anterior chamber to achieve a near-total fluid-air exchange. The infusion tubing is connected to the air pump; additional fluid is then drained through a 23-gauge needle inserted through the inferior limbus and parallel to the plane of the iris. Then the patient is rotated to supine position for retinal suturing, which will require constant air infusion in the eye.

Giant Retinal Break with Mild Proliferative Vitreoretinopathy

23.**4a** Preretinal tissue in mild degrees of PVR may cause radial folds and/or a slight roll or wrinkling of the posterior edge of the posterior retinal flap. Because the flap is mobile in mild degrees of PVR, it is difficult to peel preretinal membrane from the flap's edge. Therefore, transcleral retinal sutures are used to counteract the tendency of the posterior edge of the flap to detach postoperatively as a result of further contraction of the preretinal tissue (9).

4d

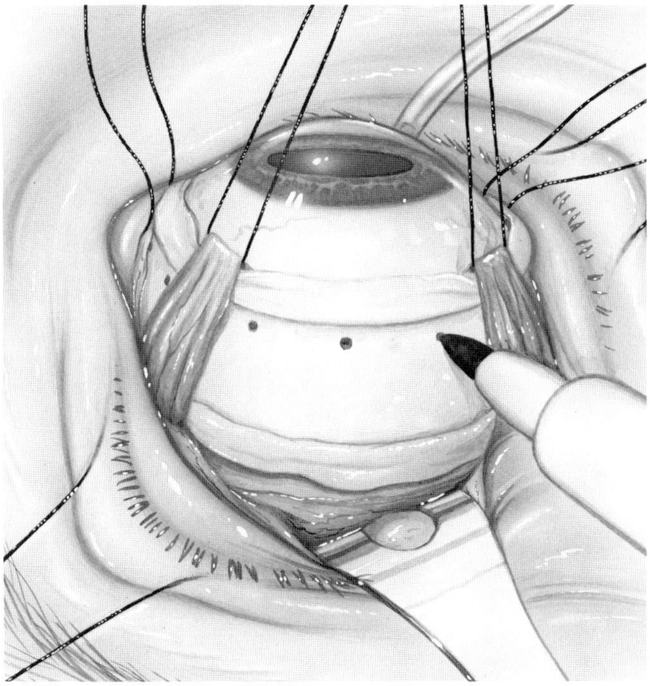

4f

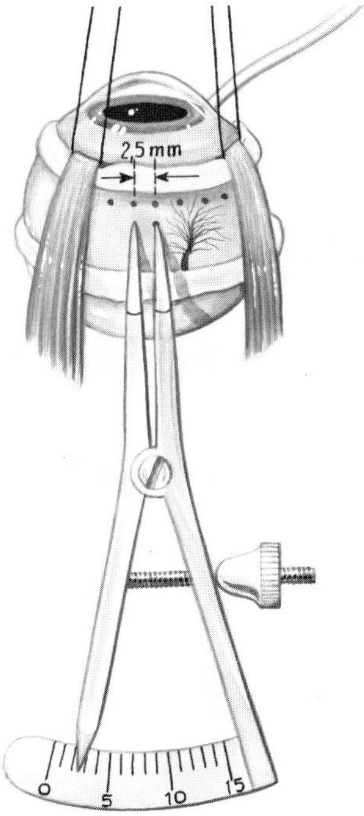

4e

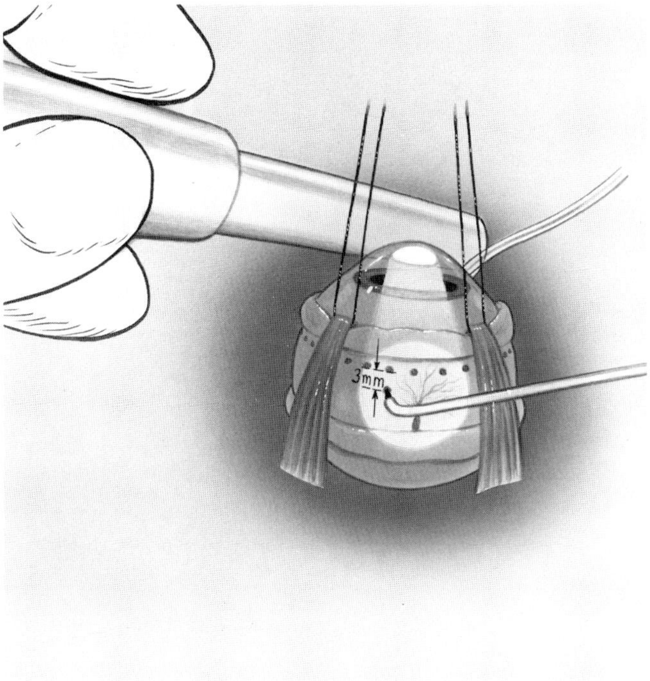

23.**4d** The posterior edge and ends of the unfolded giant retinal break are localized with indirect ophthalmoscopy and marked on the sclera using a gentian violet marking pen.

23.**4e** The sites for placement of transscleral sutures are localized by transillumination approximately every 45° along the posterior edge of the retinal flap. A hand-held transilluminator is used to transilluminate this region, to avoid perforating choroidal vessels during entry and exit of the retinal suture needle (7). A localizing mark is made with the conical electrode 3 mm posterior to the posterior edge of the flap in a meridian free of choroidal blood vessels. This marks the site where the needle of the retinal suture will enter the sclera.

23.**4f** Another mark is made 2.5 mm along the circumference of the globe from the first mark, in an area shown to be vessel-free by transillumination, where the retinal suture needle will exit from the sclera.

4g

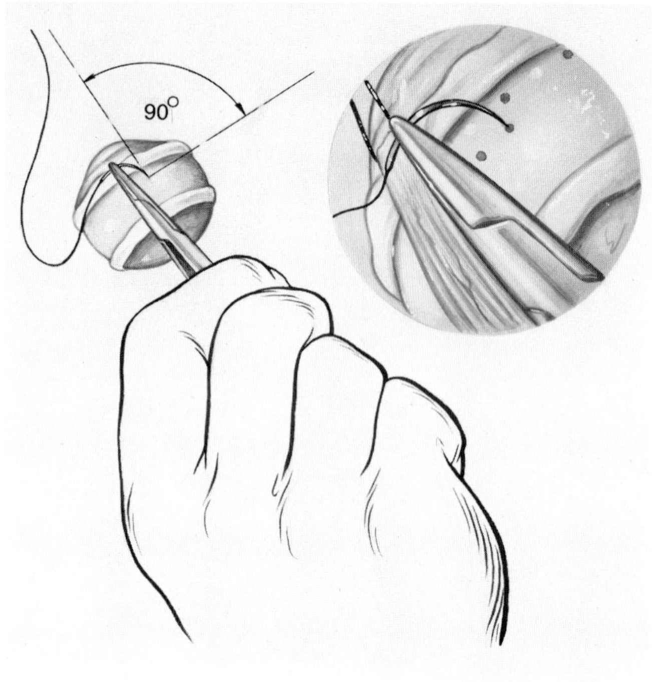

4i

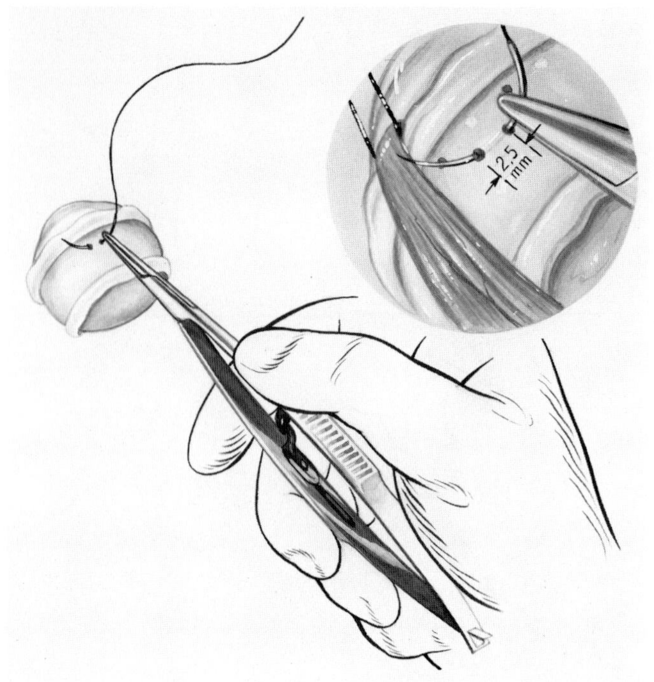

4h

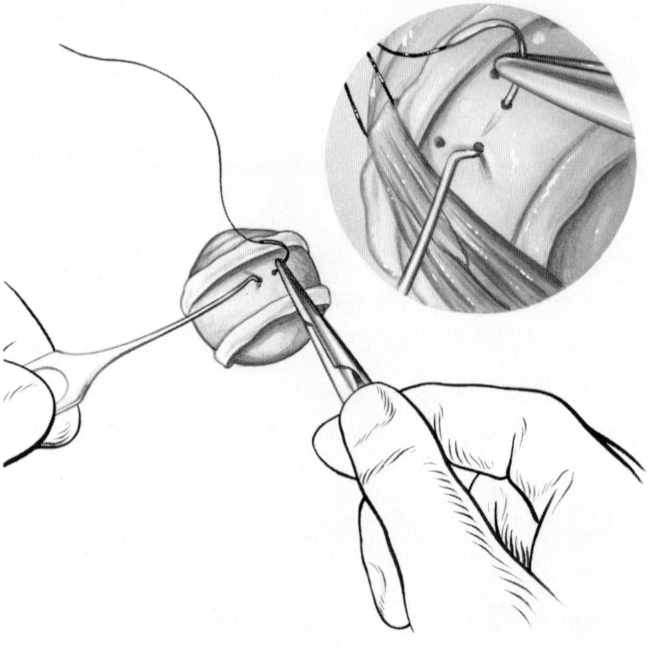

4j

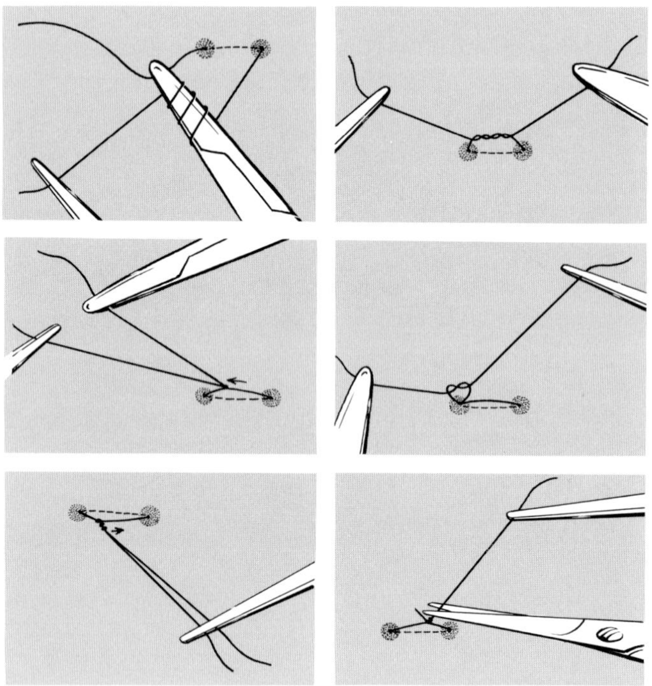

23.**4g** The needle must be held firmly at a right angle with a locking, straight-tipped needle holder. A locking needle holder is used so that the needle will pass in and out of the sclera without having to be regrasped; excessive needle movements associated with regrasping can result in the tip lacerating the retina, or in choroidal hemorrhage. To pass through rather than under the retinal flap, the needle should enter the vitreous cavity at a right angle to the scleral surface. *Inset:* The needle enters the sclera through the localizing mark.

23.**4h** The sclera adjacent to the exit site is indented slightly using a Colibri forceps, so that the needle will exit through the diathermized exit site.

23.**4i** The locking Castroviejo needle holder is rotated through 180° along its axis, so that the needle will pass in and out of the sclera in one smooth and accurate arc, exiting approximately 2.5 mm from the entry site.

23.**4j** The retinal suture is tied snugly. The first knot is locked against one suture track, tied with a double knot, and then moved toward the center.

4k

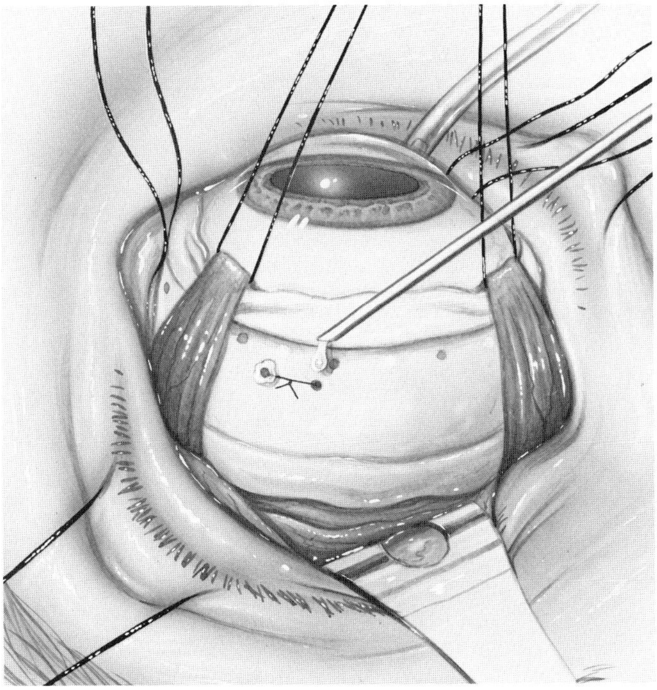

4m

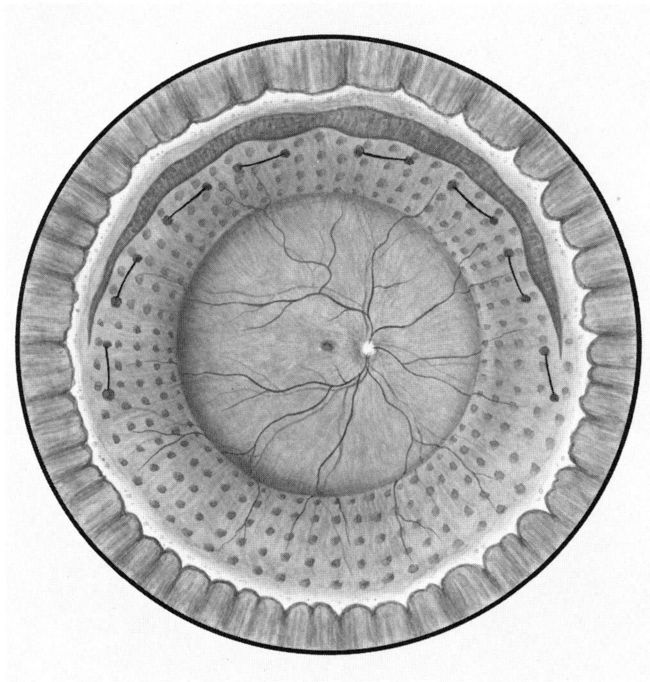

4l

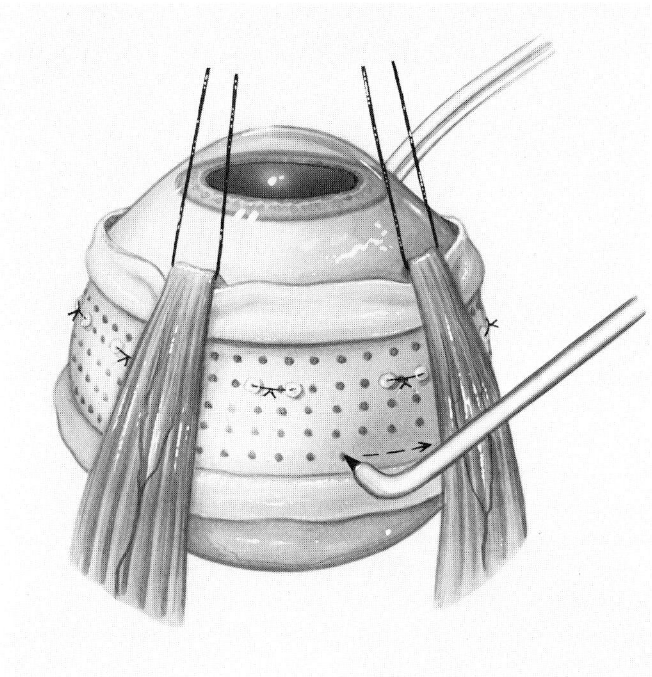

23.**4k** To prevent air leakage, the suture tracks are sealed with tissue adhesive, which is applied from a 30-gauge needle on a tuberculin syringe. Additional retinal sutures are placed approximately 30° apart along the giant retinal break. To prevent postoperative elevation of the ends of the break as a result of vitreous base traction, a suture is placed across or near the ends of the giant break (see Fig. 23.**4m**).

23.**4l** Using a blunt conical electrode, diathermy applications are spaced approximately 2.5 mm apart in the bed of the lamellar scleral resection. Frequent monitoring, with indirect ophthalmoscopy, of the intensity of the diathermy applications is important to avoid excessively strong chorioretinal diathermy burns, which can easily occur in an air-filled eye.

23.**4m** 4-0 Mersilene mattress sutures are inserted every 30° through the scleral flaps. A solid grooved silicone rubber implant is placed in the lamellar scleral bed around the globe and under a silicone rubber encircling element. A low buckling effect is desirable, because a high scleral indentation tends to shorten the diameter of the globe, producing radial folds in the retinal flap which may cause postoperative retinal detachment.

Prior to closure of the conjunctiva, air is exchanged for a 20% mixture of C_3F_8 with air, lavaging 50 ml through the vitreous cavity over a period of 2 minutes.

Postoperative prone positioning. Postoperative prone positioning of the patient is maintained for 6 hours each day for 10 days.

Postoperative laser photocoagulation. Because a strong chorioretinal adhesion in the posterior retinal flap is desirable, argon laser photocoagulation is applied along the posterior edge of the giant retinal break in two to four sessions, beginning 10 days postoperatively.

5a

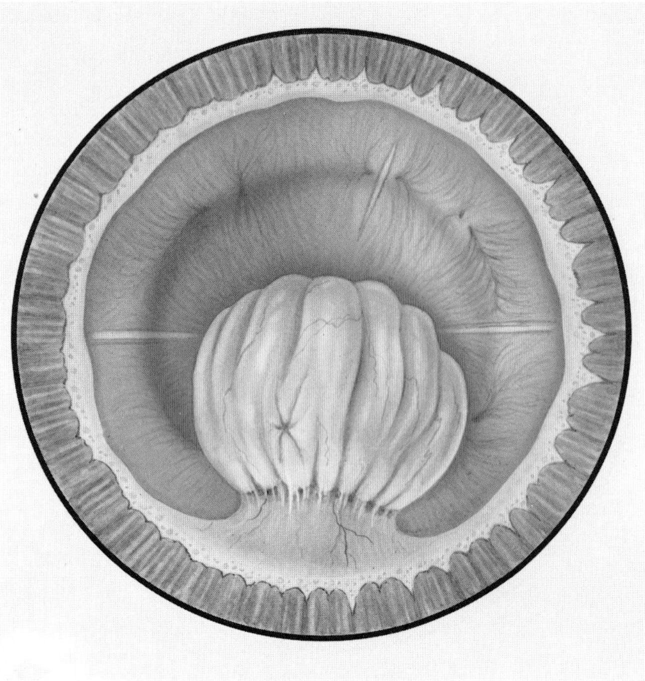

5b

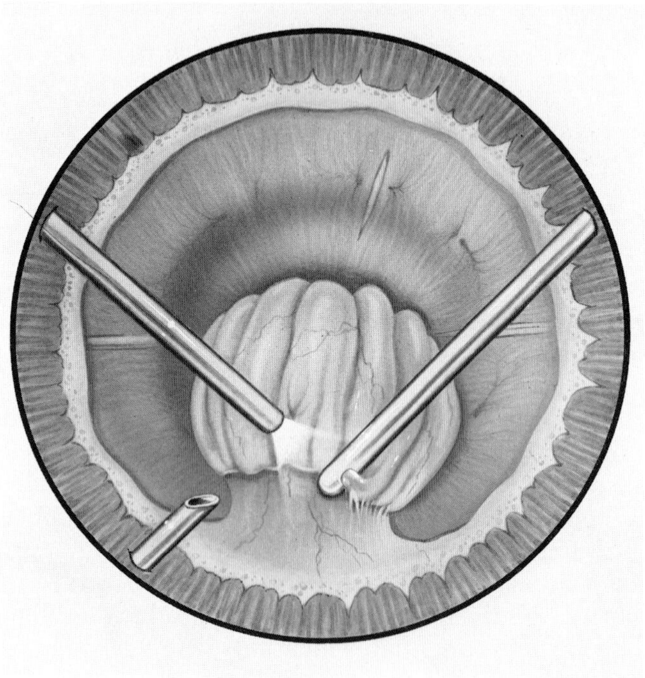

Giant Retinal Break with Severe Proliferative Vitreoretinopathy

23.**5a** In some giant retinal breaks complicated by grade D3 PVR, the posterior edge of the retinal flap becomes so contracted and rigid that preretinal or subretinal membranes cannot be peeled from it. Contraction of the preretinal tissue results in numerous radial folds in the inverted retinal flap and a purse-string contraction of its posterior edge. Transscleral retinal sutures are not effective in such cases, because the retinal flap cannot be tamponaded tightly against the pigment epithelium, and a retinal suture therefore passes under rather than through the flap.

5c

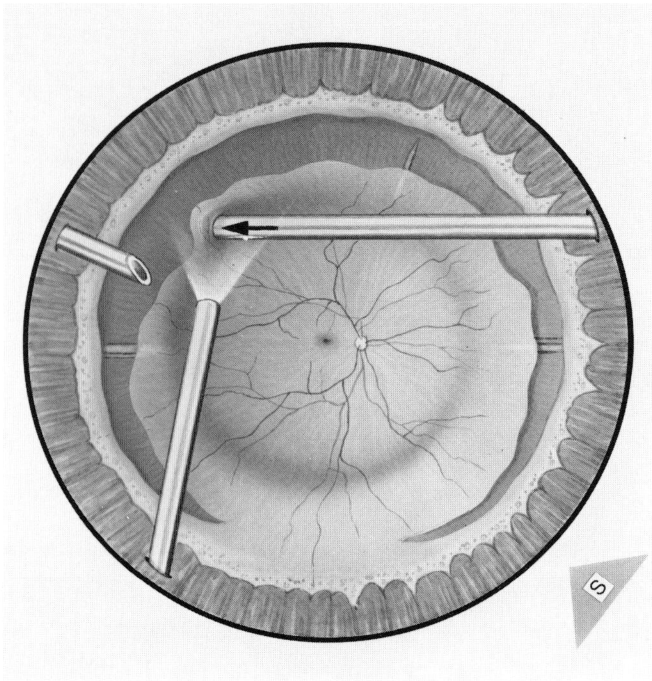

23.**5b** Thorough removal of periretinal membranes is mandatory in these desperate cases. Periretinal organization may produce thickening and pursestring contraction of the posterior edge of the retinal flap, preventing it from being unfolded. Retinectomy of this tissue may facilitate unfolding of the retinal flap.

To avoid excising an excessive amount of retina, the slowest possible cutting speed and low suction pressure are used. Retinectomy is extended posteriorly to reach retina of normal thickness. Thorough removal of periretinal membranes from both the inner and outer surfaces of the retinal flap is important. Periretinal membranes are peeled from the flap, beginning posteriorly and working anteriorly to the edge of the retinectomy.

23.**5c** A fluid-air exchange is performed, and the retinal flap is unfolded and dragged anteriorly using the back-flush needle while the retina is tamponaded with air. Preretinal membranes are then peeled under air tamponade.

To unfold the flap as far as possible anteriorly in the 11, 12, and 1 o'clock meridians, the infusion cannula is transferred to the superior sclerotomy, and the surgeon (S) sits on the side opposite the eye.

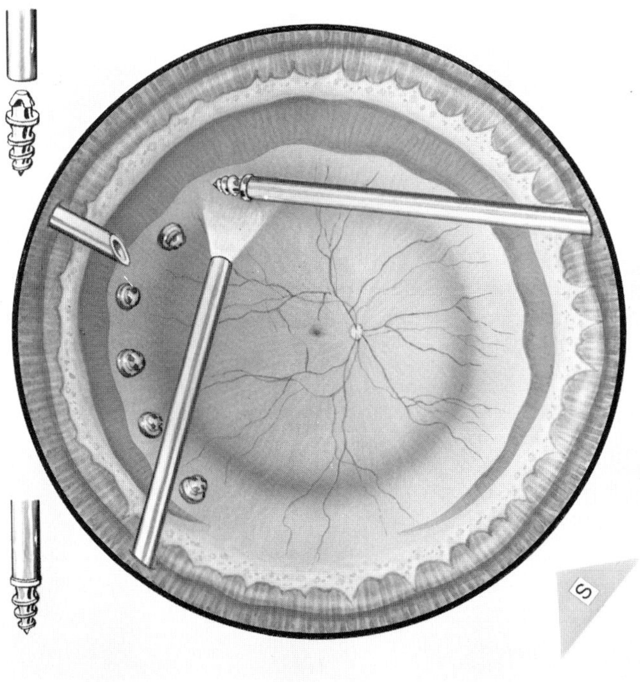

23.**5d** After the flap has been unfolded, titanium retinal screws are inserted every 30° using a screwdriver. When inserting screws in the 11, 12, and 1 o'clock meridians, the surgeon (S) sits on the side of the patient opposite the operated eye. Endolaser is applied around 360°, and the air is then replaced with fluorosilicone oil.

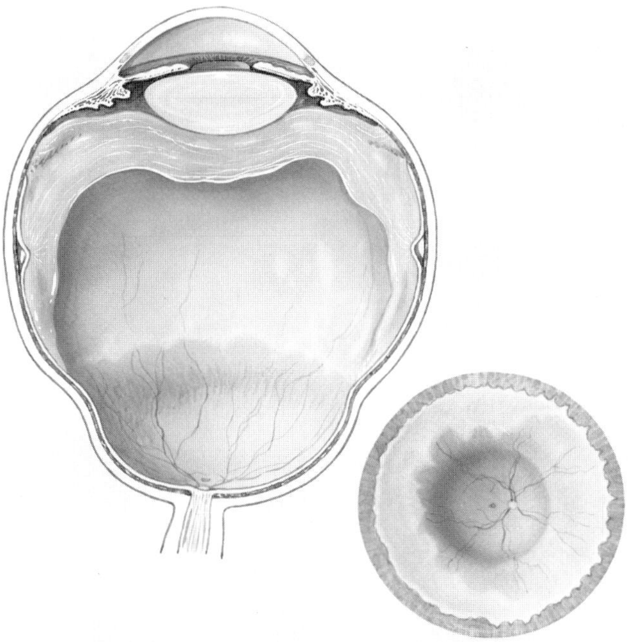

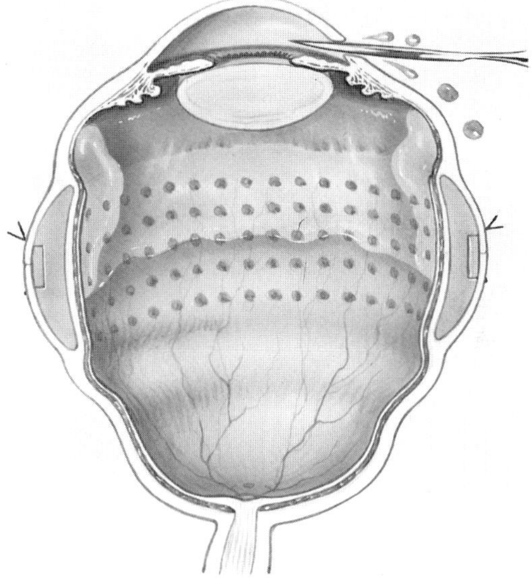

23.**6a** **Prophylactic buckling in fellow eyes of giant retinal breaks.** A high incidence of giant retinal breaks in fellow eyes with myopia in excess of 10 diopters, increasing white-without-pressure, and increasing condensation of the vitreous base, has led to the introduction prophylactic buckling in these eyes (6). Note the liquefaction of the vitreous gel in the cross section illustration and the white-without-pressure in the inset. Severe condensation of the vitreous base may produce a ridge in the retina along the posterior margin of the vitreous base. With further condensation, a giant retinal break develops along the ridge.

23.**6b** Surgical technique. A Foley catheter is inserted preoperatively to prevent distension of the bladder as a result of the use of mannitol and acetazolamide during surgery. An attempt is made to buckle approximately 180° to 210° of the globe, selecting an arc that encompasses most of the white-without-pressure and vitreous base condensation. In eyes with sclera of normal thickness, an 8 mm lamellar scleral undermining is performed in the region of the equator. Using a blunt conical electrode and low-intensity current, diathermy applications are placed 2 mm apart in the scleral bed. Since uniform and light diathermy reactions are desirable, the applications should be monitored frequently with indi- ▷

rect ophthalmoscopy. Three mattress sutures per quadrant are placed through the scleral flaps. A grooved silicone rubber implant 6 mm wide is inserted in the lamellar scleral bed. To achieve a permanent buckling effect, an encircling band is used in the groove of the implant and tied and anchored opposite the buckle.

If the combination of carbonic anhydrase inhibitor and osmotic agent fails to lower the intraocular pressure sufficiently, paracentesis is done. Inasmuch as a large portion of the vitreous gel is usually liquefied, a substantial amount of syneresis fluid may percolate into the anterior chamber and be removed by repeated paracentesis to produce a high buckling effect. The encircling band and sutures are adjusted so that the closing intraocular pressure does not exceed 20 mmHg, and indirect ophthalmoscopy reveals that the ophthalmic artery is patent (10).

References

1. Abrams GW, Williams GA, Newirth J, et al. Clinical results of titanium retinal tacks with pneumatic insertion. Am J Ophthalmol 1986; 102: 13–19.
2. Ando F, Kondo J. A plastic tack for the treatment of retinal detachment with giant tear. Am J Ophthalmol 1983; 95: 260–261.
3. Charles S. Vitreous microsurgery. Baltimore: Williams and Wilkins, 1987: 172–181.
4. de Juan E Jr, Hickingbotham D, Machemer R. Retinal tacks. Am J Ophthalmol 1985; 99: 272–274.
5. Federman JL, Shakin JL, Lanning RC. The microsurgical management of giant retinal tears with transscleral sutures. Ophthalmology 1982; 89: 832–838.
6. Freeman HM. Fellow eyes of giant retinal breaks. Trans Am Ophthalmol Soc 1978; 76: 343–382.
7. Freeman HM. Discussion of presentation by JL Federman, JL Shakin, RS Lanning: The microsurgical management of giant retinal tears with trans-scleral retinal sutures. Ophthalmology 1982; 89: 838–839.
8. Freeman HM. Current management of giant retinal breaks with an inverted retinal flap. In: Kanski JJ, Morse PH, eds. Disorders of the vitreous, retina and choroid. London: Butterworths, 1983: 210–227.
9. Freeman HM. Management of giant retinal breaks with an inverted retinal flap. In: Neetens A, ed. Modern concepts in vitreo-retinal diseases: proceedings of the vitreoretinal conference, Antwerp, 1985. Antwerp: University of Antwerp UIA Press, 1985: 183–194.
10. Freeman HM. The vitreous in idiopathic giant retinal breaks. In: Schepens CL, Neetens A, eds. The vitreous and vitreoretinal interface. New York: Springer, 1987: 229–240.
11. Freeman HM. Current management of giant retinal breaks. In: Glaser BM, Michels RG, eds. Retina, vol 3: Surgical retina. St. Louis: C V Mosby, 1989: 431–448.
12. Freeman HM, Castillejos ME. Current management of giant retinal breaks: results with vitrectomy and total air-fluid exchange in 95 cases. Trans Am Ophthalmol Soc 1981: 79: 89–102.
13. Freeman HM, Johnson MR. Giant retinal breaks. In: Spaeth G, ed. Current therapy in ophthalmic surgery. Philadelphia: Decker, 1989: 256–263.
14. Freeman HM, Schepens CL, Couvillion GC. Current management of giant retinal breaks, part II. Trans Am Acad Ophthalmol Otolaryngol 1970; 74: 59–74.
15. Glaser BM. Treatment of giant retinal tears combined with proliferative vitreoretinopathy. Ophthalmology 1986; 93: 1193–1197.
16. Gonvers, M. Giant retinal tears. In: Blankenship GW, Binder S, Gonvers M, eds. Basic and advanced vitreous surgery. New York: Springer, 1986: 177–188.
17. Hirose T, Schepens CL, Lopansri C. Subtotal open-sky vitrectomy for severe retinal detachment occurring as a late complication of ocular trauma. Ophthalmology 1981; 88: 1–9.
18. Hoffman ME, Sorr EM. Management of giant retinal tears without scleral buckling. Retina 1986; 6: 197–204.
19. Leaver PK, Cooling RJ, Feretis EB, et al. Vitrectomy and fluid/silicone-oil exchange for giant retinal tears: results at six months. Br J Ophthalmol 1984; 68: 432–438.
20. Lincoff H, Coleman J, Kreissig I, et al. The perfluorocarbon gases in the treatment of retinal detachment. Ophthalmology 1983; 90: 546–551.
21. Machemer R, Allen AW. Retinal tears 180° and greater: management with vitrectomy and intravitreal gas. Arch Ophthalmol 1976; 94: 1340–1346.
22. Michels RG. Giant retinal tears. In: Blankenship GW, Binder S, Gonvers M, eds. Basic and advanced vitreous surgery. New York: Springer, 1986: 177–188.
23. Norton EWD, Aaberg T, Fung W, Curtin VT. Giant retinal tears, I: clinical management with intravitreal air. Trans Am Ophthalmol Soc 1969; 67: 374–393.
24. Peyman GA, Redman KRV, Seetner AA. Retinal microincarceration with penetrating diathermy in the management of giant retinal tears. Arch Ophthalmol 1984; 102: 562–565.
25. Schepens CL, Freeman HM. Current management of giant retinal breaks. Trans Am Acad Ophthalmol Otolaryngol 1967; 71: 474–487.
26. Schepens CL, Dobbie JG, McMeel JW. Retinal detachments with giant breaks: preliminary report. Trans Am Acad Ophthalmol Otolaryngol 1962; 66: 471–479.
27. Schepens CL, Freeman HM, Thompson RF. A power-driven multipositional operating table. Arch Ophthalmol 1965; 73: 671–673.
28. Usui M, Hamazaki S, Takano S, Matsua H. A new surgical technique for the treatment of giant tear: transvitreoretinal fixation. Jpn J Ophthalmol 1979; 23: 206–215.
29. Živojnović R. Silicone oil in vitreoretinal surgery. Dordrecht: Nijhoff, 1987: 60–69.

24

Rhegmatogenous Retinal Detachment with Posterior or Unseen Retinal Breaks

Macular Hole

Macular holes are a rare cause of rhegmatogenous retinal detachment. The reported incidence of macular holes in retinal detachment ranges from 0.6% to 4% (1, 6, 7, 11, 12, 15, 16, 19). The higher incidence reported in Europe may be due to a higher incidence of myopia or of ocular contusion in their series. A true macular break must be distinguished from a pseudohole, which results from a macular cyst, an atrophic macula, or an incomplete macular break. Before diagnosing a macular lesion as a macular break, it is advisable to use a combination of diagnostic methods including direct or indirect ophthalmoscopy and examination with the slit lamp and contact lens. The macular area should be examined with both intense white light and red-free light, since the latter makes the thin layer of the anterior wall of a macular cyst more visible (14: 542–548).

Endolaser, vitrectomy, and long-acting gases have greatly reduced the complication rate and improved the results in cases of retinal detachment caused by macular holes (3–5, 9, 13, 17).

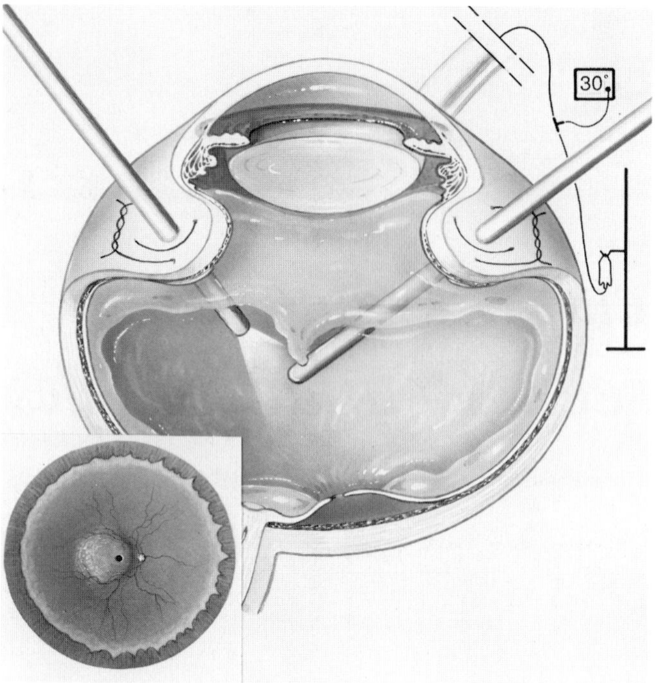

24.**1a** *Inset:* Macular hole causing a retinal detachment confined to the posterior pole.

Vitrectomy is performed to ensure that no vitreous membranes are attached to the margin of the macular hole (2). Most of the central vitreous gel posterior to the equator is removed to make room for injection of a large bubble of gas or air.

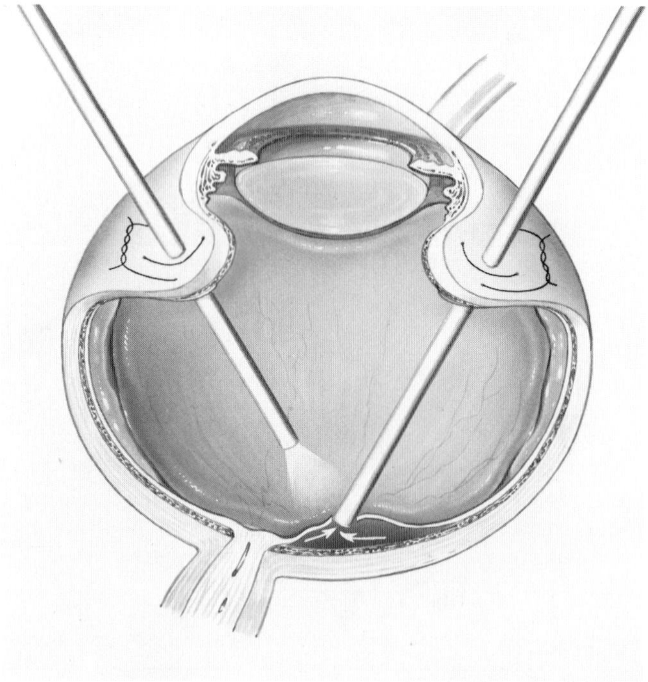

24.**1b** Subretinal fluid is drainged through the macular hole using the back-flush needle. A fluid-air exchange is then performed.

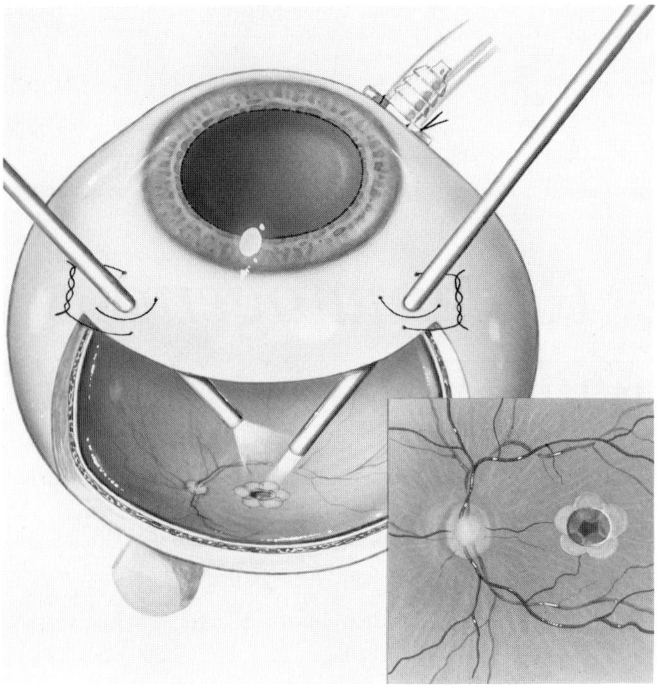

24.**1c** Following fluid-air exchange, one row of confluent applications of endolaser is placed along the edge of the macular hole. The patient is instructed to maintain the prone position for at least 8–10 hours a day for 1 week postoperatively.

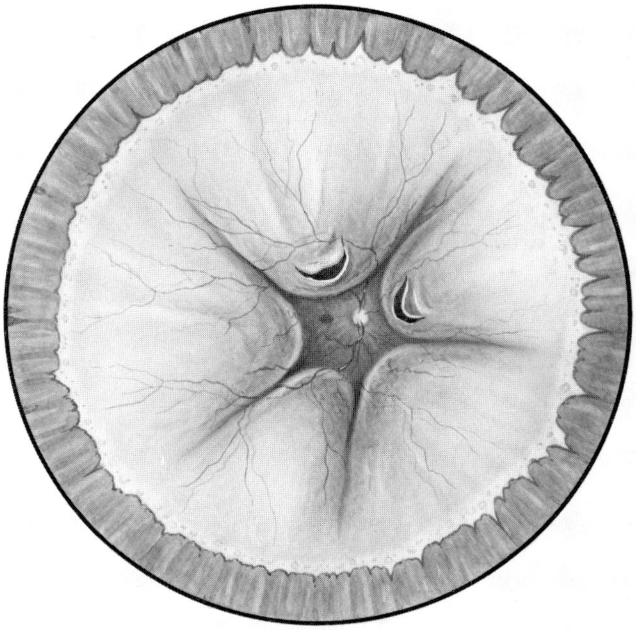

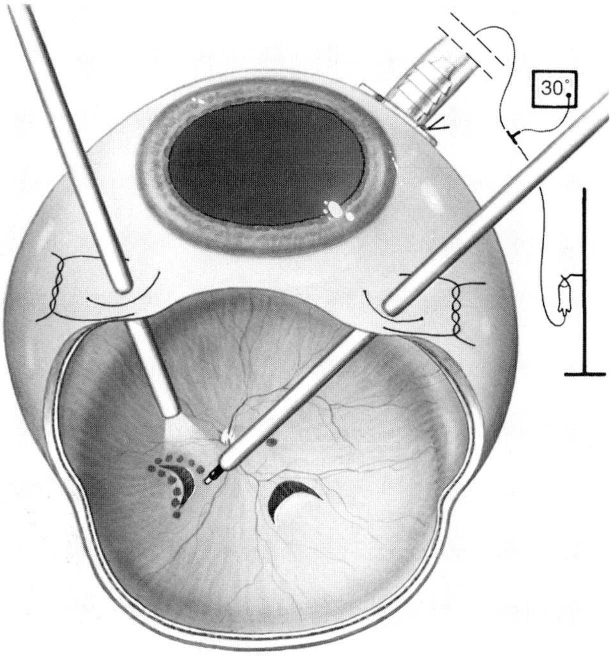

Posterior Retinal Tears

24.**2a** Retinal detachment with large, very posterior retinal breaks causing a bullous retinal detachment. The placement of a scleral buckle so far posteriorly would be extremely difficult and probably entail sacrificing two vortex veins.

24.**2b** Vitrectomy is followed by internal drainage of subretinal fluid through one of the retinal breaks, and a fluid-air exchange. Three rows of endolaser are placed around each retinal break.

Note in this highly myopic eye the posterior staphyloma with thin sclera, which would have made scleral buckling difficult and hazardous.

3a

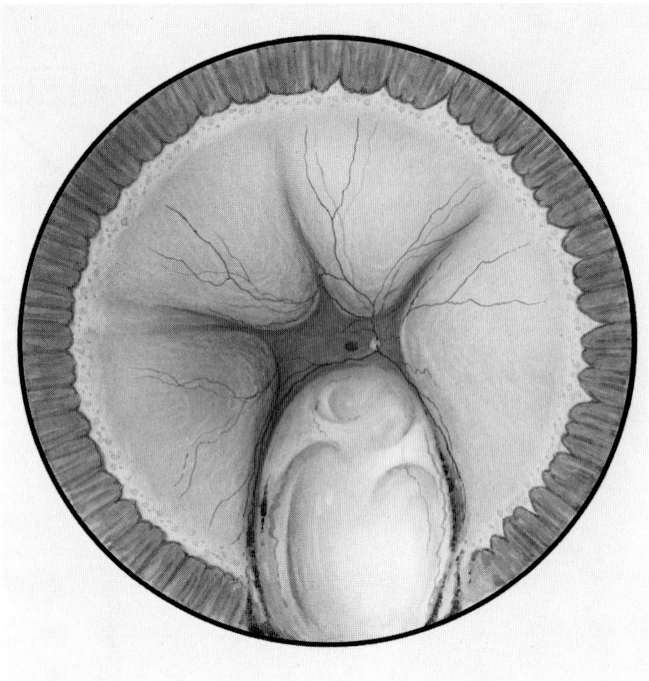

3c

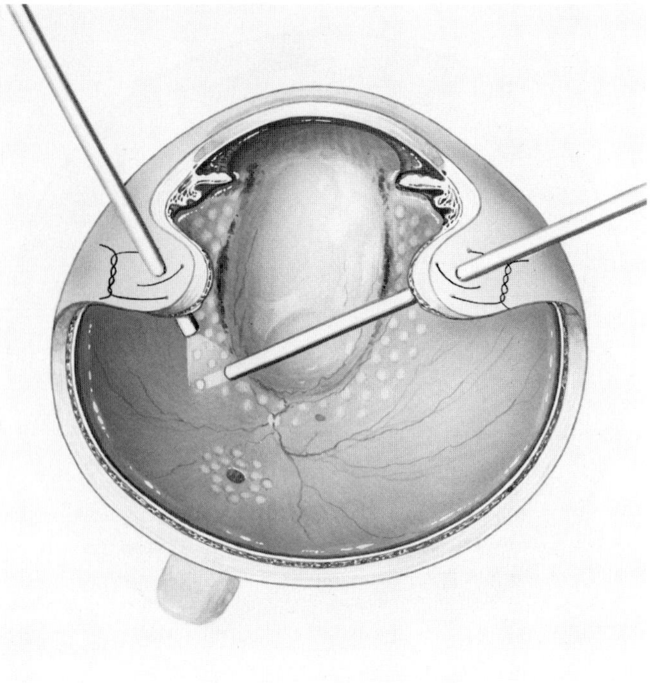

3b

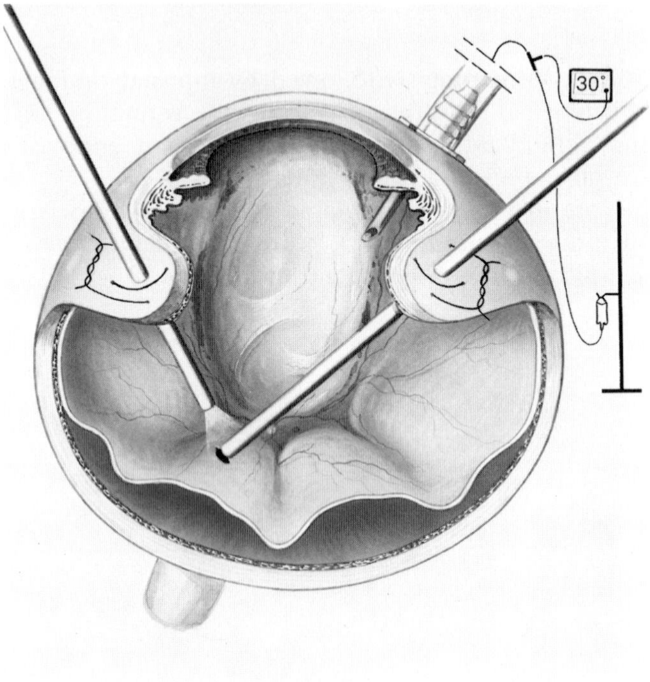

Choroidal Coloboma

24.**3a** Retinal breaks may escape detection with preoperative indirect ophthalmoscopy and biomicroscopy because of the white scleral background and the thin, diaphanous nature of the undeveloped retina within the coloboma (8, 10, 14: 615–617, 18). Prior to vitrectomy, a further search is made for retinal breaks using indirect ophthalmoscopy and scleral depression. The retina within the coloboma is reexamined intraoperatively with endoillumination and biomicroscopy using the operating microscope.

24.**3b** If no open retinal break is found, vitrectomy is performed, followed by internal drainage through a superior nasal retinotomy located midway between the equator and the optic nerve head.

24.**3c** Following fluid-air exchange, endolaser is applied around the retinotomy and in three rows along the margin of the coloboma. Low-intensity, sparser applications of small diameter are made near the optic to minimize destruction of the peripheral nerve fiber layers.

References

1. Arruga H. Ocular surgery. 3rd ed., trans. Hogan MJ, Chaparro LE. New York: McGraw-Hill, 1962: 660.
2. Avila MP, Jalkh AE, Murakami K, et al. Biomicroscopic study of the vitreous in macular breaks. Ophthalmology 1983; 90: 1277–1283.
3. Blankenship GW, Santiago IL. Treatment of myopic macular hole and detachment. Ophthalmology 1987; 94: 333–337.
4. Gonvers M. Macular hole and retinal detachment. In: Blankenship GW, Stirpe M, Gonvers M, Binder S, eds. Basic and advanced vitreous surgery. Padua: Liviana, 1986: 215–217.
5. Gonvers M, Machemer R. A new approach to treating retinal detachment with macular hole. Am J Ophthalmol 1982; 94: 468–472.
6. Havener WH, Gloeckner, S. Atlas of diagnostic techniques and treatment of retinal detachment. St. Louis: C V Mosby, 1967.
7. Howard GM, Campbell CJ. Surgical repair of retinal detachments caused by macular holes. Arch Ophthalmol 1969; 81: 317–321.
8. Jesberg DO, Schepens CL. Retinal detachment associated with coloboma of the choroid. Arch Ophthalmol 1961; 65: 163–173.
9. Leaver PK. Macular hole and retinal detachment. Trans Ophthalmol Soc UK 1975; 95: 145–147.
10. Limaye SR. Coloboma of the iris and choroid and retinal detachment in oculoauricular dysplasia (Goldenhar syndrome). Eye Ear Nose Throat Monthly 1972; 51: 384–386.
11. Margherio RR, Schepens CL. Macular breaks, 2: management. Am J Ophthalmol 1972; 74: 233–240.
12. Meyer-Schwickerath G. Macular holes and retinal detachment. In: McPherson A, ed. New and controversial aspects of retinal detachment. New York: Harper and Row, 1968: 433–447.
13. Miyakc Y. A simplified method of treating retinal detachment with macular hole: long-term follow-up. Arch Ophthalmol 1986; 104: 1234–1236.
14. Schepens CL. Retinal detachment and allied diseases. Philadelphia: W B Saunders, 1983.
15. Schiff-Wertheimer S. A propos des "trous" maculaires dans leurs rapports avec le décollement de la rétine. Bull Cox Fr Ophthalmol 1937; 49: 728–731.
16. Smolin G. Statistical analysis of retinal holes and tears. Am J Ophthalmol 1965; 60: 1055–1059.
17. Tittarelli R, Benedetti S, Leaver PK. Vitrectomy fluid-gas exchange in the treatment of macular hole. In: Blankenship GW, Stirpe M, Gonvers M, Binder S, eds. Basic and advanced vitreous surgery. Padua: Liviana, 1986: 207–208.
18. Tolentino FI, Schepens CL, Freeman HM. Vitreoretinal disorders: diagnosis and management. Philadelphia: W B Saunders, 1976: 203–204.
19. Witmer, R, Klöti R. Der heutige Stand der Netzhautchirurgie. Ophthalmologica 1965; 149: 152–160.

25

Proliferative Vitreoretinopathy

Proliferative vitreoretinopathy (PVR) is the commonest cause of failure of retinal detachment surgery. It has been reported to occur after 7% of retinal detachment operations. PVR usually occurs several weeks following retinal detachment repair. It is characterized by the growth of membranes on both surfaces of the detached retina and on the posterior surface of the detached vitreous gel.

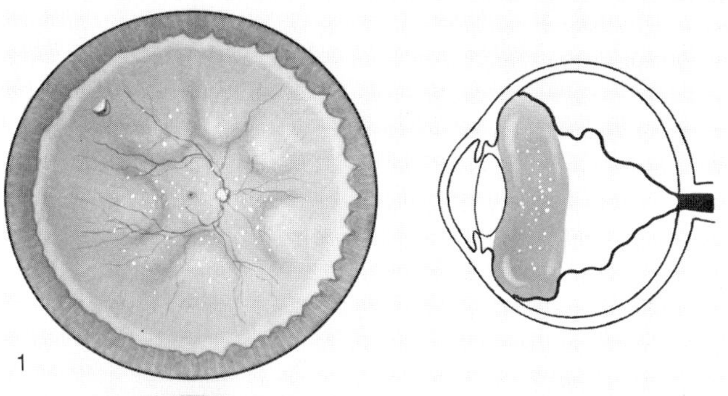

1

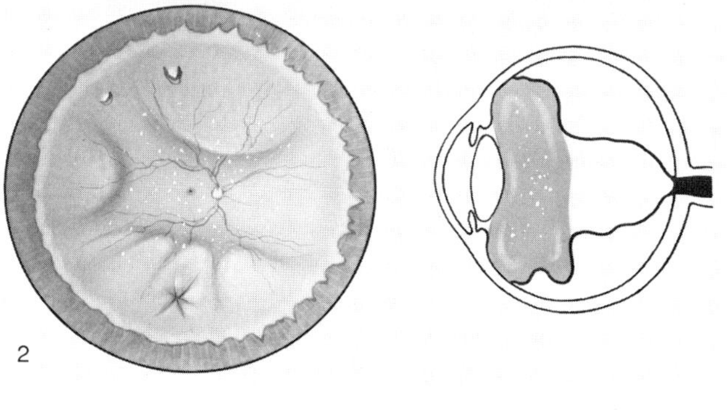

2

25.**1a** **Retina Society classification of PVR.** The clinical picture of PVR has been classified by the Retina Society into several grades of varying severity. This classification is based on the fundus and vitreous findings (16).

Grade A, or minimal, PVR has subtle findings of pigment clumps in the vitreous gel and vitreous haze (Fig. 25.**1a**, 1).

Grade B, or moderate, PVR is defined by the wrinkling of the inner retinal surface, the rolled edge of retinal breaks, or both (Fig. 25.**1a**, 2). The retina may appear to be stiff, and the retinal vessels in the wrinkled areas exhibit marked tortuosity. These features are assumed to be due to preretinal membranes. Such membranes often cannot be visualized clinically, but their presence is inferred by these findings.

1b

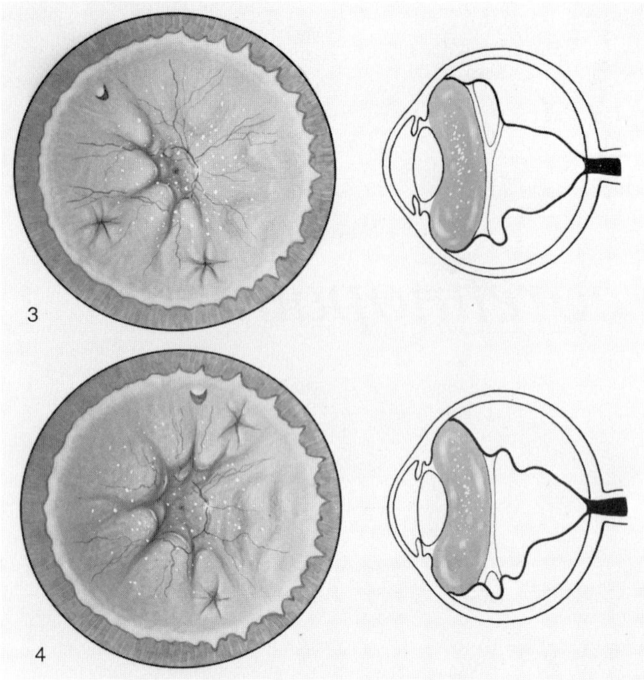

1c

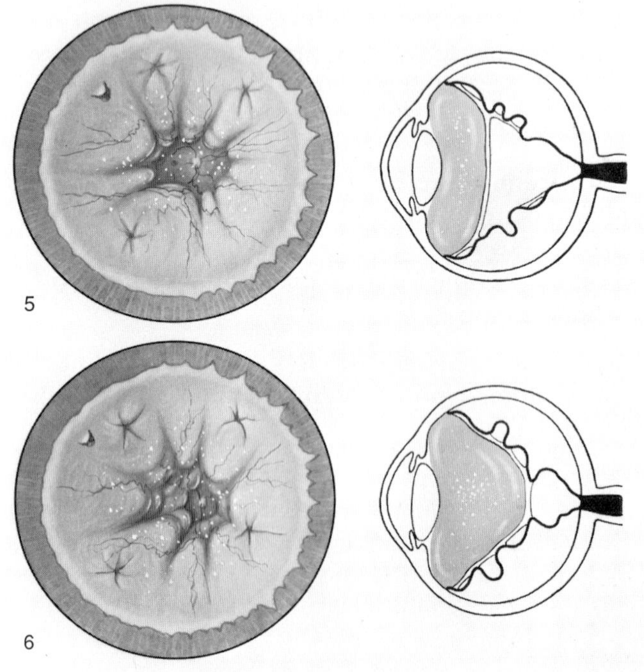

25.**1b** **Grade C, or marked, PVR** is defined by the presence of full-thickness fixed retinal folds, and is subdivided into stages C-1, C-2, and C-3.

Stage C-1 includes cases with fixed folds involving up to 3 clock hours of the retinal circumference (Fig. 25.**1b**, 3). These clock hours need not be contiguous.

Stage C-2 includes cases with fixed folds involving up to 6 clock hours (Fig. 25.**1b**, 4).

1d

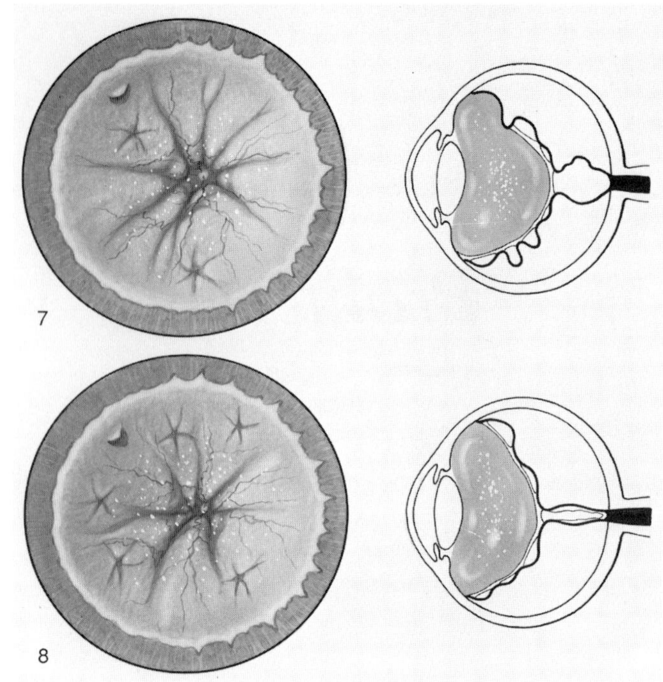

25.**1c** **Stage C-3 PVR** indicates the presence of full-thickness fixed retinal folds involving up to 9 clock hours (Fig. 25.**1c**, 5).

Grade D, or massive, PVR is characterized by full-thickness retinal folds in all four quadrants. Such cases may have the appearance of a giant starfold involving the entire retina, with radial spokes centered about the optic nerve head. This produces a funnel-like configuration of the detached retina. Grade D is subdivided into stages D-1, D-2, and D-3.

D-1 is defined as a wide funnel (Fig. 25.**1c**, 6).

25.**1d** **Stage D-2** indicates a narrow funnel whose anterior entrance can be visualized by indirect ophthalmoscopy within the 45° field of a +20D condensing lens (Fig. 25.**1d,** 7).

Stage D-3 indicates a funnel so narrow or closed that the optic nerve head cannot be seen (Fig. 25.**1d,** 8).

Surgical treatment of anterior and posterior PVR. The Retina Society classification has been criticized because it does not take into account proliferative changes in the fundus periphery that are responsible for a significant number of failures in the treatment of PVR (17, 18, 21: 16–17). For that reason, we use the term *anterior PVR* to describe cases in which the most severe proliferative changes involve the peripheral fundus and the region of the vitreous base (6, 7, 8, 11) (see Fig. 25.**3a**), and *posterior PVR* to describe cases in which the proliferative changes are most marked in the posterior fundus.

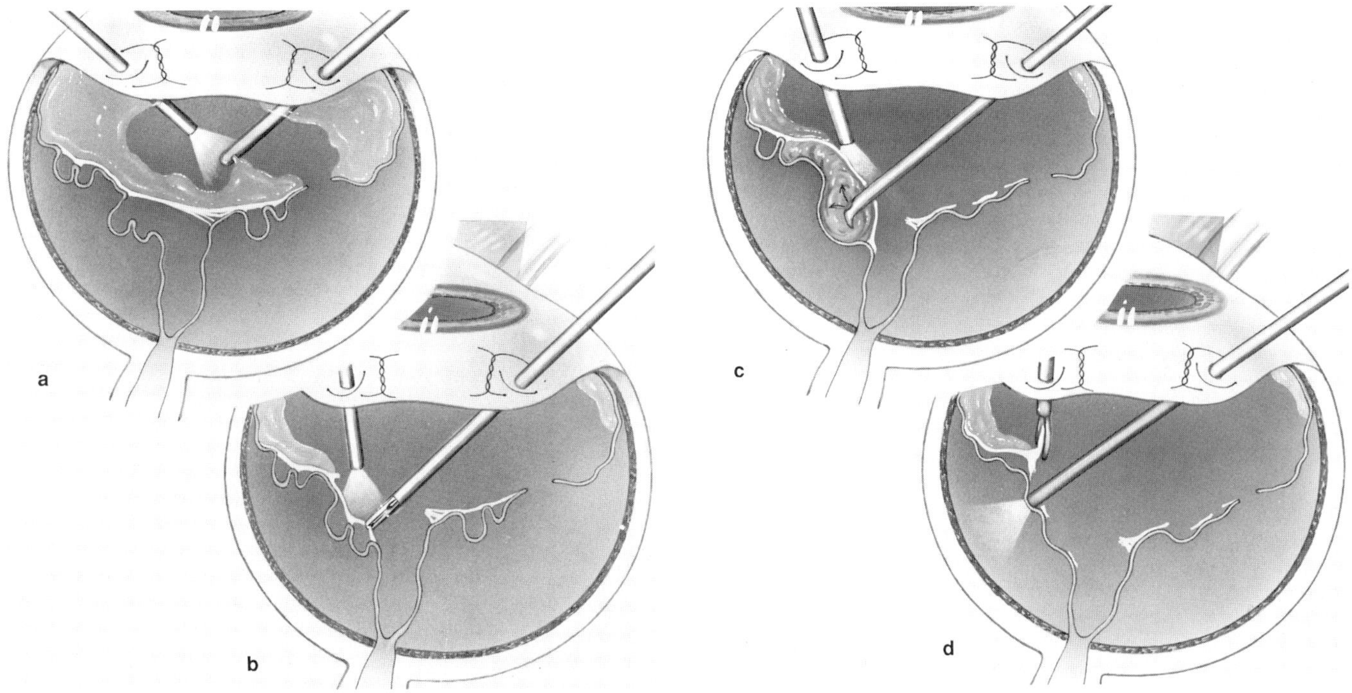

Posterior PVR

25.**2a** The surgical technique for posterior PVR utilizes the standard vitrectomy setup, including instruments for peeling membranes, such as a variety of spatulas, forceps, picks, pick-forceps, a tissue manipulator, scissors, a retinal scratcher, and hydraulic dissectors. In addition, fluid-air exchange equipment such as an air pump, extrusion needle, endodiathermy, endophotocoagulation, and long-term gases are necessary (2, 10, 12, 13, 15, 19, 20, 21: 45–61, 22).

The vitreous gel is removed carefully, starting centrally and working gradually toward the periphery. A clear crystalline lens is left intact if the PVR involves only the posterior retina.

b The elevated edge of the surface membrane is picked up with end-gripping vitreous forceps and lifted gently to separate it from the retina.

In some cases, it is necessary to employ a wide variety of instruments to separate a free edge of a membrane before it can be grasped with forceps. Scratching the surface of the retina with a retinal scratcher (Chapter 3) may separate the edge of a preretinal membrane from the retina.

The blunt membrane peeler is helpful in separating adjacent fixed, deep, radial folds when exploring for the free edge of a preretinal membrane. The hooked membrane spatula (Chapter 3) or membrane spatula knife is useful in separating firmly adherent preretinal membranes and membranes between deep radial retinal folds.

25.**2c** Extensive sheets of surface membrane may be peeled hydraulically by injecting sodium hyaluronate under the membrane using a special tip (Fig. 3.**4b**). During injection, the infusion pressure is decreased to lower the intraocular pressure and to increase the effectiveness of hydraulic dissection. The separated membrane is removed with the vitrectomy probe.

d The vitreous forceps may be combined with the light pipe for membrane peeling. The edge of the membrane is held with forceps, while the blunt tip of the light pipe is pushed gently against the retina to separate it from the membrane.

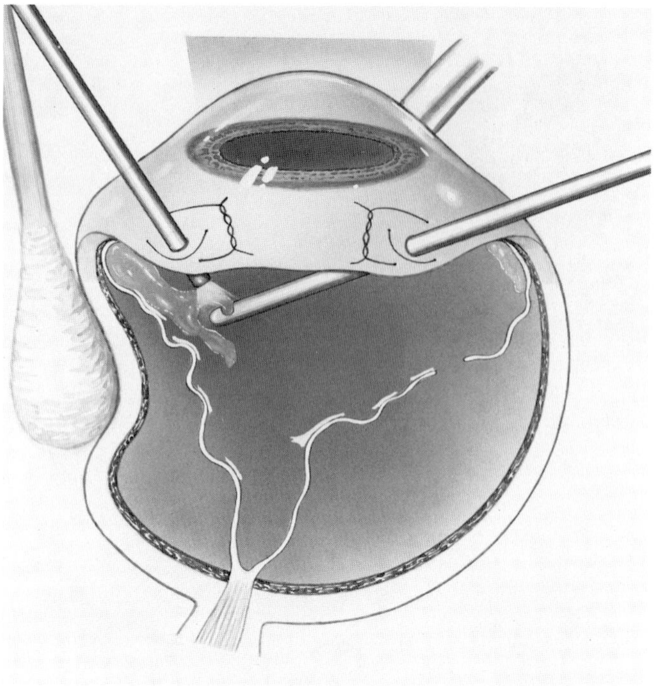

25.**2e** After membranes over fixed folds in the periphery are removed, the peripheral vitreous is trimmed using the vitrectomy probe. Scleral depression improves visualization of the region of the vitreous base.

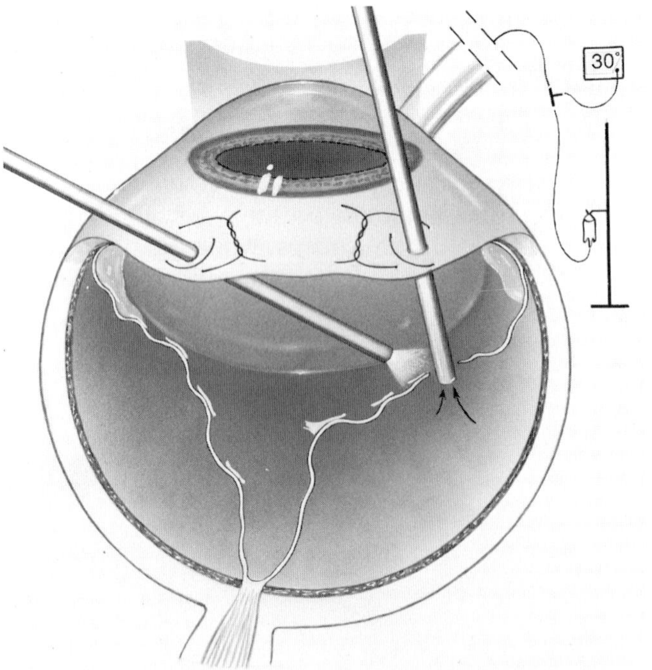

25.**2f** The retinal break is marked with endodiathermy so that it will be visualized more easily during and following fluid-air exchange. The extrusion needle or cannulated subretinal fluid aspirator (9) is inserted under direct visualization through the retinal break for the internal drainage of subretinal fluid. The infusion is switched to air, and a fluid-air exchange is carried out.

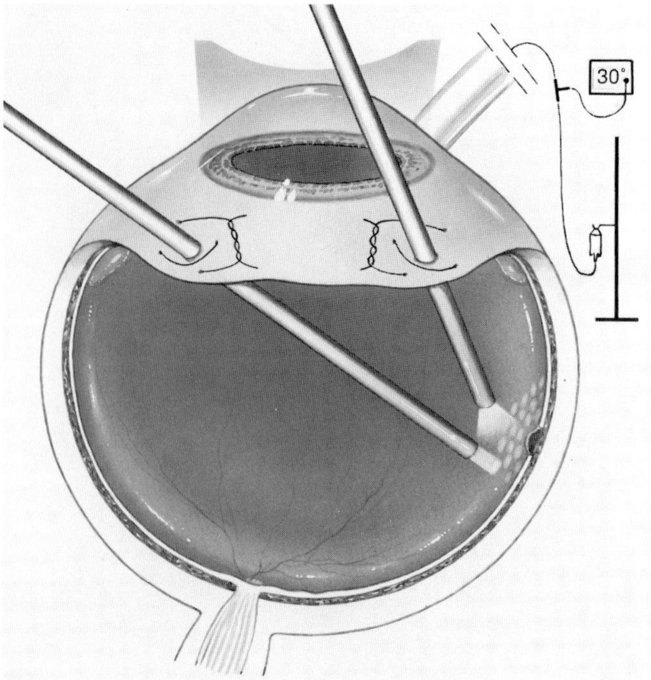

25.**2g** After the retina is reattached, all retinal breaks are surrounded by three rows of endolaser applications. A wide episcleral buckle is placed to relieve traction in the region of the vitreous base and to support peripheral retinal breaks. In many eyes, a pre-existing buckle is present, which is left undisturbed.

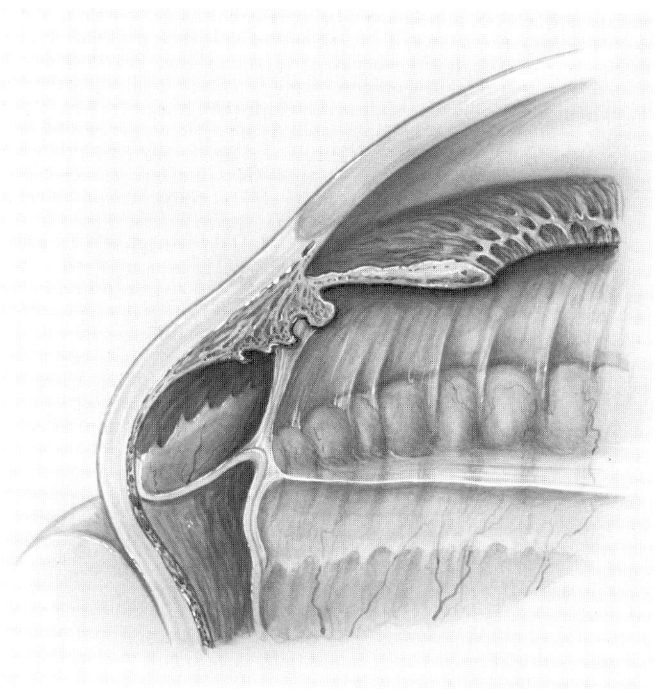

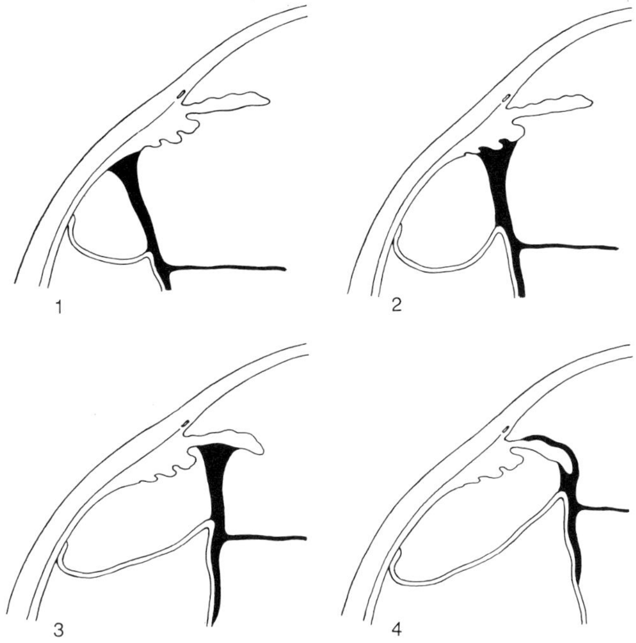

Anterior PVR

25.**3a** In eyes with anterior PVR, a sheet-like membrane is seen extending varying distances anteriorly from the peripheral retina across the ora serrata and pars plana ciliaris. Contraction of this membrane in a meridional direction pulls the peripheral retina anteriorly, producing a circumferential retinal fold that runs parallel to the ora serrata (1, 3, 5). A trough of varying width and depth develops between this fold and the pars plana ciliaris. In some eyes this membrane is continous with an equatorial membrane.

Contraction of the vitreous base and the peripheral preretinal membranes in a circumferential direction results in pleat-like retinal folds extending in a radial direction anteriorly and posteriorly from the circumferential retinal fold. These radial folds are narrow in the fundus periphery, in contrast to posterior PVR, in which radial folds are narrowed as they approach the optic nerve head.

25.**3b** The membrane may attach to the anterior border of the vitreous base and pars plicata (Fig. 25.**3b,** 1), or to the ciliary processes (Fig. 25.**3b,** 2), or to the inferior surface of the iris (Fig. 25.**3b,** 3), or, in extreme cases, to the pupillary margin (Fig. 25.**3b,** 4). In the latter case, contraction of the membrane produces a bowing of the iris posteriorly and an inversion of the pupillary margin.

3c

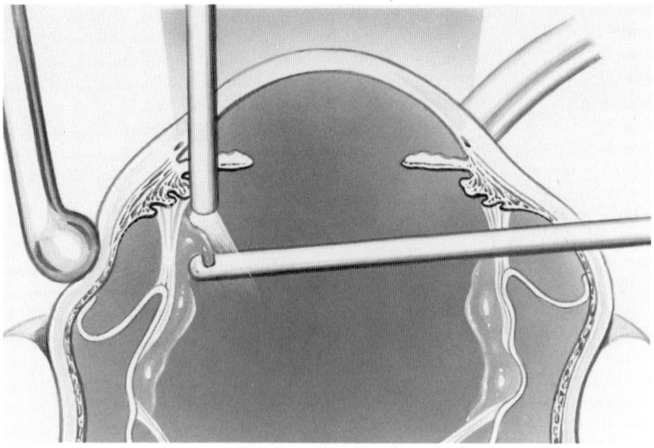

3e

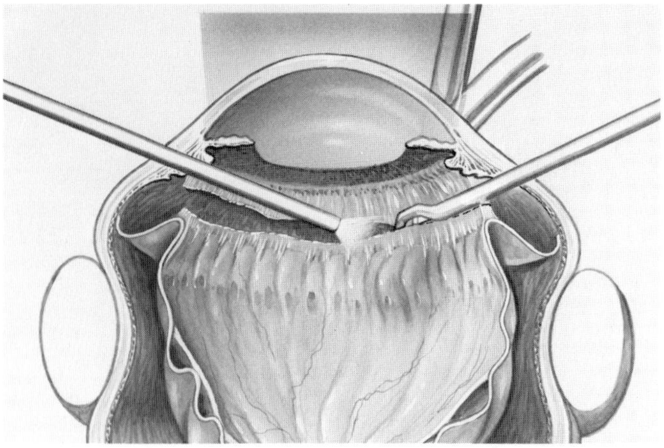

3d

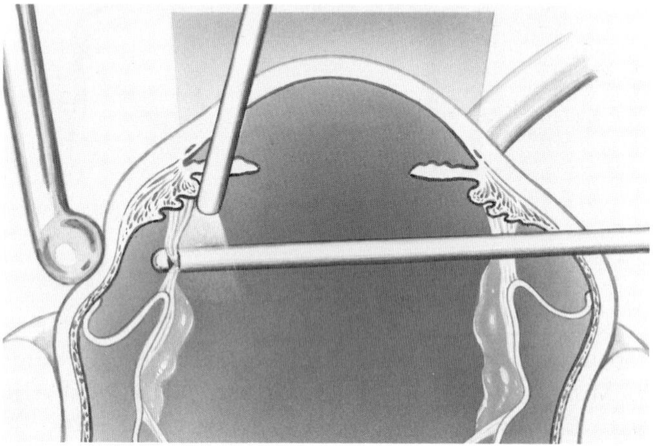

3f

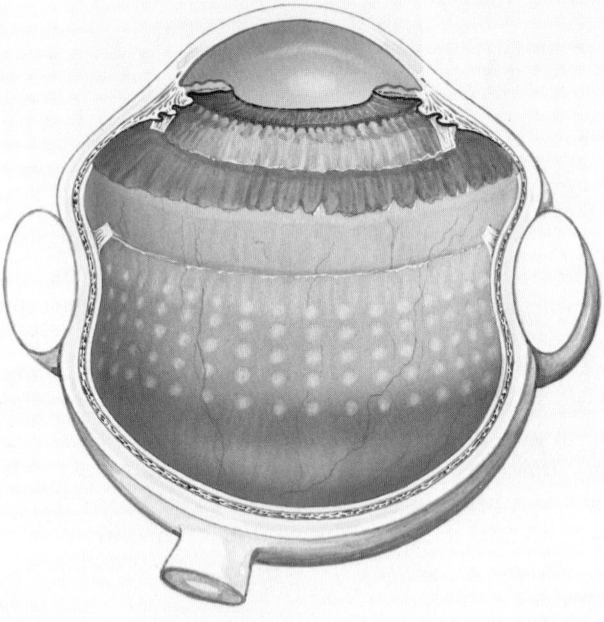

25.**3c** **Vitrectomy.** Lensectomy is performed routinely to obtain an optimum visualization of the peripheral pathology.

Scleral depression is used to improve visualization during surgery. Inasmuch as the vitreous is firmly adherent to the retina in the region of these membranes and the vitreous base, vitrectomy is performed using low suction pressure and intermittent cutting. Intermittent high-frequency cutting is used for short intervals, permitting time for careful visualization of the underlying retina.

25.**3d** The choice of scissors or vitrectomy probe to cut the anterior membrane depends on the width of the trough across which it extends. When a wide trough is present between the circumferential retinal fold and the anterior attachment of the membrane, the vitrectomy instrument is used.

25.**3e** The vitreous scissors is used to section the membranes bridging a narrow trough. When the anterior membrane is cut, traction is relieved and the trough widens, allowing the condensed and organized vitreous base within it to be partially removed with the vitrectomy probe.

25.**3f** Most eyes undergoing surgery for anterior PVR have a preexisting scleral buckle, which is not disturbed. Internal drainage of subretinal fluid and a fluid-air exchange are performed through the retinal break or a retinotomy. If the break is located in the equatorial region, the cannulated subretinal fluid aspirator is used. The instrument tip is positioned near the retinal break, and the flexible cannula is advanced through the break into the subretinal space. Subretinal fluid is vented through the handle during fluid-air exchange. The cannula is retracted from the retinal hole after retinal reattachment has been achieved. Endolaser is applied over the scleral buckle and around the fundus periphery overlying the indentation produced by the encircling band. Before closure of the conjunctiva, an air-gas exchange is done using a 20% micture of perfluoropropane gas and air, lavaging 50 ml of the mixture through the vitreous cavity over approximately 2 minutes.

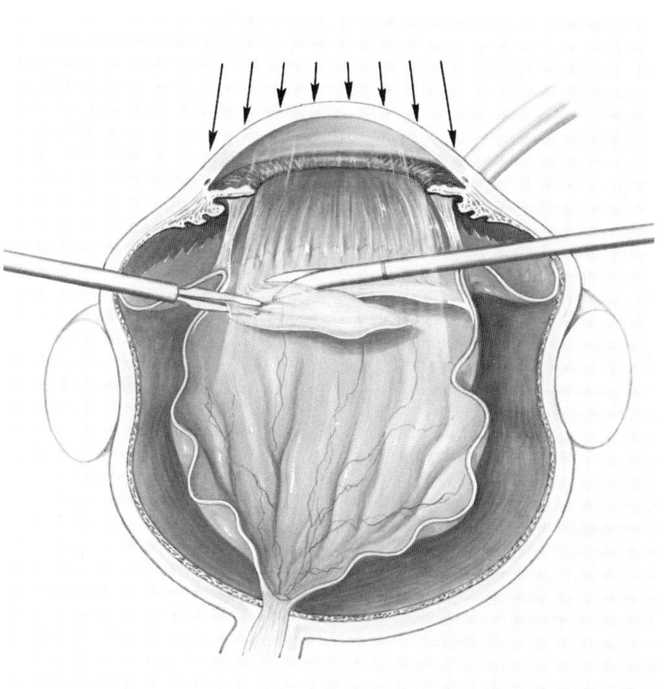

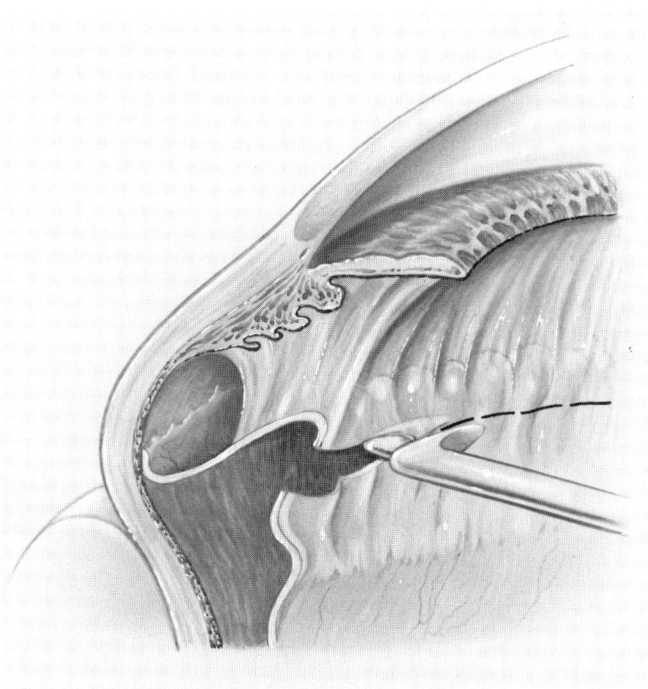

25.**4a** **Bimanual membrane peeling.** In the region of the vitreous base, preretinal membranes and the anterior hyaloid membrane are very adherent to the retina, so that attempts to peel them are frequently associated with the production of iatrogenic retinal breaks (8, 21: 50–51). In addition, traction by the anterior membrane causes the peripheral retina to become stretched, thinned, and atrophic. This atrophic retina is prone to develop retinal breaks during attempts to peel preretinal membranes from its surface. With scleral depression and a widely dilated pupil, it may be possible to illuminate the peripheral retina with the light from the operating microscope so that a bimanual technique can be used. The preretinal membrane is grasped with forceps held in the surgeon's nondominant hand, and separated from the retina with a spatula held in the dominant hand. Holding the membrane reduces excessive tractional movements during peeling attempts, and decreases the incidence of iatrogenic retinal breaks.

Focal illumination may be obtained using self-illuminating forceps or picks with a fiber-optic bundle mounted on the shaft of the instrument.

25.**4b** **Relaxing retinotomy.** A relaxing retinotomy is performed in cases in which severe preretinal organization makes it impossible to isolate the anterior membrane for sectioning (4, 14, 21: 55). The retinotomy is made slightly posterior and parallel to the vitreous base, and extended over the circumference of the unrelieved traction.

Retinotomy is followed by fluid-air exchange, internal drainage of subretinal fluid, endolaser, and air-gas exchange.

Retinectomy. Penetrating injury involving the region of the ciliary body preretinal and intraretinal organization may result in PVR with peripheral retina that is opaque, thickened, immobile, and organized into a mass of radial retinal folds. If efforts to peel preretinal and subretinal membranes, and a relaxing retinotomy, are unsuccessful, the organized retina is removed by retinectomy (8). To avoid excising an excessive amount of retinal tissue, the slowest possible cutting speed of the vitrectomy probe and low suction pressure are used. Retinectomy is continued posteriorly until smooth, relatively mobile retina of normal thickness is reached. An air-fluid exchange is performed, in conjunction with internal drainage of subretinal fluid, to tamponade the posterior retinal flap of the retinectomy against the pigment epithelium. The posterior edge of the retinectomy is mechanically fixed in position with intraocular tantalum retinal screws inserted every 30° using an intraocular screwdriver (Fig. 3.**12**). Endolaser is applied 360° around the fundus, and the air is replaced with a mixture of 20% perfluoropropane gas and air, or with fluorosilicone oil.

References

1. Abrams GW, Williams GA, Neuwirth J, McDonald HR. Clinical results of titanium retinal tacks with pneumatic insertion. Am J Ophthalmol 1986; 102: 13–19.
2. Chang S, Lincoff H, Ozmert E, et al. Management of retinal detachment with moderate PVR. In: Freeman HM, Tolentino FI, eds. Proliferative vitreoretinopathy (PVR). New York: Springer, 1988: 54–59.
3. Charles S. Vitreous microsurgery. Baltimore: Williams and Wilkins, 1981: 137.
4. Charles S. Vitreous microsurgery. 2nd ed. Baltimore: Williams and Wilkins, 1987: 142–144.
5. Charles S. Vitreous surgery for periretinal proliferation. In: Jakobiec FA, Sigelman J, eds. Advanced techniques in ocular surgery. Philadelphia: W B Saunders, 1984: 295.
6. Elner SG, Elner VM, Díaz-Rohena R, et al. Anterior PVR, part II: clinicopathologic, light microscopic, and ultrastructural findings. In: Freeman HM, Tolentino FI, eds. Proliferative vitreoretinopathy (PVR). New York: Springer, 1988: 34–45.
7. Freeman HM. Surgery of the retina and vitreous. In: Jaffe N, ed. Atlas of ophthalmic surgery. New York: Gower (in press).
8. Freeman HM, Elner SG, Tolentino FI, et al. Anterior PVR, part I: clinical findings and management. In: Freeman HM, Tolentino FI, eds. Proliferative vitreoretinoplathy (PVR). New York: Springer, 1988: 22–33.
9. Flynn HW Jr, Blumenkranz MS, Parel JM, et al. Cannulated subretinal fluid aspirator for vitreoretinal surgery. Am J Ophthalmol 1987; 103: 106–108.
10. Hanneken AM, Michels RG. Surgical treatment of PVR. In: Freeman HM, Tolentino FI, eds. Proliferative vitreoretinopathy (PVR). New York: Springer, 1988: 60–69.
11. Lewis H, Aaberg TM. Anterior proliferative vitreoretinopathy. Am J Ophthalmol 1988; 105: 277–284.
12. McCuen BW II, de Juan E Jr, Machemer R. Silicone oil in vitreoretinal surgery, part 1: surgical techniques. Retina 1985; 5: 189–197.
13. McCuen BW II, de Juan E Jr, Machemer R. Management of severe (grade D) PVR with mechanical fixation of the retina. In: Freeman HM, Tolentino FI, eds. Proliferative vitreoretinopathy (PVR). New York: Springer, 1988: 70–75.
14. Machemer R, McCuen BW, de Juan E Jr. Relaxing retinotomies and retinectomies. Am J Ophthalmol 1986; 102: 7–12.
15. Michels RG. Surgery of retinal detachment with proliferative vitreoretinopathy. Retina 1984; 4: 63–83.
16. The Retina Society Terminology Commitee. The classification of retinal detachment with proliferative vitreoretinopathy. Ophthalmology 1983; 90: 121–125.
17. Ryan SJ. The pathophysiology of proliferative vitreoretinopathy in its management. Am J Ophthalmol 1985; 100: 188-193.
18. Schepens CL. Peripheral proliferative vitreoretinopathy (P-PVR). (Letter). Ophthalmology 1987; 94: 201.
19. Stern WH, Lean JS, The Silicone Study Group. Intraocular silicone oil versus gas in the management of PVR: a multicenter clinical study. In: Freeman HM, Tolentino FI, eds. Proliferative vitreoretinopathy (PVR). New York: Springer, 1988: 88–96.
20. Tolentino FI, Freeman HM. Management of posterior PVR. In: Freeman HM, Tolentino FI, eds. Proliferative vitreoretinopathy (PVR). New York: Springer, 1988: 46–53.
21. Živojnović R. Silicone oil in vitreoretinal surgery. Dordrecht: Nijhoff, 1987.
22. Živojnović R, Mertens DAE, Peperkamp E, et al. Treatment of traumatic traction detachment in eyes with PVR and severe damage to the anterior segment. In: Freeman HM, Tolentino FI, eds. Proliferative vitreoretinopathy (PVR). New York: Springer, 1988: 76–80.

26

Macular Pucker

Macular pucker is a localized epiretinal membrane that covers, distorts, or detaches the macula. It occurs in 4–8% of eyes after uncomplicated retinal detachment surgery, or after prophylactic treatment of retinal breaks without detachment. Macular pucker is characterized by superficial wrinkling of the posterior retina, usually involving the macula and resulting in distorted or diminished vision. A localized form of preretinal fibrosis can occur spontaneously in attached retina in an eye with no other fundus abnormality. This isolated condition is termed cellophane maculopathy. Indications for surgical peeling of the membrane are reduction of visual acuity to 20/70 or worse with corrective lenses, disabling visual distortion, and a good potential for visual improvement in the absence of associated macular degeneration (1–13).

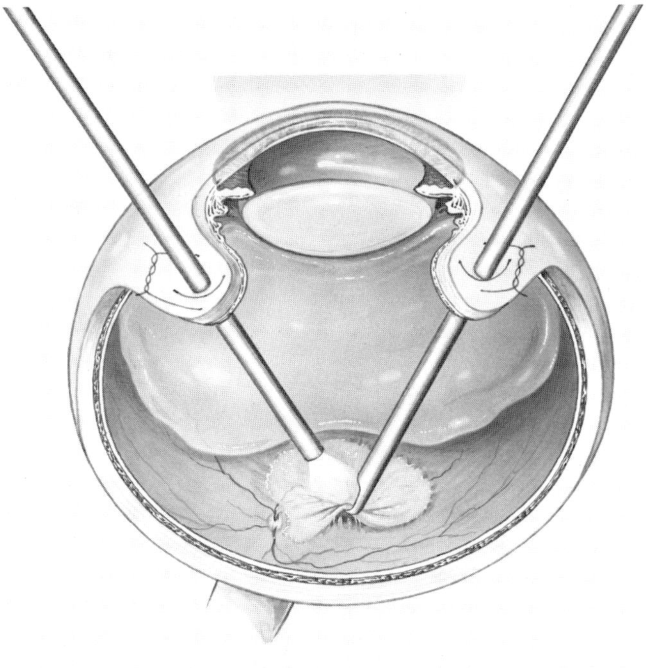

26.**1** The light pipe is introduced near the macula to find an edge of the preretinal membrane. If the membrane does not have an edge that can be grasped with forceps or isolated with one of the teeth of the retinal scratcher, a sharp pick is introduced into the thickest edge of the membrane. When the edge has been raised, it is lifted and peeled away with the end-gripping vitreous forceps. Intraretinal hemorrhage or retinal elevation during membrane peeling is an early warning sign to stop the peeling and continue with the technique described in Figure 26.**2b**.

a

b

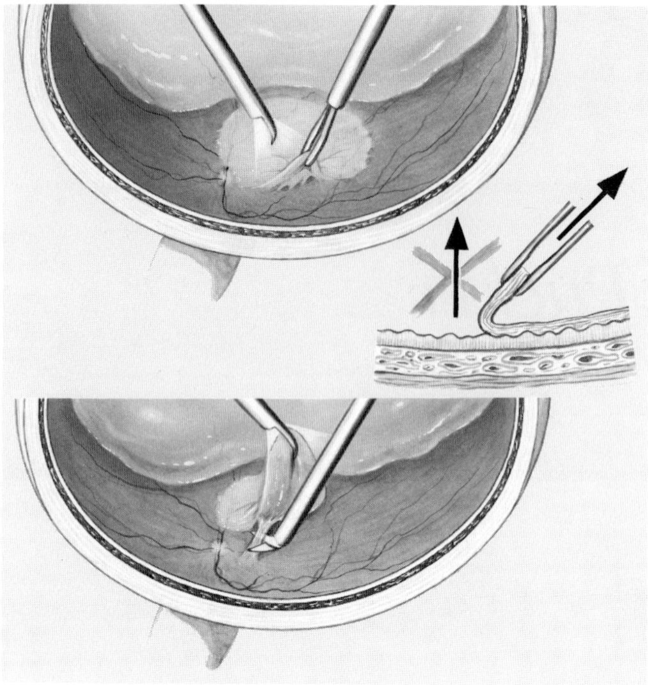

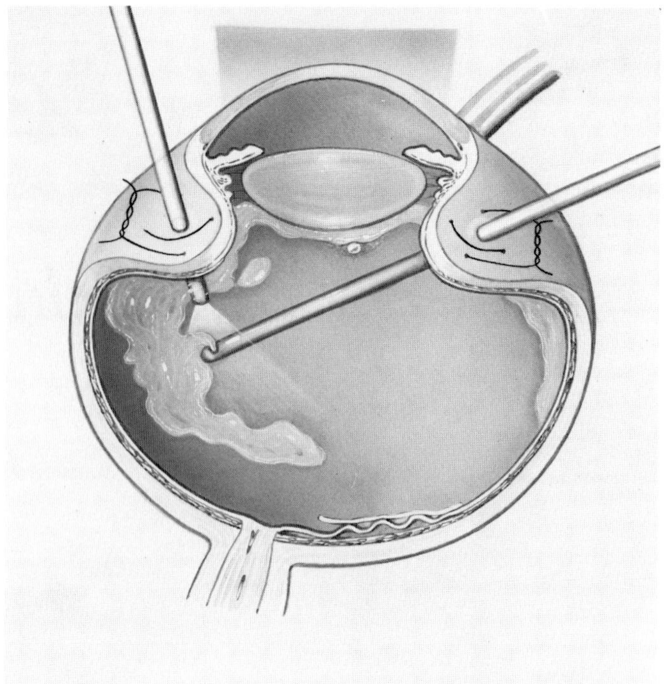

26.**2a** Macular pucker may have firm strands or adhesions joining it to the underlying macula. A lighted pick is used in combination with forceps or scissors to facilitate membrane removal. *Inset:* the forceps lifts the membrane edge, pulling it from the retinal surface at a 45° angle. The lighted pick which illuminates the area is used to tease away and break fine tissue strands connecting the membrane to the retina.

b The membrane resists separation because it is attached to the retina by a large fibrous strand. Sutherland scissors are used to segment the strand from the membrane, which is lifted up and away from the retina with the illuminated pick.

26.**3** Circulating infusion fluid has been implicated as the cause of cataractous changes following vitrectomy for macular pucker. Exposure of the lens to the circulating fluid can be minimized by not removing the anterior vitreous until after the removal of the epiretinal membrane.

After the preretinal membranes are completely separated from the macula, the vitreous gel is removed, with the exception of a layer of gel on the posterior capsule of the lens. A small, sterile air bubble is injected through the infusion line prior to anterior vitrectomy to help delineate the vitreous layer to be preserved.

References

1. Charles S. Vitreous microsurgery. 2nd ed. Baltimore: Williams and Wilkins, 1987: 153–157.
2. Clarkson JG, Green WR, Massof D. A histophatologic review of 168 cases of preretinal membrane. Am J Ophthalmol 1977; 84: 1–17.
3. Machemer R, Aaberg TM. Vitrectomy. 2nd ed. New York: Grune and Stratton, 1979: 89–91.
4. Margherio RR, Cox MS Jr, Trese MT, et al. Removal of epimacular membranes. Ophthalmology 1985; 92: 1075–1082.
5. Michels RG. A clinical and histopathologic study of epiretinal membranes affecting the macula and removed by vitreous surgery. Trans Am Ophthalmol Soc 1982; 80: 580–656.
6. Michels RG. Vitrectomy for macular pucker. Ophthalmology 1984; 91: 1384–1388.
7. Michels RG. Surgical treatment of macular pucker. In: Blankenship GW, Stirpe M, Gonvers M, Binder S, eds. Basic and advanced vitreous surgery. Padua: Liviana, 1986: 239–245.
8. Rice TA, De Bustros S, Michels RG, et al. Prognostic factors in vitrectomy for epiretinal membranes of the macula. Ophthalmology 1986; 93: 602–610.
9. Roth AM, Foos RY. Surface wrinkling retinopathy in eyes enucleated at autopsy. Trans Am Acad Ophthalmol Otolaryngol 1971; 75: 1047–1058.
10. Schepens CL. Retinal detachment and allied diseases. Philadelphia: W B Sauders, 1983: 1012–1016.
11. Tanenbaum HL, Schepens CL, Elzeneiny I, Freeman HM. Macular pucker following retinal surgery: a biomicroscopic study. Can J Ophthalmol 1969; 4: 20–23.
12. Tanenbaum HL, Schepens CL, Elezeneiny I, Freeman HM. Macular pucker following retinal detachment surgery. Arch Ophthalmol 1970; 83: 286–293.
13. Tolentino FI, Schepens CL, Freeman HM. Vitreoretinal disorders: diagnosis and management. Philadelphia: W B Saunders, 1976: 471–479.

27

Vitrectomy in Children

Vitrectomy is performed in infants and young children for persistent hyperplastic primary vitreous (PHPV), retinopathy of prematurity (ROP), acute or chronic ocular trauma, and parasitic or infectious endophthalmitis.

27.**1 a** **Pars plana approach in children.** The pars plana in infants and young children is narrow, because the eye is not fully developed (8, 14). Instruments are inserted into the vitreous through a sclerotomy 2–3 mm posterior to the limbus, stradling the pars plana and pars ciliaris. This approach avoids damaging the peripheral retina and minimizes corneal distortion during instrument manipulation. To avoid injury to nearby ciliary processes and resultant hemorrhage, the incision and insertion of vitreous instruments are directed toward the center of the globe. This approach is preferred in eyes in which it is desirable to preserve the crystalline lens.

b **Perilimbal approach.** In eyes with ROP and retinal detachment, a perilimbal approach 0.5–1 mm posterior to the limbus is preferred (1).

c Adult relationships between the ciliary body, pars plana, and retina do not develop until the age of 7 years.

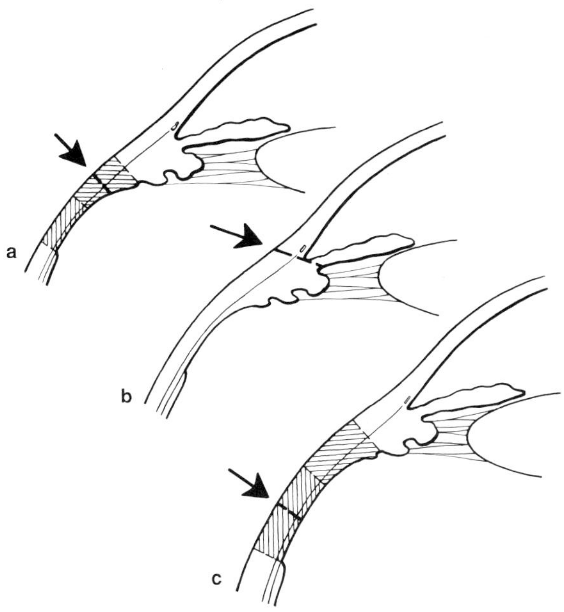

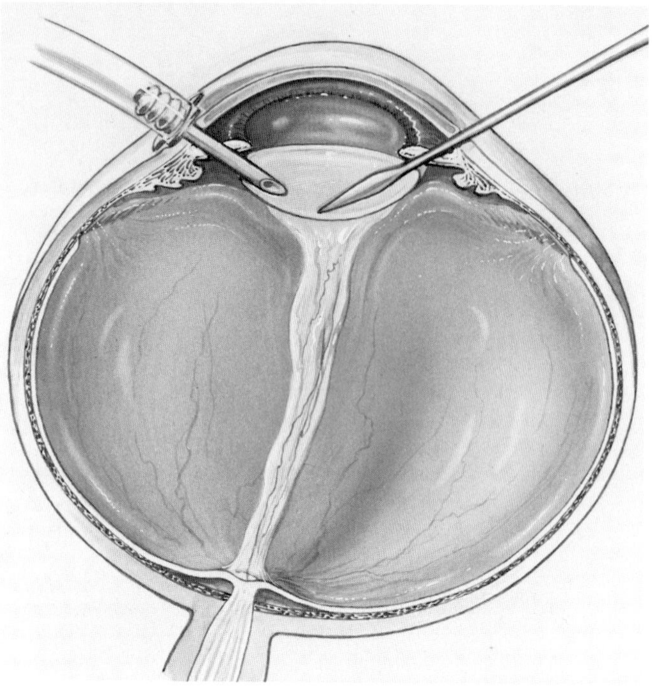

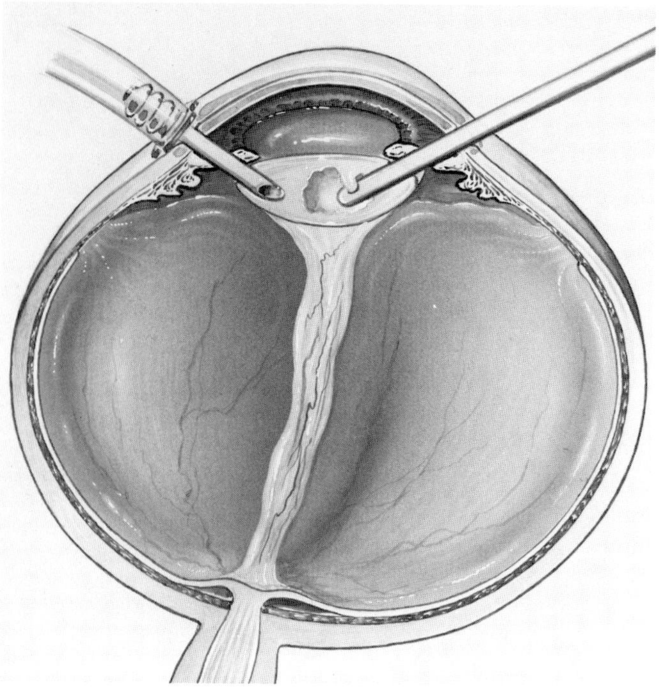

Persistent Hyperplastic Primary Vitreous

27.**2a** This congenital anomaly is found in full-term, normal-sized infants and often presents as a leukokoria. Although the clinical picture is protean, it can be classified broadly into an anterior and a posterior form. PHPV is usually unilateral (4–6, 12, 15–17, 19). The involved eye may be slightly microphthalmic. The anterior form is often associated with cataract, glaucoma, and abnormally large ciliary processes continuous with retrolental fibrovascular tissue. The posterior form is characterized by a stalk connecting the retrolental membrane to the optic disc and juxtapapillary retina, both of which may be slightly elevated. The stalk may contain a patent posterior hyaloid artery.

Limbal approach to the vitreous cavity. A specially designed 6 mm infusion cannula is inserted through an MVR blade incision through the limbus, iris, and lens equator in the inferotemporal quadrant near the horizontal meridian. The cannula is anchored with a 6-0 polyglactin suture. To facilitate complete removal of the lens cortex and nucleus, they are broken up by multiple thrusts of the blade of an MVR inserted through a superotemporal limbal incision. Infusion solution then enters the lens to hydrate the nucleus and cortex.

27.**2b** **Lensectomy.** The lens is penetrated with the MVR blade inserted through a limbal incision. To prevent rupture of the lens capsule, the infusion pressure is reduced. Using the vitrectomy probe, the lens cortex and nucleus are aspirated slowly from within the capsular bag.

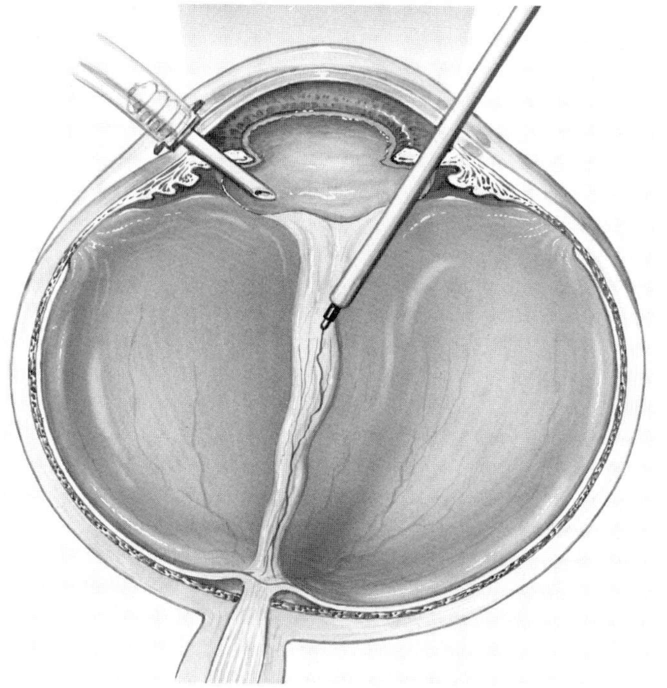

27.**2c** After lensectomy, the anterior and posterior capsules are removed using the vitrectomy probe. The fibrovascular stalk is inspected for patent blood vessels, which are coagulated with endodiathermy to prevent bleeding during removal of the stalk.

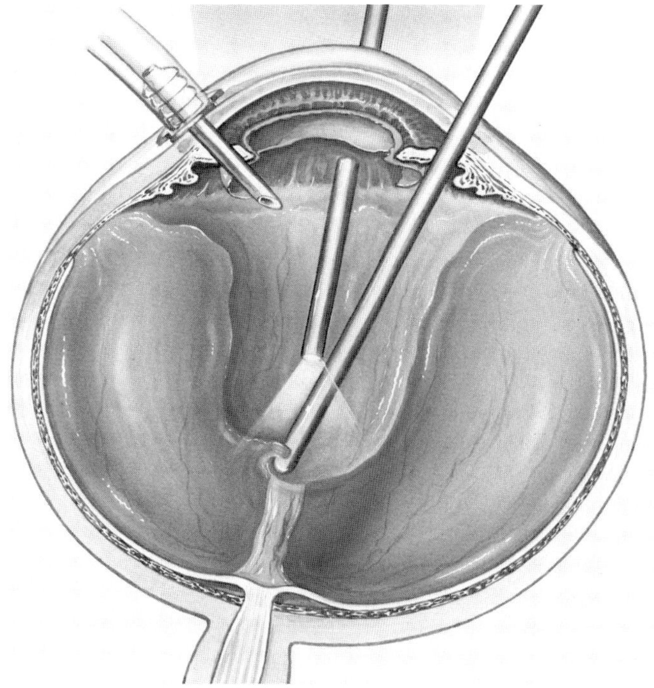

27.**2e** Vitrectomy of the central gel is carried out, leaving the cortical gel. The fibrous stalk is removed until a small stump is left near the optic disc. The sclerotomy and limbal incisions are closed with an 8-0 polyglactin suture.

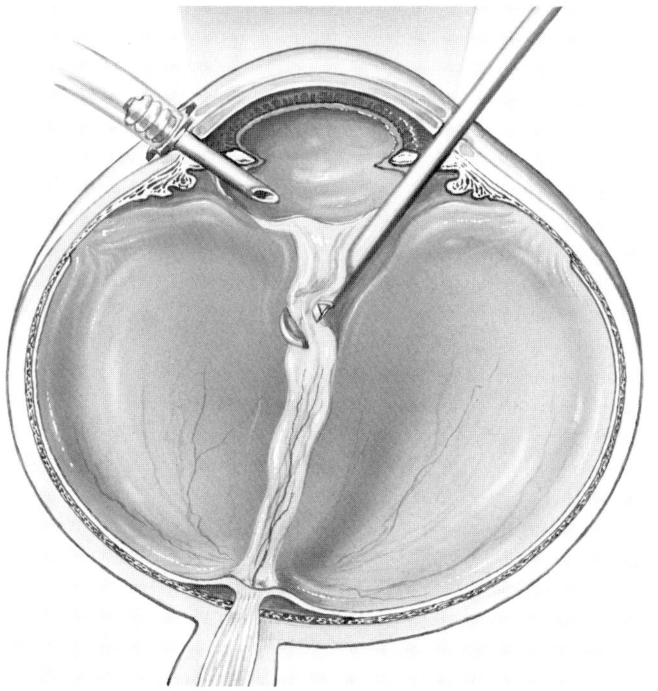

27.**2d** If the fibrovascular stalk is too dense to be engaged in the vitrectomy probe, it is sectioned into small pieces with vertical-cutting Sutherland scissors. The cut segments, which are surrounded by vitreous gel, are usually readily removed with the vitrectomy probe.

3a

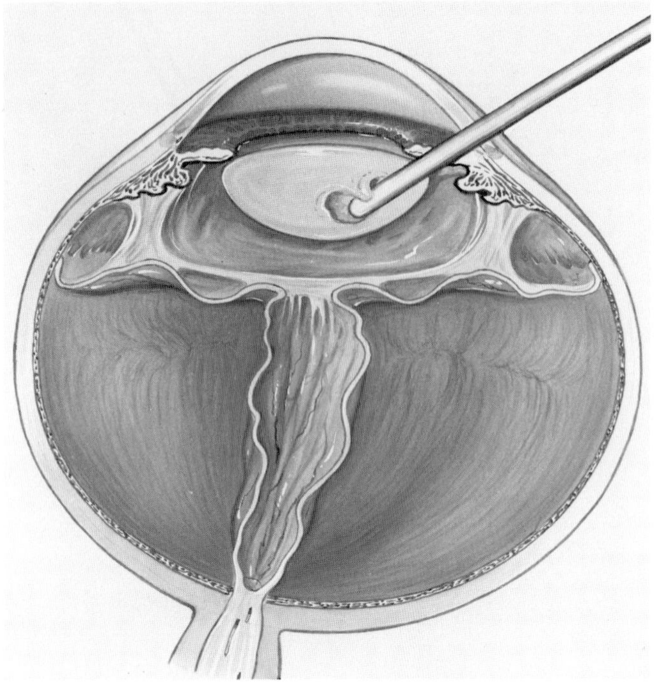

3b

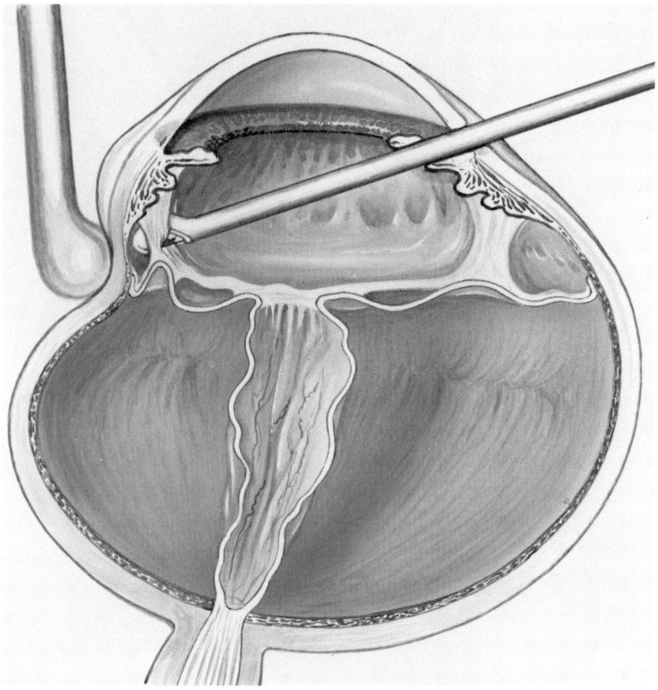

Retinopathy of Prematurity

Tractional retinal detachment in cases of retinopathy of prematurity is usually extensive, because it is associated with severe vitreous proliferation and involves both anterior and peripheral vitreous gel. Retinal detachment is characteristically funnel-shaped. The anterior portion of the funnel is wide and short, the posterior portion narrow and long (20, 21).

Two surgical approaches have been developed to remove or section retrolental tissue. One approach is through a closed system, in which instruments enter the eye through small limbal incisions and surgery is performed under controlled intraocular pressure (2, 3, 9, 10, 13, 23). The other is an "open sky" approach, in which instruments are introduced through a large corneal opening and surgery is performed under atmospheric pressure (7, 11, 22).

27.**3a** **Closed-system approach to ROP.** After the infusion cannula has been inserted, the lens is removed. Insertion of the cannula and lensectomy have been described in Figures 27.**2a** and 27.**2b**; the infusion cannula is not shown in Figures 27.**3a**–27.**3d**.

27.**3b** Following lensectomy, the vitreous gel in the anterior retinal funnel is removed with the vitrectomy probe and trimmed from the preretinal membranes. The procedure does not require a vitrectomy lens or a light pipe, because the anterior vitreous is visible with coaxial illumination from the operating microscope. The anterior peripheral portion of the vitreous cavity is examined using scleral depression. Using a spatula or vitreous dissector cutter, a tunnel is created under the anterior membrane that extends between the equatorial retinal fold and the ciliary processes or posterior surface of the iris. This anterior membrane usually extends around 360° of the anterior vitreous cavity.

3c

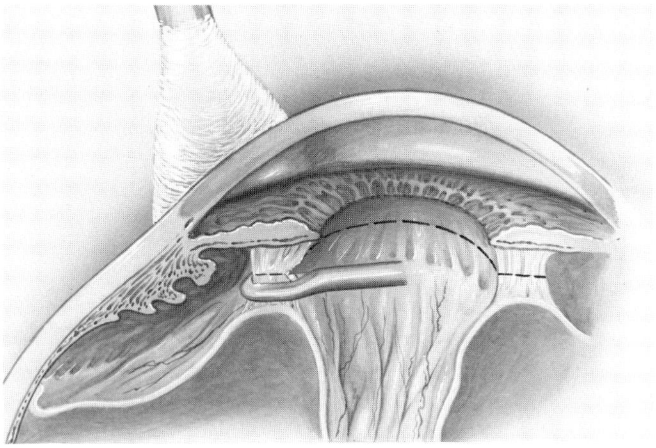

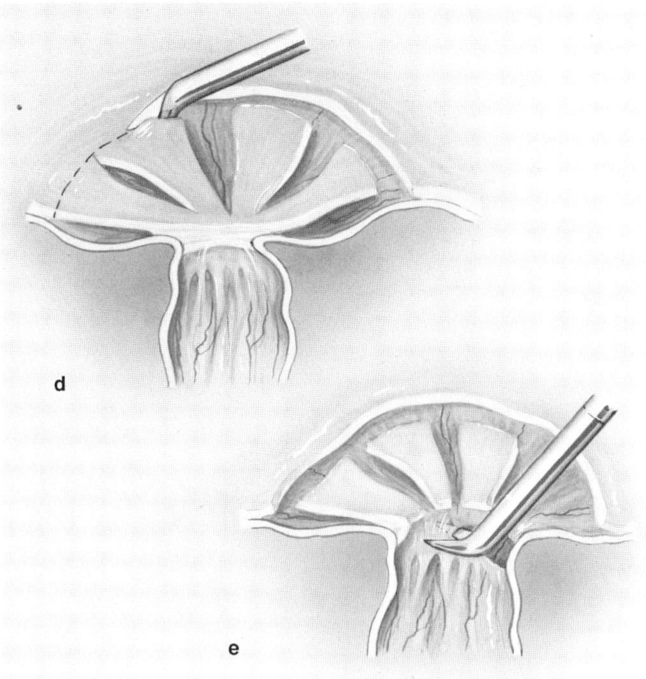

27.**3c** A trough-like fold is present peripheral to the ridge of highly elevated retina where the anterior membrane is attached. The anterior membrane is cut around 360° (broken line) to relieve anterior traction; this opens the trough and mobilizes the anterior retina.

27.**3d** After the anterior traction has been relieved, the equatorial fold may flatten to reveal a membranous plate of fibrous tissue lining the anterior part of the funnel and bridging radial retinal folds. This membranous tissue is penetrated with a bent-tip 20-gauge needle or MRV blade in an area where the membrane has separated and is elevated from the retina. The membrane is undermined with a spatula, dissector-cutter, or closed-blade Sutherland scissors, starting at the border of the vitreous base and extending posteriorly to the center of the retinal funnel. Vascularized portions of the membrane are treated with endodiathermy to prevent bleeding. Two methods may be used to remove this membrane.

As seen in the illustration, the membrane is segmented into small, pie-shaped pieces that are delaminated from the retina with Sutherland scissors and then removed with the vitrectomy probe. In some eyes, the membrane is delaminated and removed in one piece with the vitrectomy probe.

e Membrane dissection is brought to the neck of the funnel and deeper, separating thin membranes and releasing them from the radial retinal folds. The space inside the narrow portion of the funnel is usually filled with clear vitreous gel, with or without hyaloid vascular remnants that are removed with a vitrectomy probe. The detached retina usually reattaches spontaneously, as long as retinal breaks have not been created. The subretinal fluid may be left undrained, although retinal reattachment may be accomplished during the operation by external drainage of subretinal fluid and injection of BSS Plus into the vitreous cavity. If posterior retinal breaks are present, internal subretinal drainage, endolaser to the breaks, and sodium hyaluronate injection are attempted. If peripheral retinal breaks have developed, scleral buckle and external subretinal fluid drainage are attempted. However, the prognosis in such cases is poor, if not hopeless.

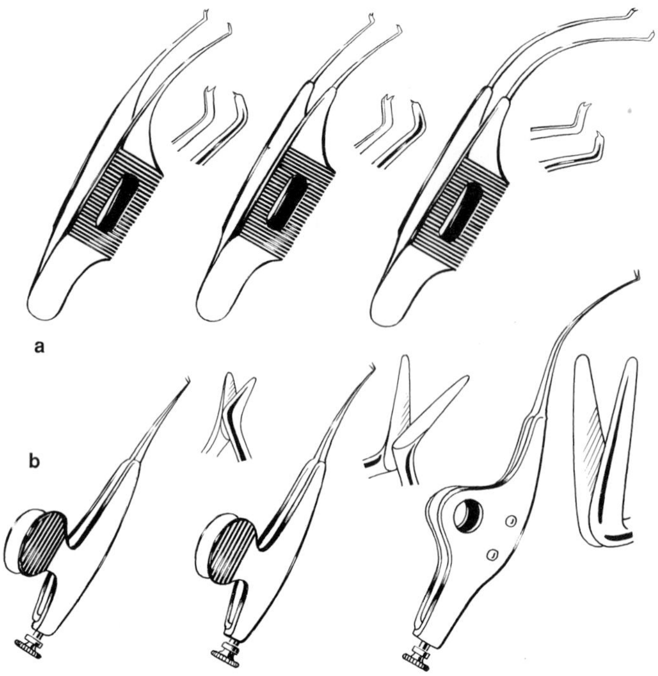

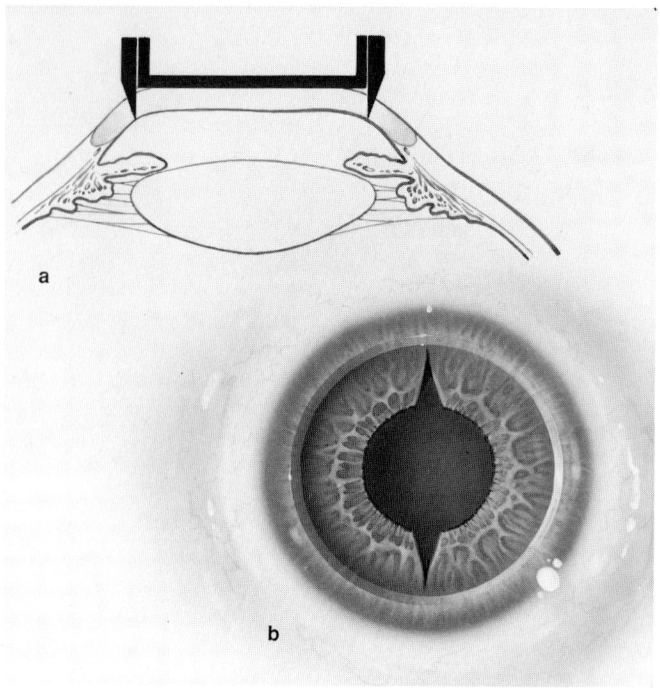

Open-Sky Vitrectomy

The transcorneal, open sky approach in the management of severe tractional retinal detachment caused by ROP provides optimum access to peripheral vitreoretinal membranes.

A fundamental advantage of the open sky approach is that it permits the surgeon not only to use two instruments in the anterior peripheral portion of the vitreous cavity, but also to switch their positions easily. In addition, visibility of the structures is better than through the cornea in the closed system of surgery. The major disadvantages of open-sky vitreous surgery is that the eye is subjected to the hypotony of atmospheric pressure during the procedure, the additional step of corneal surgery is involved, and in some instances there is increased difficulty in posterior dissection.

27.**4** Schepens and Hirose have developed special instruments for open-sky surgery. They are designed to fit under the 125 mm focal length of the operating microscope. The instruments are angulated to keep their shafts and the surgeon's hands from obstructing the surgical field (18).

a The Colibri forceps have been modified by elongating the shaft and increasing its curvature away from the tip, as shown center and right.

b The original de Wecker scissors shown on the left were modified in the same manner as the colibri forceps. The elongated and curved de Wecker scissors shown on the right are an effective dissector of fibrous membrane in the front portion of the retinal funnel.

27.**5a** **Open-sky procedure.** Sclerochoroidal incisions are made in four quadrants to drain accumulating suprachoroidal and subretinal fluid. A trephine incision, usually 7–8 mm in diameter, is made in the cornea. The cornea is penetrated in the upper quadrants by tilting the trephine and cutting the cornea more deeply in these quadrants than in the lower quadrants.

b **Corneal opening.** The trephine opening in the cornea is extended and completed 360° with corneal scissors to remove the corneal button, which is stored temporarily in a chamber filled with tissue-culture fluid. The iris is cut radially at 6 and 12 o'clock with de Wecker scissors. The lens is removed intracapsularly using the cryoprobe and a zonular stripper to break the zonules.

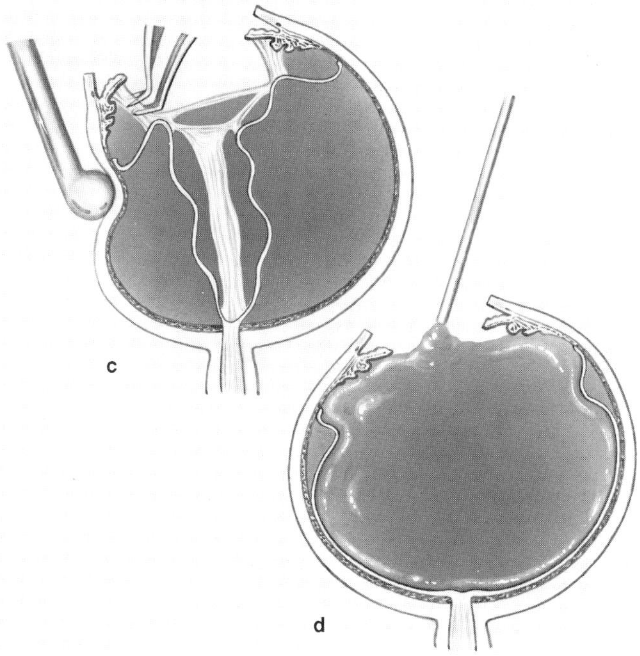

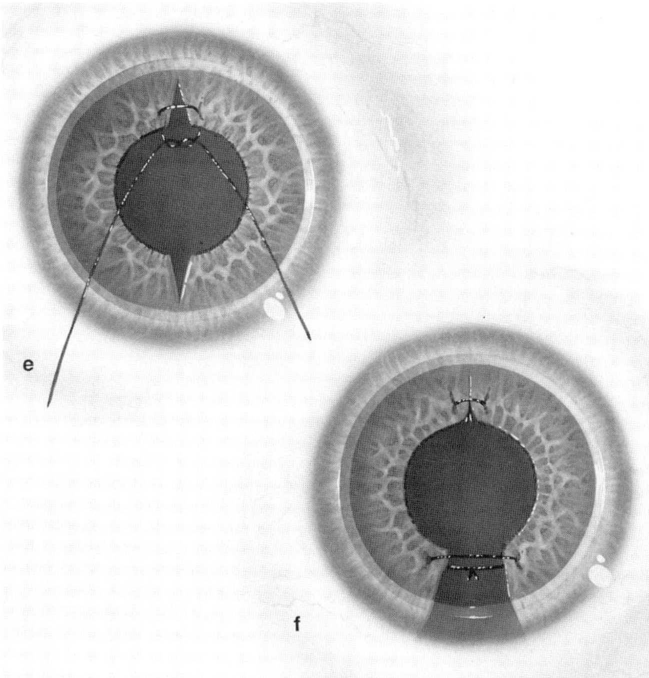

27.**5c** **Vitrectomy and membrane removal.** Anterior traction is released by dissecting the anterior membranes. The fibrous plate in front of the funnel is dissected in one piece. Blood vessels in the membrane and any bleeding retinal vessels are closed with diathermy. The posterior membrane is removed with a combination of vitrectomy probe and vitreous forceps with scissors. Visualization may be enhanced by scleral depression.

d **Subretinal fluid drainage.** When the retina is free of surface traction membranes and has become mobile, fluid vitreous is aspirated and replaced with sodium hyaluronate. The sclerochoroidotomy in one or more quadrants is retracted wide to drain subretinal fluid.

27.**5e** **Closure of iridotomies.** The iridotomies at 6 and 12 o'clock are closed with 10-0 polypropylene sutures near the pupillary margin to restore the circular shape of the pupil.

f **Closing the cornea.** The corneal button is replaced on the eye and sutured with 10-0 continuous nylon suture. Fluid in the vitreous cavity and anterior chamber is aspirated and replaced with sodium hyaluronate. The suture is pulled snugly to attain a tight anterior chamber and good approximation of the corneal wound. As more subretinal fluid is drained through the sclerotomy, additional sodium hyaluronate is injected into the eye if necessary. The sclerochoroidotomies are closed with 5-0 nylon sutures.

References

1. Charles S. Vitrectomy with ciliary body entry for retrolental fibroplasia. In: McPherson A, Hittner H, Kretzer F, eds. Retinopathy of prematurity. Toronto: B C Decker, 1986: 225–234.
2. Charles S. Vitreous microsurgery. 2nd ed. Baltimore: Williams and Wilkins, 1987: 158–171.
3. de Juan E, Machemer R. Retinopathy of prematurity. Retina 1987; 7: 63–69.
4. Federman JL, Shields JA, Altman B, et al. The surgical and nonsurgical management of persistent hyperplastic primary vitreous. Ophthalmology 1982; 89: 20–24.
5. Francois J. Persistent hyperplastic primary vitreous. Trans Can Ophthalmol Soc 1960; 23: 141–158.
6. Goldberg MF, Peyman GA. Pars plicata surgery in the child for pupillary membranes, persistent hyperplastic primary vitreous, and infantile cataract. In: Symposium on medical and surgical diseases of the retina and vitreous: transactions of the New Orleans Academy of Ophthalmology. St. Louis: C V Mosby, 1983: 228.
7. Hirose TH. Open-sky vitrectomy. In: Waltman SR, Keates RH, Hoyt CS, Frueh BR, Herschler J, Caroll DM, eds. Surgery of the eye. New York: Churchill Livingstone, 1988, vol 2: 1012–1021.
8. Kwitko M. The infant eye. In: Kwitko M, ed. Surgery of the infant eye. New York: Appleton-Century-Crofts, 1979: 1.
9. Lightfoot D, Irvine AR. Vitrectomy in infants and children with retinal detachments caused by cicatricial retrolental fibroplasia. Am J. Opthalmol 1982; 94: 305–312.
10. Machemer R. Closed vitrectomy for severe retrolental fibroplasia in infants. Ophthalmology 1983; 90: 436–441.
11. McPherson A, Hittner H, Moura R, Kretzer F. Treatment of retrolental fibroplasia with open-sky vitrectomy. In: McPherson A, Hittner H, Kretzer F, eds. Retinopathy of prematurity. Toronto: B C Decker, 1986: 193–208.
12. Marshall J. Congenital anomaly: persistence of the tunica vasculosa with subsequent buphthalmos. Trans Opthalmol Soc UK 1924; 44: 176–182.
13. Merritt JC, Lawson EE, Sprague DH, Eifrig DE. Lensectomy-vitrectomy for Stage 5 cicatricial retrolental fibroplasia. Ophthalmic Surg 1982; 13: 300–306.
14. Peyman GA, Schulman JA. Intravitreal surgery: principles and practice. New York: Appleton-Century-Crofts, 1986: 104.
15. Peyman GA, Sanders DR, Nagpal KC. Management of persistent hyperplastic primary vitreous by pars plana vitrectomy. Br J Ophthalmol 1976; 60: 756–758.
16. Pruett R, Schepens CL. Posterior hyperplastic primary vitreous. Am J Ophthalmol 1970; 69: 535–543.
17. Reese AB. Persistant hyperplastic primary vitreous. Am J Ophthalmol 1955; 40: 317–331.
18. Schepens CL. Retinal detachment and allied diseases. Philadelphia: W B Saunders, 1983, vol 2: 891–944.
19. Smith RE, Maumenee AE. Persistent hyperplastic primary vitreous: results of surgery. Trans Am Acad Ophthalmol Otolaryngol 1974; 78: 911–925.
20. Tasman W. Vitreoretinal changes in cicatricial retrolental fibroplasia. Trans Am Ophthalmol Soc 1970; 68: 548–564.
21. Tasman W. Late complications of retrolental fibroplasia. Ophthalmology 1979; 86: 1724–1740.
22. Tasman W. Retinopathy of prematurity. Ophthalmology 1985; 92: 995–999.
23. Trese MT. Surgical results of stage V retrolental fibroplasia and timing of surgical repair. Ophthalmology 1984; 91: 461–466.

28

Endophthalmitis

Endophthalmitis is a serious complication of intraocular surgery, penetrating ocular trauma, infected filtering conjunctival bleb, and immunosuppression (1, 2, 7, 9, 12). Virulent types of endophthalmitis, capable of destroying the retina within hours, are usually caused by mixed bacterial infection or gram-negative rods, and require vitrectomy without delay. Once endophthalmitis is suspected, the patient is hospitalized immediately, and broad-spectrum intravenous antibiotics should be started (4, 5, 10, 11). When potent antibiotics, including antifungal drugs, are planned, an infectious disease consultation is recommended. Preoperative and postoperative culture reports from previous surgery may provide a clue to the infecting organism (6).

In experienced hands, vitrectomy offers the best chance of saving vision and the eye with endopthalmitis. The culture specimens collected during vitrectomy facilitate early diagnosis and treatment. In addition, vitrectomy drains the abscess in the vitreous, allowing the infused broad-spectrum antibiotics to be distributed evenly in the vitreous cavity.

Immediate vitrectomy should be considered in eyes suspected of having endophthalmitis when at least one of the following conditions prevail: (a) profound and rapid visual loss, (b) absence of fundus view because of dense vitreous exudates, (c) history of recent penetrating trauma, and (d) presence of virulent bacteria in pre- and postoperative cultures.

In traumatic cases, removal of the crystalline lens with the vitrectomy probe is recommended, because the lens usually becomes cataractous. An intraocular lens implant does not have to be removed from eyes that undergo vitrectomy for endophthalmitis (3, 8). Its removal is imperative if the implant is thickly encapsulated with organized exudates that can not be aspirated with the probe.

Eyes with low-grade endophthalmitis may show minimal hypopyon, a clear vitreous, and no gross abnormal fundus findings. Nevertheless, a diagnostic tap of the anterior chamber and anterior vitreous is indicated in these eyes. The patient is sedated with 50 mg of intramuscular meperidine hydrochloride (Demerol) one hour prior to the procedure. The periorbital skin of the affected eye is swabbed with 5% povidone-iodine, and one drop is instilled topically. The cornea is anesthetized with a drop of 5% cocaine solution after 10% phenylephrine is instilled in the conjunctival cul-de-sac to minimize systemic absorption of the cocaine. The anterior chamber tap is carried out under magnification, with the patient seated in front of a slit lamp.

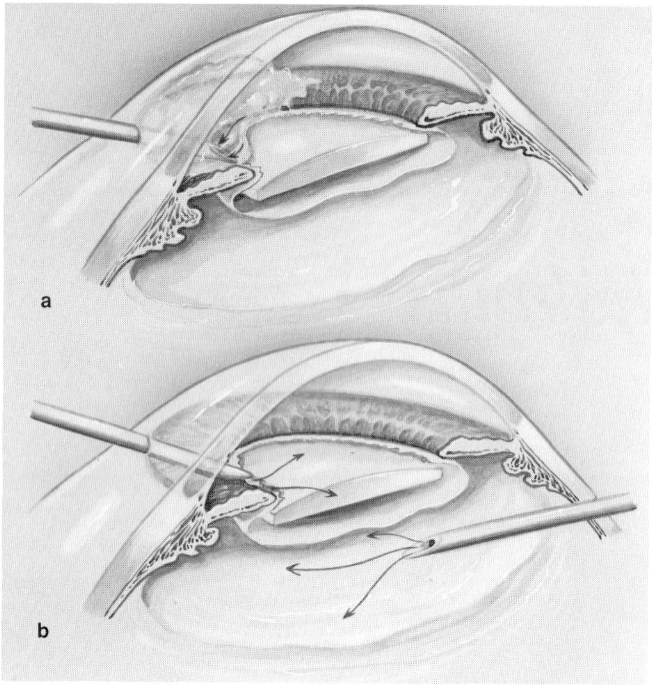

28.**1a** The setup for an anterior chamber tap includes a sterile lid speculum, a tuberculin syringe with a short 25-gauge needle, a cotton swab with a long handle, and test tubes for bacterial and fungal cultures. The long-handled cotton swab is pressed against the globe for counterpressure to stabilize it during insertion of the needle. The needle is introduced into the anterior chamber through a shelving needle incision in the cornea inferotemporally near the limbus. The anterior chamber exudate is aspirated until a 1/3 ml specimen has been obtained.

b The syringe containing the specimen is removed from the needle and replaced with a tuberculin syringe containing broad-spectrum antibiotics; 0.1 ml is injected slowly into the anterior chamber. The same amount is injected into the anterior vitreous 4 mm posterior to the limbus in the upper temporal quadrant, using a second syringe and needle containing half the dose injected into the anterior chamber. The injection site is anesthetized by applying 5% cocaine on a cotton swab. While the globe is stabilized with a cotton-tipped swab, the needle is inserted and directed toward the anterior vitreous. Antibiotic is injected slowly, with the bevel of the needle facing anteriorly.

The recommended antibiotic combinations and doses for intraocular injection in bacterial endophthalmitis are:

Gentamicin 100–200 μg/0.1 ml with cefazolin 2.25 mg/0.1 ml

Gentamicin 100–200 μg/0.1 ml with vancomycin 1.0 mg/0.1 ml

Tobramycin 100–200 μg/0.1 ml with cefazolin 2.25 mg/0.1 ml

Amikacin 400 μg/0.1 ml with vancomycin 1.0 mg/0.1 ml

The recommended antifungal agents and doses for vitreous injection in fungal endophthalmitis are:

Amphotericin 5–10 μg/0.1 ml

Miconazole 10–50 μg/0.1 ml

The recommended dose of ganciclovir for vitreous injection in viral retinitis is 200 μg/0.1 ml or 30–60 μg/ml infused with BSS Plus during vitrectomy.

If an intraocular steroid is indicated, 400 μg/0.1 ml of dexamethasone may be injected into the vitreous.

The standard vitrectomy setup for endophthalmitis includes a vitrectomy probe pack, three-way stopcock, 3 ml plastic syringe, two bottles of BSS Plus (one containing broad-spectrum antibiotics), slides for gram staining, and culture tubes. When adequate specimens have been collected, the stopcock to the syringe is closed and the syringe is removed. The evacuation line is opened to aspirate the remaining anterior chamber exudates and fibrin on the anterior surface of the intraocular lens. The limbal incision or incisions are closed.

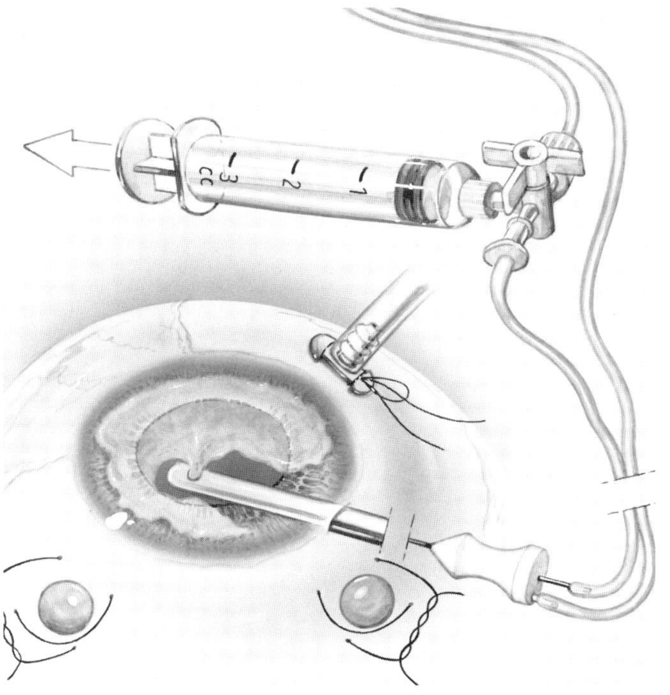

28.**2a** The infusion cannula is inserted inferotemporally. The sclerotomies are closed temporarily with plugs. The corneal wound is inspected and strengthened with additional sutures as needed.

Evacuation line: the Microvit vitrectomy system is provided with fittings along the evacuation line for a three-way stopcock attached to a Luer-Lok syringe.

Infusion line: one 500 ml bottle of BSS Plus contains the antibiotic solution, usually 20 mg of gentamicin or 1000 mg of cefazolin. This bottle is used during the vitrectomy. A 500 ml bottle of BSS Plus without antibiotic provides infusion during collection of the specimen for culture.

Removal of exudates from the anterior chamber: the vitrectomy probe is introduced into the anterior chamber through a limbal incision. Collapse of the anterior chamber during aspiration of the exudate suggests that a capsulotomy was not performed during intraocular lens implantation. If this is the case, a 20-gauge needle is inserted at the limbus for infusion of BSS Plus into the anterior chamber.

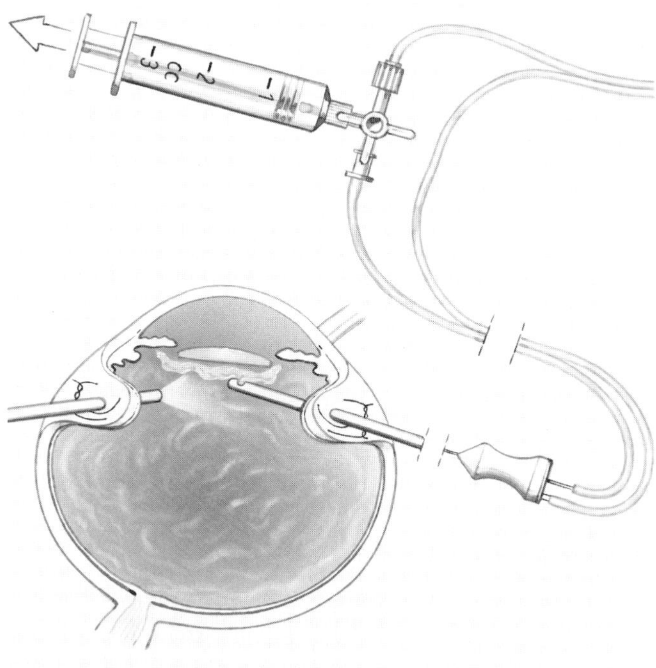

28.**2b** **Vitrectomy:** a Luer-Lok syringe is attached to the three-way stopcock connected to the evacuation line, as in Figure 28.**2a.** The endoilluminator and the vitrectomy probe are introduced into the vitreous cavity. Using the syringe for aspiration, anterior vitrectomy and removal of opacities on the posterior lens surface are done.

The syringe is removed as soon as adequate specimens have been collected. The stopcock is turned to open the evacuation line, and the bottle containing antibiotic is used to infuse the vitreous.

To preclude retinal damage, vitrectomy is confined to the central vitreous, avoiding the cortical vitreous (3).

The specimens are brought without delay to the laboratory, where slides are made for Gram staining. The specimens are planted in the following culture media:

- Blood agar (at 25 °C and 37 °C) for bacterial and fungal infection
- Chocolate agar for *Hemophilus* and *Neisseria*
- Thioglycolate media for anaerobic bacteria
- Sabouraud's media for fungi and yeast

References

1. Allen HF, Mangiaracine AB. Bacterial endophthalmitis after cataract extraction, II: incidence in 36,000 consecutive operations, with special reference to preoperative topical antibiotics. Trans Am Acad Ophthalmol Otolaryngol 1973; 77: 581–588.
2. Blankenship GW. Endophthalmitis after pars plana vitrectomy. Am J Ophthalmol 1977; 84: 815–817.
3. Charles S. Vitreous microsurgery. 2nd ed. Baltimore: Williams and Wilkins, 1987: 196.
4. Cottingham AJ, Forster RK. Vitrectomy in endophthalmitis: results of study using vitrectomy, intraocular antibiotics, or a combination of both. Arch Ophthalmol 1976; 94: 2078–2082.
5. Diamond JG. Intraocular management of endophthalmitis: a systematic approach. Arch Ophthalmol 1981; 99: 96–99.
6. Forster RK. Endophthalmitis: diagnostic cultures and visual results. Arch Ophthalmol 1974; 92: 387–392.
7. Forster RK. Endophthalmitis. In: Duane TD, ed. Clinical ophthalmology. Hagerstown, MD: Harper and Row, 1978, vol 4: 1–20.
8. Flynn HW Jr. Vitrectomy in the management of infectious endophthalmitis. In: Blankenship GW, Stirpe M, Gonvers M, Binder S, eds. Basic and advanced vitreous surgery. Padua: Liviana, 1986: 333–341.
9. Ho PC, Tolentino FI. Bacterial endophthalmitis after closed vitrectomy. Arch Ophthalmol 1984; 102: 207–210.
10. Olson JC, Flynn HW, Forster RK, Culbertson WW. Results in the treatment of postoperative endophthalmitis. Ophthalmology 1983; 90: 692–699.
11. Peyman GA. Antibiotic administration in the treatment of bacterial endophthalmitis, II: intravitreal injections. Surv Ophthalmol 1977; 21: 332–346.
12. Puliafito CA, Baker AS, Haaf J, Foster CS. Infectious endophthalmitis: review of 36 cases. Ophthalmology 1982; 89: 921–928.

29

Clotted Hyphema

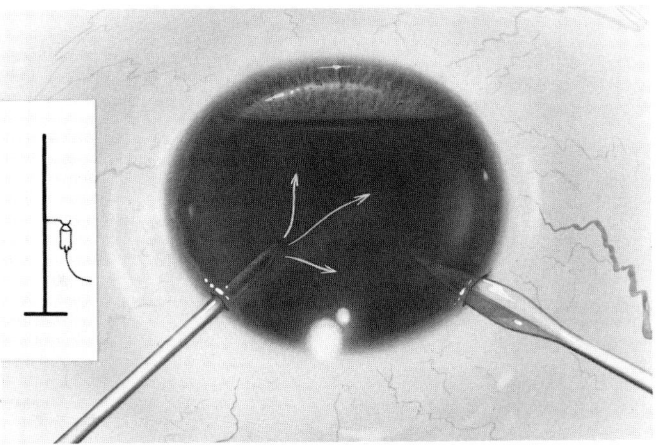

29.**1a** **Anterior chamber hemorrhage.** If a large traumatic hyphema is associated with an elevation of intraocular pressure that cannot be lowered with antiglaucomatous drops and acetazolamide, evacuation of the hyphema is indicated. It is important to rule out systemic causes of rebleeding by conducting coagulation studies and sickle cell preparation or hemoglobin electrophoresis (4, 5, 10). Preoperatively, intraocular pressure is lowered with acetazolamide and intravenous mannitol. The operation is performed under general anesthesia. To prevent hypotony and collapse of the anterior chamber, balanced saline solution is infused into the anterior chamber. A beveled limbal incision is made with the MVR knife, and a bent 20-gauge needle is inserted at the limbus with the bevel directed toward the plane of the iris. Irrigation of the blood is facilitated by depression of the outer lip of the incision (1, 2). If this fails because of an organized clot, a vitrectomy probe is used for its removal (2, 3, 6–9).

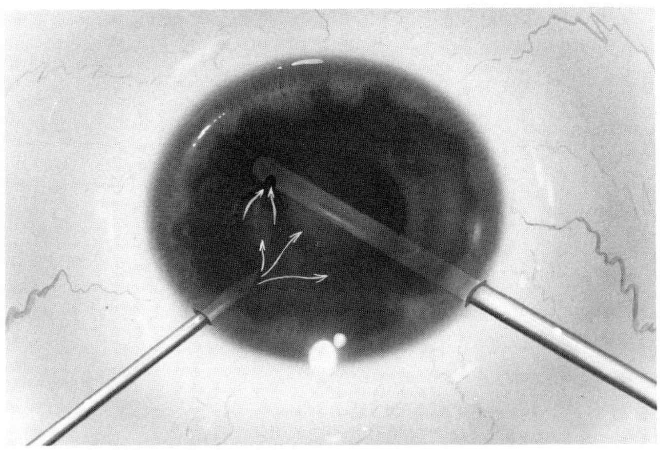

29.**1b** With the suction port at 90° to the plane of the iris, gentle suction is directed to the blood clot overlying the mid-portion of the iris. It is preferable to use the suction rather than the cutting mode of the instrument. If rebleeding occurs, or the anterior chamber shallows during suction, the infusion bottle is raised and the suction pressure reduced. The more peripheral portion of the clot, and finally the clot over the pupil, are removed. Great care should be exercised to avoid contact with iris tissue, which is hyperemic, friable, and prone to bleed. If a clot seems firmly adherent to the iris, the clot is circumcised and left in the anterior chamber.

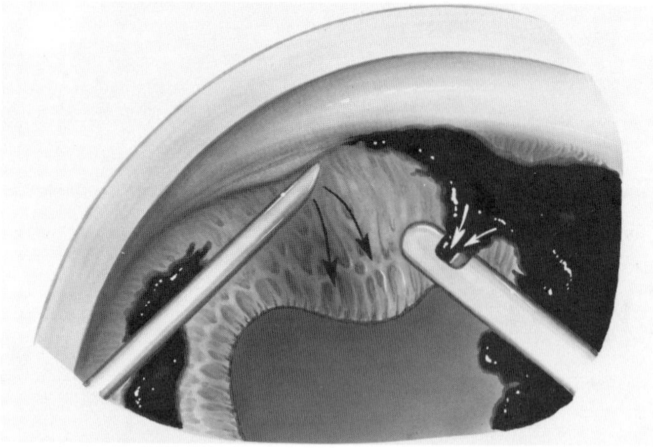

29.**1c** If a traumatic iris dialysis is suspected to be the source of hemorrhage, aspiration is continued in an effort to reveal the source of bleeding. The tip of the infusion needle is directed toward the bleeding site to improve visualization.

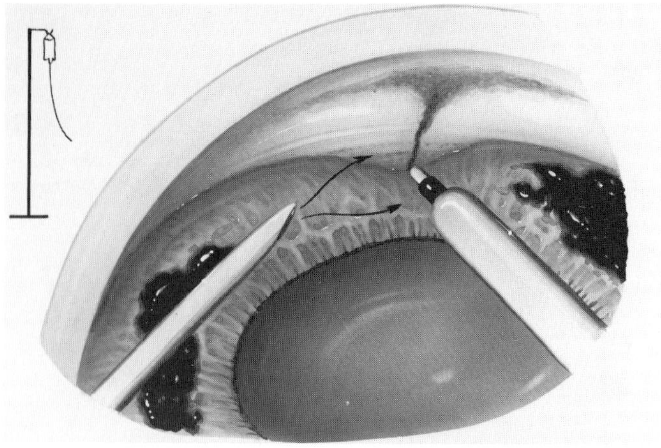

29.**1d** If a bleeding site can be visualized, it is cauterized with underwater diathermy. Following removal of the clot and blood, care should be taken to prevent prolonged hypotony either during or following removal of the instruments and cannula from the anterior chamber. A 10-0 nylon suture may be necessary to produce a watertight seal at the incision for the vitrectomy instrument.

Postoperatively, antiglaucoma medications, topical steroids, and a cycloplegic are prescribed.

References

1. Belcher CD III, Brown SVL, Simmons RJ. Anterior chamber washout for traumatic hyphema. Ophthalmic Surg 1985; 16: 475–479.
2. Deutsch TA, Feller DB. Management of ocular injuries. 2nd ed. Philadelphia: W B Saunders, 1985: 189–199.
3. Diddle, KR, Ernest JT. Rotoextractor evacuation of total hyphema. Ophthalmic Surg 1976; 7: 49–51.
4. Goldberg MF. The diagnosis and treatment of sickled erythrocytes in human hyphemas. Trans Am Ophthalmol Soc 1978; 76: 481–501.
5. Grayson M, Wilson FM II. Traumatic hyphema. In: Freeman HM, ed. Ocular trauma. New York: Appleton-Century-Crofts, 1979: 145–149.
6. McCuen BW, Fung WE. The role of vitrectomy instrumentation in the treatment of severe traumatic hyphema. Am J Ophthalmol 1979; 88: 930–934.
7. Michels RM. Blunt trauma, penetrating injuries, intraocular foreign bodies. Highlights Ophthalmol 1985; 1: 7–11.
8. Read J, Goldberg MF. Comparisons of medical treatment for traumatic hyphema. Trans Am Acad Ophthalmol Otolaryngol 1974; 78: 799–815.
9. Stern WH, Mondal KM. Vitrectomy instrumentation for surgical evacuation of total anterior chamber hyphema and control of recurrent anterior chamber hemorrhage. Ophthalmic Surg 1979; 10: 34–37.
10. Wilson FM II. Traumatic hyphema: pathogenesis and management. Ophthalmology 1980; 87: 910–919.

30

Corneoscleral Laceration, Lens Damage, and Vitreous Hemorrhage

Guidelines for Repairing Corneal Wounds

Because the repair of a corneal wound may be involved in the management of injuries of the posterior segment (11, 15), brief guidelines for the repair of corneal wounds are included in this chapter.

Vitrectomy. Vitrectomy is performed because lens material, vitreous hemorrhage, and vitreous gel may incite a marked inflammatory response in the anterior vitreous. This may result in the formation of membranes that lead to tractional or rhegmatogenous retinal detachment, or traction to the ciliary body causing hypotony and ultimately phthisis bulbi (2, 3).

Timing of Vitrectomy. Controversy exists regarding the timing of vitrectomy in certain posterior segment injuries (1, 9, 13, 16, 17). Most vitreoretinal surgeons agree that vitrectomy is indicated at the time of primary repair or a penetrating injury in eyes with endophthalmitis or reactive nonmagnetic foreign bodies such as copper, nickel, brass, or iron. In the case of a corneoscleral laceration with vitreous hemorrhage, some vitreoretinal surgeons recommend vitrectomy at the time of or within 3 days following the primary repair (4). We advocate the removal of vitreous from the anterior chamber, lensectomy, and, if visualization permits, anterior vitrectomy during the primary repair. Posterior vitrectomy is usually performed 5–14 days later, depending on the clarity of the cornea. If ultrasonography indicates a partial retinal detachment, especially a nasal one, vitrectomy is performed as soon as possible to prevent the retinal detachment from extending to involve the macula.

Tetanus prophylaxis and prophylactic antibiotics. Tetanus prophylaxis is given in patients who have not been previously immunized. We recommend prophylactic antibiotics in penetrating injuries involving the posterior segment when there is a relatively high clinical suspicion of infection due to probable contamination during or following the injury. After a specimen has been taken for culture and sensitivity, topical administration of gentamicin sulfate drops (10–20 mg/ml) and cefazolin sodium (100 mg/ml) is given hourly preoperatively. If there is a high index of suspicion of infection, and exudate is noted around the wound, 1 mg of cefazolin in 0.1 ml diluent and 0.2 mg gentamicin in 0.1 ml diluent are injected into the vitreous as the last step of the primary repair. Gentamicin sulfate (40 mg/ml) and cefazolin sodium (100 mg/ml) in 0.1 ml diluent each are injected suconjunctivally following closure of the conjunctiva.

We believe that intravitreous antibiotics are indicated during surgery and postoperatively in patients with a penetrating ocular injury. A 4-day course of intravenous therapy is probably efficacious in preventing infection. At the end of this period, all antibiotics are discontinued, and the patient is observed for 24–48 hours. If there is no sign of infection, the patient is discharged from the hospital without topical antibiotics.

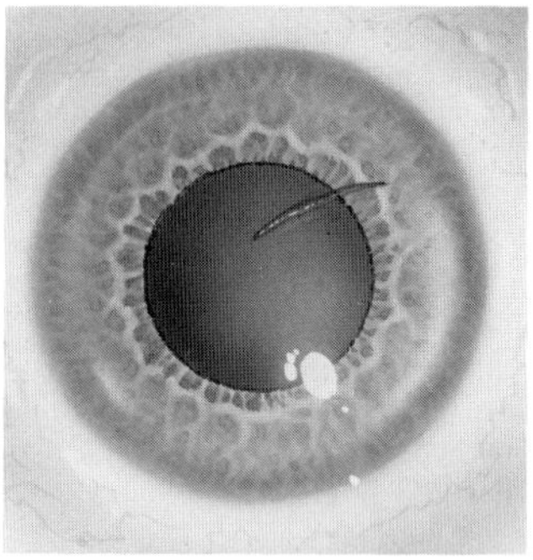

a

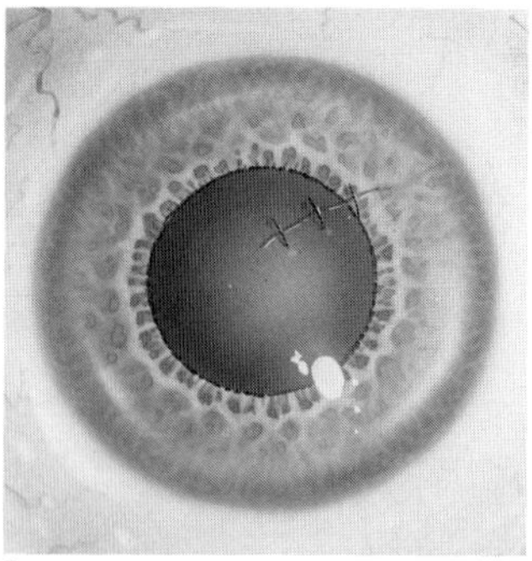

b

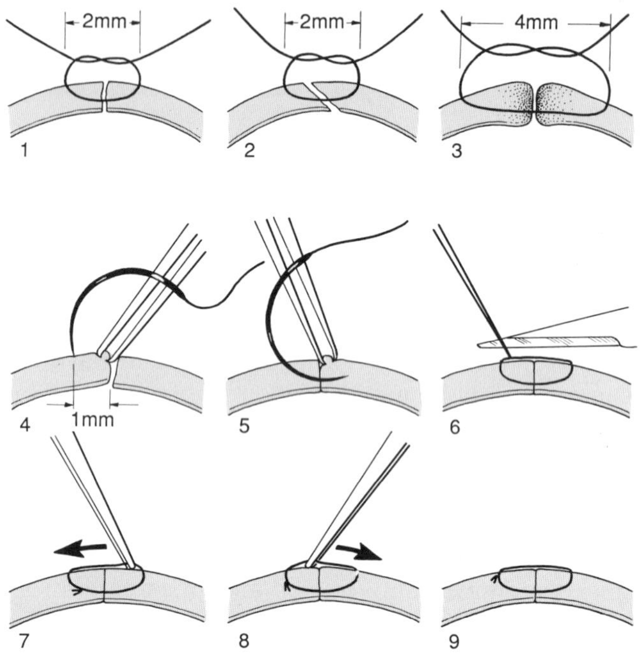

Corneal Lacerations

30.**1 a, b Repair of small corneal laceration.** To repair a small corneal laceration in an eye in which the anterior chamber is formed, the first suture is placed in the center of the wound (**a**), and subsequent sutures are placed midway between that suture and each end of the wound (**b**).

30.**1 c Corneal laceration in eyes with posterior segment trauma.**

1 Suture placement in a corneal wound with straight nonedematous edges. It is important to place the 10-0 nylon sutures deep in the cornea to avoid posterior gaping of the wound. The arms of the suture are placed 2 mm apart.

2 Suture placement in a beveled corneal wound. A larger bite is taken on the long side of the beveled edge of the wound.

3 Suture placement in a wound with edematous edges. Suture arms are placed 4 mm apart to engage stronger corneal tissue.

4 Corneal wound suturing. The edge of the wound is grasped with Castroviejo forceps with 0.12 mm teeth. The needle of the 10-0 nylon suture is entered at right angles 1 mm from the edge of the slightly everted wound.

5 During passage of the needle through the corneal stroma, slight traction to the opposite wound edge apposes the inner aspects of the wound, and helps to maintain the anterior chamber.

6 The suture is tied with a three-throw knot cinched to one side. After the knot is tightened so that no stress lines are visible in the cornea, two additional single throws are placed in opposite directions.

7 To bury the knot, the suture arm at the opposite end of the knot is grasped with tying forceps, and traction is applied in the direction of the knot.

8, 9 Slight countertraction in the opposite direction will leave the small trailing suture ends directed away from the corneal surface. This will permit easy removal of the sutures later when traction is applied to the end of the suture near the knot.

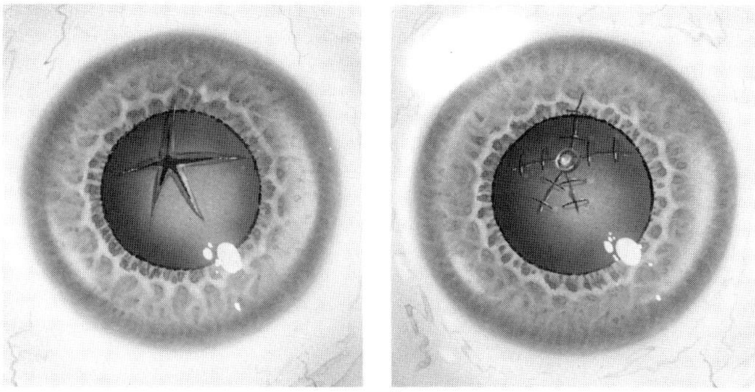

a b

30.2 Repair of stellate corneal wounds.
a A centrally-located stellate wound with loss of corneal tissue at the apex of the wound.

b We recommend the technique described by Hirst et al. (11) for the closure of stellate wounds with tissue loss. The limbs of the wound are closed with temporary 10-0 nylon sutures placed at right angles to the axis of the wound.

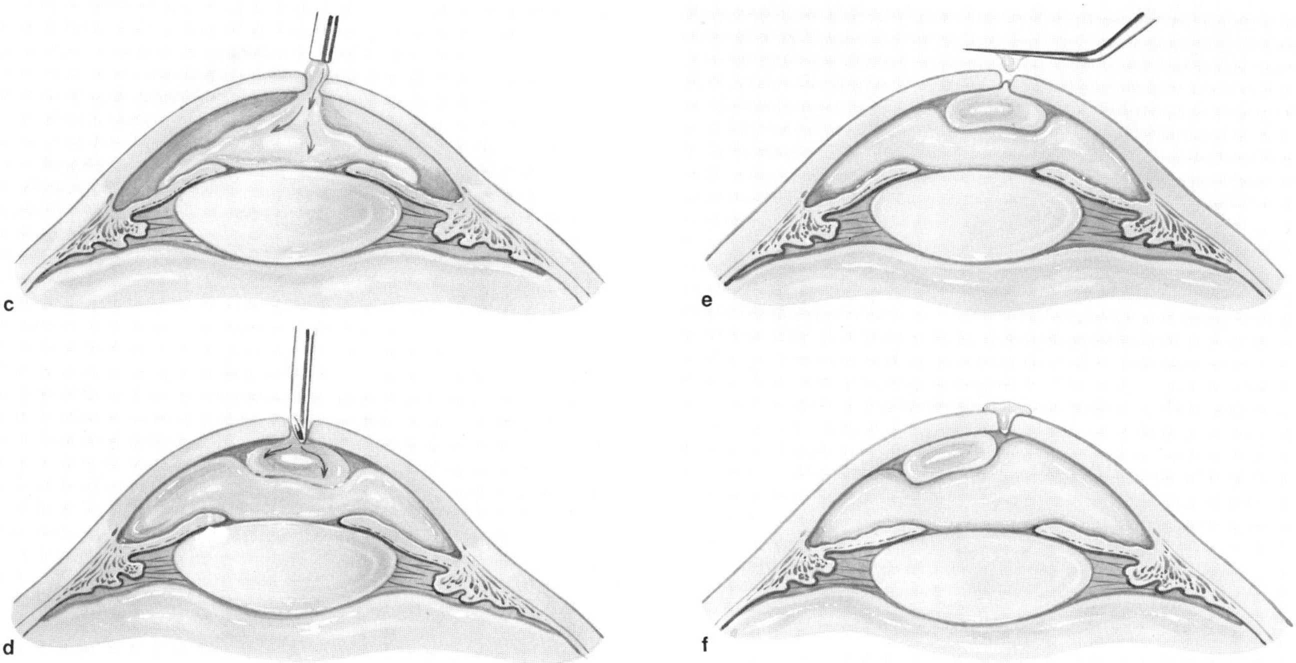

30.**2c** Sodium hyaluronate is injected through the defect in the wound to separate the iris from the posterior surface of the wound, and to partially reform the anterior chamber, which permits better placement of definitive corneal sutures (16).

d Loss of corneal tissue may require isobutyl 2-cyanoacrylate tissue adhesive to stop leakage of aqueous through the tissue defect (4). A small bubble of air is injected from a 30-gauge cannula into the sodium hyaluronate to maintain a small meniscus of air-fluid interface under the corneal tissue defect.

30.**2e** A small amount of corneal epithelium is debrided around the wound edge. The base of the perforation site is simultaneously dried with a cellulose sponge held in one hand, while the other hand applies a small drop of tissue adhesive from the undersurface of a retina or iris spatula. Care must be taken to place the glue on a completely dry surface, or it will not seal the wound.

f As the tissue adhesive dries, the anterior chamber will become watertight and spontaneously deepen.

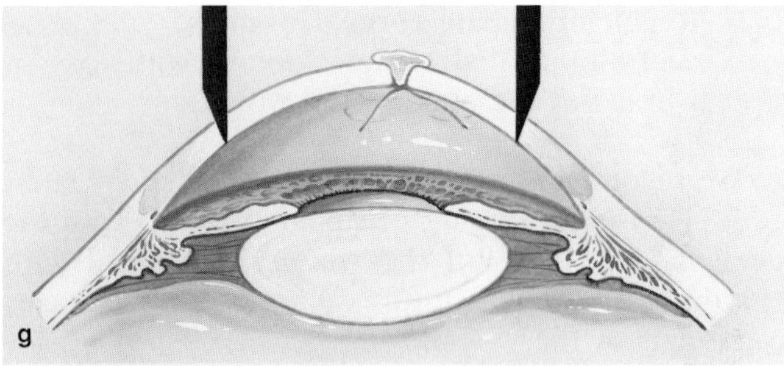

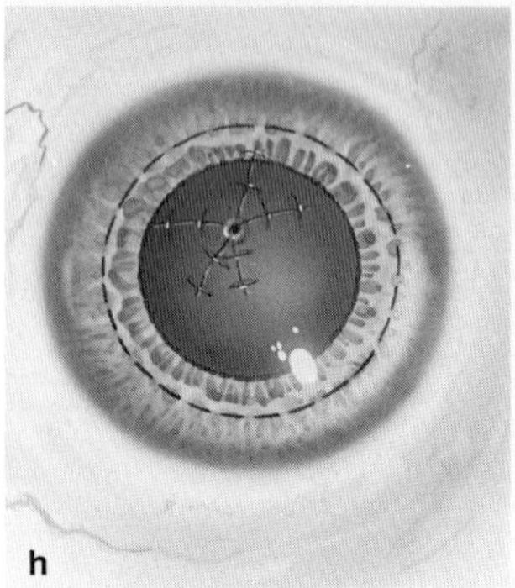

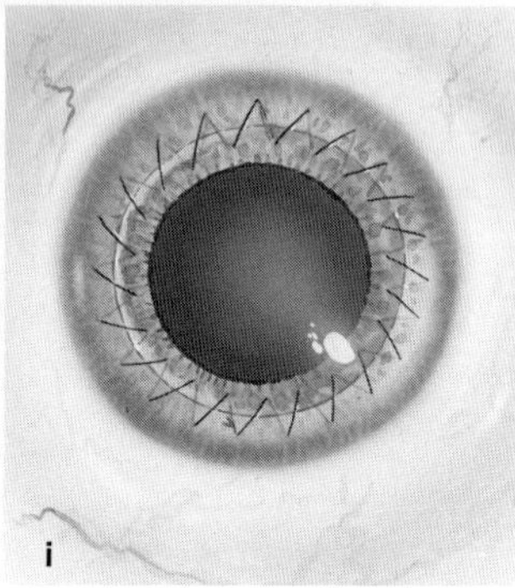

30.**2g** If the anterior chamber reforms spontaneously, further corneal surgery, such as a patch graft or keratoplasty, may be deferred. A patch graft or freehand-cut donor corneal tissue may be helpful in closing large or irregular defects resulting from tissue loss. Primary keratoplasty for corneal wounds is rarely indicated or required. Penetrating keratoplasty for extensive scars in the visual axis is performed at a subsequent session.

h In rare instances, where the central cornea is so extensively damaged that the anterior chamber cannot be reformed, a penetrating keratoplasty can be performed at the time of the primary wound repair. A corneal trephine is selected to encompass the stellate laceration. A suction trephine (Hessburg-Barron) may facilitate trephination in a soft eye (5).

i A graft from a donor eye is sutured to the cornea with continuous 10-0 nylon sutures.

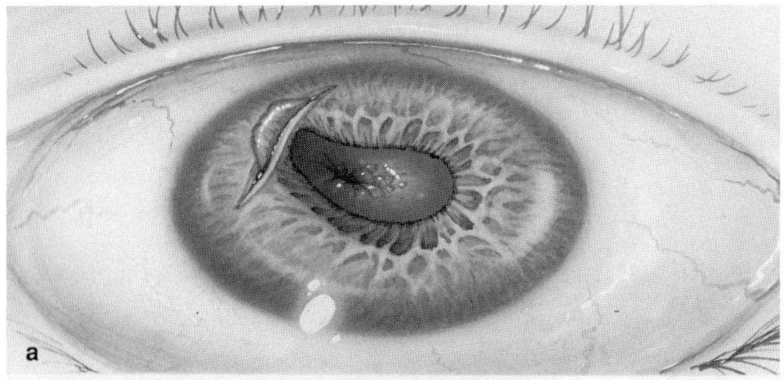

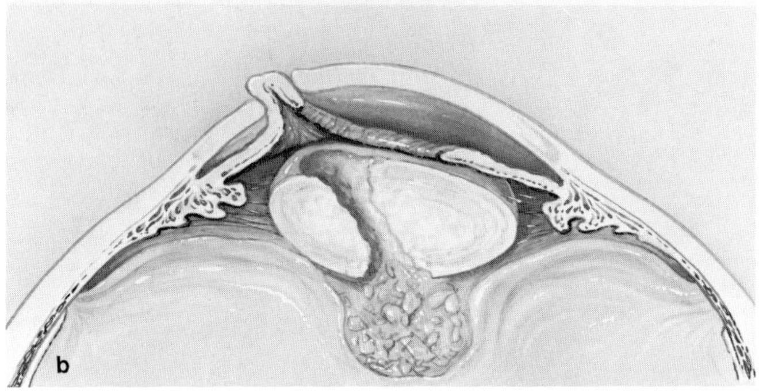

30.**3a** **Corneal laceration with iris tissue incarceration and lens damage.** Corneal laceration is associated with iris prolapse resulting in a pear-shaped pupil.

b Iris tissue is incarcerated in the wound; the anterior chamber is shallowed, and the lens ruptured. Lens material is present in the retrolental space and anterior vitreous gel.

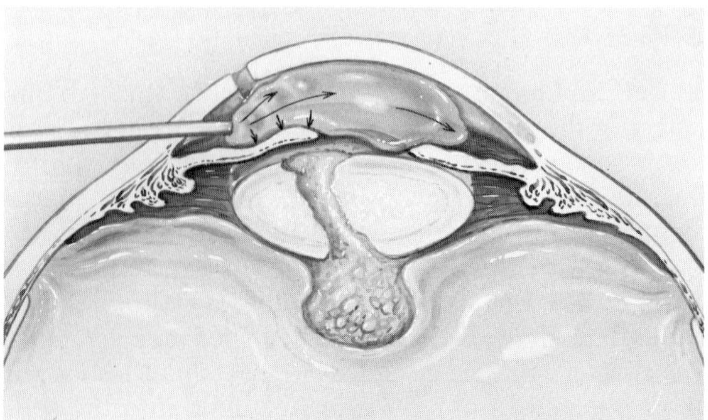

30.**3c** If the prolapse is small, an attempt may be made to reposit it using sodium hyaluronate injected through a Ziegler knife incison at the limbus. The major risk in repositing an iris prolapse is infection. Risk of infection increases with time; therefore, if repair is undertaken more than 24 hours after the injury, any prolapsed uveal or iris tissue be excised, even if it appears viable (10). Cases with extensive iris prolapse are treated by excision of the prolapse, which is cut flush with the corneal surface. Prolapsed iris should be excised if the wound is dirty, or signs of infection are present. The corneal wound then is closed with 10-0 nylon sutures.

Lens Damage

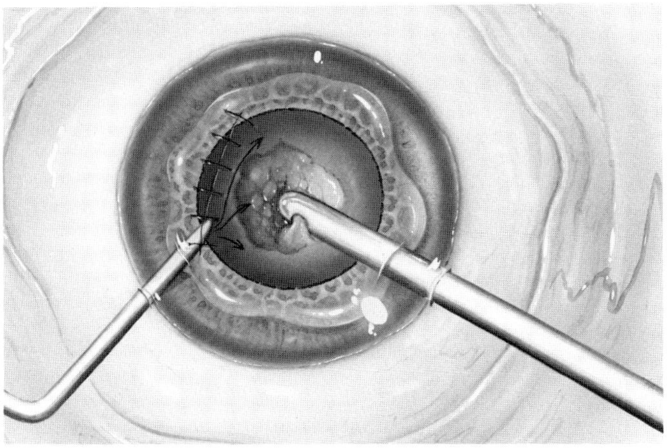

30.**3 d** **Lensectomy.** A mydriatic solution of 0.1 ml of a 1:10,000 solution of epinephrine bitartrate is injected into the anterior chamber to dilate the pupil so that lens damage can be assessed. Unless capsule rupture can be clearly identified, lensectomy should not be attempted during the primary repair. If lens damage is extensive, and one suspects that lens material is in the vitreous, a lensectomy is performed. A bent 25-gauge needle is used for infusion into the anterior chamber during lensectomy, which is performed with a vitrectomy instrument introduced through another limbal incision. The lens material can be removed by suction in young persons; in older persons, cutting action may be necessary. With a very sclerotic nucleus, ultransonic fragmentation or an extracapsular extraction may be required.

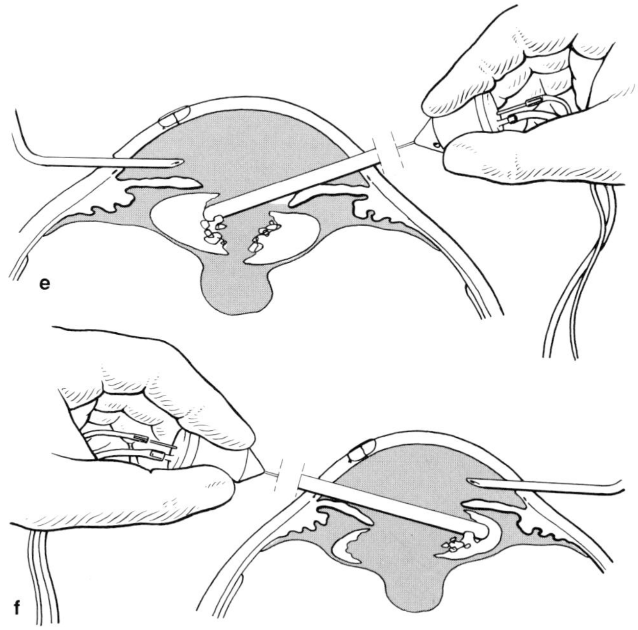

30.**3 e** It is important to remove peripheral cortical lens material. Residual lens material may incite an inflammatory response in the vitreous base, which may lead to the development of anterior proliferative vitreoretinopathy. In addition, removal of lens material will improve visualization of the region of the vitreous base.

f To remove as much peripheral cortical lens material as possible from both sides of the globe, the insertion of the infusion needle and vitrectomy probe through the limbal incisions is alternated.

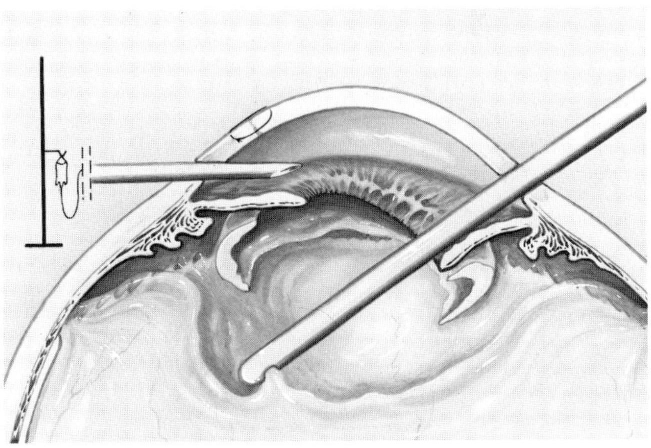

30.**3 g** **Anterior vitrectomy.** Vitrectomy is confined to the removal of the retrolental vitreous. Vitrectomy farther peripherally is fraught with risk, because of poor visualization due to inadequate illumination of the peripheral vitreous through the pupil.

4a

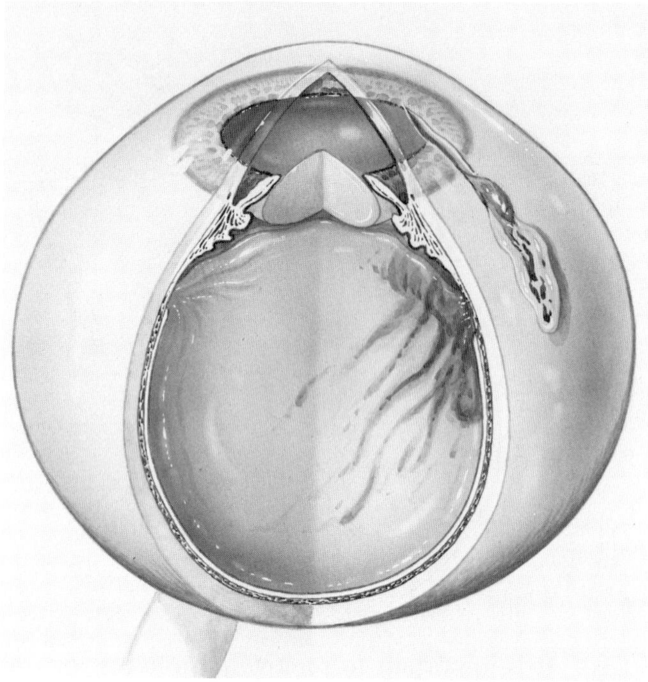

4c

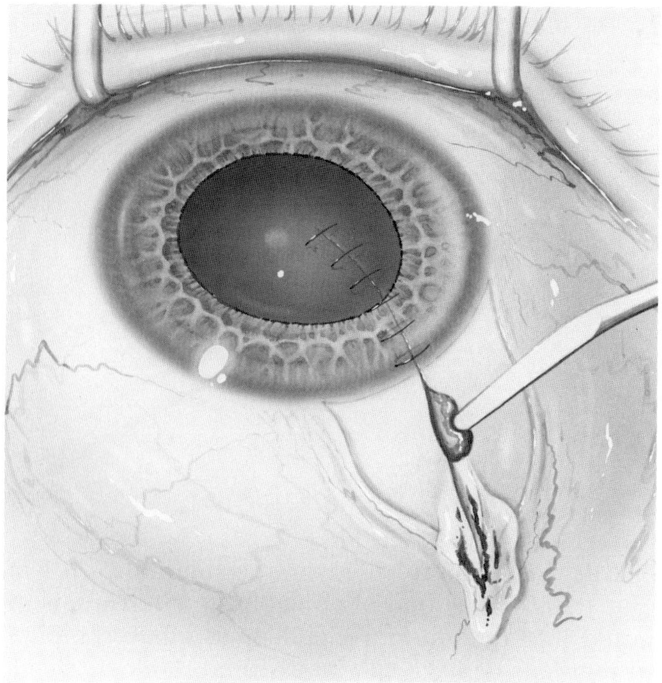

4b

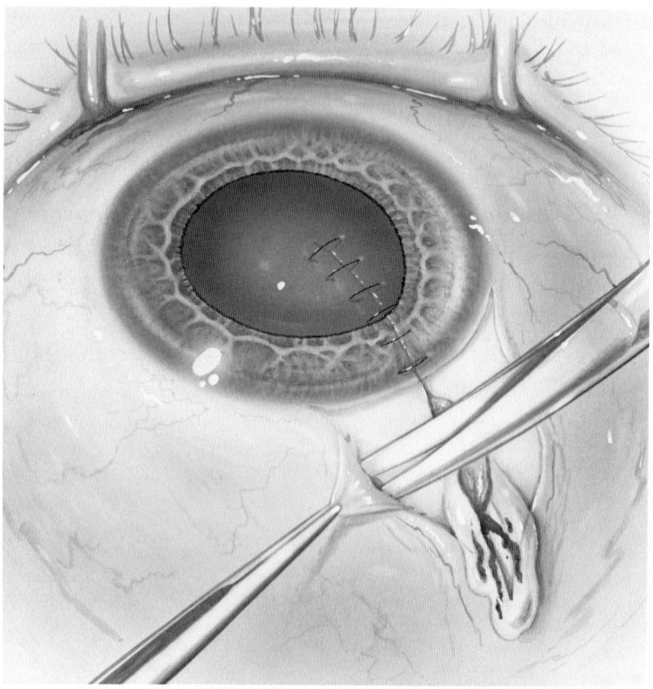

Vitreous Hemorrhage

30.**4a** Corneoscleral laceration with vitreous hemorrhage and prolapse of uveal tissue and vitreous.

30.**4b** **Exploration of extent of scleral damage.** The first corneal suture is placed at the limbus in an effort to obtain optimal approximation of the corneoscleral wound. After the corneal laceration is sutured and the anterior chamber is reformed, a peritomy is performed for a quadrant on either side of the scleral wound. To determine the posterior extent of the laceration, the conjunctiva and Tenon's capsule are reflected by sharp dissection using sharp curved iris scissors and smooth Bishop-Harmon forceps. It there is any question of a second perforation, the peritomy is extended around 360° and the globe is explored posteriorly. Using calipers to measure the distance posterior to the limbus, the posterior extent of the wound is recorded. Wounds extending more than 5 mm posteriorly will involve the vitreous base and retina.

30.**4c** **Management of prolapsing uveal tissue.** If the prolapsing uveal tissue appears viable, an attempt should be made to reposit it with an iris or retinal spatula. Uveal tissue bleeds profusely when cut; however, if it appears grossly contaminated, it is excised. The tissue is diathermized with wet-field cautery before and during excision. Excised tissue suspected of containing retina is submitted for histological examination.

4d

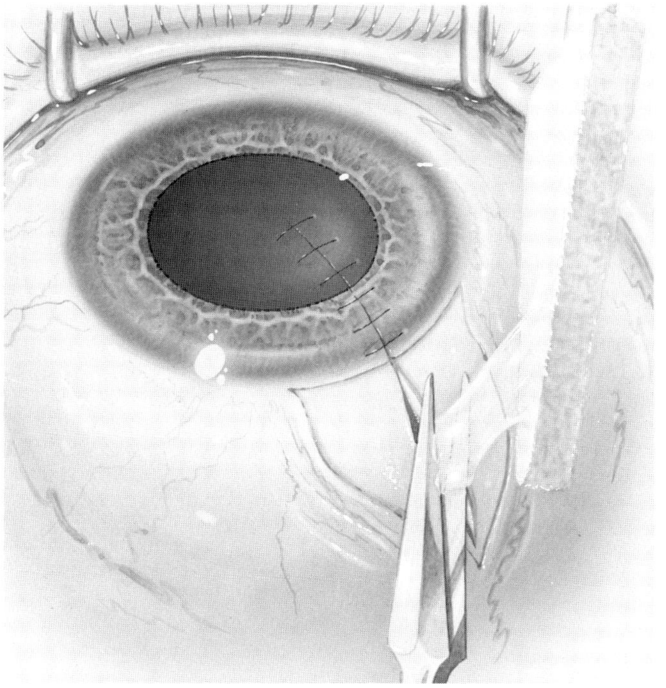

4f

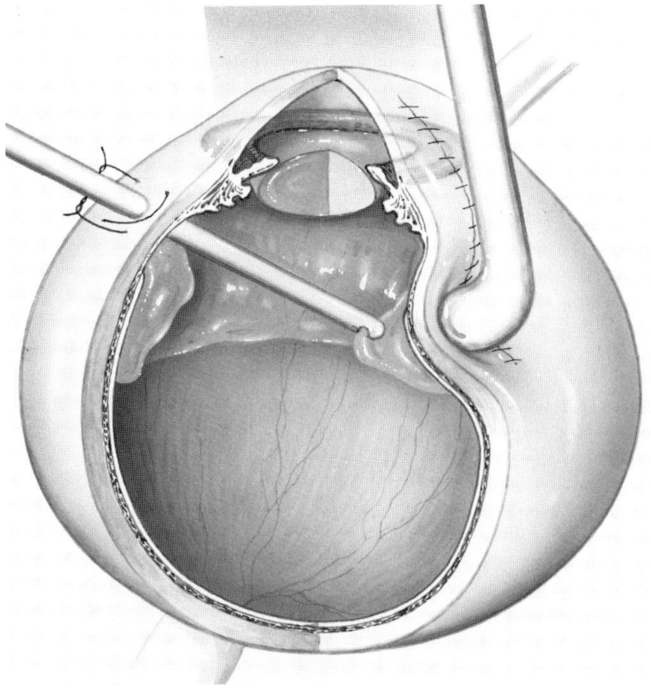

4e

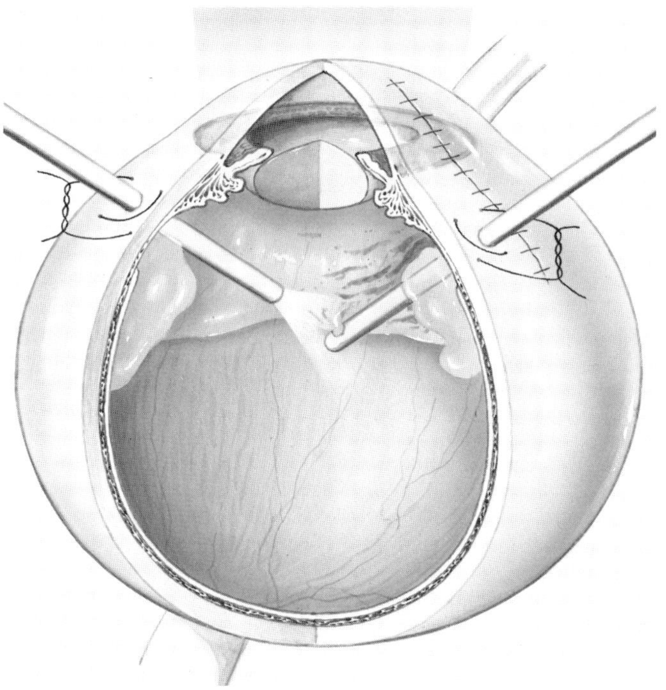

30.**4d Management of vitreous prolapse.** Using Vannas scissors, prolapsing vitreous gel is gently drawn away from the globe to cut it flush with the wound. The sponge should not be introduced deeply into the wound, because vitreous gel may be adherent to the retina, and traction by the sponge may draw retina or pars plana epithelium into the wound. The scleral wound is then closed using interrupted 8-0 nylon sutures.

If extensive damage to the lens is evident, and especially if cortical material and vitreous hemorrhage are present, a lensectomy and anterior vitrectomy are carried out, as described in Figure 30.**3g**. The conjunctiva is closed with 5-0 chromic sutures.

Postoperative follow-up. If vitreous hemorrhage obscures the fundus, ultrasonography is done 5–7 days postoperatively to determine whether a rhegmatogenous retinal or choroidal detachment has developed, and to ascertain the density and extent of the vitreous hemorrhage.

30.**4e Central and posterior vitrectomy.** Depending on the clarity of the cornea, a vitrectomy is performed 5–14 days after the primary repair. By this time the posterior vitreous is usually detached, making posterior vitrectomy easier. Ultrasonography is helpful in deciding the length of the infusion cannula to be used. A 6 mm infusion cannula is used if the eye is aphakic, and ultrasonography indicates that a choroidal or retinal detachment may be present in the quadrant selected for insertion of the infusion cannula. The 6 mm cannula has a better chance of penetrating the choroidal detachment or elevated pars plana, so that it will infuse the vitreous cavity rather than produce an extensive elevation of the uvea. Vitrectomy is begun near the midline adjacent to the equatorial plane of the vitreous cavity, and then extended posteriorly to the detached posterior hyaloid.

30.**4f Vitrectomy involving the region of the vitreous base.** The incidence of tractional retinal detachment, or the development of anterior proliferative vitreoretinopathy, may be reduced by the removal of the peripheral vitreous (7, 8). Providing visualization is good, the peripheral vitreous is cautiously removed. Scleral depression is used to detect traction to the underlying retina during vitrectomy.

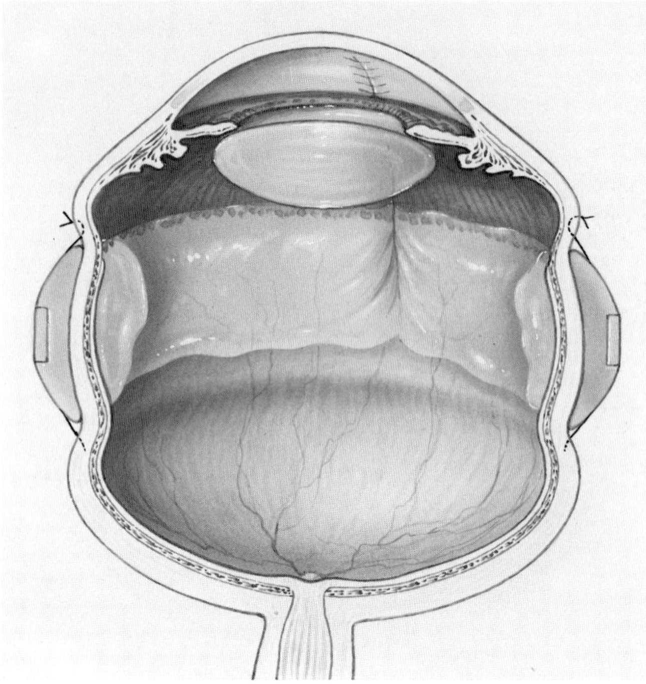

30.**4g Endolaser and episcleral buckling.** A fluid-air exchange is performed. If indirect ophthalmoscopy reveals that iatrogenic or traumatic retinal breaks are present, they are surrounded with endolaser photocoagulation. Three rows of endophotocoagulation are applied between the ora serrata and the equator the entire circumference of the fundus.

An episcleral buckling is performed to reduce postoperative vitreous traction from the remainder of the vitreous base (12). A solid silicone rubber implant (# 279), 9 mm wide, and an encircling band, are used to produce a scleral buckle. The implant is anchored so as to produce a low buckling effect from the ora serrata to include the region of the equator.

References

1. Brinton GS, Aaberg TM, Reeser FH, et al. Surgical results in ocular trauma involving the posterior segment. Am J Ophthalmol 1982; 93: 271–278.
2. Cleary PE, Ryan SJ. Histology of wound, vitreous, and retina in experimental posterior penetrating eye injury in the rhesus monkey. Am J Ophthalmol 1979; 88: 221–231.
3. Cleary PE, Ryan SJ. Method of production and natural history of experimental posterior penetrating eye injury in the rhesus monkey. Am J Ophthalmol 1979; 88: 212–220.
4. Coleman DJ. Early vitrectomy in the management of the severely traumatized eye. Am J Ophthalmol 1982; 93: 543–551.
5. Deutsch TA, Feller DB. In: Paton D, Goldberg MF, eds. Management of ocular injuries. 2nd ed. Philadelphia: W B Saunders, 1985: 143–144.
6. Eagling EM. Eye injuries. Philadelphia: J B Lippincott, 1987: 6.1–6.71.
7. Elner SG, Elner VM, Diaz-Rohena R, et al. Anterior PVR, part II: clinicopathologic, light microscopic, and ultrastructural findings. In: Freeman HM, Tolentino FI, eds. Proliferative vitreoretinopathy (PVR). New York: Springer, 1988: 34–45.
8. Freeman HM, Elner SG, Tolentino FI, et al. Anterior PVR, part I: clinical findings and management. In: Freeman HM, Tolentino FI, eds. Proliferative vitreoretinopathy (PVR). New York: Springer, 1988: 22–33.
9. Heilmann K. Indications and timing of vitrectomy in trauma. In: Blankenship GW, Stirpe M, Gonvers M, Binder S, eds. Basic and advanced vitreous surgery. Padua: Liviana, 1986: 305–309.
10. Hirst LW, de Juan E Jr. Combined use of tissue adhesive and sodium hyaluronate in treating corneal perforations. Ophthalmology 1982; 89: 1250–1253.
11. Hirst WH, Illif WJ, Michels RG. Sights and sounds in ophthalmology, vol V: ocular and periocular trauma. St. Louis: C V Mosby, 1983: 9–11.
12. Michels RG. Vitrectomy methods in penetrating ocular trauma. Ophthalmology 1980; 87: 629–645.
13. Michels RG. Penetrating injuries. In: Blankenship GW, Stirpe M, Gonvers M, Binder S, eds. Basic and advanced vitreous surgery. Padua: Liviana, 1986: 309–315.
14. Rashid ER, Waring GO III. Use of Healon in anterior segment trauma. Ophthalmic Surg 1982; 13: 201–203.
15. Rice TA, Michels RG, stark WJ, eds. Operative surgery: ophthalmic surgery. 4th ed. St. Louis: C V Mosby, 1984: 403–413. (Rob and Smith's operative surgery series.)
16. Ryan SJ. Guidelines in the management of penetrating ocular trauma, with emphasis on the role and timing of pars plana vitrectomy. Int Ophthalmol 1979; 1: 105–108.
17. Trese MT, Cox MS Jr. The role of vitreoretinal surgery in ocular trauma. In: Spoor TC, Nesi FA, eds. Management of ocular, orbital, and adnexal trauma. New York: Raven Press, 1988: 129–135.

31

Double Perforation of the Globe

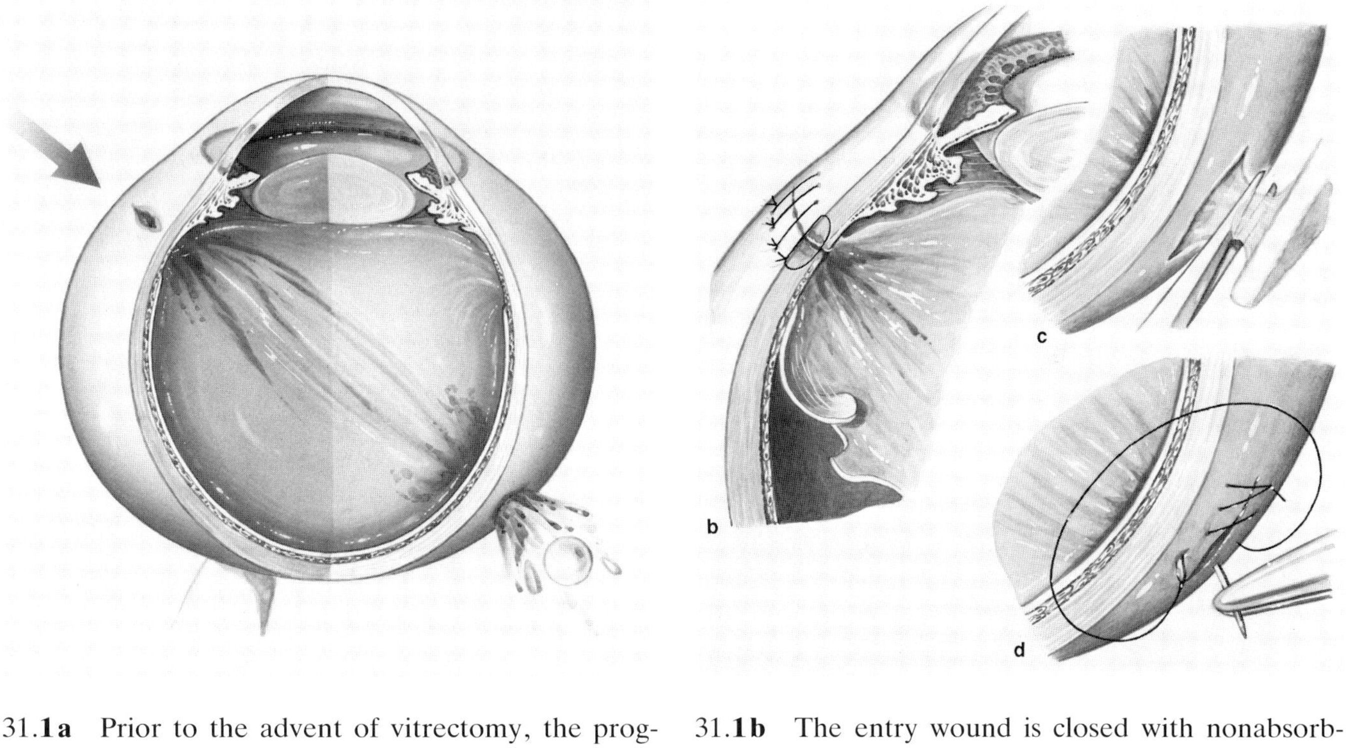

31.**1a** Prior to the advent of vitrectomy, the prognosis for double perforating injuries was very poor because of severe post-traumatic proliferative changes emanating from both the posterior and anterior wounds (1–11).

The illustration shows a double perforation of the globe by a BB (air rifle) pellet. Vitreous hemorrhage is concentrated near the pellet's entry and exit site.

31.**1b** The entry wound is closed with nonabsorbable 7-0 interrupted sutures.

c Prolapsing vitreous is excised flush with the exit wound, using a cellulose sponge and Vannas scissors. Prolapsing uveal tissue is reposited if possible, because excision may result in uncontrollable bleeding. If it becomes necessary to excise uveal tissue, it is heavily diathermized (prior to excision) using the underwater diathermy electrode.

d The exit wound is closed using a running suture. If an exit wound is small and more than 5 days old, closure is not attempted, because it is usually self-sealing.

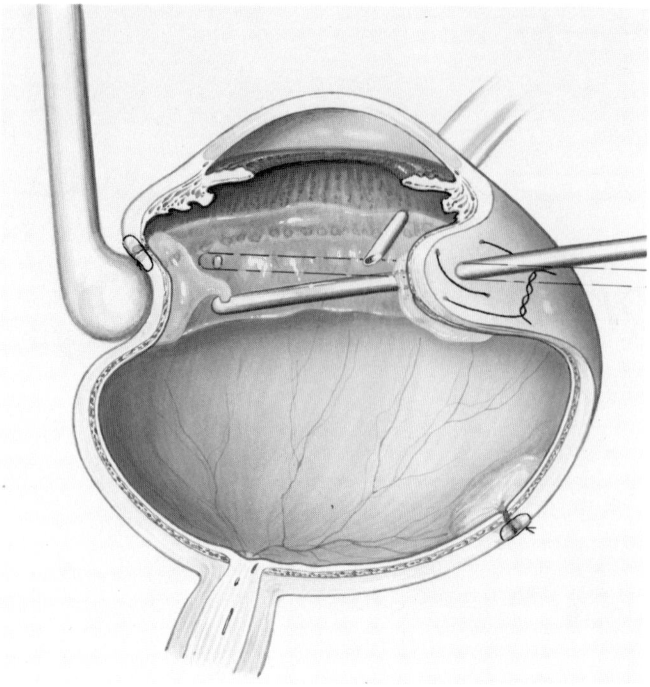

31.**1e** Vitrectomy is performed to remove the vitreous hemorrhage, cortical vitreous, and central vitreous gel. Peripheral vitreous is removed with the aid of scleral depression.

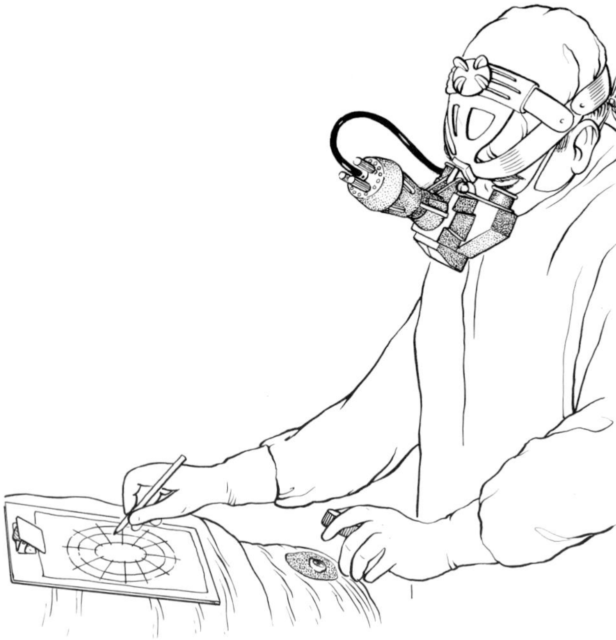

31.**1g** Indirect ophthalmoscopy and scleral depression are performed to assess the extent of the damage of the posterior segment. A search is made for the retinal break at the entry and exit sites of the foreign body, and for a traumatic retinal dialysis. A detailed large fundus drawing is made using gas-sterilized colored pencils, a drawing board, and fundus drawing paper.

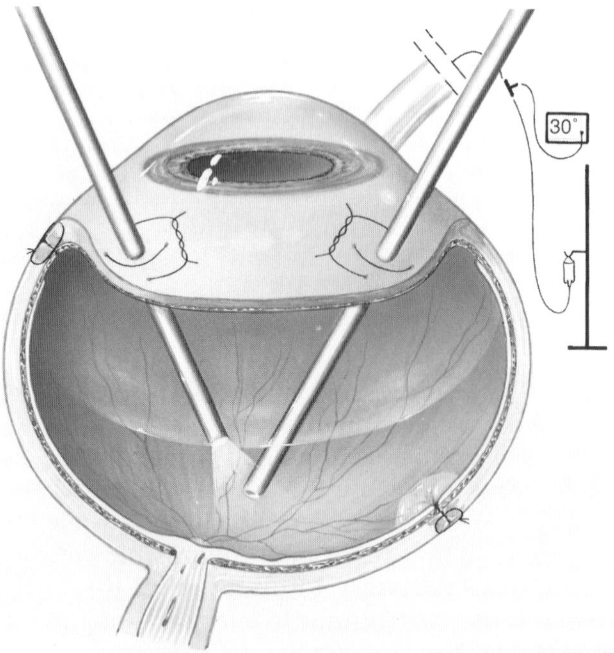

31.**1f** A fluid-air exchange is performed.

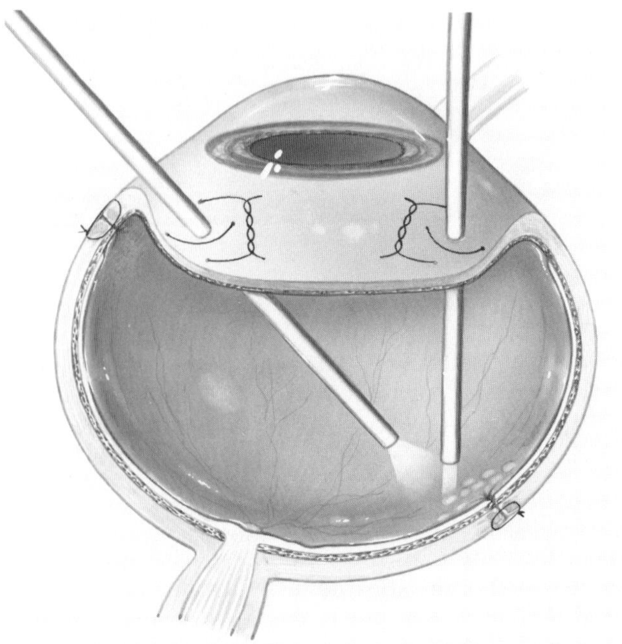

31.**1h** Three rows of endolaser are applied around the posterior perforation site.

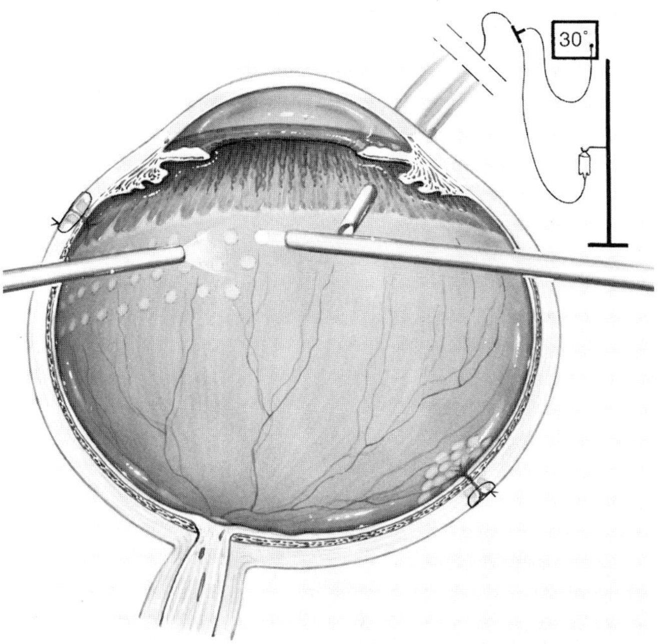

31.**1i** Three rows of endolaser are applied around 360° between the equator and ora serrata.

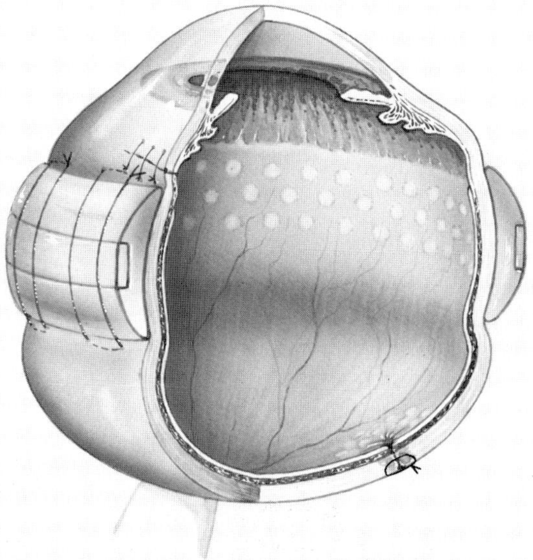

31.**1j** An episcleral buckle is placed around the equator of the globe, as described above (Chapter 20). Prior to closure of the conjunctiva, an air-gas exchange is performed using a mixture of 20% perfluorocarbon and air.

References

1. Abrams GW, Topping TM, Machemer R. Vitrectomy for injury: the effect on intraocular proliferation following perforation of the posterior segment of the rabbit eye. Arch Ophthalmol 1977; 97: 743–748.
2. Benson WE, Machemer R. Severe perforating injuries treated with pars plana vitrectomy. Am J Ophthalmol 1976; 81: 728–732.
3. Conway BP, Michels RG. Vitrectomy techniques in the management of selected penetrating ocular injuries. Ophthalmology 1980; 85: 560–583.
4. Gregor Z, Ryan SJ. Combined posterior contusion and penetrating injury in the pig eye, I: a natural history study. Br J Ophthalmol 1982; 66: 793–798.
5. Gregor Z, Ryan SJ. Combined posterior contusion and penetrating injury in the pig eye, II: histological features. Br J Ophthalmol 1982; 66: 799–804.
6. Gregor Z, Ryan SJ. Complete and core vitrectomies in the treatment of experimental posterior penetrating eye injury in the rhesus monkey, I: clinical features. Arch Ophthalmol 1983; 101: 441–445.
7. Gregor Z, Ryan SJ. Complete and core vitrectomies in the treatment of experimental posterior penetrating eye injury in the rhesus monkey, II: histologic features. Arch Ophthalmol 1983; 101: 446–450.
8. Heilmann K. Treatment of double perforating injuries. In: Blankenship GW, Stirpe M, Gonvers M, Binder S, eds. Basic and advanced vitreous surgery. Padua: Liviana, 1986: 317–321.
9. Michels RG. Vitrectomy methods in penetrating ocular trauma. Ophthalmology 1980; 87: 629–645.
10. Peyman GA, Schulman JA. Intravitreal surgery: principles and practice. New York: Appleton-Century-Crofts, 1986: 253.
11. Topping TM, Abrams GW, Machemer R. Experimental double perforating injury of the posterior segment in rabbit eyes: the natural history of intraocular proliferation. Arch Ophthalmol 1979; 97: 735–742.

32

Posterior Segment Intraocular Foreign Body

This chapter deals with the localization, routes of extraction, and removal of the following types of intraocular foreign bodies (6, 9, 11).

- Magnetic:
  - Small, anteriorly located
  - Small, posteriorly located
- Nonmagnetic:
  - Small, anteriorly located
  - Small, in an eye with vitreous hemorrhage, lens damage
  - Diameter $< 5–6$ mm
  - Diameter > 6 mm
- Encapsulated

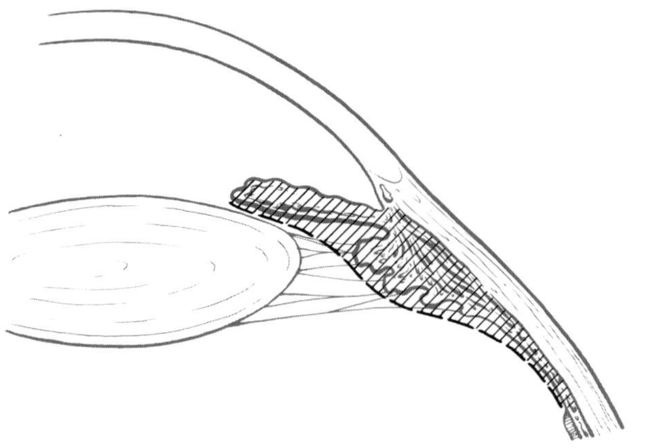

32.1 **Foreign body localization.** The combined use of X-rays, computerized axial tomography (CT scan), and ultrasonography, makes it possible ot localize most intraocular foreign bodies. When evaluating trauma cases, it should be remembered that 20% of foreign bodies penetrate the eye without causing noticeable pain (1). Whenever there is the remotest possibility of an intraocular foreign body, an X-ray should be taken. Failure to take an X-ray in a case involving a foreign body is usually indefensible, and this has held up in court since 1909 (13).

The major role of X-rays is in demonstrating the presence, number, size, and *approximate* location of foreign bodies (5). At our institution, the Sweets method of localization is used. A foreign body, or foreign material of low radiographic density, lodged in the anterior third of the globe can be located and identified by a soft-tissue technique. A dental film held by the patient is pressed posteriorly against the medial canthus, and X-rays of low kilovoltage are used to picture the anterior portion of the globe (4). This technique usually reveals tiny metallic foreign bodies, as well as glass and plastic, within the cornea, within the anterior chamber, or overlying the ciliary body (13).

A CT scan is extremely useful in precisely locating foreign bodies not clearly visible with X-rays or ultrasonography. This is largely due to the ability of the CT scan to establish relationships to various structures within the globe, such as the lens, optic nerve, and scleral coat. Because this method is so extremely sensitive to small differences in radiographic density, it is possible to show within the eye and orbit such foreign materials as plastic, glass, metals of low atomic weight, and even wood in some cases.

In a CT scan, standard axial 2 mm scans are taken through the orbit, and the data obtained in the corneal and sagittal sections are reconstructed for further localization of the foreign body. The CT scan is of special value in locating foreign bodies in the anterior part of the posterior segment, and those on the surface of the sclera. It is usually possible to determine whether a foreign body is located in the cortical vitreous, within the sclera, or externally as a result of a double perforation. In addition, the CT scan can identify soft-tissue injuries to the optic nerve, muscle entrapment, a ruptured globe, a double perforation, or an orbital hematoma.

Ultrasonography is most helpful when a foreign body is lodged in the posterior half of the posterior segment. It is particularly valuable in locating foreign bodies in relation to the retina and the inner coats of the eye wall. However, small foreign bodies can be difficult to locate by ultrasonography alone, and their approximate location should first be determined with X-ray (3).

In most cases, a foreign gody can be localized accurately, except when it is embedded in the "gray zone" between the anterior and posterior chambers (2, 7). In such cases, a combination of X-ray, ultrasonography, and CT scan should be used.

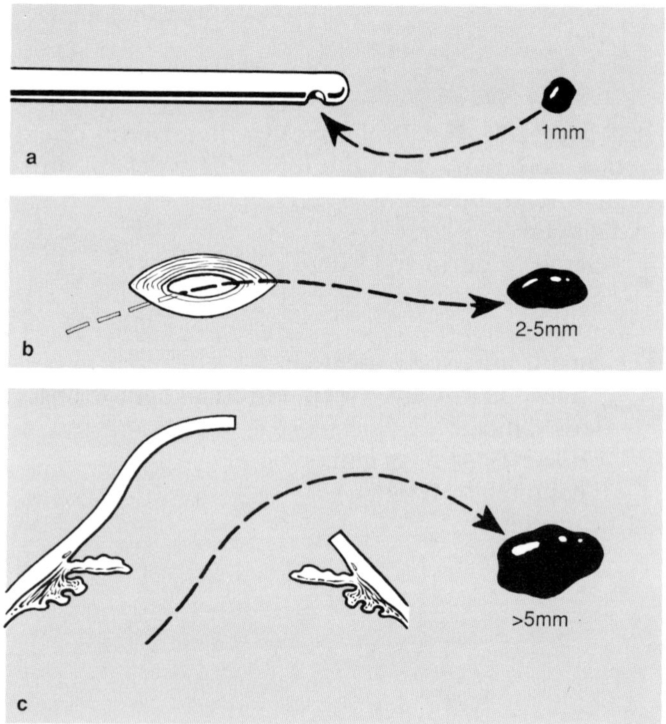

32.2 **Routes of extraction of intraocular foreign bodies.**

a Small foreign bodies are usually removed through a sclerotomy in the pars plana. If vitrectomy is performed for the removal of vitreous hemorrhage, one can estimate the size of the foreign body in relation to the diameter of the vitrectomy probe, and thus determine if the foreign body can be removed through the existing sclerotomy.

b Foreign bodies of 2–5 mm in size can be removed enlarging the sclerotomy for the vitrectomy probe.

c Foreign bodies larger than 5–6 mm are usually removed through a corneal incision.

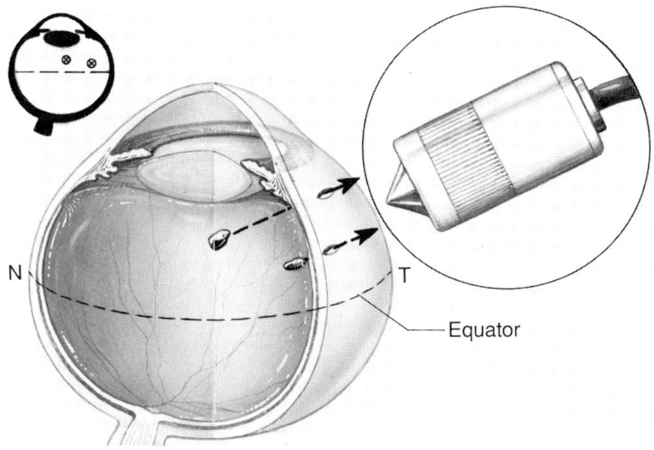

Magnetic Foreign Body

32.3 **Route of extraction of a magnetic foreign body.** Small magnetic foreign bodies in the central vitreous gel are usually extracted through a sclerotomy in the pars plana.

Inset: we prefer the broad, blunt tip of the hand-held Bronson magnet, which delivers the strongest magnetic field.

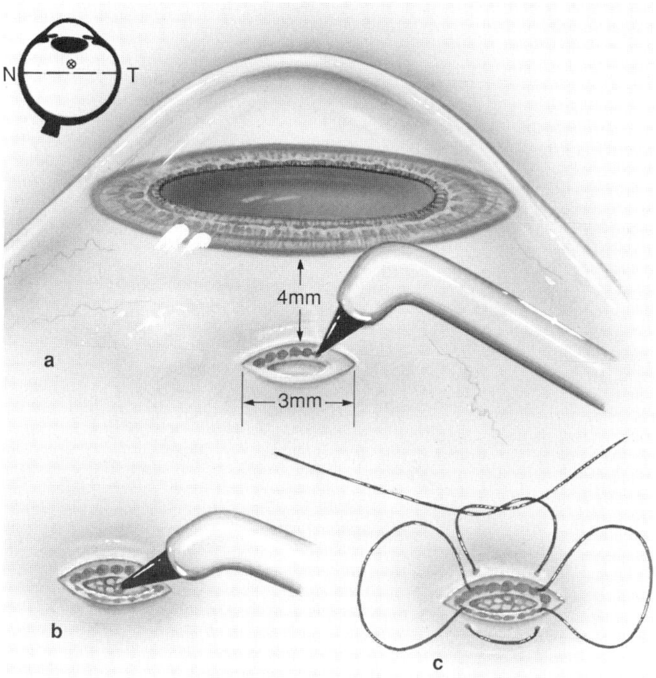

32.4 **Magnetic foreign body anterior to the equator.** *Inset,* upper left: a metallic foreign body located anterior to the equator in the mid-vitreous.

a After closing the corneal entry wound of the foreign wound body, a 3 mm sclerotomy is made 4 mm posterior to the limbus. The sclerotomy is made parallel to the limbus, so that if it has to be enlarged to accommodate the foreign body, this circumferential incision will not involve the retina or ciliary body. Using a sharp conical electrode, diathermy is applied to edges of the sclerotomy to make it gape.

b Using the blunt conical electrode, confluent applications of low-intensity diathermy are applied to the uvea to reduce the incidence of hemorrhage when the uvea is penetrated.

c A 6-0 polyglactin suture is placed across the sclerotomy, and the arms are separated to permit unencumbered removal of the foreign body.

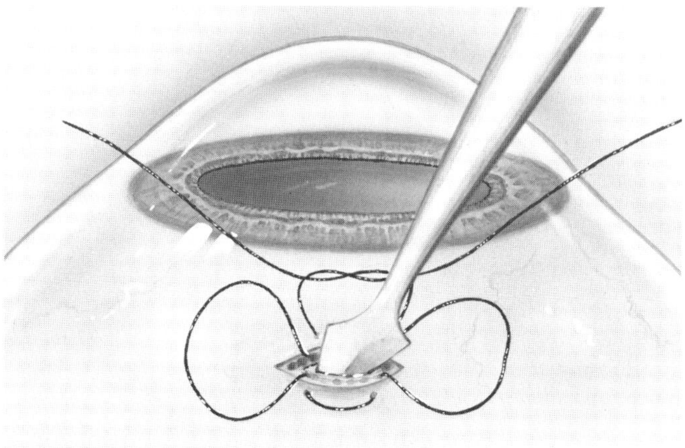

32.**4d** Prior to the application of the magnet to the sclerotomy, the uvea is penetrated using the MVR knife.

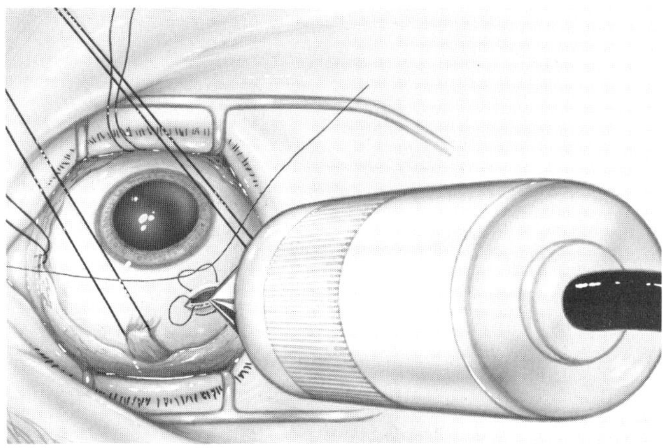

32.**4e** The tip of the magnet is placed near the lips of the sclerotomy. Short bursts of magnetic current are used, to avoid overheating the magnet; overheating makes it less efficient.

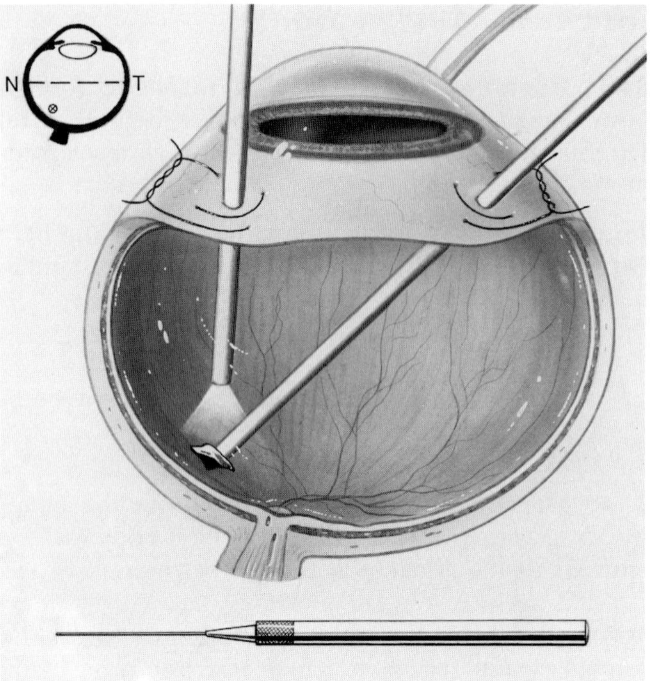

32.5 **Small posterior magnetic foreign body.** The inset shows a small posterior foreign body located near the optic nerve. When the foreign body is so small or weakly magnetic that it cannot be removed with a magnet tip held at the sclerotomy, attempts are made to remove it with an earth magnet which can be applied to its surface (10). The magnet is introduced through the pars plana and visualized with light from an endoilluminator.

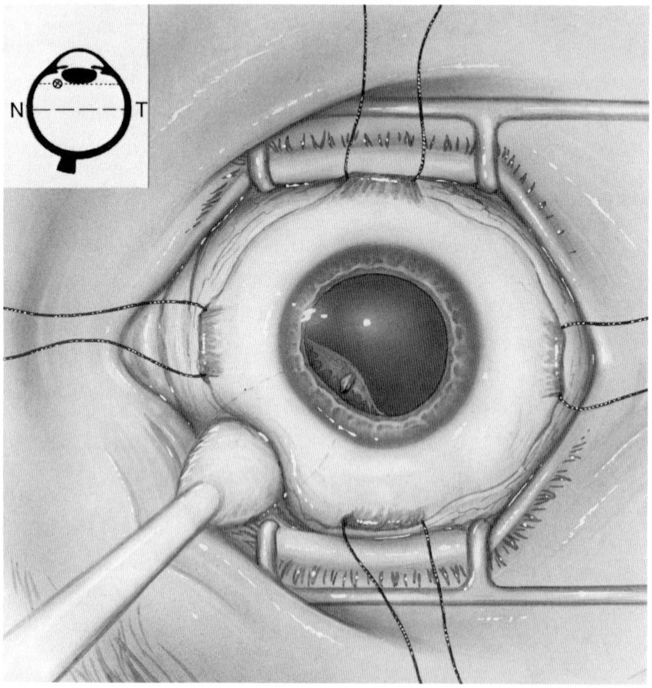

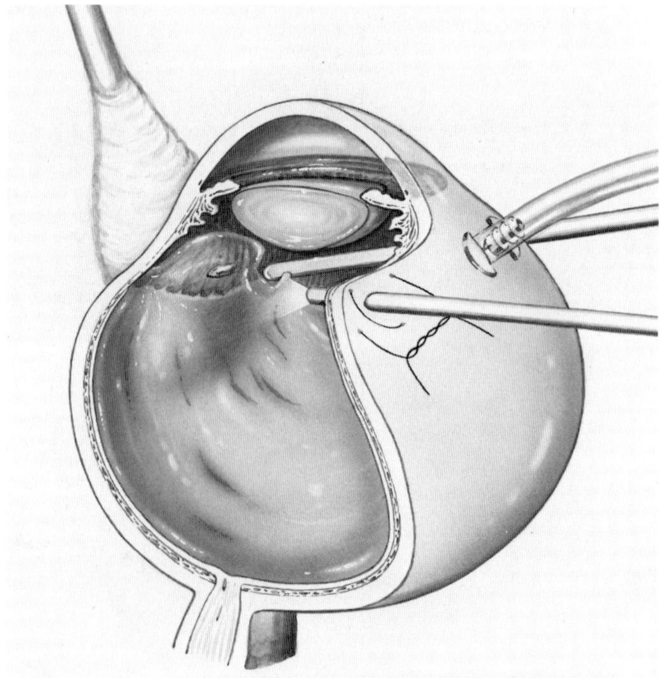

Nonmagnetic Foreign Body

32.**6a** **Small anterior nonmagnetic foreign body.** *Inset:* a small, nonmagnetic foreign body near the superonasal ora serrata at the 1:30 clock position in the right eye. Using indentation from a cotton-tipped applicator, the foreign body is visualized through the operating microscope.

32.**6b** To approach the 1:30 clock meridian with the vitrectomy probe or foreign body forceps, the surgeon sits on the temporal side of the patient's head, and the sclerotomies are made at the 2, 3:30, and 4:30 clock positions.

With the suction port directed away from the posterior surface of the lens, vitrectomy is performed to remove vitreous hemorrhage and vitreous overlying and adherent to the foreign body.

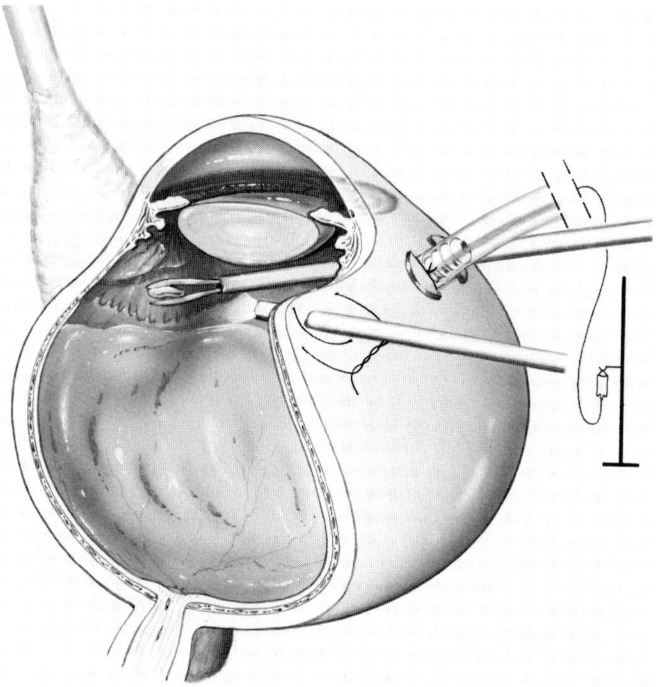

32.**6c** The infusion bottle is lowered to decrease vitreous loss through the sclerotomy during extraction of the foreign body. While the assistant depresses the sclera in the meridian of the foreign body, the foreign body is grasped with foreign body forceps.

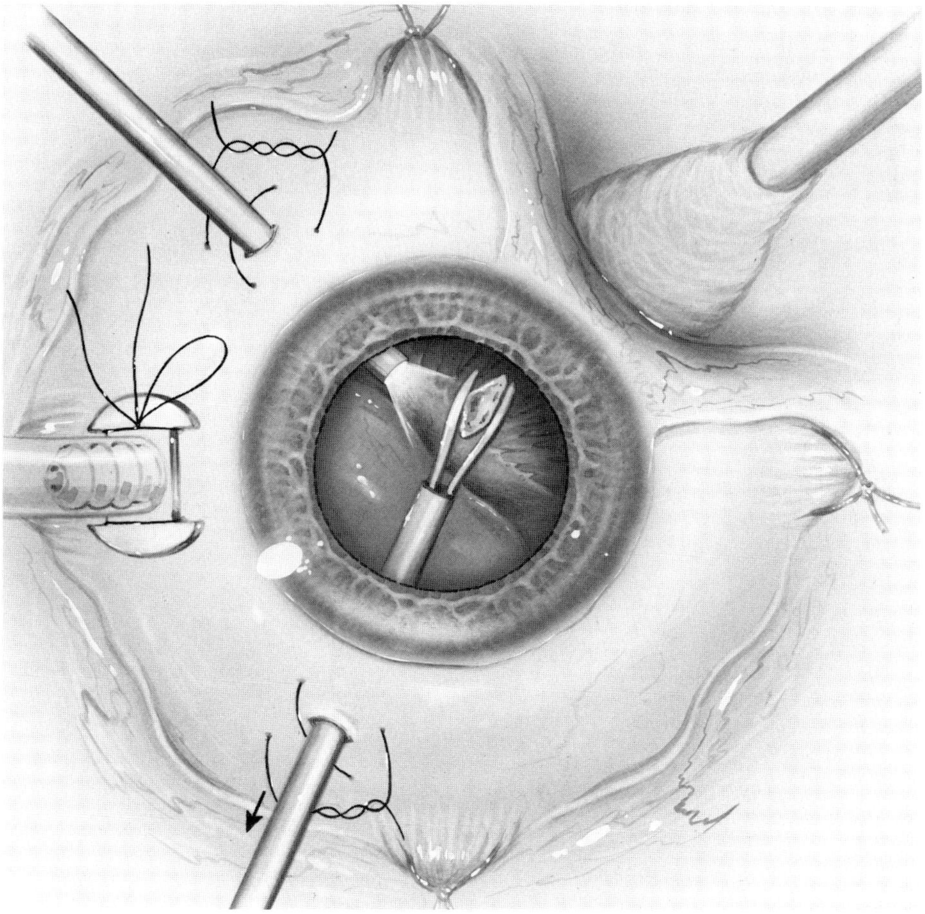

32.**6d** The foreign body is carried across the vitreous cavity in a concave arc, to avoid contact with the posterior surface of the lens. As the forceps holding the foreign body is brought near the sclerotomy, it is rotated so that its flat edges are parallel to the edges of the sclerotomy.

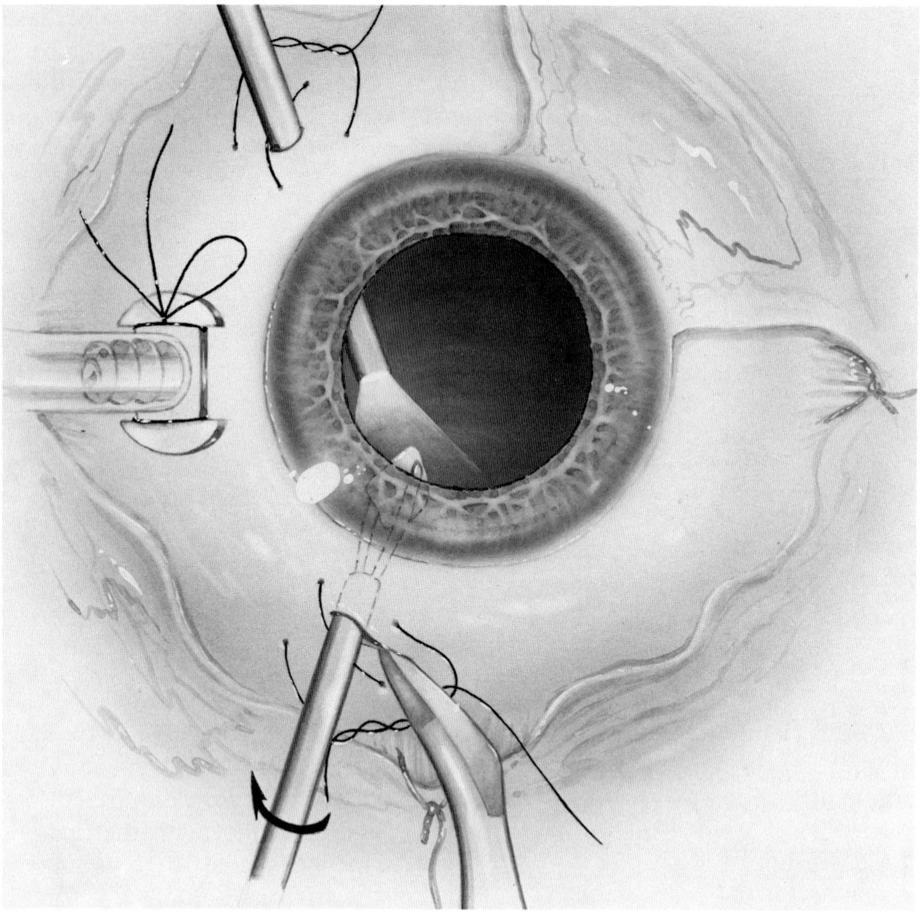

32.**6e** The sclerotomy may have to be enlarged with a scarifier if difficulty is experienced when trying to extract the foreign body.

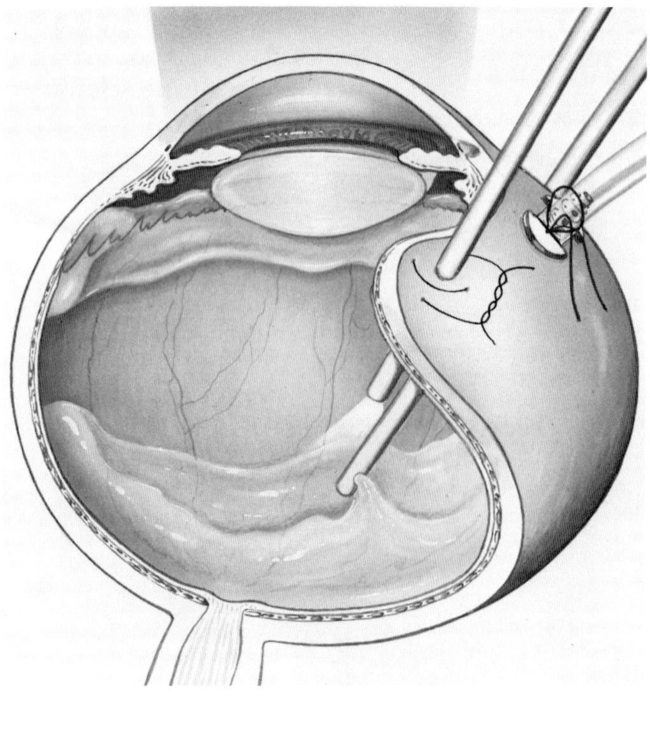

32.**6f** Following removal of the foreign body, the remaining vitreous hemorrhage is removed by vitrectomy.

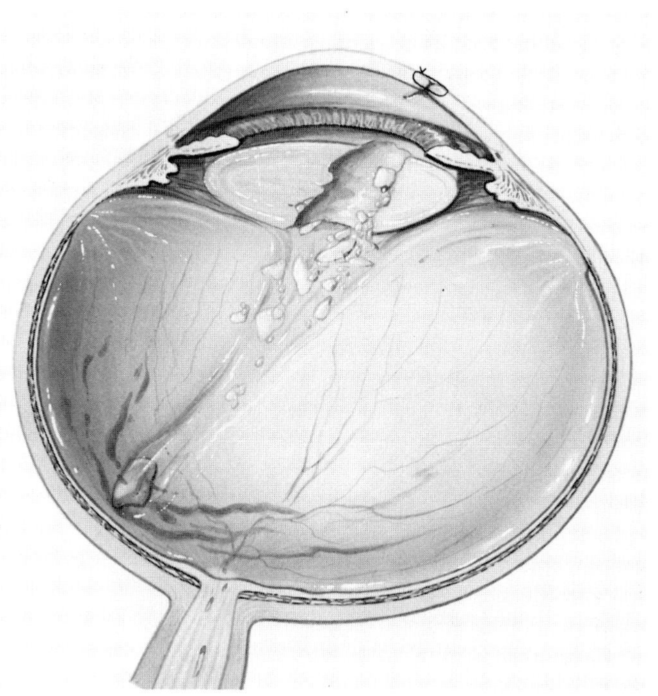

32.7a **Medium-sized nonmagnetic foreign body, lens damage, and vitreous hemorrhage.** The nonmagnetic foreign body has penetrated the cornea and lens to rest nasal to the optic nerve. Lens material and hemorrhage are mixed with the vitreous gel.

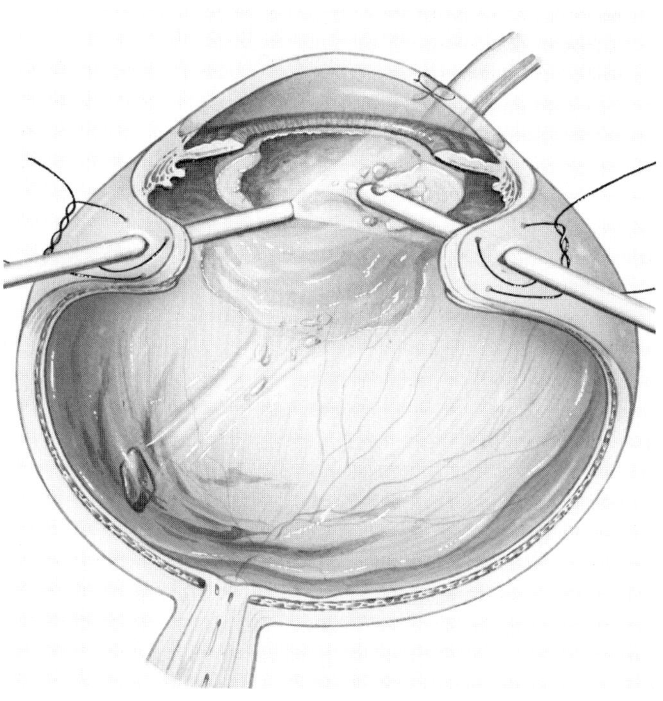

32.7b A lensectomy is performed, with removal of both anterior and posterior capsule. Suction is used to remove as much peripheral lens cortex as possible, to decrease postoperative inflammatory reaction from residual cortical lens material. Peripheral capsular remnants are removed using curved, serrated forceps.

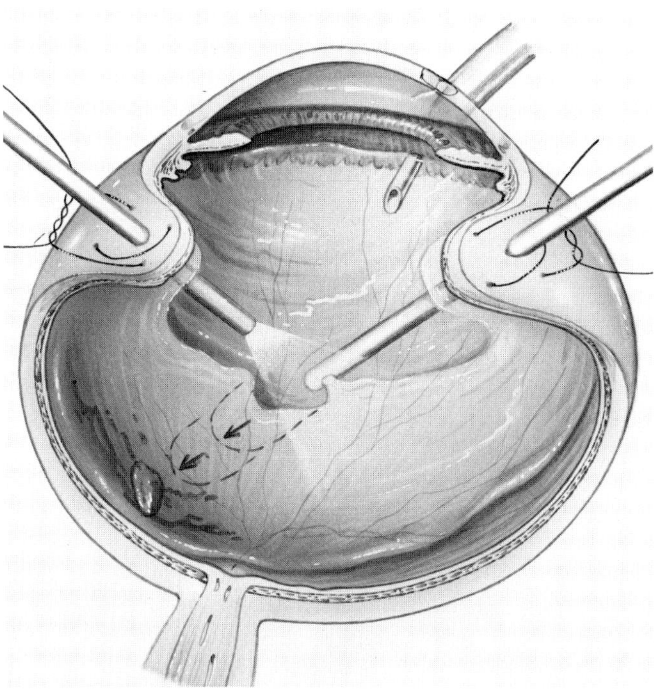

32.7c Vitrectomy is continued posteriorly by widening the tract of the foreign body. Removal of the bulk of the vitreous gel removes the scaffold upon which proliferation and cellular membranes tend to grow.

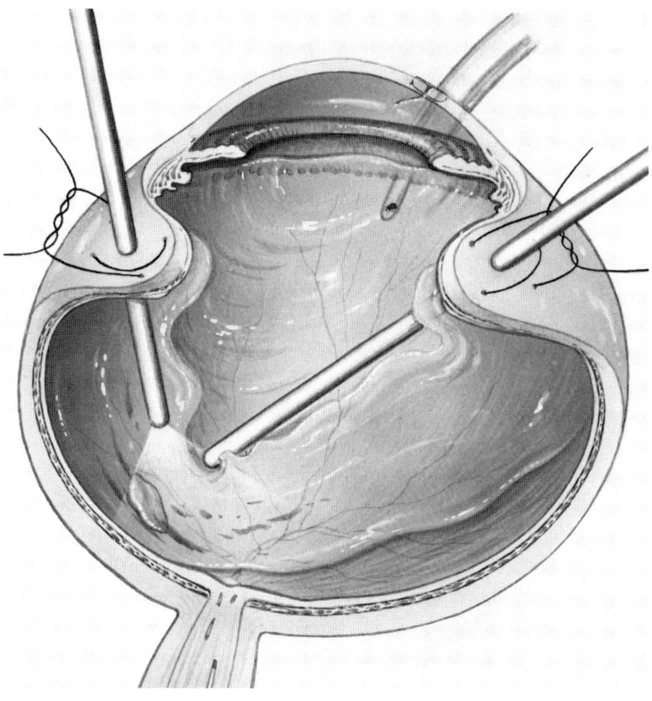

32.7d Vitrectomy is continued until the anterior surface of the foreign body is exposed. The temporal vitreous gel is left as a cushion above the retina, should the foreign body become disengaged or be dropped during extraction.

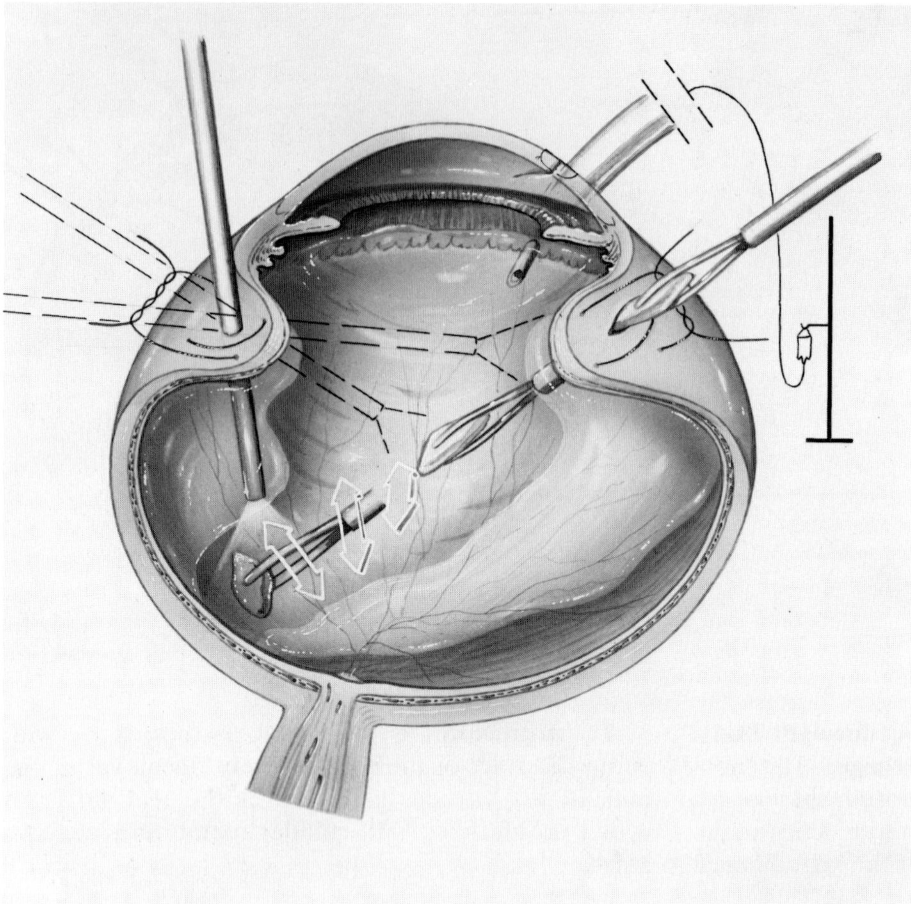

32.**7e** The foreign body is rotated so that its flat aspect parallels the equatorial axis of the sclerotomy and can more easily be removed through the sclerotomy.

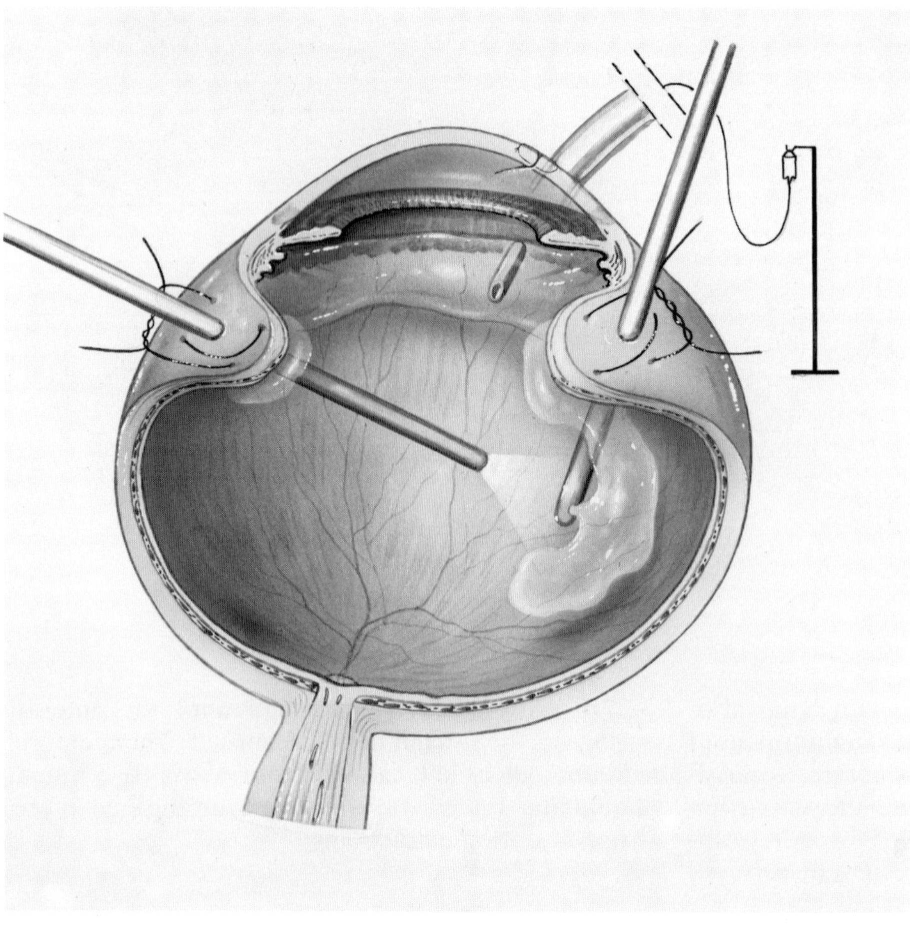

32.**7f** The temporal posterior vitreous gel is removed, so that a subtotal vitrectomy has been performed.

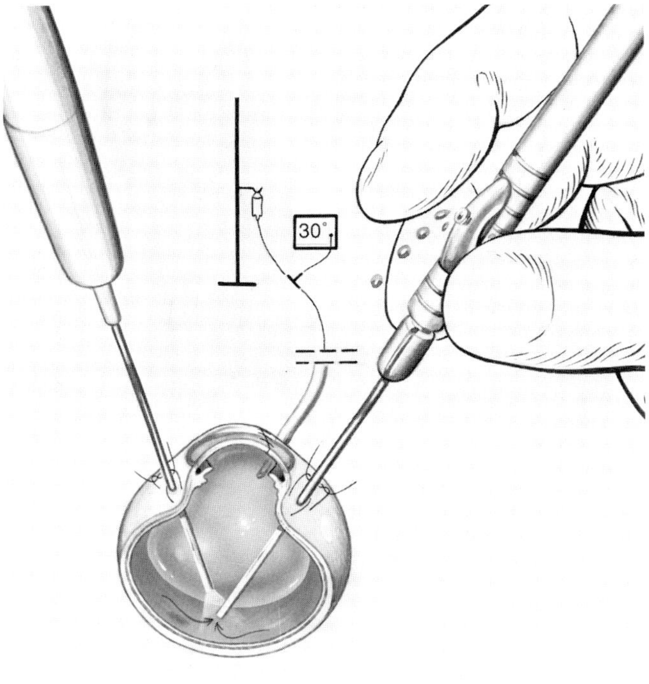

32.**7g** A fluid-air exchange is performed with an air pump setting of 30 mmHg.

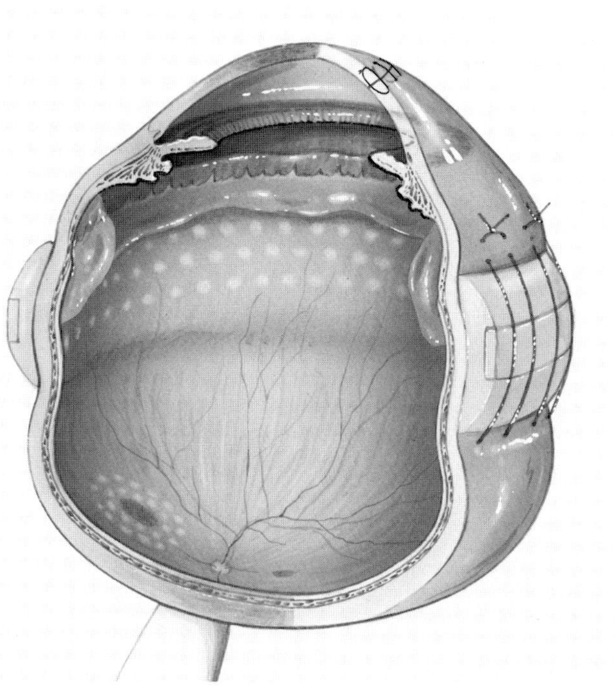

32.**7i** An equatorial episcleral buckle is made using a 9 mm solid silicone rubber implant and a 2.5 mm encircling silicone rubber band.

An air-gas exchange is performed using a 20% mixture of perfluorocarbon gas and air lavaged through the vitreous cavity over 2–3 minutes.

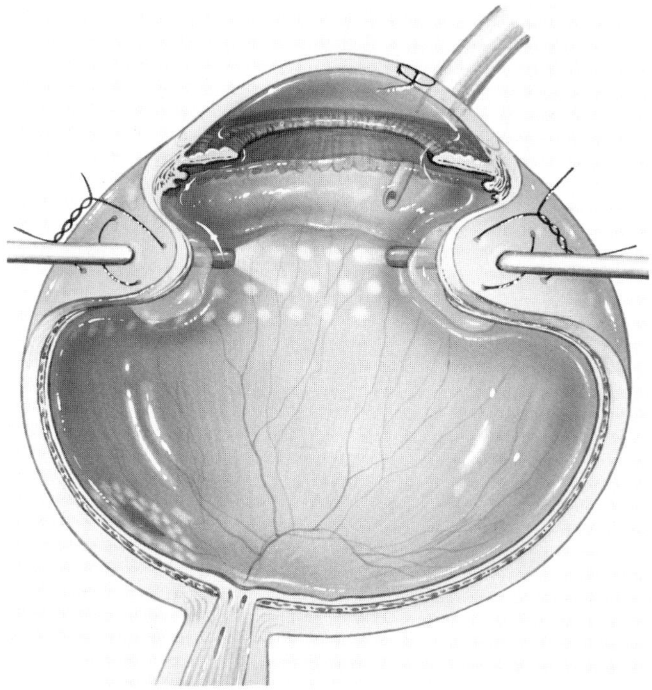

32.**7h** Endolaser is applied in three rows around 360° of the fundus from the ora serrata to the equator, and in two rows around the foreign body's point of impact on the retina.

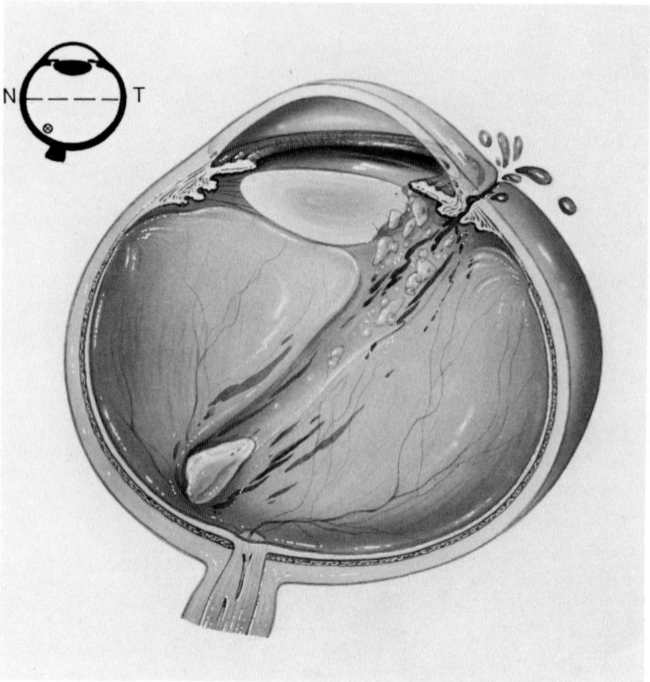

32.**8a** **Large nonmagnetic foreign body.** The inset shows a large intraocular foreign body located nasal to the optic nerve in the right eye.

The scleral laceration involves the ciliary body, and is associated with lens damage and vitreous hemorrhage.

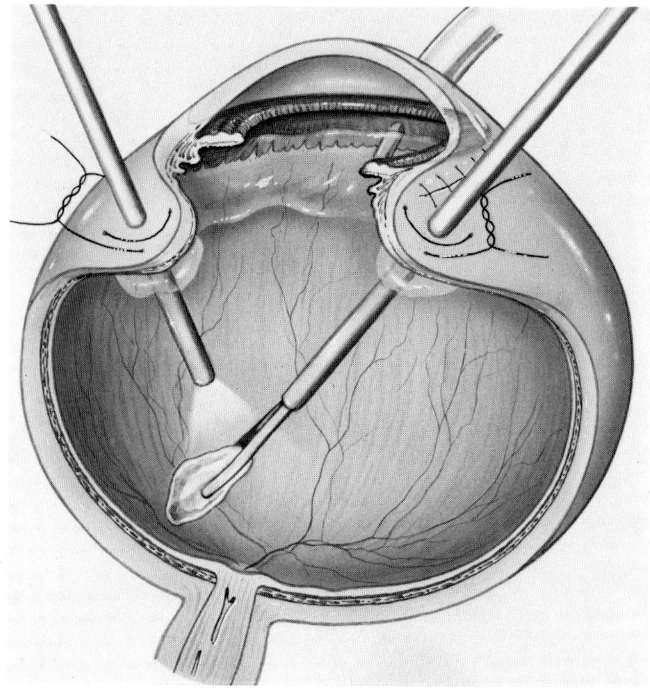

32.**8c** The foreign body is grasped with foreign body forceps.

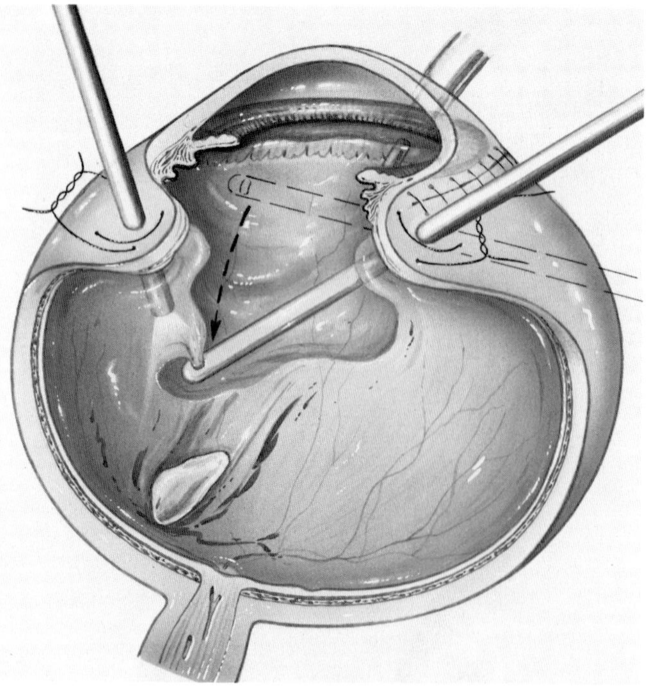

32.**8b** The scleral laceration is sutured using interrupted sutures. If the nonmagnetic foreign body is suspected of containing copper (which incites a severe vitreous reaction), lensectomy and vitrectomy are performed to expose the foreign body, and removal should be attempted at the time of laceration repair.

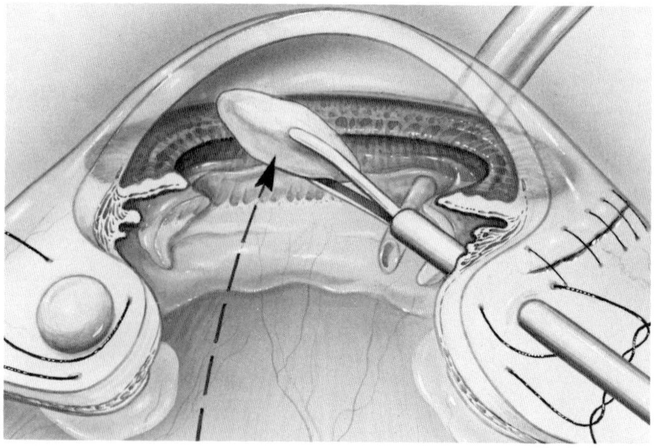

32.**8d** The foreign body is brought through the pupil into the anterior chamber.

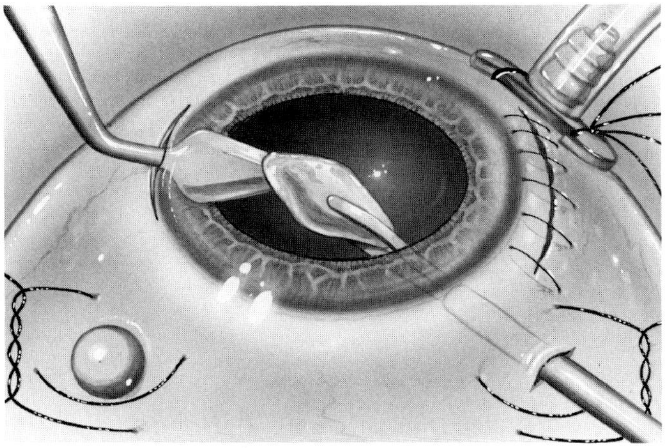

32.**8e** A foreign body larger than 5 mm is removed through the anterior chamber. While the surgeon holds the foreign body in the pupillary plane with his right hand, a keratome incision is made at the limbus with his left hand. The keratome blade is used to displace the iris posteriorly to facilitate removal of the foreign body (8).

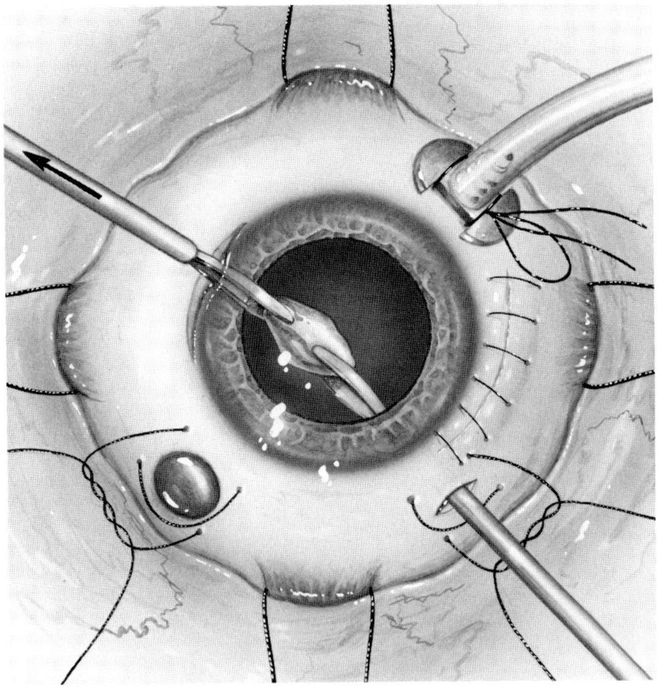

32.**8g** An alternative method of removing a relatively large foreign body through the anterior chamber is the "shaking hands" maneuver (7). Once the foreign body has been brought into the anterior chamber, it is grasped by a second forceps introduced through a limbal incision.

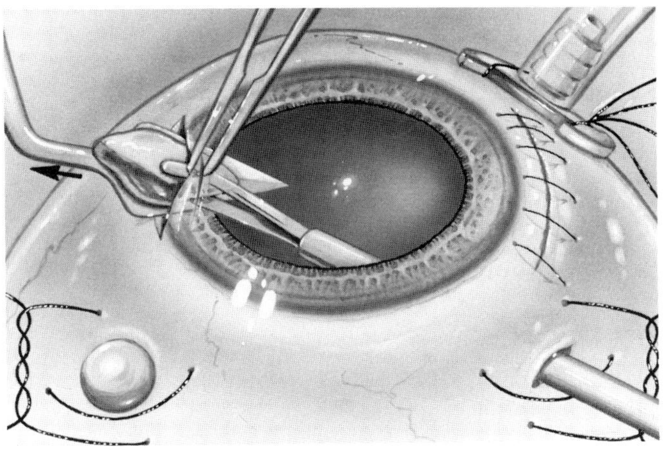

32.**8f** To facilitate delivery of the foreign body from the anterior chamber, the anterior lip of the limbal incision is raised by the assistant using a Colibri forceps. The wound is closed with interrupted sutures, and the remaining posterior vitreous gel and hemorrhage are removed. Endolaser, episcleral buckling, and a fluid-gas exchange are performed.

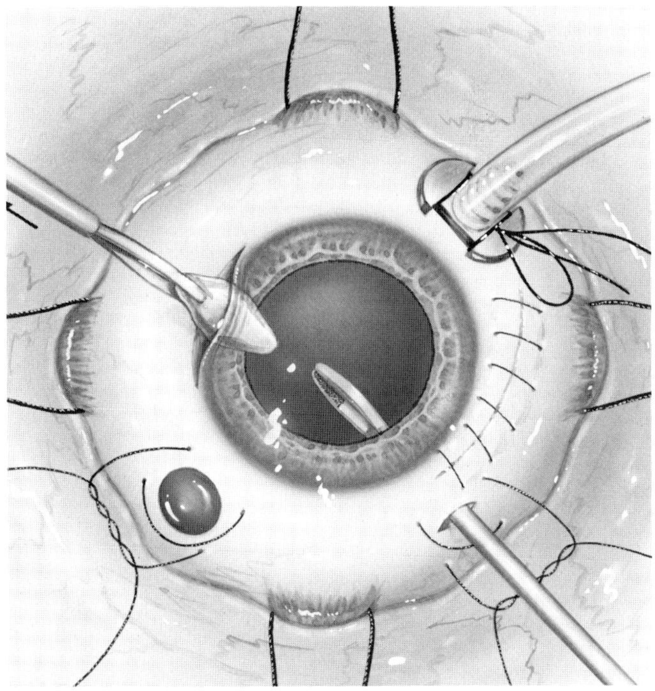

32.**8h** When it is felt that the foreign body is firmly grasped by the forceps in the surgeon's left hand, the transfer is complete, and the foreign body is extracted through the limbal incision.

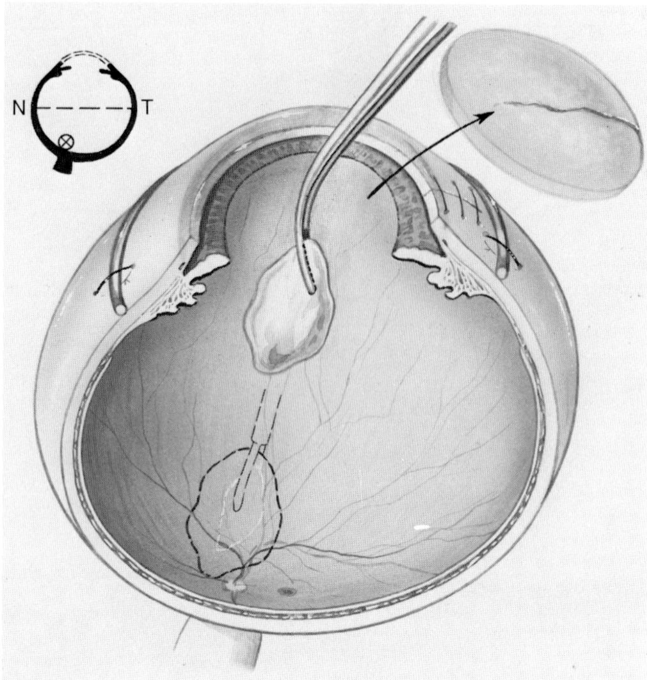

32.**9** **Large intraocular foreign body.** Foreign bodies up to 8 mm in diameter can be removed by the open-sky approach (7, 12), using Schweiger forceps. If marked corneal scarring is present, foreign body removal can be combined with a penetrating keratoplasty.

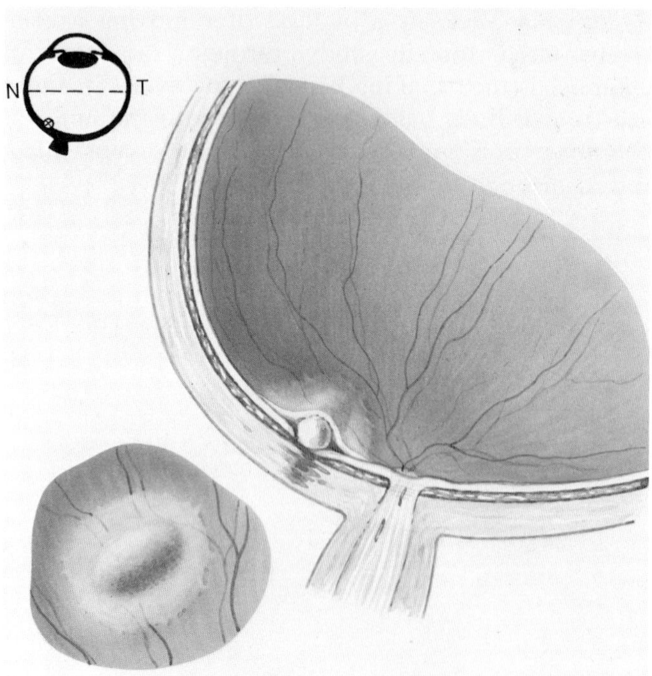

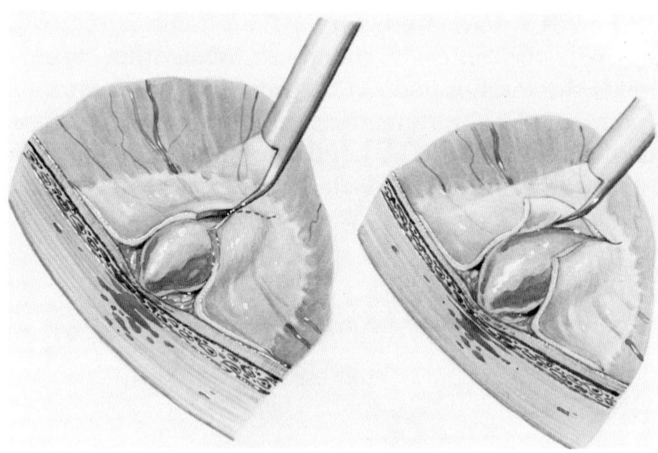

b **c**

Encapsulated Foreign Body

32.**10a** *Inset,* above: a foreign body near the optic nerve papilla. It is covered by a thin, membranous capsule.

Inset, below: a small semi-opaque capsule overlying the foreign body.

32.**10b** An incision is made through the capsule using a self-illuminating pick.

c The capsule is separated from the surface of the foreign body.

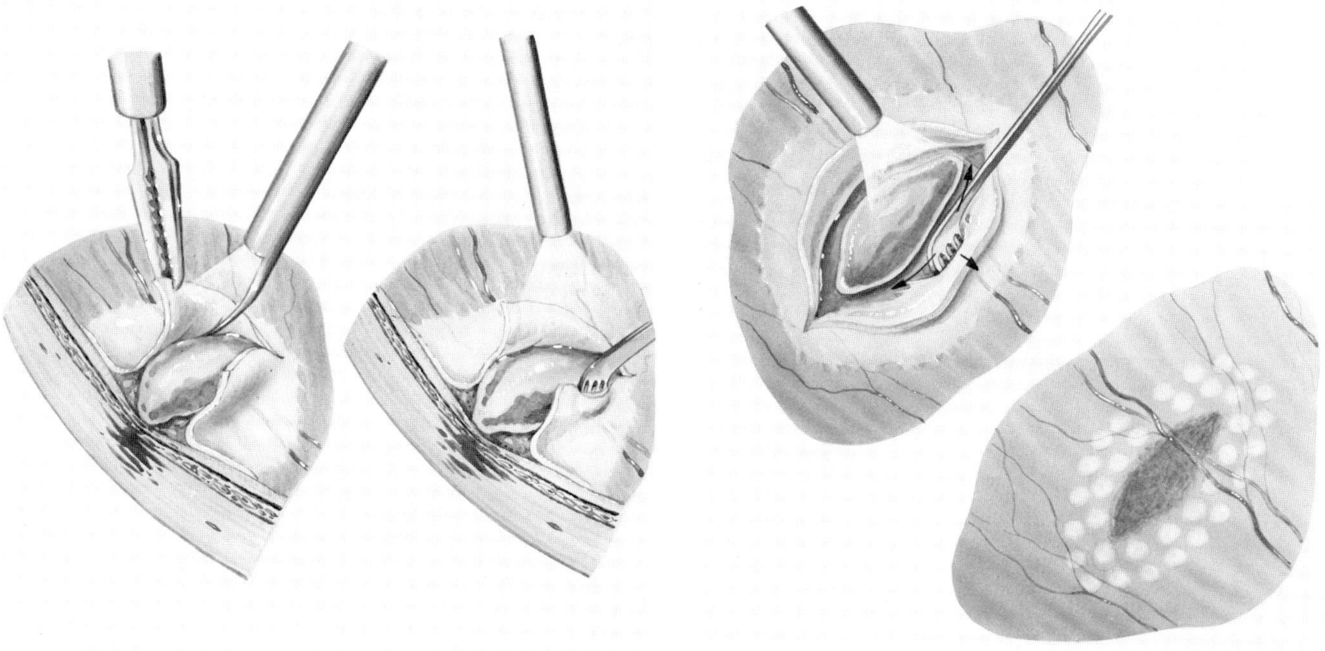

d e f g

32.**10d** Using a bimanual technique, the membrane is grapsed with forceps held in the nondominant hand, and separated from the foreign body using the light pick.

e The right-angled teeth of the retinal scratcher are useful in separating the capsule from the foreign body.

32.**10f** The edges of the foreign body are isolated so that it can be grasped with forceps or removed with an earth magnet.

g Following removal of the foreign body, two rows of endolaser applications are made around the site of encapsulation.

References

1. Bettman JW. The medicolegal implications of the management of trauma. In: Freeman HM, ed. Ocular trauma. New York: Appleton-Century-Crofts, 1979: 63–69.
2. Coleman DJ, Lizzi LL, Jack RI. Ultrasonography of the eye and orbit. Philadelphia: Lea and Febiger, 1977: 255–264.
3. Coleman DJ, Smith ME. Ultrasound in the preoperative evaluation of trauma. In: Freeman HM, ed. Ocular trauma. New York: Appleton-Century-Crofts, 1979: 23–30.
4. Freeman HM. Examination of the traumatized eye. In: Miller D, Stegman R, eds. Treatment of anterior segment ocular trauma. Montreal: Medicopea, 1986: 95–119.
5. Hirst LW, Illiff WJ, Michels RG. Sights and sounds in ophthalmology, vol V: ocular and periocular trauma. St. Louis: C V Mosby, 1983: 23–24.
6. Hutton WL. Management of intraocular foreign bodies by pars plana vitrectomy. In: Freeman HM, ed. Ocular trauma. New York: Appleton-Century-Crofts, 1979: 197–204.
7. Malbran ES. Modern methods of management of intraocular foreign bodies. Highlights Ophthalmol 1985; 1: 62–108.
8. Michels RM. Blunt trauma, penetrating injuries, intraocular foreign bodies. Highlights Ophthalmol 1985; 1: 56–59.
9. Neubauer H. Management of nonmagnetic intraocular foreign bodies. In: Freeman HM, ed. Ocular trauma. New York: Appleton-Century-Crofts, 1979: 187–196.
10. Parel JM. Progress in foreign body extractors. In: Blankenship GW, Stirpe M, Gonvers M, Binder S, eds. Basic and advanced vitreous surgery. Padua: Liviana, 1986: 321–332.
11. Rice TA, Michels RG, Stark WJ, eds. Operative surgery: ophthalmic surgery. 4th ed. St. Louis: C V Mosby, 1984: 419–423. (Rob and Smith's operative surgery series.).
12. Schepens CL. Retinal detachment and allied disease. Philadelphia: W B Saunders, 1983: 930–931.
13. Trokel SI. Radiologic evaluation of ophthalmologic trauma. In: Freeman HM, ed. Ocular trauma. New York: Appleton-Century-Crofts, 1979: 15–22.

Index